Essentials of Personality Disorders

Edited by

John M. Oldham, M.D., M.S.
Andrew E. Skodol, M.D.
Donna S. Bender, Ph.D.

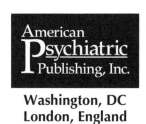

American Psychiatric Publishing, Inc.

Washington, DC
London, England

Copyright © 2009 American Psychiatric Publishing, Inc.
ALL RIGHTS RESERVED

Manufactured in the United States of America on acid-free paper
13 12 11 10 09   5 4 3 2 1
First Edition

Typeset in Adobe's Palatino and Optima.

American Psychiatric Publishing, Inc.
1000 Wilson Boulevard
Arlington, VA 22209-3901
www.appi.org

Library of Congress Cataloging-in-Publication Data
Essentials of personality disorders / edited by John M. Oldham, Andrew E. Skodol, Donna S. Bender ; associate editors, Glen O. Gabbard ... [et al.]. — 1st ed.
    p. ; cm.
Companion to: The American Psychiatric Publishing textbook of personality disorders / edited by John M. Oldham, Andrew E. Skodol, Donna S. Bender ; associate editors, Glen O. Gabbard ... [et al.]. 1st ed. c2005.
  Includes bibliographical references and index.
  ISBN 978-1-58562-358-7 (alk. paper)
1. Personality disorders. I. Oldham, John M. II. Skodol, Andrew E. III. Bender, Donna S., 1960– IV. American Psychiatric Publishing textbook of personality disorders.
[DNLM: 1. Personality Disorders. WM 190 E784 2009]
  RC554.E883 2009
  616.85'81–dc22

                                                                          2008044430

British Library Cataloguing in Publication Data
A CIP record is available from the British Library.

To our families, who have supported us:

Karen, Madeleine, and Michael Oldham;
Laura, Dan, and Ali Skodol; and
John and Joseph Rosegrant.

To our colleagues, who have helped us.

To our patients, who have taught us.

And to each other, for the friendship that has enriched our work together.

Contents

PART I

Basic Concepts

PART II

Clinical Evaluation

PART III

Etiology

PART IV

Treatment

PART V

New Developments and Future Directions

Contributors

Samuel A. Ball, Ph.D.
Professor of Psychiatry, Department of Psychiatry, Yale University School of Medicine; Director of Research, the APT Foundation, Inc., New Haven, Connecticut

Anthony W. Bateman, M.A., F.R.C.Psych.
Visiting Professor, Sub-Department of Clinical Health Psychology, University College London; Consultant Psychotherapist, Barnet, Enfield, and Haringey Mental Health Trust, London, England

Donna S. Bender, Ph.D.
Research Associate Professor of Psychiatry, University of Arizona College of Medicine; Chief Executive Officer and Director, Sunbelt Collaborative, Tucson, Arizona

Beth S. Brodsky, Ph.D.
Assistant Clinical Professor of Medical Psychology, Department of Psychiatry, Columbia University College of Physicians and Surgeons; Research Scientist, Department of Molecular Imaging and Neuropathology, New York State Psychiatric Institute, New York, New York

Elizabeth Bromley, M.D.
Assistant Professor in Residence, Department of Psychiatry and Biobehavioral Sciences, Semel Institute Health Services Research Center, University of California, Los Angeles, California

Emil F. Coccaro, M.D.
Ellen C. Manning Professor and Chairman, Department of Psychiatry, University of Chicago, Chicago, Illinois

Patricia Cohen, Ph.D.
Professor of Clinical Epidemiology in Psychiatry, Columbia University College of Physicians and Surgeons, New York, New York

Thomas Crawford, Ph.D.
Assistant Clinical Professor of Medical Psychology, Columbia University College of Physicians and Surgeons, New York, New York

Peter Fonagy, Ph.D., F.B.A.
Freud Memorial Professor of Psychoanalysis and Head of the Research Department of Clinical, Educational, and Health Psychology, University College London; Chief Executive of the Anna Freud Centre, London, England; Consultant to the Child and Family Program, Menninger Department of Psychiatry, Baylor College of Medicine, Houston, Texas

Glen O. Gabbard, M.D.
Brown Foundation Chair of Psychoanalysis and Professor, Department of Psychiatry, Baylor College of Medicine; Training and Supervising Analyst, Houston-Galveston Psychoanalytic Institute, Houston, Texas

Kim L. Gratz, Ph.D.
Assistant Professor and Director, Personality Disorders Research, Department of Psychiatry and Human Behavior, University of Mississippi Medical Center, Jackson, Mississippi

Carlos M. Grilo, Ph.D.
Professor of Psychiatry, Department of Psychiatry, Yale University School of Medicine; Professor of Psychology, Yale University, New Haven, Connecticut

John G. Gunderson, M.D.
Professor of Psychiatry, Harvard Medical School, Boston, Massachusetts; Director, Psychosocial and Personality Research, and Director, Borderline Personality Disorder Center, McLean Hospital, Belmont, Massachusetts

Thomas G. Gutheil, M.D.
Professor of Psychiatry, Department of Psychiatry, Beth Israel Deaconess Medical Center, Harvard Medical School, and Co-Founder, Program in Psychiatry and the Law, Massachusetts Mental Health Center, Boston, Massachusetts

Amy Heim, Ph.D.
Private practice, Lexington, Massachusetts

Jeffrey G. Johnson, Ph.D.
Associate Professor of Clinical Psychology, Department of Psychiatry, College of Physicians and Surgeons, Columbia University; Research Scientist IV, Epidemiology of Mental Disorders Department, New York State Psychiatric Institute, New York, New York

Nathan Kolla, M.D.
Psychiatry Resident, Department of Psychiatry, University of Toronto, Toronto, Ontario, Canada

Paul S. Links, M.D., F.R.C.P.C.
Arthur Sommer Rotenberg Chair in Suicide Studies, Professor of Psychiatry, Department of Psychiatry, St. Michael's Hospital, University of Toronto, Toronto, Ontario, Canada

Pamela G. McGeoch, M.A.
Graduate Faculty, Department of Psychology, The New School University, New York, New York

Thomas H. McGlashan, M.D.
Professor of Psychiatry, Department of Psychiatry, Yale University School of Medicine, New Haven, Connecticut

Edmund C. Neuhaus, Ph.D.
Director, Behavioral Health Partial Hospital Program, Co-Director of Psychology Training, McLean Hospital, Belmont, Massachusetts; Assistant Clinical Professor, Harvard Medical School, Boston, Massachusetts

John S. Ogrodniczuk, Ph.D.
Associate Professor, Department of Psychiatry, University of British Columbia, Vancouver, British Columbia, Canada

John M. Oldham, M.D., M.S.
Senior Vice President and Chief of Staff, The Menninger Clinic; Professor and Executive Vice Chairman, Menninger Department of Psychiatry and Behavioral Sciences, Baylor College of Medicine, Houston, Texas

William E. Piper, Ph.D.
Professor and Head, Division of Behavioural Science; Director, Psychotherapy Program, Department of Psychiatry, University of British Columbia, Vancouver, British Columbia, Canada

Abigail Schlesinger, M.D.
Assistant Professor, Western Psychiatric Institute and Clinic, University of Pittsburgh School of Medicine, Pittsburgh, Pennsylvania

Larry J. Siever, M.D.
Executive Director, Mental Illness Research, Education and Clinical Center, Bronx Veterans Administration Medical Center, Bronx, New York; Professor of Psychiatry, Department of Psychiatry, The Mount Sinai School of Medicine, New York, New York

Kenneth R. Silk, M.D.
Professor and Director, Personality Disorders Program, Department of Psychiatry, University of Michigan Health System, Ann Arbor, Michigan

Andrew E. Skodol, M.D.
Research Professor of Psychiatry, University of Arizona College of Medicine; President, Sunbelt Collaborative, Tucson, Arizona

George W. Smith, M.S.W.
Director, Outpatient Personality Disorder Services, McLean Hospital, Boston, Massachusetts

Paul H. Soloff, M.D.
Professor of Psychiatry, Western Psychiatric Institute and Clinic, University of Pittsburgh, Pittsburgh, Pennsylvania

Barbara Stanley, Ph.D.
Professor of Clinical Psychiatry, Department of Psychiatry, Columbia University College of Physicians and Surgeons; Research Scientist, Department of Molecular Imaging and Neuropathology, New York State Psychiatric Institute, New York, New York

Svenn Torgersen, Ph.D.
Professor, Department of Psychology, University of Oslo, Oslo, Norway

Louisa M.C. van den Bosch, Ph.D.
Clinical Psychologist/Psychotherapist, CSP Leiden; Administrative Executive, Dialexis, Noordwijkerhout, The Netherlands

Roel Verheul, Ph.D.
Professor of Personality Disorders, Viersprong Institute for Studies on Personality Disorders (VISPD); University of Amsterdam, Department of Clinical Psychology; Amsterdam, Chief Executive Officer, Center for Psychotherapy De Viersprong, Halsteren, The Netherlands

Drew Westen, Ph.D.
Professor, Department of Psychiatry and Behavioral Sciences and Department of Psychology, Emory University, Atlanta, Georgia

DISCLOSURE OF INTERESTS

The following contributor to this book has indicated a financial interest in or other affiliation with a commercial supporter, a manufacturer of a commercial product, a provider of a commercial service, a nongovernmental organization, and/or a government agency, as listed below.

Paul S. Links, M.D., F.R.C.P.C.—*Educational grant*: Eli Lilly

The following contributors have no competing interests to report:

Samuel A. Ball, Ph.D.
Anthony W. Bateman, M.A., F.R.C.Psych.
Donna S. Bender, Ph.D.
Beth S. Brodsky, Ph.D.
Elizabeth Bromley, M.D.
Patricia Cohen, Ph.D.
Thomas Crawford, Ph.D.
Glen O. Gabbard, M.D.
Carlos M. Grilo, Ph.D.
John G. Gunderson, M.D.
Thomas G. Gutheil, M.D.
Amy Heim, Ph.D.
Jeffrey G. Johnson, Ph.D.
Nathan Kolla, M.D.
Pamela G. McGeoch, M.A.
Thomas H. McGlashan, M.D.
Edmund C. Neuhaus, Ph.D.
John S. Ogrodniczuk, Ph.D.
William E. Piper, Ph.D.
Larry J. Siever, M.D.
Kenneth R. Silk, M.D.
George W. Smith, M.S.W.
Paul H. Soloff, M.D.
Barbara Stanley, Ph.D.
Svenn Torgersen, Ph.D.
Roel Verheul, Ph.D.
John M. Oldham, M.D., M.S.
Andrew E. Skodol, M.D.

Introduction

From as early as the fifth century B.C., it has been recognized that every human being develops an individualized signature pattern of behavior that is reasonably persistent and predictable throughout life. Hippocrates proposed that the varieties of human behavior could be organized into what we might now call prototypes—broad descriptive patterns of behavior characterized by typical, predominant, easily recognizable features—and that most individuals could be sorted into these broad categories. Sanguine, melancholic, choleric, and phlegmatic types of behavior were, in turn, thought to derive from "body humors," such as blood, black bile, yellow bile, and phlegm, and the predominance of a given body humor in an individual was thought to correlate with a particular behavior pattern. Although we now call body humors by different names (neurotransmitters, transcription factors, second messengers), the ancient principle that fundamental differences in biology correlate with relatively predictable patterns of behavior is strikingly familiar.

In spite of long-standing worldwide interest in personality types, however, remarkably little progress has been made, until recently, in our understanding of those severe and persistent patterns of inner experience and behavior that result in enduring emotional distress and impairment in occupational functioning and interpersonal relationships—the conditions we now refer to as personality disorders. For decades, it was widely recognized that some severely disturbed individuals just seemed to have been "born that way," a view we now know to be true in some cases involving significant genetic loading or risk. In the twentieth century, however, we became more interested in the role of the environment during early development in determining the shape of lasting adult behavior—a view that for a while extended well beyond the realm of the personality disorders to include most major mental disorders. We know, of course, that the early life environment is indeed critically important—from health-promoting, highly nurturing environments to stressful and neglectful environments from which only the most resilient emerge unscathed. But we also know that variable degrees of genetic risk predispose many of us to become ill in very specific ways, should we unluckily encounter more stress than we can tolerate.

In recent years, we have begun to see an upsurge of empirical and clinical interest in personality disorders. Improved standardized diagnostic systems have led to semistructured research interviews that are being used not only in studies of clinical populations but also in community-based studies, to give us, for the first time, good data about the epidemiology of these disorders. Personality disorders occur in about 10% of the general population, and their public health significance has been documented by studies showing their extreme social dysfunction and high health care utilization. As clinical populations are becoming better defined, new and more rigorous treatment studies are being carried out, with increasingly promising results. No longer are personality disorders swept into the "hopeless cases" bin. An explosion of knowledge and technology in the neurosciences has made the formerly black box, the brain, more and more transparent. Mapping the human genome paved the way for new gene-finding technologies that are being put to work to tackle complex psychiatric disorders, including the personality disorders. New transgenic animal models are providing important hints about the genetic loci driving certain behavior types, such as attachment and bonding behavior. Brain imaging studies are allowing researchers to zero in on malfunctioning areas of the brain in specific personality disorders.

A great deal of work must still be done. Fundamental questions remain, such as what is the relationship between traits of general, or normal, personality functioning and personality psychopathology. Directly related to this issue is the ongoing debate about whether dimensional or categorical systems best capture the full scope of personality differences and personality pathology. Extensive impairment can be associated with personality disorders, but we are gaining new knowledge regarding their longer-term course and increased understanding of factors contributing to variations in course. There is a strong momentum of interest internationally in these issues, as new research findings emerge daily to inform the process.

In light of the continuing and increased activity and progress in the field of personality studies and personality disorders, we judged the time to be right to develop a companion volume to *The American Psychiatric Publishing Textbook of Personality Disorders,* published in 2005 to cover and update the essentials of this topic. Because of space constraints, it was necessary to be selective regarding what material to include in the *Essentials* volume, and we have tried to focus on material that is up-to-date and useful to practicing clinicians. This new volume is organized into several parts: 1) Basic Concepts, 2) Clinical Evaluation, 3) Etiology, 4) Treat-

ment, and 5) New Developments and Future Directions.

PART I: BASIC CONCEPTS

Basic Concepts, the first part of *Essentials of Personality Disorders,* might be thought of as setting the stage for the parts that follow. In Chapter 1, Oldham presents a brief overview of the recent history of the personality disorders, along with a summary look at the evolution of the personality disorders component in successive editions of the *American Psychiatric Association Diagnostic and Statistical Manual of Mental Disorders.* Heim and Westen, in the next chapter, review the major theories that have influenced our thinking about the nature of personality and personality disorders.

PART II: CLINICAL EVALUATION

In the section on clinical evaluation beginning with Chapter 3, Skodol reviews the defining features of DSM-IV-TR personality disorders, discusses complementary approaches to the clinical assessment of a patient with a possible personality disorder, provides guidance on general problems encountered in the routine clinical evaluation, and describes patterns of Axis I and Axis II disorder comorbidity. In Chapter 4, Grilo and McGlashan provide an overview of the clinical course and outcome of personality disorders, synthesizing the empirical literature on the stability of personality disorder psychopathology.

PART III: ETIOLOGY

The section on etiology of the personality disorders begins with Chapter 5. Torgersen presents the best data we have to date on the population-based epidemiology of the personality disorders. Although there are relatively few well-designed population-based studies, Torgersen reviews a number of studies, including his own Norwegian study, and tabulates prevalence ranges and averages for individual DSM-defined personality disorders as well as for all personality disorders taken together (showing an overall average prevalence rate for the personality disorders of over 12%). Of particular interest in these data are cross-cultural comparisons, suggesting significant cultural differences in the prevalence of selected personality disorders. Substantial progress has been made in our understanding of the neurobiology of the personality disorders, as reviewed in Chapter 6 by Coccaro and Siever. Although a great deal more is known about the neurobiology of some personality disorders (e.g., schizotypal personality disorder and borderline personality disorder) than others (e.g., Cluster C personality disorders), the underlying neurobiological dysfunction involved in personality disorders characterized by cognitive symptomatology, impulsivity, and mood dysregulation is becoming increasingly clear.

Understanding the etiology of the personality disorders involves not just cross-sectional genetic and neurobiological analysis; environmental influences shaping personality must be understood as well. In Chapter 7, Cohen and Crawford provide a developmental perspective. Although, by convention, DSM-IV-TR personality disorders are generally not diagnosed until late adolescence, there is increasing recognition of early patterns of behavior that are thought to be precursors to certain personality disorders. The challenge to identify true early precursors of personality disorders, versus the risk of inaccurate labeling of transient symptoms, is central to the work ahead of us as we focus more and more on prevention strategies. Complementing this developmental approach, the authors of Chapter 8, Johnson, Bromley, and McGeoch, review the relevance of childhood experiences to the development of adaptive and maladaptive personality traits. They emphasize the importance of stress, but also of protective factors that can offset and even prevent the development of maladaptive traits in vulnerable individuals.

PART IV: TREATMENT

The treatment section begins with Chapter 9, a discussion of the levels of care available for patients with personality disorders. Gunderson, Gratz, Neuhaus, and Smith offer guidelines for determining the appropriate intensity of treatment services for individual patients. Four levels of care are addressed: hospitalization, partial hospitalization/day treatment, intensive outpatient, and outpatient.

Chapters 10 through 14 offer a range of treatment options. Gabbard (Chapter 10) summarizes the salient features of psychoanalysis and psychodynamic psychotherapy as applied to patients with character pathology. One psychodynamic model, mentalization-based therapy, is of special interest in the treatment of patients with borderline personality disorder, as described in Chapter 11 by Fonagy and Bateman. In this model, borderline personality disorder is seen as dysfunction in self-regulation, critically related to interpersonal dynamics. In Chapter 12, Stanley and Brodsky outline the core elements of dialectical behavior therapy, which includes individual and group interventions, and is chiefly used to treat parasuicidal behaviors in patients with borderline personality disorder.

Apart from the realm of individual treatments, there are other venues for therapeutic interventions. In Chapter 13, Piper and Ogrodniczuk demonstrate the application of group therapy to personality disorders. Soloff (Chapter 14) takes up the issue of pharmacotherapy and other somatic treatments, because many patients with personality disorders may benefit by complementing their psychosocial treatments with medication.

The final five chapters of this section address issues of great importance pertaining to most, if not all, treatments. Bender (Chapter 15) underscores the necessity of explicitly considering alliance building across all treatment modalities, while Gutheil (Chapter 16) cautions practitioners about dynamics that can lead treaters to boundary violations when working with certain patients with personality disorders. Schlesinger and Silk, in Chapter 17, provide recommendations about the best way of negotiating collaborative treatments, since many patients with personality disorders are engaged in several modalities with several clinicians at the same time.

In recognition of the fact that patients with personality disorders can be particularly challenging, we have included two chapters devoted to the issues often faced when treating these individuals. Of prime importance is the risk for suicide. In Chapter 18, Links and Kolla provide evidence on the association of suicidal behavior and personality disorders, examine modifiable risk factors, and discuss clinical approaches to the assessment and management of suicide risk. In Chapter 19, Verheul, van den Bosch, and Ball focus on pathways to substance abuse in patients with personality disorders, and discuss issues of differential diagnosis and treatment.

PART V: NEW DEVELOPMENTS AND FUTURE DIRECTIONS

In the final section of *Essentials of Personality Disorders*, Skodol, Bender, and Oldham summarize current controversies and speculate about future directions, as the work gets under way to consider the best strategies to classify and understand the personality disorders in DSM-V.

We are grateful to all of the authors of each chapter for their careful and thoughtful contributions, and we hope that we have succeeded in providing a current, definitive review of the field. We would particularly like to thank Liz Bednarowicz for her organized and steadfast administrative support, without which this volume would not have been possible.

John M. Oldham, M.D., M.S.
Houston, Texas

Andrew E. Skodol, M.D.
Phoenix, Arizona

Donna S. Bender, Ph.D.
Tucson, Arizona

Part I

Basic Concepts

1

Personality Disorders

Recent History and the DSM System

John M. Oldham, M.D., M.S.

PERSONALITY TYPES AND PERSONALITY DISORDERS

Charting a historical review of efforts to understand personality types and the differences among them would involve exploring centuries of scholarly archives, worldwide, on the varieties of human behavior. For it is human behavior, in the end, that serves as the most valid measurable and observable benchmark of personality. In many important ways, we are what we do. The "what" of personality is easier to come by than the "why," and each of us has a personality style that is unique, almost like a fingerprint. At a school reunion, recognition of classmates not seen for decades derives as much from familiar behavior as from physical appearance.

As to why we behave the way we do, we know now that a fair amount of the reason relates to our "hardwiring." To varying degrees, heritable temperaments that vary widely from one individual to another determine the amazing range of behavior in the newborn nursery, from cranky to placid. Each individual's temperament remains a key component of that person's developing personality, to which is added the shaping and molding influences of family, caretakers, and environmental experiences. This process is, we now know, bidirectional, so that the "inborn" behavior of the infant can elicit behavior in parents or caretakers that can, in turn, reinforce infant behavior: placid, happy babies may elicit warm and nurturing behaviors; irritable babies may elicit impatient and neglectful behaviors.

Sections of this chapter have been modified from Oldham JM, Skodol AE: "Charting the Future of Axis II." *Journal of Personality Disorders* 14:17–29, 2000. Reprinted with permission of Guilford Press.

However, even-tempered, easy-to-care-for babies can have bad luck and land in a nonsupportive or even abusive environment that may set the stage for a personality disorder, and difficult-to-care-for babies can have good luck and be protected from future personality pathology by specially talented and attentive caretakers. Once these highly individualized dynamics have had their main effects and an individual has reached late adolescence or young adulthood, his or her personality will usually have been pretty well established. We know that this is not an ironclad rule; there are "late bloomers," and high-impact life events can derail or reroute any of us. How much we can change if we need and want to is variable, but change is possible. How we define the differences between personality styles and personality disorders, how the two relate to each other, what systems best capture the magnificent variety of nonpathological human behavior, and how we think about and deal with extremes of behavior that we call personality disorders are all spelled out in great detail in the chapters of this textbook. In this first chapter, I briefly describe how psychiatrists in the United States have approached the definition and classification of the personality disorders, building on broader international concepts and theories of psychopathology.

TWENTIETH-CENTURY CONCEPTS OF PERSONALITY PSYCHOPATHOLOGY

Personality pathology has been recognized in most influential systems of classifying psychopathology. The well-known contributions by European pioneers of descriptive psychiatry, such as Kraepelin (1904), Bleuler (1924), Kretschmer (1926), and Schneider (1923/1950) had an important impact on early twentieth-century American psychiatry. For the most part, Kraepelin, Bleuler, and Kretschmer described personality types or temperaments, such as aesthenic, autistic, schizoid, cyclothymic, or cycloid, that were thought to be pre-cursors or less extreme forms of psychotic conditions, such as schizophrenia or manic-depressive illness—systems that can clearly be seen as forerunners of current Axis I/Axis II "spectrum" models. Schneider, on the other hand, described a set of "psychopathic personalities" that he viewed as separate disorders co-occurring with other psychiatric disorders. Although these classical systems of descriptive psychopathology resonate strongly with the framework eventually adopted by the American Psychiatric Association (APA) and published in its *Diagnostic and Statistical Manual of Mental Disorders* (DSM), they were widely overshadowed in American psychiatry during the mid-twentieth century by theory-based psychoanalytic concepts stimulated by the work of Sigmund Freud and his followers.

Freud emphasized the presence of a dynamic unconscious, a realm that, by definition, is mostly unavailable to conscious thought but is a powerful motivator of human behavior (key ingredients of his topographical model). His emphasis on a dynamic unconscious was augmented by his well-known tripartite structural theory, a conflict model serving as the bedrock of his psychosexual theory of pathology (Freud 1926). Freud theorized that certain unconscious sexual wishes or impulses (id) could threaten to emerge into consciousness (ego), thus colliding with conscience-driven prohibitions (superego) and producing "signal" anxiety, precipitating unconscious defense mechanisms and, when these coping strategies prove insufficient, leading to frank symptom formation. For the most part, this system was proposed as an explanation for what were called at the time the *symptom neuroses*, such as hysterical neurosis or obsessive-compulsive neurosis. During the 1940s, 1950s, and 1960s, these ideas became dominant in American psychiatry, followed later by interest in other psychoanalytic principles, such as object relations theory.

Freud's concentration on the symptom neuroses involved the central notion of anxiety as the engine that led to defense mechanisms and to symptom formation, and as a critical factor in motivating patients to work hard in psychoanalysis to face painful realizations and to tolerate stress within the treatment itself (such as that involved in the "transference neurosis"). Less prominently articulated were Freud's notions of character pathology, but generally character disorders were seen to represent "pre-oedipal" pathology. As such, patients with these conditions were judged less likely to be motivated to change. Instead of experiencing anxiety related to the potential gratification of an unacceptable sexual impulse, patients with "fixations" at the oral-dependent stage, for example, experienced anxiety when *not* gratifying the impulse—in this case, the need to be fed. Relief of anxiety thus could be accomplished by some combination of real and symbolic feeding—attention from a parent or parent figure or consumption of alcohol or drugs. Deprivations within the psychoanalytic situation, then—inevitable by its very nature—could lead to patient flight and interrupted treatment.

In a way, social attitudes mirrored and extended these beliefs such that although personality pathology was well known, it was often thought to reflect weakness of character or willfully offensive or socially deviant behavior produced by faulty upbringing, rather than understood as "legitimate" psychopathology. A good example of this view could be seen in military psychiatry in the mid-1900s, where those discharged from active duty for mental illness, with eligibility for disability and medical benefits, did not include individuals with "character disorders" (or alcoholism and substance abuse) because these conditions were seen as "bad behavior" and led to administrative, nonmedical separation from the military.

In spite of these common attitudes, clinicians recognized that many patients with significant impairment in social or occupational functioning, or with significant emotional distress, needed treatment for psychopathology that did not involve frank psychosis or other syndromes characterized by discrete, persistent symptom patterns such as major depressive episodes, persistent anxiety, or dementia. General clinical experience and wisdom guided treatment recommendations for these patients, at least for those who sought treatment. Patients with paranoid, schizoid, or antisocial patterns of thinking and behaving often did not seek treatment. Others, however, often resembled patients with symptom neuroses and did seek help for problems ranging from self-destructive behavior to chronic misery. The most severely and persistently disabled of these patients were often referred for intensive, psychoanalytically oriented long-term inpatient treatment at treatment centers such as Austen Riggs, Chestnut Lodge, Menninger Clinic, McLean Hospital, New York Hospital Westchester Division, New York State Psychiatric Institute, Sheppard Pratt, and other long-term inpatient facilities available at the time. Other patients, able to function outside of a hospital setting and often hard to distinguish from patients with neuroses, were referred for outpatient psychoanalysis or intensive psychoanalytically oriented psychotherapy. As Gunderson (2001) described, the fact that many such patients in psychoanalysis regressed and seemed to get worse, rather than showing improvement in treatment, was one factor that contributed to the emerging concept of borderline personality disorder (BPD), thought initially to be in the border zone between the psychoses and the neuroses. Patients in this general category included some who had previously been labeled as having latent schizophrenia (Bleuler 1924), ambulatory schizophrenia (Zillborg 1941), pseudoneurotic schizophrenia (Hoch and Polatin 1949), psychotic character (Frosch 1964), or "as-if" personality (Deutsch 1942).

These developments coincided with new approaches based on alternative theoretical models that were emerging within the psychoanalytic framework, such as the British object relations school. New conceptual frameworks, such as Kernberg's (1975) model of borderline personality organization or Kohut's (1971) concept of the central importance of empathic failure in the histories of narcissistic patients, served as the basis for an intensive psychodynamic treatment approach for selected patients with personality disorders. These strategies and others are reviewed in detail in Chapter 10, "Psychoanalysis and Psychodynamic Psychotherapy."

THE DSM SYSTEM

Contrary to assumptions commonly encountered, personality disorders have been included in every edition of DSM. Largely driven by the need for standardized psychiatric diagnosis in the context of World War II, the U.S. War Department in 1943 developed a document labeled "Technical Bulletin 203," representing a psychoanalytically oriented system of terminology for classifying mental illness precipitated by stress (Barton 1987). The APA charged its Committee on Nomenclature and Statistics to solicit expert opinion and to develop a diagnostic manual that would codify and standardize psychiatric diagnoses. This diagnostic system became the framework for the first edition of DSM (DSM-I; American Psychiatric Association 1952). This manual was widely utilized, and it was subsequently revised on several occasions, leading to DSM-II (American Psychiatric Association 1968), DSM-III (American Psychiatric Association 1980), DSM-III-R (American Psychiatric Association 1987), DSM-IV (American Psychiatric Association 1994), and DSM-IV-TR (American Psychiatric Association 2000). Figure 1–1 (Skodol 1997) portrays the ontogeny of diagnostic terms relevant to the personality disorders from DSM-I through DSM-IV (DSM-IV-TR involved only text revisions; it used the same diagnostic terms as DSM-IV).

Although not explicit in the narrative text, DSM-I reflected the general view of personality disorders at the time, elements of which persist to the present. Generally, personality disorders were viewed as more or less permanent patterns of behavior and human interaction that were established by early adulthood and were unlikely to change throughout the life cycle. Thorny issues such as how to differentiate personality disorders from personality styles or traits, which remain actively debated today, were clearly identified at the time. Personality disorders were contrasted with the symptom neuroses in a number of ways, particularly that the neuroses were characterized by anxiety and distress, whereas the personality disorders were often ego-syntonic and thus not recognized by those who had them. Some personality disorders are currently referred to as "externalizing" disorders—that is, disorders in which the patient disavows any problem but blames all discomfort on the real or perceived unreasonableness of others.

In DSM-I, personality disorders were generally viewed as deficit conditions reflecting partial developmental arrests or distortions in development secondary to inadequate or pathological early caretaking. The personality disorders were grouped primarily into "personality pattern disturbances," "personality trait disturbances," and "sociopathic personality disturbances." *Personality pattern disturbances* were viewed as the most entrenched conditions and likely to be recalcitrant to change, even with treatment; these included inadequate personality, schizoid personality, cyclothymic personality, and paranoid personality. *Personality trait disturbances* were thought to be less pervasive and disabling, so that in the absence of stress these patients could function relatively well. If under significant stress, however, patients with emotionally unstable, passive-aggressive, or compulsive personalities were thought to show emotional distress and deterioration in functioning, and they were variably motivated for and amenable to treatment. The category of *sociopathic personality disturbances* reflected what were generally seen as types of social deviance at the time, including antiso-

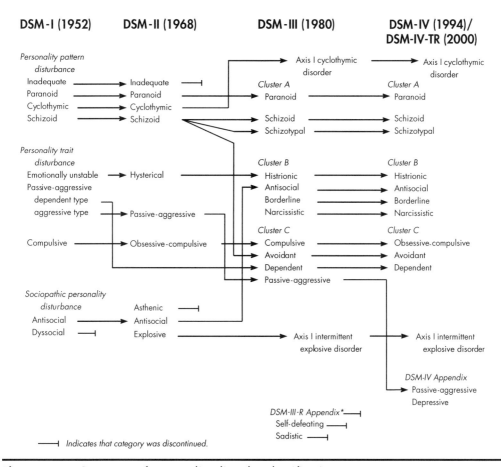

Figure 1–1.   Ontogeny of personality disorder classification.

*No changes were made to the personality disorder classification in DSM-III-R except for the inclusion of self-defeating and sadistic personality disorders in Appendix A: Proposed Diagnostic Categories Needing Further Study. These two categories were not included in DSM-IV or in DSM-IV-TR.

Source.   Reprinted with permission from Skodol AE: "Classification, Assessment, and Differential Diagnosis of Personality Disorders." *Journal of Practical Psychiatry and Behavioral Health* 3:261–274, 1997.

cial reaction, dyssocial reaction, sexual deviation, and addiction (subcategorized into alcoholism and drug addiction).

The primary stimulus leading to the development of a new, second edition of DSM was the publication of the eighth edition of the International Classification of Diseases (World Health Organization 1967) and the wish of the APA to reconcile its diagnostic terminology with this international system. In the DSM revision process, an effort was made to move away from theory-derived diagnoses and to attempt to reach consensus on the main constellations of personality that

were observable, measurable, enduring, and consistent over time. The earlier view that patients with personality disorders did not experience emotional distress was discarded, as were the DSM-I subcategories of personality pattern, personality trait, and sociopathic personality disturbances. One new personality disorder was added, called asthenic personality disorder, only to be deleted in the next edition of the DSM.

By the mid-1970s, greater emphasis was placed on increasing the reliability of all diagnoses; whenever possible, diagnostic criteria that were observable and measurable were developed to define each diagnosis. DSM-III, the third edition of the diagnostic manual, introduced a multiaxial system. Disorders classified on Axis I included those generally seen as episodic, characterized by exacerbations and remissions, such as psychoses, mood disorders, and anxiety disorders. Axis II was established to include the personality disorders as well as mental retardation; both groups were seen as composed of early-onset, persistent conditions, but mental retardation was understood to be "biological" in origin, in contrast to the personality disorders, which were generally regarded as "psychological" in origin. The stated reason for placing the personality disorders on Axis II was to ensure that "consideration is given to the possible presence of disorders that are frequently overlooked when attention is directed to the usually more florid Axis I disorders" (American Psychiatric Association 1980, p. 23). It is generally agreed that the decision to place the personality disorders on Axis II led to greater recognition of the personality disorders and stimulated extensive research and progress in our understanding of these conditions.

As shown in Figure 1–1, the DSM-II diagnoses of inadequate personality disorder and asthenic personality disorder were discontinued in DSM-III. The diagnosis of explosive personality disorder was changed to intermittent explosive disorder, cyclothymic personality disorder was renamed cyclothymic disorder, and both of these diagnoses were moved to Axis I. Schizoid personality disorder was felt to be too broad a category in DSM-II, and it was recrafted into three personality disorders: *schizoid personality disorder*, reflecting "loners" who are uninterested in close personal relationships; *schizotypal personality disorder*, understood to be on the schizophrenia spectrum of disorders and characterized by eccentric beliefs and nontraditional behavior; and *avoidant personality disorder*, typified by self-imposed interpersonal isolation driven by self-consciousness and anxiety. Two new personality disorder

diagnoses were added in DSM-III: BPD and narcissistic personality disorder. In contrast to initial notions that patients called "borderline" were on the border between the psychoses and the neuroses, the criteria defining BPD in DSM-III emphasized emotional dysregulation, unstable interpersonal relationships, and loss of impulse control more than cognitive distortions and marginal reality testing, which were more characteristic of schizotypal personality disorder. Among many scholars whose work greatly influenced and shaped our understanding of borderline pathology were Kernberg (1975) and Gunderson (1984, 2001, 2008). Although concepts of narcissism had been described by Freud, Reich, and others, the essence of the current views of narcissistic personality disorder emerged from the work of Millon (1969), Kohut (1971), and Kernberg (1975).

DSM-III-R was published in 1987 after an intensive process to revise DSM-III involving widely solicited input from researchers and clinicians and following similar principles to those articulated in DSM-III, such as assuring reliable diagnostic categories that were clinically useful and consistent with research findings, thus minimizing reliance on theory. Efforts were made for diagnoses to be "descriptive" and to require a minimum of inference, although the introductory text of DSM-III-R acknowledged that for some disorders, "particularly the Personality Disorders, the criteria require much more inference on the part of the observer" (American Psychiatric Association 1987, p. xxiii). No changes were made in DSM-III-R diagnostic categories of personality disorders, although some adjustments were made in certain criteria sets, for example, making them uniformly polythetic instead of defining some personality disorders with monothetic criteria sets (e.g., dependent personality disorder) and others with polythetic criteria sets (e.g., BPD). In addition, two personality disorders were included in DSM-III-R in Appendix A ("Proposed Diagnostic Categories Needing Further Study")—self-defeating personality disorder and sadistic personality disorder—based on prior clinical recommendations to the DSM-III-R personality disorder subcommittee. These diagnoses were considered provisional, pending further review and research.

DSM-IV was derived after an extensive process of literature review, data analysis, field trials, and feedback from the profession. Because of the increase in research stimulated by the criteria-based multiaxial system of DSM-III, a substantial body of evidence existed to guide the DSM-IV process. As a result, the threshold for approval of revisions for DSM-IV was higher than that used in DSM-III or DSM-III-R. DSM-IV introduced, for the first time, a set of general diagnostic criteria for any personality disorder (Table 1–1), underscoring qualities such as early onset, long duration, inflexibility, and pervasiveness. Diagnostic categories and dimensional organization of the personality disorders into clusters remained the same in DSM-IV as in DSM-III-R, with the exception of the relocation of passive-aggressive personality disorder from the "official" diagnostic list to Appendix B ("Criteria Sets and Axes Provided for Further Study"). Passive-aggressive personality disorder, as defined by DSM-III and DSM-III-R, was thought to be too unidimensional and generic; it was tentatively retitled "negativistic personality disorder," and the criteria were revised. In addition, the two provisional Axis II diagnoses in DSM-III-R, self-defeating personality disorder and sadistic personality disorder, were dropped because of insufficient research data and clinical consensus to support their retention. One other personality disorder was proposed and added to Appendix B: depressive personality disorder. Although substantially controversial, this provisional diagnosis was proposed as a pessimistic cognitive style; its validity and its distinction from passive-aggressive personality disorder on Axis II or dysthymic disorder on Axis I, however, remain to be established.

DSM-IV-TR, published in 2000, did not change the diagnostic terms or criteria of DSM-IV. The intent of DSM-IV-TR was to revise the descriptive, narrative text accompanying each diagnosis where it seemed indicated and to update the information provided. Only minimal revisions were made in the text material accompanying the personality disorders.

CURRENT CONTROVERSIES AND FUTURE DIRECTIONS

There is a general consensus, at least in the United States, that the placement of the personality disorders on Axis II has stimulated research and focused clinical and educational attention on these disabling conditions. However, there is growing debate about the continued appropriateness of maintaining the personality disorders on a separate axis in future editions of the diagnostic manual and about whether a dimensional or a categorical system of classification is preferable. As new knowledge has rapidly accumulated about the personality disorders, these controversies take their places among many ongoing constructive dialogues, such as the relationship of normal personality to personality disorder, the pros and cons of polythetic criteria sets, how to determine the appropriate number of criteria (i.e., threshold) required for each diagnosis, which personality disorder categories have construct validity, which dimensions best cover the scope of normal and abnormal personality, and others. Many of these discussions overlap with and inform each other, and these considerations for the future are discussed in detail in Chapter 20 of this volume, "Future Directions: Toward DSM-V."

CONCLUSION

This brief review of recent notions of personality pathology serves as a window on the rapid progress in our field and in our understanding of psychiatric disorders. Increas-

---

Table 1–1. General diagnostic criteria for a personality disorder

---

A. An enduring pattern of inner experience and behavior that deviates markedly from the expectations of the individual's culture. This pattern is manifested in two (or more) of the following areas:

    (1) cognition (i.e., ways of perceiving and interpreting self, other people, and events)

    (2) affectivity (i.e., the range, intensity, lability, and appropriateness of emotional response)

    (3) interpersonal functioning

    (4) impulse control

B. The enduring pattern is inflexible and pervasive across a broad range of personal and social situations.

C. The enduring pattern leads to clinically significant distress or impairment in social, occupational, or other important areas of functioning.

D. The pattern is stable and of long duration, and its onset can be traced back at least to adolescence or early adulthood.

E. The enduring pattern is not better accounted for as a manifestation or consequence of another mental disorder.

F. The enduring pattern is not due to the direct physiological effects of a substance (e.g., a drug of abuse, a medication) or a general medical condition (e.g., head trauma).

Source. Reprinted with permission from American Psychiatric Association: *Diagnostic and Statistical Manual of Mental Disorders*, 4th Edition, Text Revision. Washington, DC, American Psychiatric Association, 2000.

---

ingly, a stress/diathesis framework seems applicable in medicine in general as a unifying model of illness—a model that can easily encompass the personality disorders (Paris 1999). Variable genetic vulnerabilities predispose us all to potential future illness that may or may not develop depending on the balance of specific stressors and protective factors.

The personality disorders represent maladaptive exaggerations of nonpathological personality styles resulting from predisposing temperaments combined with stressful circumstances. Neurobiology can be altered in at least some Axis II disorders, as it can be in Axis I disorders. Our challenge for the future is to recognize that not all personality disorders are alike, nor are personality disorders fundamentally different from many other psychiatric disorders. What may be somewhat unique to the personality disorders is their correlation and continuity with normal functioning, which could be an important consideration in future revisions of our diagnostic system. As we learn more about the etiologies and pathology of the personality disorders, it will no longer be necessary, or even desirable, to limit our diagnostic schemes to atheoretical, descriptive phenomena, and we can look forward to an enriched understanding of these disorders.

REFERENCES

American Psychiatric Association: Diagnostic and Statistical Manual of Mental Disorders. Washington, DC, American Psychiatric Association, 1952

American Psychiatric Association: Diagnostic and Statistical Manual of Mental Disorders, 2nd

Edition. Washington, DC, American Psychiatric Association, 1968

American Psychiatric Association: Diagnostic and Statistical Manual of Mental Disorders, 3rd Edition. Washington, DC, American Psychiatric Association, 1980

American Psychiatric Association: Diagnostic and Statistical Manual of Mental Disorders, 3rd Edition, Revised. Washington, DC, American Psychiatric Association, 1987

American Psychiatric Association: Diagnostic and Statistical Manual of Mental Disorders, 4th Edition. Washington, DC, American Psychiatric Association, 1994

American Psychiatric Association: Diagnostic and Statistical Manual of Mental Disorders, 4th Edition, Text Revision. Washington, DC, American Psychiatric Association, 2000

Barton WE: The History and Influence of the American Psychiatric Association. Washington, DC, American Psychiatric Press, 1987

Bleuler E: Textbook of Psychiatry (English translation). New York, Macmillan, 1924

Deutsch H: Some forms of emotional disturbance and their relationship to schizophrenia. Psychoanal Q 11:301–321, 1942

Freud S: Inhibitions, Symptoms and Anxiety, Standard Edition. London, Hogarth Press, 1926

Frosch J: The psychotic character: clinical psychiatric considerations. Psychiatr Q 38:81–96, 1964

Gunderson JG: Borderline Personality Disorder. Washington, DC, American Psychiatric Press, 1984

Gunderson JG: Borderline Personality Disorder: A Clinical Guide. Washington, DC, American Psychiatric Publishing, 2001

Gunderson JG: Borderline Personality Disorder. Washington, DC, American Psychiatric Publishing, 2008

Hoch PH, Polatin P: Pseudoneurotic forms of schizophrenia. Psychiatr Q 23:248–276, 1949

Kernberg OF: Borderline Conditions and Pathological Narcissism. New York, Jason Aronson, 1975

Kohut H: The Analysis of the Self: A Systematic Approach to the Treatment of Narcissistic Personality Disorder. New York, International Universities Press, 1971

Kraepelin E: Lectures on Clinical Psychiatry (English translation). New York, Wood Press, 1904

Kretschmer E: Hysteria (English translation). New York, Nervous and Mental Disease Publishers, 1926

Millon T: Modern Psychopathology: A Biosocial Approach to Maladaptive Learning and Functioning. Philadelphia, PA, WB Saunders, 1969

Paris J: Nature and Nurture in Psychiatry: A Predisposition-Stress Model of Mental Disorders. Washington, DC, American Psychiatric Press, 1999

Schneider K: Psychopathic Personalities (1923). London, Cassell, 1950

Skodol AE: Classification, assessment, and differential diagnosis of personality disorders. Journal of Practical Psychology and Behavioral Health 3:261–274, 1997

World Health Organization: International Classification of Diseases, 8th Revision. Geneva, World Health Organization, 1968

Zillborg G: Ambulatory schizophrenia. Psychiatry 4:149–155, 1941

2

Theories of Personality and Personality Disorders

Amy Heim, Ph.D.
Drew Westen, Ph.D.

Personality refers to enduring patterns of cognition, emotion, motivation, and behavior that are activated in particular circumstances (see Mischel and Shoda 1995; Westen 1995). This minimalist definition (i.e., one that most personality psychologists would accept, despite widely differing theories) underscores two important aspects of personality. First, personality is dynamic, characterized by an ongoing interaction of mental, behavioral, and environmental events. Second, inherent in personality is the potential for variation and flexibility of responding (activation of specific processes under particular circumstances). Enduring ways of responding need not be broadly generalized to be considered aspects of personality (or to lead to dysfunction), because many aspects of personality are triggered by specific situations, thoughts, or feelings. For example, a tendency to bristle and respond with opposition, anger, or passive resistance to perceived demands of male authority figures may or may not occur with female authorities, peers, lovers, or subordinates. Nevertheless, this response tendency represents an enduring way of thinking, attending to information, feeling, and responding that is clearly an aspect of personality (and one that can substantially affect adaptation).

Preparation of this manuscript was supported in part by National Institute of Mental Health grants MH62377 and MH62378 (Westen).

Among the dozens of approaches to personality advanced over the past century, two are of the most widespread use in clinical practice: the psychodynamic and the cognitive-social or cognitive-behavioral. Two other approaches have gained increased interest among personality disorder researchers: trait psychology, one of the oldest and most enduring empirical approaches to the study of normal personality; and biological approaches, which reflect a long-standing tradition in descriptive psychiatry as well as more recent developments in behavioral genetics and neuroscience. Although most theories have traditionally fallen into a single "camp," several other approaches are best viewed as integrative. These include Benjamin's (1996a, 1996b) interpersonal approach, which integrates interpersonal, psychodynamic, and social learning theories; Millon's (1990) evolutionary–social learning approach, which has assimilated broadly from multiple traditions (e.g., psychoanalytic object relations theory); and Westen's (1995, 1998) functional-domains model, which draws on psychodynamic, evolutionary, behavioral, cognitive, and developmental research. In this chapter we briefly consider how each approach conceptualizes personality disorders.

PSYCHODYNAMIC THEORIES

Psychoanalytic theorists were the first to generate a concept of personality disorder (also called *character disorder*, reflecting the idea that personality disorders involve character problems not isolated to a specific symptom or set of independent symptoms). Personality disorders began to draw considerable theoretical attention in psychoanalysis by the middle of the twentieth century (e.g., Fairbairn 1952; Reich 1933/1978), in part because they were common and difficult to treat, and in part because they defied understanding using the psychoanalytic models prevalent at the time. For years, analysts

had understood psychological problems in terms of conflict and defense using Freud's topographic model (conscious, preconscious, unconscious) or his structural model (id, ego, superego). In classical psychoanalytic terms, most symptoms reflect maladaptive compromises, forged outside of awareness, among conflicting wishes, fears, and moral standards. For example, a patient with anorexia nervosa who is uncomfortable with her impulses and who fears losing control over them may begin to starve herself as a way of demonstrating that she can control even the most persistent of desires, hunger. Some of the personality disorders currently identified in DSM-IV (American Psychiatric Association 1994) and its update, DSM-IV-TR (American Psychiatric Association 2000), have their roots in early psychoanalytic theorizing about conflict—notably dependent, obsessive-compulsive, and to some extent histrionic personality disorders (presumed to reflect fixations at the oral, anal, and phallic stages, respectively).

Although some psychoanalysts have argued that a conflict model can account for severe personality pathology (e.g., Abend et al. 1983), most analytic theorists have turned to ego psychology, object relations theory, self psychology, and relational theories to help understand patients with personality disorders. According to these approaches, the problems seen in patients with character disorders run deeper than maladaptive compromises among conflicting motives, and reflect derailments in personality development regarding temperament, early attachment experiences, and their interaction (e.g., Balint 1969; Kernberg 1975b). Many of the DSM-IV personality disorders have roots in these later approaches, notably schizoid, borderline, and narcissistic personality disorders.

Psychoanalytic ego psychology focuses on the psychological functions (in contemporary cognitive terms, the skills, procedures, and processes involved in self-regulation) that must be in place for people to behave adaptively, attain their goals, and meet external demands (see Bellak et al. 1973; Blanck and Blanck 1974; Redl and Wineman 1951). From this perspective, patients with personality disorders may have various deficits in functioning, such as poor impulse control, difficulty regulating affects, and deficits in the capacity for self-reflection. These deficits may render them incapable of behaving consistently in their own best interest or of taking the interests of others appropriately into account (e.g., they lash out aggressively without forethought or cut themselves when they become upset).

Object relations, relational, and self psychological theories focus on the cognitive, affective, and motivational processes presumed to underlie functioning in close relationships (Aron 1996; Greenberg and Mitchell 1983; Mitchell 1988; Westen 1991b). From this point of view, personality disorders reflect a number of processes. Internalization of attitudes of hostile, abusive, critical, inconsistent, or neglectful parents may leave patients with personality disorder vulnerable to fears of abandonment, self-hatred, a tendency to treat themselves as their parents treated them, and so forth (Benjamin 1996a, 1996b; Masterson 1976; McWilliams 1998). Patients with personality disorder often fail to develop mature, constant, multifaceted representations of the self and others. As a result, they may be vulnerable to emotional swings when significant others are momentarily disappointing, and they may have difficulty understanding or imagining what might be in the minds of the people with whom they interact (Fonagy and Target 1997; Fonagy et al. 1991, 2003). Those with personality disorder often appear to have difficulty forming a realistic, balanced view of themselves that can weather momentary failures or criticisms and may have a corresponding inability to activate procedures (hypothesized to be based on loving, soothing experiences with early caregivers) that would be useful for self-soothing in the face of loss, failure, or threats to safety or self-esteem (e.g., Adler and Buie 1979). A sub-

stantial body of research supports many of these propositions, particularly vis-à-vis borderline personality disorder (BPD), the most extensively studied personality disorder (e.g., Baker et al. 1992; Gunderson 2001; Westen 1990a, 1991a).

From a psychodynamic point of view, perhaps the most important features of personality disorders are the following: a) they represent constellations of psychological processes, not distinct symptoms that can be understood in isolation; b) they can be located on a continuum of personality pathology from relative health to relative sickness; c) they can be characterized in terms of character style, which is orthogonal to level of disturbance (e.g., a patient can have an obsessional style but be relatively sick or relatively healthy); d) they involve both implicit and explicit personality processes, only some of which are available to introspection (and thus amenable to self-report); and e) they reflect processes that are deeply entrenched, often serve multiple functions, and/or have become associated with regulation of affects and are hence resistant to change.

The most comprehensive theory that embodies these principles is the theory of personality structure or organization developed by Otto Kernberg (1975a, 1984, 1996). In his theory, Kernberg proposed a continuum of pathology, from chronically psychotic levels of functioning, through borderline functioning (severe personality disorders), through neurotic to normal functioning. In Kernberg's view, people with severe personality pathology are distinguished from people whose personality is organized at a psychotic level by their relatively intact capacity for reality testing (the absence of hallucinations or psychotic delusions) and their relative ability to distinguish between their own thoughts and feelings and those of others (the absence of beliefs that their thoughts are being broadcast on the radio; their recognition, although sometimes less than complete, that the persecutory thoughts in their heads are voices from the past rather than true hal-

lucinations, etc.). What distinguishes individuals with severe personality pathology
from people with "neurotic" (that is, healthier) character structures includes 1) their
more maladaptive modes of regulating their
emotions through immature, reality-distort-
ing defenses such as denial and projection
(e.g., refusing to recognize the part they play
in generating some of the hostility they engender from others); and 2) their difficulty in
forming mature, multifaceted representations of themselves and significant others
(e.g., believing that a person they once loved
is really all bad, with no redeeming features,
and is motivated only by the desire to hurt
them). Kernberg refers to these two aspects
of borderline personality organization as
"primitive defenses" and "identity diffusion." This level of severe personality disturbance shares some features with the DSM-
IV's BPD diagnosis. However, borderline
personality organization is a broader construct, encompassing patients with paranoid, schizoid, schizotypal, and antisocial
personality disorders as well as some patients who would receive a DSM-IV diagnosis of narcissistic, histrionic, or dependent
personality disorder. (Some schizotypal and
borderline patients may at times fall "south
of the border" into the psychotic range.)
Some research supports the notion that patients fall on a continuum of severity of personality pathology (see Millon and Davis
1995; Tyrer and Johnson 1996), with disorders such as paranoid and borderline personality disorder representing more severe
forms, and disorders such as obsessive-
compulsive personality disorder less severe
(Westen and Shedler 1999a).

Although many of Kernberg's major contributions have been in the understanding of
borderline phenomena, his theory of narcissistic disturbance contributed substantially
to the development of the diagnosis of narcissistic personality disorder in DSM-III
(American Psychiatric Association 1980), just
as his understanding of borderline phenomena contributed to the borderline diagnosis.

According to Kernberg, whereas borderline
patients lack an integrated identity, narcissistic patients are typically developmentally
more advanced, in that they have been able
to develop a coherent (if distorted) view of
themselves. Narcissistic phenomena, in
Kernberg's view, lie on a continuum from
normal (characterized by adequate self-
esteem regulation) to pathological (narcissistic personality disorder) (Kernberg 1984,
1998). Individuals with narcissistic personality disorder need to construct a grossly inflated view of themselves to maintain self-
esteem and may appear grandiose, sensitive
to the slightest attacks on their self-esteem
(and hence vulnerable to rage or depression),
or both. Not only are the conscious self-representations of narcissistic patients inflated
but so too are the representations that constitute their ideal selves. Actual and ideal self-
representations stand in dynamic relation to
one another. Thus, one reason narcissistic patients must maintain an idealized view of self
is that they have a correspondingly grandiose view of who they should be, a divergence
that leads to tremendous feelings of shame,
failure, and humiliation.

The concept of a grandiose self is central to
the self psychology of Heinz Kohut, a major
theorist of narcissistic personality pathology
whose ideas, like those of Kernberg, contributed to the DSM-III diagnosis of narcissistic
personality disorder (Goldstein 1985). Kohut's theory grew out of his own and others'
clinical experiences with patients whose problems (such as feelings of emptiness or unstable
self-esteem) did not respond well to existing
(psychoanalytic) models. Narcissistic pathology, according to Kohut, results from faulty
self-development. Kohut's concept of the *self*
refers to the nucleus of a person's central ambitions and ideals and the talents and skills
used to actualize them (Kohut 1971, 1977;
Wolf 1988). It develops through two pathways
("poles") that provide the basis for self-esteem. The first is the *grandiose self*—an idealized representation of self that emerges in children through empathic mirroring by their

parents ("Mommy, watch!") and provides the nucleus for later ambitions and strivings. The second is the *idealized parent imago*—an idealized representation of the parents that provides the foundation for ideals and standards for the self. Parental mirroring allows the child to see his or her reflection in the eyes of a loving and admiring parent; idealizing a parent or parents allows the child to identify with and become like them. In the absence of adequate experiences with parents who can mirror the child or serve as appropriate targets of idealization (for example, when the parents are self-involved or abusive), the child's self-structure cannot develop, preventing the achievement of cohesion, vigor, and normal self-esteem (described by Kohut as "healthy narcissism"). As a result, the child develops a disorder of the self, of which pathological narcissism is a prototypic example.

COGNITIVE-SOCIAL THEORIES

Cognitive-social theories (Bandura 1986; Mischel 1973, 1979) offered the first comprehensive alternative to psychodynamic approaches to personality. First developed in the 1960s, these approaches are sometimes called social learning theories, cognitive-social learning theory, social cognitive theories, and cognitive-behavioral theories. Cognitive-social theories developed from behaviorist and cognitive roots. From a behaviorist perspective, personality consists of learned behaviors and emotional reactions that tend to be relatively specific (rather than highly generalized) and tied to particular environmental contingencies. Cognitive-social theories share the behaviorist belief that learning is the basis of personality and that personality dispositions tend to be relatively specific and shaped by their consequences. They share the cognitive view that the way people encode, transform, and retrieve information, particularly about themselves and others, is central to personality. From a cognitive-social perspective, personality reflects a constant interplay between environmental demands and the way the individual processes information about the self and the world (Bandura 1986).

Cognitive-social theorists have only recently begun to write about personality disorders (e.g., Beck et al. 2003; Linehan 1993a; Pretzer and Beck 1996; Young 1990). In large part this late entrance into the study of personality disorders reflects the assumption, initially inherited from behaviorism, that personality is composed of relatively discrete, learned processes that are more malleable and situation specific than implied by the concept of personality disorder. Cognitive-social theories focus on a number of variables presumed to be most important in understanding personality disorders, including schemas, expectancies, goals, skills and competencies, and self-regulation (Bandura 1986, 1999; Cantor and Kihlstrom 1987; Mischel 1973, 1979; Mischel and Shoda 1995). Although particular theorists have tended to emphasize one or two of these variables in explaining personality disorders, such as the schemas involved in encoding and processing information about the self and others (Beck et al. 2003) or the deficits in affect regulation seen in borderline patients (Linehan 1993a), a comprehensive cognitive-social account of personality disorders would likely address all of them.

For example, patients with personality disorders have dysfunctional schemas that lead them to misinterpret information (as when patients with BPD misread and misattribute people's intentions); attend to and encode information in biased ways (as when patients with paranoid personality disorder maintain vigilance for perceived slights or attacks); or view themselves as bad or incompetent (pathological self-schemas). Related to these schemas are problematic expectancies, such as pessimistic expectations about the world, beliefs about the malevolence of others, and fears of being mocked. Patients with personality disorders may have pathological self-efficacy expectancies, such as the dependent patient's belief that she or he cannot survive on his or own, the avoidant patient's belief that he or she is likely to fail in social circumstances, or the narcissistic patient's grandiose expectations about what she or he can accomplish. Equally important are competencies—that is, skills and abilities used for solving problems. In social-cognitive terms, social intelligence includes a variety of competencies that help people navigate interpersonal waters (Cantor and Harlow 1994; Cantor and Kihlstrom 1987), and patients with personality disorders tend to be notoriously poor interpersonal problem solvers.

Of particular relevance to severe personality disorders is self-regulation, which refers to the process of setting goals and subgoals, evaluating one's performance in meeting these goals, and adjusting one's behavior to achieve these goals in the context of ongoing feedback (Bandura 1986; Mischel 1990). Problems in self-regulation, including a deficit in specific skills, form a central aspect of Linehan's (1993a, 1993b) work on BPD. Linehan regards emotion dysregulation as the essential feature of BPD. The key characteristics of emotion dysregulation include difficulty 1) inhibiting inappropriate behavior related to intense affect, 2) organizing oneself to meet behavioral goals, 3) regulating physiological arousal associated with intense emotional arousal, and 4) refocusing attention when emotionally stimulated (Linehan 1993b). Many of the behavioral manifestations of BPD (e.g., cutting) can be viewed as consequences of emotional dysregulation. Deficits in emotion regulation lead to other problems, such as difficulties with interpersonal functioning and with the development of a stable sense of self.

According to another cognitive-behavioral approach, Beck's cognitive theory (Beck 1999; Beck et al. 2003; Pretzer and Beck 1996), dysfunctional beliefs constitute the primary pathology involved in the personality disorders (Beck et al. 2001), which are viewed as "pervasive, self-perpetuating cognitive-interpersonal cycles" (Pretzer and Beck 1996,

p. 55). Beck's theory highlights three aspects of cognition: 1) automatic thoughts (beliefs and assumptions about the world, the self, and others); 2) interpersonal strategies; and 3) cognitive distortions (systematic errors in rational thinking). Beck and colleagues have described a unique cognitive profile characteristic of each of the DSM-IV personality disorders. For example, an individual diagnosed with schizoid personality disorder would have a view of himself as a self-sufficient loner, a view of others as unrewarding and intrusive, and a view of relationships as messy and undesirable, and his primary interpersonal strategy would involve keeping his distance from other people (Pretzer and Beck 1996). He would use cognitive distortions that minimize his recognition of how relationships with others can be sources of pleasure. A study of dysfunctional beliefs (as assessed by the Personal Beliefs Questionnaire [A.T. Beck, J.S. Beck, unpublished assessment instrument, The Beck Institute for Cognitive Therapy and Research, Bala Cynwyd, Pennsylvania, 1991]) provides some initial support for the link between particular beliefs and the DSM-IV personality disorders (Beck et al. 2001).

Building on Beck's cognitive theory, Young and colleagues (Young and Gluhoski 1996; Young and Lindemann 2002; Young et al. 2003) have added a fourth level of cognition: early maladaptive schemas, which they have defined as "broad and pervasive themes regarding oneself and one's relationships with others, developed during childhood and elaborated throughout one's life" (Young and Lindemann 2002, p. 95). The authors distinguish these schemas from automatic thoughts and underlying assumptions, noting that the schemas are associated with greater levels of affect, are more pervasive, and involve a strong interpersonal aspect. Young and colleagues have identified 16 early maladaptive schemas, each of which comprises cognitive, affective, and behavioral components. They have also identified three cognitive processes involving schemas that define key features of personality disorders: *schema maintenance*, which refers to the processes by which maladaptive schemas are rigidly upheld (e.g., cognitive distortions, self-defeating behaviors); *schema avoidance*, which refers to the cognitive, affective, and behavioral ways individuals avoid the negative affect associated with the schema; and *schema compensation*, which refers to ways of overcompensating for the schema (e.g., becoming a workaholic in response to a schema of self as failure).

Mischel and Shoda (1995) have offered a compelling social-cognitive account of personality that focuses on if–then contingencies—that is, conditions that activate particular thoughts, feelings, and behaviors. Although they have not linked this model to personality disorders, one could view personality disorders as involving a host of rigid, maladaptive if–then contingencies. For example, for some patients, the first hints of trouble in a relationship may activate concerns about abandonment. These in turn may elicit anxiety or rage, to which the patient responds with desperate attempts to lure the person back that often backfire (such as manipulative statements and suicidal gestures). From an integrative psychodynamic-cognitive viewpoint, Horowitz (1988, 1998) offered a model that similarly focused on the conditions under which certain states of mind become active, which he has tied more directly to a model of personality disorders; and Wachtel (1977, 1997) has similarly described cyclical psychodynamics, in which people manage to elicit from others precisely the kind of reactions of which they are the most vigilant and afraid.

TRAIT THEORIES

Trait psychology focuses less on personality processes or functions than do psychodynamic or cognitive-social approaches, and hence has not generated an approach to treatment, although it has generated highly pro-

ductive empirical research programs. *Traits* are emotional, cognitive, and behavioral tendencies on which individuals vary (e.g., the tendency to experience negative emotions). According to Gordon Allport (1937), who pioneered the trait approach to personality, the concept of *trait* has two separate but complementary meanings: it is both an observed tendency to behave in a particular way and an inferred underlying personality disposition that generates this behavioral tendency. In the empirical literature, traits have largely been defined operationally, as the average of a set of self-report items designed to assess a given trait (e.g., items indicating a tendency to feel anxious, sad, ashamed, guilty, self-doubting, and angry that all share a common core of negative affectivity or neuroticism).

Researchers have begun recasting personality disorders in terms of the most prominent contemporary trait theory, the Five-Factor Model (FFM) of personality (McCrae and Costa 1997; Widiger 2000; Widiger and Costa 1994). (We address other trait models that have been more closely associated with biological theories later.) The FFM is a description of the way personality descriptors tend to covary and hence can be understood in terms of latent factors (traits) identified via factor analysis. Based on the lexical hypothesis of personality—that important personality attributes will naturally find expression in words used in everyday language—the FFM emerged from factor analysis of adjectival descriptions of personality originally selected from *Webster's Unabridged Dictionary* (Allport and Odbert 1936). Numerous studies, including cross-cultural investigations, have found that when participants in nonclinical (normal) samples are asked to rate themselves on dozens or hundreds of adjectives or brief sentences, the pattern of self-descriptions can often be reduced to five overarching constructs (Costa and McCrae 1997; Goldberg 1993): 1) neuroticism or negative affect (how much they tend to be distressed); 2) extraversion or positive affect (the extent to which they tend to be gregarious, high-energy, and happy);

3) conscientiousness; 4) agreeableness; and 5) openness to experience (the extent to which they are open to emotional, aesthetic, and intellectual experiences).

McCrae and Costa (1990, 1997) proposed a set of lower-order traits, or facets, within each of these broadband traits that can allow a more discriminating portrait of personality. Thus, an individual's personality profile is represented by a score on each of the five factors plus scores on six lower-order facets or subfactors within each of these broader constructs (e.g., anxiety and depression as facets of neuroticism). Advocates of the FFM argue that personality disorders reflect extreme versions of normal personality traits, so that the same system can be used for diagnosing normal and pathological personality. From the perspective of the FFM, personality disorders are not discrete entities separate and distinct from normal personality. Rather, they represent extreme variants of normal personality traits or blends thereof.

In principle, one could classify personality disorders in one of two ways using the FFM. The first, and that more consistent with the theoretical and psychometric tradition within which the FFM developed, is simply to identify personality pathology by extreme values on each of the five factors (and perhaps on their facets). For example, extremely high scores on the neuroticism factor and its facets (anxiety, hostility, depression, self-consciousness, impulsivity, and vulnerability) all represent aspects of personality pathology. Whether this strategy is appropriate for all factors and facets, and when to consider extreme responses on one or both poles of a dimension pathological, are matters of debate. Extreme extraversion, for example, may or may not be pathological, depending on the social milieu and the person's other traits. Similarly, extreme openness to experience could imply a genuinely open attitude toward emotions, art, and so forth or an uncritical, "flaky," or schizotypal cognitive style. The advantages of this approach, however, are that it integrates the understanding and assessment of normal and pathological personality and that it establishes dimensions of personality pathology using well-understood empirical procedures (factor analysis).

Another way to proceed using the FFM is to translate clinically derived categories into five-factor language (Coker et al. 2002; Lynam and Widiger 2001; Widiger and Costa 1994). For example, Widiger et al. (2002) described antisocial personality disorder (ASPD) as combining low agreeableness with low conscientiousness. Because analysis at the level of five factors often lacks the specificity to characterize complex disorders such as BPD (high neuroticism plus high extraversion), proponents of the FFM have often moved to the facet level. Thus, whereas all six neuroticism facets (anxiety, hostility, depression, self-consciousness, impulsivity, and vulnerability) are characteristic of patients with BPD, patients with avoidant personality disorder are characterized by only four of these facets (anxiety, depression, self-consciousness, and vulnerability).

Similarly, Widiger et al. (1994, 2002) described obsessive-compulsive personality disorder as primarily an extreme, maladaptive variant of conscientiousness. They add, however, that obsessive-compulsive patients tend to be low on the compliance and altruism facets of agreeableness (i.e., they are oppositional and stingy) and low on some of the facets of openness to experience as reflected in being closed to feelings and closed to values (i.e., morally inflexible). Numerous studies have shown predicted links between DSM-IV Axis II disorders and FFM factors and facets (Axelrod et al. 1997; Ross et al. 2002; Trull et al. 2001), although other studies have found substantial overlap among the FFM profiles of patients with very different disorders (e.g., borderline and obsessive-compulsive) using major FFM self-report inventories (Morey et al. 2002).

BIOLOGICAL PERSPECTIVES

The first biological perspectives on personality disorders, which influenced the current Axis II classification, stemmed from the observations of the pioneering psychiatric taxonomists in the early twentieth century, notably Bleuler (1911/1950) and Kraepelin (1896/1919). These authors and others noticed, for example, that the relatives of schizophrenic patients sometimes appeared to have attenuated symptoms of the disorder that endured as personality traits, such as interpersonal and cognitive peculiarity. More recently, researchers have used the methods of trait psychology (particularly the reliance on self-report questionnaires and factor analysis) to study personality disorders from a biological viewpoint. In some cases, they have developed item sets with biological variables in mind (e.g., neurotransmitters and their functions) or have reconsidered patterns of covariation among different traits in light of hypothesized neurobiological systems or circuits. In other cases, they have applied behavior-genetic approaches to study personality traits (as well as DSM-IV disorders). We explore each of these approaches in turn. (Researchers are just beginning to use neuroimaging to study personality disorders, particularly BPD [e.g., Herpertz et al. 2001], but the results at this point are preliminary, and hence we do not address them further here.)

Traits and Neural Systems

Siever and Davis (1991) provided one of the first attempts to reconsider the personality disorders from a neurobiology perspective. They proposed a model based on core characteristics of Axis I disorders relevant to personality disorders and related these characteristics to emerging knowledge of their underlying neurobiology. They focused on cognitive/perceptual organization (schizophrenia and other psychotic disorders); impulsivity/aggression (impulse control disorders); affective instability (mood disorders); and anxiety/inhibition (anxiety disorders). Conceptualized in dimensional terms, Axis I disorders such as schizophrenia represent the extreme end of a continuum. Milder abnormalities can be seen in patients with personality disorder, either directly (as subthreshold variants) or through their influence on adaptive strategies (coping and defense).

Siever and Davis linked each dimension to biological correlates and indicators, some presumed to be causal and others to provide markers of underlying biological dysfunction (e.g., eye movement dysfunction in schizophrenia, which is also seen in individuals with schizotypal personality disorder and in nonpsychotic relatives of schizophrenic probands). They also pointed to suggestive data on neurotransmitter functioning that might link Axis II disorders with Axis I syndromes such as depression. More recently, Siever and colleagues (New and Siever 2002; Siever et al. 2002) proposed an approach to BPD that tries to circumvent the problems created by the heterogeneity of the diagnosis by examining the neurobiology of specific dimensions thought to underlie the disorder (endophenotypes), especially impulsive aggression and affective instability.

The major attempt thus far to develop a trait model of personality disorders based on a neurobiological model is Cloninger's seven-factor model of personality (Cloninger 1998; Cloninger et al. 1993). In his model, Cloninger divided personality structure into two domains: *temperament* ("automatic associative responses to basic emotional stimuli that determine habits and skills") and *character* ("self-aware concepts that influence voluntary intentions and attitudes") (Cloninger 1998, p. 64). According to Cloninger, each of these domains is defined by a mode of learning and the underlying neural systems involved in that learning: temperament is associated with associative/procedural learning, and character is associated with insight learning. The temperament domain includes four dimensions, each theoretically linked to particular neurotransmitter systems: 1) novelty seeking (exploration, extravagance, impulsivity), associated with dopamine; 2) harm avoidance (characterized by pessimism, fear, timidity), associated with serotonin and γ-aminobutyric acid (GABA); 3) reward dependence (sentimentality, social attachment, openness), associated with norepinephrine and serotonin; and 4) persistence (industriousness, determination, ambitiousness, perfectionism), associated with glutamate and serotonin (Cloninger 1998, p. 70). The character domain includes three dimensions: 1) self-directedness (responsibility, purposefulness, self-acceptance), considered the "major determinant of the presence or absence of personality disorder" (Cloninger et al. 1993, p. 979); 2) cooperativeness (empathy, compassion, helpfulness); and 3) self-transcendence (spirituality, idealism, enlightenment).

Cloninger (1998) proposed that all personality disorders are low on the character dimensions of self-directedness and cooperativeness. What distinguishes patients with different disorders are their more specific profiles. In broad strokes, the Cluster A personality disorders (schizotypal, schizoid, paranoid) are associated with low reward dependence; the Cluster B personality disorders (borderline, antisocial, narcissistic, histrionic) are associated with high novelty seeking; and the Cluster C personality disorders (dependent, avoidant, obsessive-compulsive) are associated with high harm avoidance. Individual personality disorders may be described more fully by profiles obtained from Cloninger's self-report Temperament and Character Inventory (Cloninger and Svrakic 1994). For example, BPD would consist of high harm avoidance, high novelty seeking, and low reward dependence as well as low scores on the character dimensions.

More recently, a dimensional neurobehavioral model was offered by Depue, Lenzenweger, and colleagues (e.g., Depue and Collins 1999; Depue and Lenzenweger 2001). Their model regards personality disorders as emergent phenotypes arising from the interaction of basic neurobehavioral systems that underlie major personality traits (Depue and Lenzenweger 2001, p. 165). Through an extensive examination of the psychometric literature on the structure of personality traits as well as a theoretical analysis of the neurobehavioral systems likely to be relevant to personality and personality dysfunction, they identified five trait dimensions that may account for the range of personality disorder phenotypes. They labeled these five traits 1) agentic extraversion (reflecting both the activity and gregariousness components of extraversion); 2) neuroticism; 3) affiliation; 4) nonaffective constraint (the opposite pole of which is impulsivity); and 5) fear. For example, the neurobehavioral system underlying the trait of agentic extraversion is positive incentive motivation, which is common to all mammalian species and involves positive affect and approach motivation. The dopaminergic system has been strongly implicated in incentive-motivated behavior, such that individual differences in the former predict differences in the latter. Research on this model is just beginning, but the model is promising in its integration of research on neural systems involved in fundamental functions common to many animal species (such as approach, avoidance, affiliation with conspecifics, and inhibition of punished behavior) with individual differences research in personality psychology.

Behavior-Genetic Approaches

The vast majority of behavior-genetic studies of personality have focused on normal personality traits, such as those that compose the FFM and Eysenck's (1967, 1981) three-factor model (extraversion, neuroticism, and psychoticism). These studies have generally shown moderate to high heritability (30%–60%) for a range of personality traits (Livesley et al. 1993; Plomin and Caspi 1999) relevant to personality disorders. The most frequently studied traits, extraversion and neuroticism, have produced heritability estimates of 54%–74% and 42%–64%, respectively (Eysenck 1990).

Behavior-genetic data are proving increasingly useful in both etiological and taxonomic work (e.g., Krueger 1999; Livesley et al. 1998). Livesley et al. (2003) noted that behavior-genetic data can help address the persistent lack of consensus among trait psychologists regarding which traits to study by helping them study the causes of trait covariation (as opposed to simply describing it). Establishing congruence between a proposed phenotypic model of personality traits and the genetic structure underlying it would support the validity of a proposed factor model. The same holds true for models of personality disorders.

To test this approach, Livesley et al. (1998) administered the Dimensional Assessment of Personality Pathology—Basic Questionnaire to a large sample of individuals with and without personality disorders, including twin pairs. This self-report measure consists of 18 traits considered to underlie personality disorder diagnoses (e.g., identity problems, oppositionality, social avoidance). Factor analysis indicated a four-factor solution: emotional dysregulation, dissocial behavior, inhibition, and compulsivity. Results also showed high congruence for all four factors between the phenotypic and behavior-genetic analyses, indicating strong support for the proposed factor solution. In addition, the data showed substantial residual heritability for many lower-order traits, suggesting that these traits likely are not simply components of the higher-order factors but include unique components (specific factors) as well. Krueger and colleagues (e.g., Krueger 1999) have similarly found, using structural equation modeling with a large twin sample, that broadband internalizing and externalizing personality factors account for much of the variance in many common Axis I disorders (e.g., mood, anxiety, and substance use) and that genetic and environmental sources of variance are associated with many of both

the higher- and lower-order factors they identified.

Compared with research on normal personality traits (as well as many Axis I disorders), behavior-genetic studies of personality disorders are relatively rare. The most common designs have been family studies in which researchers begin with the personality disorder proband and then assess other family members. The major limitation of this method is that familial aggregation of disorders can support either genetic or environmental causes. As in all behavior-genetic research, twin and adoption studies provide more definitive data. Most of these studies have examined only a subset of the DSM personality disorders, particularly schizotypal, antisocial, and borderline personality disorders. These disorders appear to reflect a continuum of heritability, with schizotypal most strongly linked to genetic influences, antisocial linked both to environmental and genetic variables, and borderline showing the smallest estimates of heritability in the majority of studies (see Nigg and Goldsmith 1994).

Research on the heritability of schizotypal personality disorder provides the clearest evidence of a genetic component to a personality disorder. (Schizotypal personality disorder is defined by criteria such as odd beliefs or magical thinking, unusual perceptual experiences, odd thinking and speech, suspiciousness, inappropriate or constricted affect, and behavior or appearance that is odd or eccentric.) As mentioned earlier, Bleuler and Kraepelin noted peculiarities in language and behavior among some relatives of their schizophrenic patients. Bleuler called this presentation "latent schizophrenia" and considered it to be a less severe and more widespread form of schizophrenia. Further research into the constellation of symptoms characteristic of relatives of schizophrenic patients ultimately resulted in the creation of the DSM diagnosis of schizotypal personality disorder (Spitzer et al. 1979). A genetic relationship between schizophrenia and schizotypal personality disorder is now well established (Kendler and Walsh 1995; Lenzenweger 1998). In one study, Torgersen (1984) found that 33% (7 of 21) of identical co-twins had schizotypal personality disorder, whereas only 4% (1 of 23) of fraternal co-twins shared the diagnosis. Data from a later twin study (Torgersen et al. 2000), which used structural equation modeling, estimated heritability at 0.61.

ASPD, in contrast, appears to have both genetic and environmental roots, as documented in adoption studies (Cadoret et al. 1995). An adult adoptee whose biological parent has an arrest record for antisocial behavior is four times more likely to have problems with aggressive behavior than a person without a biological vulnerability. At the same time, a person whose adoptive parent has ASPD is more than three times more likely to develop the disorder, regardless of biological history. As is the case with other behavior-genetic findings, twin studies suggest that environmental and genetic factors grow more predictive as individuals get older (Lyons et al. 1995). In considering the data on ASPD and other personality disorders, however, it is important to remember that all estimates of heritability are sample dependent. Turkheimer et al. (2003) found, for example, that genes account for most of the variability in IQ among middle-class children but that over 60% of the variance in IQ in samples from low socioeconomic backgrounds reflects shared environment. Socioeconomic status may similarly moderate the relation between genes and environment and antisocial behavior.

Data on the behavioral genetics of BPD are mixed. Several studies have found only modest evidence of heritability (e.g., Dahl 1993; Nigg and Goldsmith 1994; Reich 1989). A rare twin study conducted by Torgersen (1984) failed to find evidence for the genetic transmission of the disorder, although the sample was relatively small. A more recent twin study by Torgersen et al. (2000) focused on the heritability of several personality disorders, finding a substantial genetic compo-

nent to several personality disorders, with most heritability estimates between 0.50 and 0.60, including BPD. Increasingly, researchers are suggesting that specific components of BPD may have higher heritability than the BPD diagnosis taken as a whole. For example, several authors (Nigg and Goldsmith 1994; Widiger and Frances 1994) suggest that neuroticism, which is highly heritable, is at the core of many borderline features (e.g., negative affect and stress sensitivity). Other components of BPD have shown substantial heritability as well (e.g., problems with identity, impulsivity, affective lability) (Livesley et al. 1993; Skodol et al. 2002).

A caveat worth mentioning, however, is that behavior-genetic studies that systematically measure environmental influences directly (e.g., measuring developmental toxins such as sexual abuse), rather than deriving estimates of shared and nonshared environment statistically from residual terms, often obtain very different estimates of environmental effects, and this may well be the case with many personality disorders. For example, if one child in a family responds to sexual abuse by becoming avoidant and constricted and another responds to the same experience by becoming borderline and impulsive, researchers will mistakenly conclude—unless they actually measured developmental variables—that shared environment has no effect, because a shared environmental event led to nonshared responses (see Turkheimer and Waldron 2000; Westen 1998). Recent work by Caspi et al. (2002) showing genes and environmental events (e.g., sexual abuse) interacting in predicting subsequent personality and psychopathology emphasize the same point.

INTEGRATIVE THEORIES

Of all the disorders identified in DSM-IV-TR, the personality disorders are likely to be among those that most require biopsychosocial perspectives. They are also disorders for which we may gain substantially by integrating data from both clinical observation and research, from classical theories of personality that delineate personality functions, and from more contemporary research that emphasizes traits. The emergence of several integrative models is thus perhaps not surprising. We briefly describe three such models in the following discussion: Millon's evolutionary–social learning model, Benjamin's interpersonal model, and Westen's functional-domains model.

Millon's Evolutionary–Social Learning Model

Millon developed a comprehensive model of personality and personality disorders that he initially framed in social learning terms (Millon 1969), describing personality in terms of three polarities: pleasure/pain, self/other, and passive/active. These polarities reflect the nature of reinforcement that controls the person's behavior (rewarding or aversive), the source or sources that provide reinforcement (oneself or others), and the instrumental behaviors and coping strategies used to pursue reinforcement (active or passive). Millon (Davis and Millon 1999; Millon 1990; Millon and Davis 1996; Millon and Grossman 2005) eventually reconceptualized his original theory in evolutionary terms. In doing so, he added a fourth polarity, thinking/feeling, which reflects the extent to which people rely on abstract thinking or intuition.

Millon's reconceptualized theory outlined four basic evolutionary principles consistent with the polarities described by his earlier theory: 1) aims of existence, which refer to life enhancement and life preservation, and which are reflected in the pleasure/pain polarity; 2) modes of adaptation, which he described in terms of accommodation to, versus modification of, the environment (whether one adjusts or tries to adjust the world, particularly other people) and which are reflected in the passive/active polarity; 3) strategies of replication or reproduction,

which refer to the extent to which the person focuses on individuation or nurturance of others and which are reflected in the self/other polarity; and 4) processes of abstraction, which refer to the ability for symbolic thought and which are represented by the thinking/feeling polarity.

Millon identified 14 personality prototypes that can be understood in terms of the basic polarities. For example, patients with schizoid personality disorder tend to have little pleasure, to have little involvement with others, to be relatively passive in their stance to the world, and to rely on abstract thinking over intuition. In contrast, patients with histrionic personality disorder are pleasure seeking, interpersonally focused (although in a self-centered way), highly active, and short on abstract thinking. Millon's theory led to the distinction between avoidant and schizoid personality disorder in DSM-III. Whereas schizoid personality disorder represents a passive-detached personality style, avoidant personality disorder represents an active-detached style characterized by active avoidance motivated by avoidance of anxiety. Millon also developed both a comprehensive measure to assess the DSM personality disorders and his own theory-driven personality disorder classification, the Millon Clinical Multiaxial Inventory (Millon and Davis 1997). The instrument, now in its third edition, has been used in hundreds of studies and is widely used as an assessment tool in clinical practice (e.g., Espelage et al. 2002; Kristensen and Torgersen 2001).

Benjamin's Interpersonal Model

Benjamin's (1993, 1996a, 1996b) interpersonal theory, called Structural Analysis of Social Behavior (SASB), focuses on interpersonal processes in personality and psychopathology and their intrapsychic causes, correlates, and sequelae. Influenced by Sullivan's (1953) interpersonal theory of psychiatry, by object relations approaches, and by research using the interpersonal circumplex (e.g., Kiesler 1983; Leary 1957; Schaefer 1965), the SASB is a three-dimensional circumplex model with three "surfaces," each of which represents a specific focus. The first surface focuses on actions directed at a person (e.g., abuse by a parent toward the patient). The second surface focuses on the person's response to real or perceived actions by the other (e.g., recoiling from the abusive parent). The third surface focuses on the person's actions toward him- or herself, or what Benjamin calls the "introject" (e.g., self-abuse). The notion behind the surfaces is that the first two are interpersonal and describe the kinds of interaction patterns (self with other) in which the patient engages with significant others (e.g., parents, attachment figures, therapists). The third surface represents internalized attitudes and actions toward the self (e.g., self-criticism that began as criticism from parents). According to Benjamin, children learn to respond to themselves and others by identifying with significant others (acting like them), recapitulating what they experienced with significant others (e.g., eliciting from others what they experienced before), and introjecting others (treating themselves as others have treated them).

As with all circumplex models, each surface has two axes that define its quadrants. In the SASB (as in other interpersonal circumplex models), love and hate represent the two poles of the horizontal axis. Enmeshment and differentiation are the endpoints of the vertical axis. The SASB offers a translation of each of the DSM Axis II criteria (and disorders) into interpersonal terms (Benjamin 1993, 1996b). In this respect, it has two advantages. First, it can reduce the number of co-occurring conditions that need to be identified in a given patient by specifying the interpersonal antecedents that elicit the patient's responses. For example, maladaptive anger is characteristic of many of the DSM-IV personality disorders but has different interpersonal triggers and meanings (Benjamin 1993). Anger in patients with BPD often reflects perceived

neglect or abandonment. Anger in narcissistic personality disorder tends to follow from perceived slights or failures of other people to give the patient everything he or she wants (entitlement). Anger in patients with ASPD is often cold, detached, and aimed at controlling the other person. Second, the SASB model is able to represent multiple, often conflicting aspects of the way patients with a given disorder behave (or complex, multifaceted aspects of a single interpersonal interaction) simultaneously. Thus, a single angry outburst by a borderline patient could reflect an effort to get distance from the other, to hurt the other, and to get the other to respond and hence be drawn back into the relationship. Benjamin has devised several ways of operationalizing a person's dynamics or an interpersonal interaction (e.g., in a therapy hour), ranging from direct observation and coding of behavior to self-report questionnaires, all of which yield descriptions using the same circumplex model.

Westen's Functional-Domains Model

Westen (1995, 1996, 1998) described a model of domains of personality functioning that draws substantially on psychoanalytic clinical theory and observation as well as on empirical research in personality, cognitive, developmental, and clinical psychology. Although some aspects of the model are linked to research on etiology, the model is less a theory of personality disorders than an attempt to delineate and systematize the major elements of personality that define a patient's personality, whether or not the patient has a personality disorder. The model differs from trait approaches in its focus on personality processes and functions (e.g., the kinds of affect regulation strategies the person uses, the ways she represents the self and others mentally, as well as more behavioral dispositions, such as whether she engages in impulsive or self-destructive behavior). However, it shares with trait approaches the view that a single model should be able to accommodate relatively healthy as well as relatively disturbed personality styles and dynamics.

The model suggests that a systematic personality case formulation must answer three questions, each composed of a series of subquestions or variables that require assessment: 1) What does the person wish for, fear, and value, and to what extent are these motives conscious or unconscious, collaborating or conflicting? 2) What psychological resources—including cognitive processes (e.g., intelligence, memory, intactness of thinking processes), affects, affect regulation strategies (conscious coping strategies and unconscious defenses), and behavioral skills—does the person have at his or her disposal to meet internal and external demands? 3) What is the person's experience of the self and others, and how able is the individual—cognitively, emotionally, motivationally, and behaviorally—to sustain meaningful and pleasurable relationships?

From a psychodynamic perspective, these questions correspond roughly to the issues raised by classical psychoanalytic theories of motivation and conflict (Brenner 1982); ego-psychological approaches to adaptive functioning; and object-relational, self-psychological, attachment, and contemporary relational (Aron 1996; Mitchell 1988) approaches to understanding people's experience of self with others. Each of these questions and subdimensions, however, is also associated with a number of research traditions in personality, clinical, cognitive, and developmental psychology (e.g., on the development of children's representations of self, representations of others, moral judgment, attachment styles, ability to tell coherent narratives) (see Damon and Hart 1988; Fonagy et al. 2002; Harter 1999; Livesley and Bromley 1973; Main 1995; Westen 1990a, 1990b, 1991b, 1994). Westen and Shedler (1999a) used this model as a rough theoretical guide to ensure comprehensive coverage of personality domains in developing items for the Shedler-Westen Assessment Proce-

dure Q-Sort, a personality pathology measure for use by expert informants, although the model and the measure are not closely linked (i.e., one does not require the other).

From this point of view, individuals with particular personality disorders are likely to be characterized by 1) distinct constellations of motives and conflicts, such as chronic worries about abandonment in BPD or a conflict between the wish for and fear of connectedness to others in avoidant personality disorder; 2) deficits in adaptive functioning, such as poor impulse control, lack of self-reflective capacities (see Fonagy and Target 1997), and difficulty regulating affect (Linehan 1993a; Westen 1991a) in BPD or subclinical cognitive disturbances in schizotypal personality disorder; and 3) problematic ways of thinking, feeling, and behaving toward themselves and significant others, such as a tendency to form simplistic, one-dimensional representations of the self and others, to misunderstand why people (including the self) behave as they do, and to expect malevolence from other people (characteristics seen in patients with many personality disorders, such as paranoid, schizoid, and borderline) (Kernberg 1975a, 1984; Westen 1991a). In this model, a person's level of personality health–sickness (from severe personality disorder to relatively healthy functioning), which can be assessed reliably using a personality health prototype or a simple rating of level of personality organization derived from Kernberg's work (Westen and Muderrisoglu 2003; Westen and Shedler 1999b), reflects his or her functioning in each of these three domains.

People who do not have severe enough pathology to receive a personality disorder diagnosis can similarly be described using this approach. For example, a successful male executive presented for treatment with troubles in his marriage and his relationships at work, as well as low-level feelings of anxiety and depression. None of these characteristics approached criteria for a personality disorder (or any Axis I disorders, except the relatively nondescript diagnosis of adjustment disorder with mixed anxious and depressed mood). Using this model, one would note that he was competitive with other people, a fact of which he was unaware (Question 1); had impressive capacities for self-regulation but was intellectualized and afraid of feelings and often used his enjoyment of his work as a way of retreating from his family (Question 2); and had surprisingly noncomplex representations of others' minds (for a person who could solve noninterpersonal problems in complex ways) and consequently would often became angry and attack at work without stopping to empathize with the other person's perspective (Question 3). This description is, of course, highly oversimplified, but it gives a sense of how the model can be used to describe personality dynamics in patients without a diagnosable personality disorder (Westen 1998; Westen and Shedler 1999b).

CASE EXAMPLE

To see how some of the models discussed here operate in practice, consider the following brief case description:

> Mr. A was a man in his early 20s who came to treatment for lifelong problems with depression, anxiety, and feelings of inadequacy. He was a kind, introspective, sensitive man who nevertheless had tremendous difficulty making friends and interacting comfortably with people. He was constantly worried that he would misspeak, he would ruminate after conversations about what he had said and the way he was perceived, and he had only one or two friends with whom he felt comfortable. He wanted to be closer to people, but he was frightened that he would be rejected and was afraid of his own anger in relationships. While interacting with people (including his therapist), he would often have a running commentary with them in his mind, typically filled with aggressive content. He was in a 2-year relationship with a woman who was emotionally and physically

very distant, whom he saw twice a month and with whom he rarely had sex. Prior to her, his sexual experiences had all been anxiety provoking and short lived, in every sense.

> Mr. A tended to be inhibited in many areas of his life. He was emotionally constricted and seemed particularly uncomfortable with pleasurable feelings. He tended to speak in intellectualized terms about his life and history and seemed afraid of affect. He felt stifled in his chosen profession, which did not allow him to express many of his intellectual abilities or creative impulses. He alternated between overcontrol of his impulses, which was his modal stance in life, and occasional breakthroughs of poorly thought-out, impulsive actions (as when he bought an expensive piece of equipment with little forethought about how he would pay for it).

> Mr. A came from a working-class family in Boston and had lost his father, a policeman, as a young boy. He was reared by his mother and later by a stepfather with whom he had a positive relationship. He also described a good relationship with his mother, although she, like several members of her extended family, struggled with depression, and she apparently suffered a lengthy major depressive episode after her husband's death.

For purposes of brevity, we briefly explicate this case from two theoretical standpoints that provide very different approaches to case formulation: the FFM and the functional-domains viewpoint. (In clinical practice, a functional-domains account and a psychodynamic account are similar, because the former reflects an attempt to systematize and integrate with empirical research [and minimal jargon] the major domains emphasized by classical psychoanalytic, ego-psychological, and object-relational/self-psychological/relational approaches.)

From a five-factor perspective, the most salient features of Mr. A's personality profile were his strong elevations in neuroticism and introversion (low extraversion). He was high on most of the facets of neuroticism, notably anxiety, depression, anger, self-consciousness, and vulnerability. He was low on most facets of extraversion as well, particularly gregariousness, assertiveness, activity, and happiness. This combination of high negative affectivity and low positive affectivity, which left him vulnerable to feelings of depression, captures his anxious, self-conscious social avoidance.

No other broadband factors describe Mr. A adequately, although specific FFM facets provide insight into his personality. He was moderately high in agreeableness, being compliant, modest, and tender-minded; however, he was not particularly high on trust, altruism, or straightforwardness (reflecting his tendency to behave passive-aggressively). He was moderately conscientious, showing moderate scores on the facets of orderliness and discipline. He similarly showed moderate openness to experience, being artistically oriented but low on comfort with feelings. His scores on facets such as intellectual curiosity would likely be moderate, reflecting both an interest and an inhibition. Indeed, a tendency to receive moderate scores because of opposing dynamics would be true of his facet scores on several traits, such as achievement orientation.

A functional-domains perspective would offer a similar summary diagnosis to that of a psychodynamic approach, along with a description of his functioning on the three major domains outlined in the model. In broadest outline, from this point of view Mr. A had a depressive, avoidant, and obsessional personality style organized at a low-functioning neurotic level. In other words, he did not have a personality disorder, as evidenced by his ability to maintain friendships and stable employment, but he had considerable psychological impediments to love, work, and life satisfaction, with a predominance of depressive, avoidant, and obsessional dynamics.

With respect to motives and conflicts (and interpersonal issues, around which many of his conflicts centered), Mr. A had a number of conflicts that impinged on his ca-

pacity to lead a fulfilling life. He wanted to connect with people, but he was inhibited by social anxiety, feelings of inadequacy, and an undercurrent of anger toward people that he could not directly express (which emerged in his "running commentaries" in his mind). Although he worried that he would fail others, he always felt somehow unfulfilled in his relationships with them and could be subtly critical. He likely had high standards with which he compared himself and others and against which both frequently fell short. He also had trouble handling his anger, aggressive impulses, and desires for self-assertion. He would frequently behave in passive or self-punitive ways rather than appropriately asserting his desires or expressing his anger. This pattern contributed in turn to a lingering hostile fantasy life and a tendency at times to behave passive-aggressively.

Sex was particularly conflictual for Mr. A, not only because it forced him into an intimate relationship with another person but because of his feelings of inadequacy, his discomfort in looking directly at a woman's body (because of his associations to sex and women's bodies), and his worries that he was homosexual. When with a woman, he frequently worried that he would "accidentally" touch her anus and be repulsed, although interestingly, his sexual fantasies (and humor) had a decidedly anal tone. Homosexual images would also jump into his mind in the middle of sexual activity, which led to considerable anxiety.

With respect to adaptive resources, Mr. A had a number of strengths, notably his impressive intellect, a dry sense of humor, a capacity to introspect, and an ability to persevere. Nevertheless, his overregulation of his feelings and impulses left him vulnerable to breakthroughs of anger, anxiety, and impulsive action. He distanced himself from emotion, in an effort to regulate anxiety, depression, excitement, and pleasure, which seemed to him both undeserved and threatening.

With respect to his experience of self and relationships, Mr. A's dominant interpersonal concerns centered around rejection, shame, and aloneness. He was able to think about himself and others in complex ways and to show genuine care and concern toward other people, although these strengths were often not manifest because of his interpersonal avoidance. He had low self-esteem, although he had some intellectual awareness that his feelings toward himself were unrealistically negative. He often voiced identity concerns, wondering what he was going to do with his life and where he would fit in and feeling adrift without either meaningful work or love relationships that were sustaining. (This is, of course, a very skeletal description of functional domains in Mr. A; for a more thorough description, and an empirical description using the Shedler-Westen Assessment Procedure Q-Sort, see Westen 1998.)

CONCLUSION

Clearly, there are a number of ways to conceptualize personality disorders. The case example applied, in a highly schematic way, two specific approaches: the FFM and the functional-domains (or psychodynamic) model. Using these two very different methods provides some sense of how one might formulate a case from two very different theoretical perspectives—notably a case on which Axis II personality disorder diagnostic thresholds would not be met because the patient's pathology is not severe enough for a diagnosis of personality disorder. Nevertheless, some of the patient's problematic personality attributes obviously affected his well-being and Axis I symptoms and contributed to his seeking treatment. Theory, research, and this brief case example all suggest that including a broader range of personality functioning is crucial as the field evolves and should be one of the primary goals guiding the revision of Axis II in DSM-V to increase its clinical utility and improve the delivery of care.

REFERENCES

Abend SM, Porder MS, Willick MS: Borderline Patients: Psychoanalytic Perspectives. New York, International Universities Press, 1983

Adler G, Buie D: Aloneness and borderline psychopathology: the possible relevance of child development issues. Int J Psychoanal 60:83–96, 1979

Allport G: Personality: A Psychological Interpretation. New York, Henry Holt, 1937

Allport G, Odbert H: Trait-names: a psycho-lexical study, in Psychological Monographs, Vol 47. Princeton, NJ, Psychological Review, 1936

American Psychiatric Association: Diagnostic and Statistical Manual of Mental Disorders, 3rd Edition. Washington, DC, American Psychiatric Association, 1980

American Psychiatric Association: Diagnostic and Statistical Manual of Mental Disorders, 4th Edition. Washington, DC, American Psychiatric Association, 1994

American Psychiatric Association: Diagnostic and Statistical Manual of Mental Disorders, 4th Edition, Text Revision. Washington, DC, American Psychiatric Association, 2000

Aron L: A Meeting of Minds: Mutuality in Psychoanalysis, Vol 4. New York, Analytic Press, 1996

Axelrod S, Widiger T, Trull T, et al: Relations of five-factor model antagonism facets with personality disorder symptomatology. J Pers Assess 69:297–313, 1997

Baker L, Silk KR, Westen D, et al: Malevolence, splitting, and parental ratings by borderlines. J Nerv Ment Dis 180:258–264, 1992

Balint M: The Basic Fault: Therapeutic Aspects of Regression. Evanston, IL, Northwestern University Press, 1969

Bandura A: Social Foundations of Thought and Action. Englewood Cliffs, NJ, Prentice Hall, 1986

Bandura A: Social cognitive theory of personality, in Handbook of Personality: Theory and Research, 2nd Edition. Edited by Pervin L, John O. New York, Guilford, 1999, pp 154–196

Beck A: Cognitive aspects of personality disorders and their relation to syndromal disorders: a psychoevolutionary approach, in Personality and Psychopathology. Edited by Cloninger CR. Washington, DC, American Psychiatric Association, 1999, pp 411–429

Beck A, Butler A, Brown G, et al: Dysfunctional beliefs discriminate personality disorders. Behav Res Ther 39:1213–1225, 2001

Beck AT, Freeman A, Davis DD, et al: Cognitive Therapy of Personality Disorders, 2nd Edition. New York, Guilford, 2003

Bellak L, Chassan JB, Gediman HK, et al: Ego function assessment of analytic psychotherapy combined with drug therapy. J Nerv Ment Dis 157:465–469, 1973

Benjamin L[S]: Interpersonal Diagnosis and Treatment of Personality Disorders. New York, Guilford, 1993

Benjamin LS: Interpersonal Diagnosis and Treatment of Personality Disorders, 2nd Edition. New York, Guilford, 1996a

Benjamin LS: An interpersonal theory of personality disorders, in Major Theories of Personality Disorder. Edited by Clarkin JF, Lenzenweger MF. New York, Guilford, 1996b, pp 141–220

Blanck G, Blanck R: Ego Psychology: Theory and Practice. New York, Columbia University Press, 1974

Bleuler E: Dementia Praecox or the Group of Schizophrenias (1911). New York, International Universities Press, 1950

Brenner C: The Mind in Conflict. New York, International Universities Press, 1982

Cadoret RJ, Yates WR, Troughton E, et al: Genetic–environmental interaction in the genesis of aggressivity and conduct disorders. Arch Gen Psychiatry 52:916–924, 1995

Cantor N, Harlow RE: Personality, strategic behavior, and daily life problem solving. Cur Dir Psychol Sci 3:169–172, 1994

Cantor N, Kihlstrom JF: Personality and Social Intelligence. Englewood Cliffs, NJ, Prentice-Hall, 1987

Caspi A, McClay J, Moffitt T, et al: Role of genotype in the cycle of violence in maltreated children. Science 297:851–854, 2002

Cloninger CR: The genetics and psychobiology of the seven-factor model of personality, in Biology of Personality Disorders. Edited by Silk KR (Review of Psychiatry Series, Vol 17; Oldham JM, Riba MB, series eds). Washington, DC, American Psychiatric Press, 1998, pp 63–92

Cloninger CR, Svrakic D: Differentiating normal and deviant personality by the seven-factor personality model, in Differentiating Normal and Abnormal Personality. Edited by Strack S, Lorr M. New York, Springer, 1994, pp 40–64

Cloninger CR, Svrakic DM, Przybeck TR: A psychobiological model of temperament and character. Arch Gen Psychiatry 50:975–990, 1993

Coker L, Samuel D, Widiger T: Maladaptive personality functioning within the Big Five and the five-factor model. J Personal Disord 16:385–401, 2002

Costa P, McCrae R: Longitudinal stability of adult personality, in Handbook of Personality Psychology. Edited by Hogan R, Johnson J. San Diego, CA, Academic Press, 1997, pp 269–290

Dahl A: The personality disorders: a critical review of family, twin, and adoption studies. J Personal Disord 7 (suppl):86–99, 1993

Damon W, Hart D: Self-Understanding in Childhood and Adolescence. New York, Cambridge University Press, 1988

Davis R: Millon: Essentials of his science, theory, classification, assessment, and therapy. J Pers Assess 72:330–352, 1999

Depue R, Collins P: Neurobiology of the structure of personality: dopamine, facilitation of incentive motivation, and extraversion. Behav Brain Sci 22:491–569, 1999

Depue R, Lenzenweger M: A neurobehavioral dimensional model, in Handbook of Personality Disorders: Theory, Research, and Treatment. Edited by Livesley J. New York, Guilford, 2001, pp 136–176

Espelage DL, Mazzeo SE, Sherman R, et al: MCMI-II profiles of women with eating disorders: a cluster analytic investigation. J Personal Disord 16:453–463, 2002

Eysenck H: The Biological Basis of Personality. Springfield, IL, Charles C Thomas, 1967

Eysenck H: A Model for Personality. New York, Springer-Verlag, 1981

Eysenck HJ: Biological dimensions of personality, in Handbook of Personality: Theory and Research. Edited by Pervin LA. New York, Guilford, 1990, pp 244–276

Fairbairn WR: Psychoanalytic Studies of the Personality. London, Tavistock, 1952

Fonagy P, Target M: Attachment and reflective function: their role in self-organization. Dev Psychopathol 9:679–700, 1997

Fonagy P, Steele H, Steele M: Maternal representations of attachment during pregnancy predict the organization of infant-mother attachment at one year of age. Child Dev 62:891–905, 1991

Fonagy P, Gergely G, Jurist EL, et al: Affect Regulation, Mentalization, and the Development of the Self. New York, Other Press, 2002

Fonagy P, Target M, Gergely G, et al: The developmental roots of borderline personality disorder in early attachment relationships: a theory and some evidence. Psychoanalytic Inquiry 23:412–459, 2003

Goldberg L: The structure of phenotypic personality traits. Am Psychol 48:26–34, 1993

Goldstein W: DSM-III and the narcissistic personality. Am J Psychother 39:4–16, 1985

Greenberg JR, Mitchell S: Object Relations in Psychoanalytic Theory. Cambridge, MA, Harvard University Press, 1983

Gunderson JG: Borderline Personality Disorder: A Clinical Guide. Washington, DC, American Psychiatric Publishing, 2001

Harter S: The Construction of the Self: A Develop
mental Perspective. New York, Guilford, 1999

Herpertz SC, Dietrich TM, Wenning B, et al: Evidence of abnormal amygdala functioning in
borderline personality disorder: a functional
MRI study. Biol Psychiatry 50: 292–298, 2001

Horowitz M: Introduction to Psychodynamics: A
Synthesis. New York, Basic Books, 1988

Horowitz MJ: Cognitive Psychodynamics: From
Conflict to Character. New York, Wiley, 1998

Kendler K, Walsh D: Schizotypal personality disorder in parents and the risk for schizophrenia
in siblings. Schizophr Bull 21:47–52, 1995

Kernberg OF: Borderline Conditions and Pathological Narcissism. New York, Jason Aronson,
1975a

Kernberg OF: Transference and countertransference in the treatment of borderline patients.
J Natl Assoc Priv Psychiatr Hosp 7:14–24, 1975b

Kernberg OF: Severe Personality Disorders: Psychotherapeutic Strategies. New Haven, CT,
Yale University Press, 1984

Kernberg O: A psychoanalytic theory of personal-
ity disorders, in Major Theories of Personality
Disorder. Edited by Clarkin J, Lenzenweger
M. New York, Guilford, 1996, pp 106–140

Kernberg O: Pathological narcissism and narcissistic personality disorder: theoretical background and diagnostic classification, in Disorders of Narcissism: Diagnostic, Clinical, and
Empirical Implications. Edited by Ronningstam E. Washington, DC, American Psychiatric Association, 1998, pp 29–51

Kiesler D: The 1982 interpersonal circle: a taxonomy for complementarity in human transac-
tions. Psychol Rev 90:185–214, 1983

Kohut H: The Analysis of the Self: A Systematic
Approach to the Treatment of Narcissistic Per-
sonality Disorders. New York, International
Universities Press, 1971

Kohut H: The Restoration of the Self. New York,
International Universities Press, 1977

Kraepelin E: Dementia Praecox and Paraphrenia
(1896). Chicago, IL, Chicago Medical Book Co,
1919

Kristensen H, Torgersen S: MCMI-II personality
traits and symptom traits in parents of children with selective mutism: a case-control
study. J Abnorm Psychol 110:648–652, 2001

Krueger RF: The structure of common mental disorders. Arch Gen Psychiatry 56:921–926, 1999

Leary T: Interpersonal Diagnosis of Personality: A
Functional Theory and Methodology for Per-
sonality Evaluation. Oxford, England, Ronald
Press, 1957

Lenzenweger M: Schizotypy and schizotypic psychopathology, in Origins and Development of
Schizophrenia: Advances in Experimental

Psychopathology. Edited by Lenzenweger M,
Dworkin R. Washington, DC, American Psychological Association, 1998, pp 93–122

Linehan MM: Cognitive-Behavioral Treatment of
Borderline Personality Disorder. New York,
Guilford, 1993a

Linehan MM: Skills-Training Manual for Treatment of Borderline Personality Disorder. New
York, Guilford, 1993b

Livesley WJ, Bromley DB: Person Perception in
Childhood and Adolescence. London, Wiley,
1973

Livesley WJ, Jang KZ, Jackson DN, et al: Genetic
and environmental contributions to dimensions
of personality disorder. Am J Psychiatry
150:1826–1831, 1993

Livesley WJ, Jang KL, Vernon PA: Phenotypic and
genetic structure of traits delineating personality disorder. Arch Gen Psychiatry 55:941–
948, 1998

Livesley WJ, Jang K, Vernon P: Genetic basis of
personality structure, in Handbook of Psychology: Personality and Social Psychology,
Vol 5. Edited by Millon T, Lerner M. New
York, Wiley, 2003, pp 59–83

Lynam DR, Widiger TA: Using the five-factor
model to represent the DSM-IV personality
disorders: an expert consensus approach.
J Abnorm Psychol 110:401–412, 2001

Lyons M, Toomey R, Faraone S, et al: Correlates of
psychosis proneness in relatives of schizophrenic patients. Journal of Abnormal Psychology and Psychotherapy: Theory, Research
and Practice 104:390–394, 1995

Main M: Recent studies in attachment: overview,
with selected implications for clinical work, in
Attachment Theory: Social, Developmental,
and Clinical Perspectives. Edited by Goldberg
S, Muir R, Kerr J. Hillsdale, NJ, Analytic Press,
1995, pp 407–474

Masterson J: Psychotherapy of the Borderline
Adult: A Developmental Approach. New
York, Brunner/Mazel, 1976

McCrae R, Costa P: Personality in Adulthood.
New York, Guilford, 1990

McCrae R, Costa PL: Personality trait structure as a
human universal. Am Psychol 52:509–516, 1997

McWilliams N: Relationship, subjectivity, and inference in diagnosis, in Making Diagnosis
Meaningful: Enhancing Evaluation and Treatment of Psychological Disorders. Edited by
Barron JW. Washington, DC, American Psychological Association, 1998, pp 197–226

Millon T: Modern Psychopathology: A Biosocial
Approach to Maladaptive Learning and Functioning. Philadelphia, PA, WB Saunders, 1969

Millon T: Toward a New Psychology. New York,
Wiley, 1990

Millon T, Davis R: Conceptions of personality disorders: historical perspectives, the DSMs, and future directions, in The DSM-IV Personality Disorders: Diagnosis and Treatment of Mental Disorders. Edited by Livesley WJ. New York, Guilford, 1995, pp 3–28

Millon T, Davis R: An evolutionary theory of personality disorders, in Major Theories of Personality Disorder. Edited by Clarkin J, Lenzenweger M. New York, Guilford, 1996, pp 221–346

Millon T, Davis R: The MCMI-III: present and future directions. J Pers Assess 68:69–85, 1997

Millon T, Grossman SD: Sociocultural factors, in The American Psychiatric Publishing Textbook of Personality Disorders. Edited by Oldham JM, Skodol AE, Bender DS. Washington, DC, American Psychiatric Publishing, 2005, pp 223–235

Mischel W: Toward a cognitive social learning reconceptualization of personality. Psychol Rev 39:351–364, 1973

Mischel W: On the interface of cognition and personality: beyond the person-situation debate. Am Psychol 34:740–754, 1979

Mischel W: Personality dispositions revisited and revised: a view after three decades, in Handbook of Personality: Theory and Research. Edited by Pervin L. New York, Guilford, 1990, pp 111–134

Mischel W, Shoda Y: A cognitive-affective system theory of personality: reconceptualizing situations, dispositions, dynamics, and invariance in personality structure. Psychol Rev 102:246–268, 1995

Mitchell SA: Relational Concepts in Psychoanalysis: An Integration. Cambridge, MA, Harvard University Press, 1988

Morey LC, Gunderson JG, Quigley BD, et al: The representation of borderline, avoidant, obsessive-compulsive, and schizotypal personality disorders by the five-factor model. J Personal Disord 16:215–234, 2002

New A, Siever L: Neurobiology and genetics of borderline personality disorder. Psychiatric Annals of Clinical Psychiatry 32:329–336, 2002

Nigg JT, Goldsmith H: Genetics of personality disorders: perspectives from personality and psychopathology research. Psychol Bull 115:346–380, 1994

Plomin R, Caspi A: Behavioral Genetics and Personality. New York, Guilford, 1999

Pretzer JL, Beck AT: A cognitive theory of personality disorders, in Major Theories of Personality Disorder. Edited by Clarkin J, Lenzenweger M. New York, Guilford, 1996, pp 36–105

Redl F, Wineman D: Children Who Hate: The Disorganization and Breakdown of Behavior Controls. Glencoe, IL, Free Press, 1951

Reich JH: Familiality of DSM-III dramatic and anxious personality clusters. J Nerv Ment Dis 177:96–100, 1989

Reich W: Character Analysis, 3rd Edition (1933). New York, Simon and Schuster, 1978

Ross S, Lutz C, Bailley S: Positive and negative symptoms of schizotypy and the five-factor model: a domain and facet level analysis. J Pers Assess 79:53–72, 2002

Schaefer E: Configurational analysis of children's reports of parent behavior. J Consult Psychol 29:552–557, 1965

Siever LJ, Davis KL: A psychobiological perspective on the personality disorders. Am J Psychiatry 148:1647–1658, 1991

Siever LJ, Torgersen S, Gunderson JG, et al: The borderline diagnosis, III: identifying endophenotypes for genetic studies. Biol Psychiatry 51:964–968, 2002

Skodol AE, Siever LJ, Livesley WJ, et al: The borderline diagnosis II: biology, genetics, and clinical course. Biol Psychiatry 51:951–963, 2002

Spitzer RL, Endicott J, Gibbon M: Crossing the border into borderline personality and borderline schizophrenia. Arch Gen Psychiatry 36:17–24, 1979

Sullivan HS: The Interpersonal Theory of Psychiatry. New York, Norton, 1953

Torgersen S: Genetic and nosological aspects of schizotypal and borderline personality disorders. Arch Gen Psychiatry 41:546–554, 1984

Torgersen S, Lygren S, Oien PA, et al: A twin study of personality disorders. Compr Psychiatry 41:416–425, 2000

Trull T, Widiger T, Burr R: A structured interview for the assessment of the Five-Factor Model of personality: facet-level relations to the Axis II personality disorders. J Pers 69:175–198, 2001

Turkheimer E, Waldron M: Nonshared environment: a theoretical, methodological, and quantitative review. Psychol Bull 126:78–108, 2000

Turkheimer E, Haley A, Waldron M, et al: Socioeconomic status modifies heritability of IQ in young children. Psychol Sci 14:623–628, 2003

Tyrer P, Johnson T: Establishing the severity of personality disorder. Am J Psychiatry 153:1593–1597, 1996

Wachtel P: Psychoanalysis and Behavior Therapy. New York, Basic Books, 1977

Wachtel P: Psychoanalysis, Behavior Therapy, and the Relational World. Washington, DC, American Psychological Association, 1997

Westen D: The relations among narcissism, egocentrism, self-concept, and self-esteem: experimental, clinical and theoretical considerations. Psychoanalysis and Contemporary Thought 13:183–239, 1990a

Westen D: Towards a revised theory of borderline object relations: contributions of empirical research. Int J Psychoanal 71:661–693, 1990b

Westen D: Cognitive-behavioral interventions in the psychoanalytic psychotherapy of borderline personality disorders. Clin Psychol Rev 11:211–230, 1991a

Westen D: Social cognition and object relations. Psychol Bull 109:429–455, 1991b

Westen D: Toward an integrative model of affect regulation: applications to social-psychological research. J Pers 62:641–667, 1994

Westen D: A clinical-empirical model of personality: life after the Mischelian ice age and the NEO-lithic era. J Pers 63:495–524, 1995

Westen D: A model and a method for uncovering the nomothetic from the idiographic: an alternative to the five-factor model? J Res Pers 30:400–413, 1996

Westen D: Case formulation and personality diagnosis: two processes or one? In Making Diagnosis Meaningful: Enhancing Evaluation and Treatment of Psychological Disorders. Edited by Barron JW. Washington, DC, American Psychological Association, 1998, pp 111–138

Westen D, Muderrisoglu S: Assessing personality disorders using a systematic clinical interview: evaluation of an alternative to structured interviews. J Personal Disord 17:351–369, 2003

Westen D, Shedler J: Revising and assessing Axis II, part I: developing a clinically and empirically valid assessment method. Am J Psychiatry 156:258–272, 1999a

Westen D, Shedler J: Revising and assessing Axis II, part II: toward an empirically based and clinically useful classification of personality disorders. Am J Psychiatry 156:273–285, 1999b

Widiger T: Personality disorders in the 21st century. J Personal Disord 14:3–16, 2000

Widiger T, Costa P: Personality and personality disorders. Journal of Abnormal Psychology and Psychotherapy: Theory, Research, and Practice 103:78–91, 1994

Widiger T, Frances A: Towards a dimensional model for the personality disorders, in Personality Disorders and the Five-Factor Model of Personality. Edited by Costa P, Widiger T. Washington, DC, American Psychological Association, 1994, pp 19–39

Widiger T, Trull TJ, Clarkin JF, et al: A description of the DSM-IV personality disorders with the five-factor model of personality, in Personality Disorders and the Five-Factor Model of Personality, 2nd Edition. Edited by Costa PT Jr, Widiger TA. Washington, DC, American Psychological Association, 2002, pp 89–99

Wolf E: Treating the Self: Elements of Clinical Self-Psychology. New York, Guilford, 1988

Young J: Cognitive Therapy for Personality Disorders: A Schema-Focused Approach. Sarasota, FL, Professional Resource Exchange, 1990

Young J, Gluhoski V: Schema-focused diagnosis for personality disorders, in Handbook of Relational Diagnosis and Dysfunctional Family Patterns. Edited by Kaslow F. Oxford, England, Wiley, 1996, pp 300–321

Young J, Lindemann M: An integrative schema-focused model for personality disorders, in Clinical Advances in Cognitive Psychotherapy: Theory and Application. Edited by Leahy R, Dowd T. New York, Springer, 2002, pp 93–109

Young J, Klosko J, Weishaar M: Schema therapy for borderline personality disorder, in Schema Therapy: A Practitioner's Guide. New York, Guilford, 2003

Part II

Clinical Evaluation

3

Manifestations, Clinical Diagnosis, and Comorbidity

Andrew E. Skodol, M.D.

A *personality disorder* is defined in DSM-IV-TR as an "enduring pattern of inner experience and behavior that deviates markedly from the expectations of the individual's culture, is pervasive and inflexible, has an onset in adolescence or early adulthood, is stable over time, and leads to distress or impairment" (American Psychiatric Association 2000, p. 685). Personality disorders are reported on Axis II of the DSM-IV-TR multiaxial system to ensure that consideration is given to their presence in all patient evaluations, even when Axis I disorder psychopathology is present and prominent.

DSM-IV-TR includes criteria for the diagnosis of 10 specific personality disorders, arranged into three clusters based on descriptive similarities. Cluster A is commonly referred to as the "odd or eccentric" cluster and includes paranoid, schizoid, and schizotypal personality disorders. Cluster B, the "dramatic, emotional, or erratic" cluster, includes antisocial, borderline, histrionic, and narcissistic personality disorders. Cluster C, the "anxious and fearful" cluster, includes avoidant, dependent, and obsessive-compulsive personality disorders. DSM-IV-TR also provides for a residual category of personality disorder not otherwise specified (PDNOS). This category is to be used when a patient meets the general criteria for a personality disorder and has features of several different types but does not meet criteria for any specific personality disorder (i.e., "mixed" personality disorder) or is considered to have a personality disorder not included in the official classification (e.g., self-defeating or depressive personality disorders).

Sections of this chapter have been modified with permission from Skodol AE: *Problems in Differential Diagnosis: From DSM-III to DSM-III-R in Clinical Practice*. Washington, DC, American Psychiatric Press, 1989

This chapter considers the manifestations, problems in differential diagnosis, and patterns of comorbidity of the DSM-IV-TR personality disorders. Included in this chapter are descriptions of the clinical characteristics of the 10 DSM-IV-TR personality disorders; discussions of problems in interviewing the patient with a suspected personality disorder in state versus trait discrimination, trait versus disorder distinctions, categorical versus alternative classificatory approaches to personality disorder diagnosis, and diagnosis based on inferential judgments; and an overview of personality disorder comorbidity. Despite limitations in the DSM approach, personality disorders diagnosed by this system have been shown since the 1980s to have considerable clinical utility in predicting functional impairment over and above that associated with comorbid Axis I disorders, extensive and intensive utilization of treatment resources, and in many cases, adverse outcomes.

DEFINING FEATURES OF PERSONALITY DISORDERS

Patterns of Inner Experience and Behavior

The general diagnostic criteria for a personality disorder in DSM-IV-TR (see Table 1–1) indicate that a pattern of inner experience and behavior is manifest by characteristic patterns of 1) cognition (i.e., ways of perceiving and interpreting self, other people, and events); 2) affectivity (i.e., the range, intensity, lability, and appropriateness of emotional response); 3) interpersonal functioning; and 4) impulse control. Patients with personality disorders are expected to have manifestations in at least two of these areas.

Cognitive Features

Personality disorders commonly affect the ways patients think about their relationships with other people and about themselves. Most of the DSM-IV-TR diagnostic criteria for paranoid personality disorder reflect a disturbance in cognition, characterized by pervasive distrust and suspiciousness of others. Patients with paranoid personality disorder suspect that others are exploiting, harming, or deceiving them; doubt the loyalty or trustworthiness of others; read hidden, demeaning, or threatening meanings into benign remarks or events; and perceive attacks on their character or reputation. Among the major symptoms of schizotypal personality disorder are characteristic cognitive and perceptual distortions, such as ideas of reference; odd beliefs and magical thinking (e.g., superstitiousness, belief in clairvoyance or telepathy); bodily illusions; and suspiciousness and paranoia similar to that observed in patients with paranoid personality disorder.

Patients with borderline personality disorder (BPD) may also experience transient paranoid ideation when under stress, but the characteristic cognitive manifestations of borderline patients are dramatic shifts in their views toward people with whom they are intensely emotionally involved. These shifts emanate from disturbances in mental representations of self and others (Bender and Skodol 2007) and result in their overidealizing others at one point and then devaluating them at another point, when they feel disappointed, neglected, or uncared for. This phenomenon is commonly referred to as "splitting." Patients with narcissistic personality disorder exhibit a grandiose sense of self; have fantasies of unlimited success, power, brilliance, beauty, or ideal love; and believe that they are special or unique.

Patients with avoidant personality disorder have excessively negative opinions of themselves, in contrast to patients with narcissistic personality disorder. They see themselves as inept, unappealing, and inferior, and they constantly perceive that they are being criticized or rejected. Patients with dependent personality disorder also lack self-confidence and believe that they are unable to make decisions or to take care of themselves. Patients with obsessive-compulsive personality disorder (OCPD) are perfectionistic and rigid in their thinking and are often preoccupied with details, rules, lists, and order.

Affective Features

Some patients with personality disorders are emotionally constricted, whereas others are excessively emotional. Among the constricted types are patients with schizoid personality disorder, who experience little pleasure in life, appear indifferent to praise or criticism, and are generally emotionally cold, detached, and unexpressive. Patients with schizotypal personality disorder also often have constricted or inappropriate affect, although they can exhibit anxiety in relation to their paranoid fears. Patients with OCPD have considerable difficulty expressing loving feelings toward others, and when they do express affection, they do so in a highly controlled or stilted manner.

Among the most emotionally expressive patients with personality disorders are those with borderline and histrionic personality disorders. Patients with BPD are emotionally labile and react very strongly, particularly in interpersonal contexts, with a variety of intensely dysphoric emotions, such as depression, anxiety, or irritability. They are also prone to inappropriate, intense outbursts of anger and are often preoccupied with fears of being abandoned by those they are attached to and reliant upon. Patients with histrionic personality disorder often display rapidly shifting emotions that seem to be dramatic and exaggerated but are shallow in comparison to the intense emotional expression seen in BPD. Patients with antisocial personality disorder (ASPD) characteristically have problems with irritability and aggressive feelings toward others, which are expressed in the context of threat or intimidation. Patients with narcissistic personality disorder display arrogant, haughty attitudes and have no empathy for other people. Patients with avoidant personality disorder are dominated by anxiety in social situations; those with dependent personality disorder are preoccupied by anxiety over the prospects of separation from caregivers and the need to be independent.

Interpersonal Features

Interpersonal problems are probably the most typical of personality disorders (Benjamin 1996; Gunderson 2007; Hill et al. 2008; Kiesler 1996). Other mental disorders are characterized by prominent cognitive or affective features or by problems with impulse control. All personality disorders, however, also have interpersonal manifestations that can be described along the two orthogonal poles of the so-called interpersonal circumplex: dominance versus submission and affiliation versus detachment.

Personality disorders characterized by a need for or a tendency toward dominance in interpersonal relationships include antisocial, histrionic, narcissistic, and obsessive-compulsive. ASPD patients deceive and intimidate others for personal gain. Patients with histrionic and narcissistic personality disorders need to be the center of attention and require excessive admiration, respectively. OCPD patients need to control others and have them submit to their ways of doing things. On the submissive side are patients with avoidant and dependent personality disorders. Patients with avoidant personality disorder are inhibited in interpersonal relationships because they are afraid of being shamed or ridiculed. Patients with dependent personality disorder will not disagree with important others for fear of losing their support or approval and will actually do things that are unpleasant, demeaning, or self-defeating in order to receive nurturance from them. BPD patients may alternate between submissiveness and dominance, seeming to become deeply involved and dependent only to turn manipulative and demanding when their needs are not met.

In the domain of affiliation versus detachment, patients with histrionic, narcissistic, and dependent personality disorders have the greatest degrees of affiliative behavior, whereas patients with paranoid, schizoid, schizotypal, avoidant, and obsessive-compulsive personality disorders are the most detached. Patients with histrionic, narcissistic, and dependent personality disorders are pro-social because of their needs for attention, admiration, and support, respectively. Patients with paranoid personality disorder do not trust others enough to become deeply involved; patients with schizotypal personality disorder have few friends or confidants, in part from a lack of trust and in part as a result of poor communication and inadequate relatedness. Patients with avoidant personality disorder are socially isolated because of their feelings of inadequacy and their fears of rejection, whereas those with schizoid personality disorder neither desire nor enjoy relationships. Patients with OCPD opt for work and productivity over friendships and interpersonal activity because they feel more in control in the former than the latter. Patients with BPD again can vacillate between being overly attached and dependent on someone (often one who is not the best match) and being isolated, distant, and aloof.

Problems With Impulse Control

Problems with impulse control can also be viewed as extremes on a continuum. Personality disorders characterized by a lack of impulse control include ASPD and BPD. Disorders involving problems with overcontrol include avoidant, dependent, and obsessive-compulsive personality disorders. ASPD is a prototype of a personality disorder characterized by impulsivity. Patients with ASPD break laws, exploit others, fail to plan ahead, get into fights, ignore commitments and obligations, and exhibit generally reckless behaviors without regard to consequences, such as speeding, driving while intoxicated, having impulsive sex, or abusing drugs. Patients with BPD also show many problems with impulse control, including impulsive spending, indiscriminate sex, substance abuse, reckless driving, and binge eating. In addition, patients with BPD engage in recurrent suicidal threats, gestures, or attempts and in self-mutilating behavior such as cutting or burning. Finally, patients with BPD have problems with anger management, have frequent temper outbursts, and at times may even engage in physical fights.

In contrast, patients with avoidant personality disorder are generally inhibited, especially in relation to people, and are reluctant to take risks or to undertake new activities. Patients with dependent personality disorder cannot even make decisions and do not take initiative to start things. Patients with OCPD are overly conscientious and scrupulous about morality, ethics, and values; they cannot bring themselves to throw away even worthless objects and are miserly.

The DSM-IV-TR personality disorder clusters, specific personality disorder types, and their principal defining clinical features are presented in Table 3–1.

Pervasiveness and Inflexibility

For a personality disorder to be present, the disturbances reviewed earlier have to be manifest frequently over a wide range of behaviors, feelings, and perceptions and in many different contexts. In DSM-IV-TR, attempts are made to stress the pervasiveness of the behaviors caused by personality disorders. Added to the basic definition of each personality disorder, serving as the "stem" to which individual features apply, is the phrase "present in a variety of contexts." For example, the essential features of paranoid personality disorder in DSM-IV-TR, preceding the specific criteria, begin: "A pervasive distrust and suspiciousness of others such that their motives are interpreted as malevolent, beginning by early adulthood and present in a variety of contexts, as indicated by four (or more) of the following" (American Psychiatric Association 2000, p. 694). Similarly, for dependent personality disorder, the criteria are preceded by the description: "A pervasive and excessive need to be

Table 3–1. DSM-IV-TR personality clusters, specific types, and their defining clinical features

Cluster	Type	Characteristic features
A		**Odd or eccentric**
	Paranoid	Pervasive distrust and suspiciousness of others such that their motives are interpreted as malevolent
	Schizoid	Pervasive pattern of detachment from social relationships and restricted range of expression of emotions in interpersonal settings
	Schizotypal	Pervasive pattern of social and interpersonal deficits marked by acute discomfort with, and reduced capacity for, close relationships as well as by cognitive or perceptual distortions and eccentricities of behavior
B		**Dramatic, emotional, or erratic**
	Antisocial	History of conduct disorder before age 15; pervasive pattern of disregard for and violation of the rights of others; current age at least 18
	Borderline	Pervasive pattern of instability of interpersonal relationships, self-image, and affects, and marked impulsivity
	Histrionic	Pervasive pattern of excessive emotionality and attention seeking
	Narcissistic	Pervasive pattern of grandiosity (in fantasy or behavior), need for admiration, and lack of empathy
C		**Anxious or fearful**
	Avoidant	Pervasive pattern of social inhibition, feelings of inadequacy, and hypersensitivity to negative evaluation
	Dependent	Pervasive and excessive need to be taken care of that leads to submissive and clinging behavior and fears of separation
	Obsessive-compulsive	Pervasive pattern of preoccupation with orderliness, perfectionism, and mental and interpersonal control at the expense of flexibility, openness, and efficiency

Source. Adapted from American Psychiatric Association: *Diagnostic and Statistical Manual of Mental Disorders,* Fourth Edition, Text Revision. Washington, DC, American Psychiatric Association, 2000, p. 685. Used with permission. Copyright 2000 American Psychiatric Association.

taken care of that leads to submissive and clinging behavior and fears of separation, beginning by early adulthood and present in a variety of contexts, as indicated by five (or more) of the following" (American Psychiatric Association 2000, p. 725).

Inflexibility is a feature that helps to distinguish personality traits or styles and personality disorders. Inflexibility is indicated by a narrow repertoire of responses that are repeated even when the situation calls for an alternative behavior or in the face of clear evidence that a behavior is inappropriate or not working. For example, an obsessive-compulsive person rigidly adheres to rules and organization even in recreation and loses enjoyment as a consequence. An avoidant person is so fearful of being scrutinized or criticized, even in group situations in which he or she could hardly be the focus of such attention, that life becomes painfully lonely.

Onset and Clinical Course

Personality and personality disorders have traditionally been assumed to reflect stable descriptions of a person, at least after a certain age. Thus, the patterns of inner experience and behaviors described earlier are called "enduring." Personality disorder is also described as "of long duration," with an onset that "can be traced back at least to adolescence or early adulthood" (American Psychiatric Association 2000, p. 686). These concepts persist as integral to the definition of personality disorder despite a large body of empirical evidence that suggests that personality disorder psychopathology is not as stable as the DSM definition would indicate. Longitudinal studies indicate that personality disorders tend to improve over time, at least from the point of view of their overt clinical signs and symptoms (Grilo et al. 2004; Johnson et al. 2000; Lenzenweger 1999; Zanarini et al. 2006). Furthermore, personality disorder criteria sets consist of combinations of pathological personality traits and symptomatic behaviors (McGlashan et al. 2005; Zanarini et al. 2007). Some behaviors, such as self-mutilating behavior (BPD), may be evidenced much less frequently than traits such as "views self as socially inept, personally unappealing or inferior to others" (avoidant personality disorder). How stable individual manifestations of personality disorders actually are and what the stable components of personality disorders are have become areas of active empirical research. It may be that personality psychopathology waxes and wanes depending on the circumstances of a person's life (see Chapter 4, "Course and Outcome").

Distress or Impairment in Functioning

Another important aspect of personality disorders that distinguishes them from traits or styles is that personality disorders lead to distress or impairment in functioning. By their nature, some personality disorders may not be accompanied by obvious subjective distress on the part of the patient. Examples would include schizoid personality disorder, in which a patient is ostensibly satisfied with his or her social isolation and does not seem to need or desire the companionship of others, and ASPD, in which the patient has utter disdain and disregard for social norms and will not experience distress unless his activities are thwarted. On the other side of the coin are patients with BPD, who are likely to experience and express considerable distress, especially when disappointed in a significant other, or patients with avoidant personality disorder, who, in contrast with schizoid patients, are usually very uncomfortable and unhappy with their lack of close friends and companions.

All personality disorders are maladaptive, however, and are accompanied by functional problems in school or at work, in social relationships, or at leisure. The requirement for impairment in psychosocial functioning is codified in DSM-IV-TR in its criterion C of the general diagnostic criteria for a personality disorder, which states that "the enduring pattern [of inner experience and behavior, i.e., personality] leads to clinically significant distress or impairment in social, occupational, or other important areas of functioning" (American Psychiatric Association 2000, p. 689).

A number of studies have compared patients with personality disorders to patients with no personality disorder or with Axis I disorders and have found that patients with personality disorders were more likely to be functionally impaired (Skodol and Gunderson 2008). Specifically, they are more likely to be separated, divorced, or never married and to have had more unemployment, frequent job changes, or periods of disability. It is interesting that only rarely have patients with personality disorders been found to be less well educated. Fewer studies have examined quality of functioning, but in those that have, poorer social functioning or interpersonal relationships and poorer work functioning or occupational achievement and satisfaction have been found among patients with personality disorders than with other disorders. When patients with different personality disorders were compared with each other on levels of functional impairment, those with severe personality disorders such as schizotypal and borderline were found to have significantly more impairment at work, in social relationships, and at leisure than patients with less severe personality disorders, such as OCPD, or with an impairing Axis I disorder, such as major depressive disorder (MDD) without personality disorder. Patients with avoidant personality disorder had intermediate levels of impairment. Even the less impaired patients with personality disorders (e.g., OCPD), however, had moderate to severe impairment in at least one area of functioning (or a Global Assessment of Functioning rating of 60 or less) (Skodol et al. 2002). The finding that significant impairment may be in only one area suggests that patients with personality disorders differ not only in the degree of associated functional impairment but also in the breadth of impairment across functional domains.

Another important aspect of the impairment in functioning in patients with personality disorders is that it tends to be persistent even beyond apparent improvement in personality disorder psychopathology itself (Seivewright et al. 2004; Skodol et al. 2005). The persistence of impairment is understandable if one considers that personality disorder psychopathology has usually been long-standing and, therefore, has disrupted a person's work and social development over a period of time (Roberts et al. 2003). The "scars" or residua of personality disorder pathology take time to heal or be overcome. With time (and treatment), however, improvements in functioning can occur.

APPROACHES TO CLINICAL INTERVIEWING

Interviewing a patient to assess for a possible personality disorder presents certain challenges that are somewhat unique. Thus, the interviewer is likely to need to rely on a variety of techniques for gathering information to arrive at a clinical diagnosis, including observation and interaction with the patient, direct questioning, and interviewing informants.

Observation and Interaction

One problem in evaluating a patient for a personality disorder arises from the fact that most people are not able to view their own personality objectively (Zimmerman 1994). Because personality is, by definition, the way a person sees, relates to, and thinks about himself or herself and the environment, a person's assessment of his or her own personality must be colored by it. The expression of Axis I psychopathology may also be colored by Axis II personality style—for example, symptoms exaggerated by the histrionic or minimized by the compulsive personality—but the symptoms of Axis I disorders are usually more clearly alien to the patient and more easily identified as problematic. People usually learn about their own problem behavior and their patterns of interaction with others through the reactions or observations of other people in their environments.

Traditionally, clinicians have not conducted the same kind of interview in assessing patients suspected of having a personality disturbance as they do with persons suspected of having, for example, a mood or an anxiety disorder. Rather than directly questioning the patient about characteristics of his or her personality, the clinician, assuming that the patient cannot accurately describe these traits, looks for patterns in the way the patient describes social relations and work functioning. These two areas usually give the clearest picture of personality style in general and personality problems specifically. Clinicians have also relied heavily on their observations of how patients interact with them during an evaluation interview or in treatment as manifestations of their patients' personalities (Westen 1997).

These approaches have the advantage of circumventing the lack of objectivity patients might have about their personalities, but they also create problems. The clinician usually comes away with a global impression of the patient's personality but frequently is not aware of many of that patient's specific personality characteristics because he or she has not made a systematic assessment of the signs and symptoms of the wide range of personality disorders (Blashfield and Herkov 1996; Morey and Ochoa 1989; Zimmerman and Mattia 1999). In routine clinical practice, clinicians tend to use the nonspecific DSM-IV-TR diagnosis of PDNOS when they believe that a patient meets the general criteria for a personality disorder, because they often do not have enough information to make a specific diagnosis (Verheul and Widiger 2004). Alternatively, clinicians will diagnose personality disorders hierarchically: once a patient is seen as having one (usually severe) personality disorder, the clinician will not assess whether traits of other personality disorders are present (Adler et al. 1990; Herkov and Blashfield 1995).

Reliance on interaction with the clinician for personality diagnosis runs the risk of generalizing a mode of interpersonal relating that may be limited to a particular situation or context—that is, the evaluation itself. Although the interaction of patient and clinician can be a useful and objective observation, caution should be used in interpreting its significance, and attempts must be made to integrate this information into a broader overall picture of patient functioning.

Direct Questioning

In psychiatric research, a portion of the poor reliability of personality disorder diagnosis has been assumed to be due to the variance in information resulting from unsystematic assessment of personality traits. Therefore, efforts have been made to develop various structured methods for assessing personality disorders (McDermut and Zimmerman 2008) comparable with those that have been successful in reducing information variance in assessing Axis I disorders (Kobak et al. 2008). These methods include both 1) self-report measures such as the Personality Diagnostic Questionnaire—4 (Hyler 1994), the Millon Clinical Multiaxial Inventory—III (Millon et al. 1997), and the Minnesota Multiphasic Personality Inventory–2 (Somwaru and Ben-Porath 1995); and 2) clinical interviews such as the Structured Interview for DSM-IV Personality (Pfohl et al. 1997), the International Personality Disorder Examination (Loranger 1999), the Structured Clinical Interview for DSM-IV Axis II Personality Disorders (First et al. 1997), the Diagnostic Interview for DSM-IV Personality Disorders (Zanarini et al. 1996), and the Personality Disorder Interview–IV (Widiger et al. 1995).

The interviews are based on the general premise that the patient can be asked specific questions that will indicate the presence or absence of each of the criteria of each of the 10 DSM-IV-TR personality disorder types. The self-report instruments are generally considered to require a follow-up interview because of a very high rate of apparently false-positive responses, but data from studies comparing self-report measures with clinical interviews suggest that the former aid in identification of personality disturbances

(Hyler et al. 1990, 1992). Thus, the clinician can keep in mind that patients do not necessarily deny negative personality attributes: in fact, the evidence suggests that they may even overreport traits that clinicians might not think are very important, and that patients can, if asked, consistently describe a wide range of personality traits to multiple interviewers. A self-report inventory might be an efficient way to help focus a clinical interview on a narrower range of personality disorder psychopathology. A semistructured interview is useful clinically when the results of an assessment might be subject to close scrutiny, such as in child custody, disability, or forensic evaluations (Widiger and Coker 2002).

Interviewing Informants

Frequently, a patient with a personality disorder consults a mental health professional for evaluation or treatment because another person has found his or her behavior problematic. This person may be a boss, spouse, boyfriend or girlfriend, teacher, parent, or representative of a social agency. Indeed, some people with personality disorders do not even recognize the problematic aspects of their manner of relating or perceiving except as it has a negative effect on someone with whom they interact.

Because of these "blind spots" that people with personality disorders may have, the use of a third-party informant in the evaluation can be useful (Zimmerman et al. 1986). In some treatment settings, such as a private individual psychotherapy practice, it may be considered counterproductive or contraindicated to include a third party, but in many inpatient and outpatient settings, certainly during the evaluation process, it may be appropriate and desirable to see some person close to the patient to corroborate both the patient's report and one's own clinical impressions.

Of course, there is no reason to assume that the informant is bias-free or not coloring a report about the patient with his or her own personality style. In fact, the correspondence between patient self-assessments of personality disorder psychopathology and informant assessments has been generally found to be modest at best (Klonsky et al. 2002). Agreement on pathological personality traits, temperament, and interpersonal problems appears to be somewhat better than on DSM personality disorders. Informants usually report more personality psychopathology than patients. Self/informant agreement on personality disorders is highest for Cluster B disorders (excluding narcissistic personality disorder), lower for Clusters A and C, and lowest for traits related to narcissism and entitlement, as might be expected. So the clinician must make a judgment about the objectivity of the informant and use this as a part, but not a sufficient part, of the overall data on which to base a personality disorder diagnosis (Zimmerman et al. 1988). Which source, the patient or the informant, provides information that is more useful for clinical purposes, such as choosing a treatment or predicting outcome (e.g., Klein 2003), is yet to be definitively determined.

PROBLEMS IN CLINICAL ASSESSMENT

Assessing Pervasiveness

The pervasiveness of personality disturbance can be difficult to determine. When a clinician inquires if a person "often" has a particular experience, a patient will frequently reply "sometimes," which then has to be judged for clinical significance. What constitutes a necessary frequency for a particular trait or behavior (Widiger 2002) and in how many different contexts or with how many different people the trait or behavior needs to be expressed has not been well worked out. Clinicians are forced to rely on their own judgment, keeping in mind also that maladaptivity and inflexibility are hallmarks of pathological traits.

For the clinician interviewing a patient with a possible personality disorder, data about the many areas of functioning, the interpersonal relationships with people interacting in different social roles with the patient, and the nature of the patient–clinician relationship should be integrated into a comprehensive assessment of pervasiveness. Too often, clinicians place disproportionate importance on a patient's functioning at a particular job or with a particular boss or significant other person.

State Versus Trait

An issue that cuts across all personality disorder diagnoses and presents practical problems in differential diagnosis is the distinction between clinical state and personality trait. Personality is presumed to be an enduring aspect of a person, yet assessment of personality ordinarily takes place cross-sectionally—that is, over a brief interval in time. Thus, the clinician is challenged to separate out long-term dispositions of the patient from other more immediate or situationally determined characteristics. This task is more complicated by the fact that the patient often comes for evaluation when there is some particularly acute problem, which may be a social or job-related crisis or the onset of an Axis I disorder (Shea 1997). In either case, the situation in which the patient is being evaluated is frequently a state that is not completely characteristic of the patient's life over the longer run.

Assessing an Enduring Pattern

DSM-IV-TR indicates that personality disorders are of long duration and are not "better accounted for as a manifestation or consequence of another mental disorder" (American Psychiatric Association 2000, p. 689). Making these determinations in practice is not easy. First of all, an accurate assessment requires recognition of current state. An assessment of current state, in turn, includes knowledge of the circumstances that have

prompted the person to seek treatment, the consequences in terms of the decision to seek treatment, the current level of stress, and any actual Axis I psychopathology, if present.

The DSM-IV-TR multiaxial system is of considerable aid in the assessment of these problems because of its separation of Axis I disorders from Axis II disorders and its individual axes for physical disorders and psychosocial stressors. A multiaxial system forces clinicians to think about the effects of aspects of patients' current state on long-term patterns of behavior, but it does not make the distinctions for them.

It is not clear from the diagnostic criteria of DSM-IV-TR how long a pattern of personality disturbance needs to be present, or when it should become evident, for a personality disorder to be diagnosed. Earlier iterations of the DSM stated that patients were usually age 18 years or older when personality disorder was diagnosed because it can be argued that, up to that age, a personality pattern could neither have been manifest long enough nor have become significantly entrenched to be considered a stable constellation of behavior. DSM-IV-TR states, however, that some manifestations of personality disorder are usually recognizable by adolescence or earlier and that personality disorders can be diagnosed in persons younger than age 18 years who have manifestated symptoms for at least 1 year. Longitudinal research has shown that personality disorder symptoms evident in childhood or early adolescence may not persist into adult life (Johnson et al. 2000). Longitudinal research has also shown that there is continuity between certain disorders of childhood and adolescence and personality disorders in early adulthood (Kasen et al. 1999, 2001). Thus, a young boy with oppositional defiant or attention-deficit/hyperactivity disorder in childhood may go on to develop conduct disorder as an adolescent, which can progress to full-blown ASPD in adulthood (Bernstein et al. 1996; Lewinsohn et al. 1997; Rey et al. 1995; Zoccolillo et al. 1992). ASPD is the only diagnosis not given before age 18; an adolescent exhibiting significant antisocial behavior before age 18 years is diagnosed with conduct disorder.

Regarding the course of a personality disorder, DSM-IV-TR states that personality disorders are relatively stable over time, although certain of them (e.g., ASPD and BPD) may become somewhat attenuated with age, whereas others may not or may, in fact, become more pronounced (e.g., obsessive-compulsive and schizotypal personality disorders). As mentioned earlier and discussed in greater detail in Chapter 4, "Course and Outcome," this degree of stability may not necessarily pertain to all of the features of all DSM-IV-TR personality disorders equally.

To assess stability retrospectively, the clinician must ask questions about periods of a person's life that are of various degrees of remoteness from the current situation. Retrospective reporting is subject to distortion, however, and the only sure way of demonstrating stability over time is, therefore, to do prospective follow-up evaluations. Thus from a practical, clinical point of view, personality disorder diagnoses made cross-sectionally and on the basis of retrospectively collected data would be tentative or provisional pending confirmation by longitudinal evaluation. On an inpatient service, a period of intense observation by many professionals from diverse perspectives may suffice to establish a pattern over time (Skodol et al. 1988, 1991). In a typical outpatient setting in which encounters with the patients are much less frequent, more time may be required. Ideally, features of a personality disorder should be evident over years, but it is not practical to wait inordinate amounts of time before coming to a diagnostic conclusion.

Assessing the Effect of an Axis I Disorder

An Axis I disorder can complicate the diagnosis of a personality disorder in several ways (Widiger and Sanderson 1995; Zimmerman 1994). An Axis I disorder may cause changes in a person's behavior or attitudes that can appear to be signs of a personality disorder. Depression, for example, may cause a person to seem excessively dependent, avoidant, or self-defeating. Cyclothymia or bipolar disorder (not otherwise specified; bipolar II) may lead to periods of grandiosity, impulsivity, poor judgment, and depression that might be confused with manifestations of narcissistic or borderline personality disorders.

The clinician must be aware of the Axis I psychopathology and attempt to assess Axis II independently. This assessment can be attempted in one of two ways. First, the clinician can ask about aspects of personality functioning at times when the patient is not experiencing Axis I symptoms. This approach is feasible when the Axis I disorder is of recent onset and short duration or, if more chronic, if the course of the disorder has been characterized by relatively clear-cut episodes with complete remission and symptom-free periods of long duration. When the Axis I disorder is chronic and unremitting, then the Axis I psychopathology and personality functioning blend together to an extent that makes differentiating between them clearly artificial.

A second approach to distinguishing signs of Axis I pathology from signs of Axis II personality is longitudinal and would defer an Axis II diagnosis pending the outcome of a trial of treatment for the Axis I disorder. This strategy may be the preferred approach in the case of a long-standing and chronic Axis I disorder, like cyclothymia, that has never been previously recognized or treated. Although one always runs the risk of a partial response to treatment and some residual symptoms, this tactic may bring the clinician as close, practically speaking, as he or she will get to observing the patient's baseline functioning. The following case is adapted from Skodol (1989).

Case Example

A 24-year-old unemployed man sought psychiatric hospitalization because of a serious problem with depression. The man reported that he had felt mildly, but continuously, depressed since the age of 16. When he reached his twenties, he had begun to have more severe bouts that made him suicidal and unable to function.

During the most recent episode, beginning about 6 months previously, he had quit his job as a taxi driver and isolated himself from his friends. He spent his time "lying around and eating a lot" and, in fact, had gained 60 pounds. He had difficulty falling asleep, felt fatigued all day long, could not concentrate, felt worthless ("There's no purpose to my life") and guilty ("I missed my chances; I've put my family through hell"), and had taken an overdose of sleeping pills.

The man received a semistructured interview assessment of Axis II psychopathology. In describing his personality, he said that he once thought of himself as lively and good-natured, but that over the past 4 or 5 years, he felt he had changed. He said that he was very sensitive to criticism, afraid to get involved with people, fearful of new places and experiences, convinced he was making a fool of himself, and afraid of losing control. He felt very dependent on others for decision making and for initiative. He said that he was so "needy" of others that they "could do anything" to him and he would "take it." He felt helpless when alone, was sure he would end up "alone and in the streets," and was constantly looking to others, especially family members, for comfort and reassurance.

The man also thought that people took advantage of him now and that he "let them" because he never stood up for his own self-interest. He felt like a total failure with no redeeming virtues. He said he either deliberately passed up opportunities to improve his situation because he felt "I don't deserve any better" or else undermined himself "without thinking" by failing to follow through, for example, on a job interview. He believed that no one could really be trusted, that old friends probably talked about him behind his back ("They think I'm a slob"), that he could not open up with new people because they too would eventually turn on him and reject

him, and that he now carried a chip on his shoulder because he had been "burned" by others so often. He admitted that he was not blame-free in relationships because he had also used people, especially members of his family.

The patient felt that he was not improving in his outpatient treatment of the last 3 years. His reason for seeking hospitalization, in addition to the fact that he continually thought of suicide and was frightened he might actually succeed in killing himself, was that he felt "totally lost" in his life, without direction, goals, or knowing what mattered to him. He said he felt "hollow." "If they cut me open after I was dead," he said, "they'd probably find out I was all shriveled up inside."

This man's description of his "personality," the ways in which he characteristically thought about himself, saw others and his relationships to them, and behaved, actually met DSM-IV-TR criteria for avoidant, dependent, paranoid, and borderline personality disorders. He was hospitalized for long-term treatment, which was available at the time. In addition to receiving individual, psychoanalytically oriented psychotherapy sessions and participating in a variety of therapeutic groups, he was given fluoxetine, up to 80 mg/day, for treatment of Axis I MDD and dysthymia.

Six months after admission, the patient reported that he felt significantly less depressed. Measured in terms of the Hamilton Rating Scale for Depression, the initial severity of his depression was 30, and his posttreatment score was 10. A repeat semistructured assessment of his personality functioning revealed that he no longer met DSM-IV-TR criteria for any personality disorder, although he continued to exhibit some dependent traits.

Another example of the way in which Axis I and II disorders interact to obscure differential diagnosis is the case of apparent Axis II psychopathology that, in fact, is the prodrome of an Axis I disorder. Distinguishing Cluster A personality disorders, such as paranoid, schizoid, and schizotypal, from the early signs of Axis I disorders in the schizophrenia and other psychotic disorders class can be particularly difficult. If a clinician is evaluating a patient early in the course of the initial onset of a psychotic disorder, he or she may be confronted with changes in the person toward increasing suspiciousness, social withdrawal, eccentricity, or reduced functioning. Because the diagnosis of psychotic disorders, including schizophrenia, requires that the patient have an episode of active psychosis with delusions and hallucinations, it is not possible to diagnose this prodrome as a psychotic disorder. In fact, until the full-blown disorder is present, the clinician cannot be certain if it is, indeed, a prodrome.

If a change in behavior is of recent onset, then it does not meet the stability criteria for a personality disorder. In such cases, the clinician is forced to diagnose an unspecified mental disorder (nonpsychotic; DSM-IV-TR code 300.9). If, however, the pattern of suspiciousness or social withdrawal with or without eccentricities has been well established, it may legitimately be a personality disorder and be diagnosed as such.

If the clinician follows such a patient over time and the patient develops a full-fledged psychotic disorder, the personality disturbance is no longer adequate for a complete diagnosis because none of the Axis II disorders includes frankly psychotic symptoms. This fairly obvious point is frequently overlooked in practice. All of the personality disorders that have counterpart psychotic disorders on Axis I have milder symptoms in which reality testing is, at least in part, intact. For instance, a patient with paranoid personality disorder may have referential ideas but not frank delusions of reference, and a patient with schizotypal personality disorder may have illusions but not hallucinations. A possible exception is BPD, in which brief psychotic experiences (lasting minutes to an hour or two at most) are included in the diagnostic criteria. In all cases, however, when the patient becomes psychotic for even a day or two, an additional Axis I diagnosis is necessary.

For the patient with a diagnosis of schizotypal personality disorder, the occurrence of a 1-month-long psychotic episode almost certainly means the disturbance will meet the criteria for schizophrenia, the symptoms of schizotypal personality disorder "counting" as prodromal symptoms toward the 6-month duration requirement. Under these circumstances, the diagnosis of schizophrenia, with its pervasive effects on cognition, perception, functional ability, and so on, is sufficient, and a diagnosis of schizotypal personality disorder is redundant. When the patient becomes nonpsychotic again, he or she would be considered to have residual schizophrenia instead of schizotypal personality disorder.

Personality Traits Versus Personality Disorders

Another difficult distinction is between personality traits or styles and personality disorders. All patients—all people for that matter—can be described in terms of distinctive patterns of personality, but all do not necessarily warrant a diagnosis of personality disorder. This error is particularly common among inexperienced evaluators. The important features that distinguish pathological personality traits from normal traits are their inflexibility and maladaptiveness, as discussed earlier.

DSM-IV-TR recognizes that it is important to describe personality style as well as to diagnose personality disorder on Axis II. Therefore, instructions are included to list personality features on Axis II even when a personality disorder is absent, or to include them as modifiers of one or more diagnosed personality disorders (e.g., BPD with histrionic features). In practice, however, this option has been seldom utilized (Skodol et al. 1984), even though research has shown that, in addition to the approximately 50% of clinic patients who meet criteria for a personality disorder, another 35% warrant information descriptive of their personality styles on Axis II (Kass et al. 1985). The overlap among

the features of personality disorders also becomes very evident when emphasis is placed
on the assessment of traits of all personality
disorders, even when one is predominant.

The following case example (adapted
from Skodol 1989) describes a patient with an
Axis I disorder whose ongoing treatment
was very much affected by Axis II personality traits, none of which met criteria for a personality disorder.

Case Example

A 25-year-old, single female receptionist
was referred for outpatient therapy following hospitalization for her first
manic episode. The patient had attended
college for 1 year but dropped out in order to "go into advertising." Over the
next 5 years, she had held a series of receptionist, secretarial, and sales jobs,
each of which she quit because she
wasn't "getting ahead in the world." She
lived in an apartment on the north side
of Chicago, by herself, that her parents
had furnished for her. She ate all of her
meals, however, at her mother's house
and claimed not even to have a box of
crackers in her cupboard. Between her
jobs, her parents paid her rent.

Her "career" problems stemmed
from the fact that, although she felt
quite ordinary and without talent for
the most part, she had fantasies of a career as a movie star or high fashion
model. She took acting classes and sing-
ing lessons but had never had even a
small role in a play or show. What she
desired was not so much the careers
themselves but the glamour associated
with them. Although she wanted to
move in the circles of the "beautiful
people," she was certain that she had
nothing to offer them. She sometimes
referred to herself as nothing but a shell
and scorned herself because of it. She
was unable to picture herself working
her way up along any realistic career
line, feeling both that it would take too
long and that she would probably fail.

She had had three close relationships with men that were characterized
by an intense interdependency that ini-

tially was agreeable to both parties. She
craved affection and attention and fell
deeply in love with these men. However, she eventually became overtly
self-centered, demanding, and manipulative, and the man would break off the
relationship. After breaking up, she
would almost immediately start claiming that the particular man was "going
nowhere," was not for her, and would
not be missed. In between these relationships, she often had periods in
which she engaged in a succession of
one-night stands, having sex with a
half-dozen partners in a month. Alternatively, she would frequent rock clubs
and bars, "in-spots," as she called them,
merely on the chance of meeting someone who would introduce her to the
glamorous world she dreamed of.

The patient had no female friends
other than her sister. She could see little
use for such friendships. She preferred
spending her time shopping for stylish
clothes or watching television alone at
home. She liked to dress fashionably
and seductively but often felt that she
was too fat or that her hair was the
wrong color. She had trouble controlling her weight and would periodically
go on eating binges for a few days that
might result in a 10-pound weight gain.
She read popular novels but had very
few other interests. She admitted she
was bored much of the time but would
not admit that cultural or athletic pur-
suits were other than a waste of time.

This patient was referred for outpatient follow-up without an Axis II personality disorder diagnosis. In fact, her
long-term functioning failed to meet
DSM-IV-TR criteria for any specific type
of personality disorder. On the other
hand, she almost met the criteria for
several, especially BPD: the patient
showed signs of impulsivity (overeat-
ing, sexual promiscuity), intense interpersonal relationships (manipulative,
overidealization/devaluation), identity
disturbance, and chronic feelings of
emptiness. She did not, however, display intense anger, intolerance of being
alone, physically self-damaging behavior, stress-related paranoia or dissociation, or affective instability indepen-

dent of her mood disorder. Similarly, she had symptoms of histrionic personality disorder: she was inappropriately sexually seductive and used her physical appearance to draw attention to herself, but she was not emotionally overdramatic. She had shallow expression of emotions and was uncomfortable when she was not the center of attention, but was not overly suggestible. She also had some features of narcissistic, avoidant, and dependent personality disorders. The attention paid to personality traits in her outpatient clinic evaluation conveyed a vivid picture of the patient's complicated personality pathology, which became the focus of her subsequent therapy.

Effects of Gender, Culture, and Age

Gender

Although definitive estimates about the sex ratio of personality disorders cannot be made because ideal epidemiological studies do not exist, some personality disorders are believed to be more common in clinical settings among men and others among women. Personality disorders listed in DSM-IV-TR as occurring more often among men are paranoid, schizoid, schizotypal, antisocial, narcissistic, and obsessive-compulsive personality disorders. Those occurring more often in women are borderline, histrionic, and dependent personality disorders. Avoidant is said to be equally common in men and women. Apparently elevated sex ratios that do not reflect true prevalence rates can be the result of sampling or diagnostic biases in clinical settings (Widiger 1998). True differences may be due to biological factors such as hormones, social factors such as child-rearing practices, and their interactions (Morey et al. 2005).

Culture

Apparent manifestations of personality disorders must be considered in the context of a patient's cultural reference group and the degree to which behaviors such as diffidence,

passivity, emotionality, emphasis on work and productivity, and unusual beliefs and rituals are culturally sanctioned. Only when such behaviors are clearly in excess or discordant with the standards of a person's cultural milieu would the diagnosis of a personality disorder be considered. Certain sociocultural contexts may lend themselves to eliciting and reinforcing behaviors that might be mistaken for personality disorder psychopathology. Members of minority groups, immigrants, or refugees, for example, might appear overly guarded or mistrustful, avoidant, or hostile in response to experiences of discrimination, language barriers, or problems in acculturation (Alarcon 2005).

Age

Although personality disorders are usually not diagnosed prior to age 18 years, certain thoughts, feelings, and behaviors suggestive of personality psychopathology may be apparent in childhood. For example, dependency, social anxiety and hypersensitivity, disruptive behavior, or identity problems may be developmentally expected. Follow-up studies of children have shown decreases in such behaviors over time (Johnson et al. 2000), although children with elevated rates of personality disorder–type signs and symptoms do appear to be at higher risk for both Axis I and Axis II disorders in young adulthood (Johnson et al. 1999; Kasen et al. 1999). Thus, some childhood problems may not turn out to be transitory, and personality disorder may be viewed developmentally as a failure to mature out of certain age-appropriate or phase-specific feelings or behaviors. A developmental perspective on personality disorders is presented more fully in Chapter 7, "Developmental Issues."

Other Aspects of Personality Functioning

A problem with the DSM conceptualizations of personality disorders is that the individual categories do not correspond well with existing treatment approaches. Thus, whether a clinician is a psychodynamically oriented therapist, a cognitive-behavioral therapist, or a psychopharmacologist, information in addition to that necessary for a DSM personality disorder diagnosis is needed to formulate a treatment plan. Usually, this additional information is based on the theory of why a patient has a personality disorder and/or the mechanisms responsible for perpetuating the dysfunctional patterns.

Conflicts, Ego Functions, Object Relations, and Defense Mechanisms

Psychodynamically oriented clinicians have expressed dissatisfaction with the DSM system of axes, including Axis II, since its inception. The DSM multiaxial system fails, in their opinion, to discriminate between patients according to clinical variables important for planning treatment with psychodynamic psychotherapy (Karasu and Skodol 1980). Thus, they may be more interested in exploring conflicts between wishes, fears, and moral standards; ego functions such as impulse control or affect regulation; or self and other (object) representations based on early attachment experiences than on the signs and symptoms of personality disorders. Elaborations of psychodynamic theories of personality disorders can be found in Chapter 2, "Theories of Personality and Personality Disorders," and Chapter 10, "Psychoanalysis and Psychodynamic Psychotherapy," along with discussions of relevant clinical variables.

Several groups of researchers (Bond and Vaillant 1986; Perry and Cooper 1989; Vaillant et al. 1986) have been able to document empirically the clinical utility of categorizing a patient's defensive functioning. *Defense mechanisms* are automatic psychological processes that protect people against anxiety and against awareness of internal or external stressors or dangers. Although this work was considered too early in its development to justify including a separate official axis based on it, Appendix B in DSM-IV-TR ("Criteria Sets and Axes Provided for Further Study")

includes a Defensive Functioning Scale and a Glossary of Specific Defense Mechanisms and Coping Styles. The 27 defense mechanisms defined in this glossary are acting-out, affiliation, altruism, anticipation, autistic fantasy, denial, devaluation, displacement, dissociation, help-rejecting complaining, humor, idealization, intellectualization, isolation of affect, omnipotence, passive aggression, projection, projective identification, rationalization, reaction formation, repression, self-assertion, self-observation, splitting, sublimation, suppression, and undoing. Some defense mechanisms, such as projection, splitting, or acting-out, are always maladaptive, whereas others, such as sublimation or humor, are adaptive. Patients with personality disorders have characteristic predominant defensive patterns. Thus patients with paranoid personality disorder use denial and projection, those with BPD typically rely on acting-out and splitting (among others), and those with OCPD use isolation of affect and undoing (Perry and Bond 2005). Clinicians may note current defenses or coping styles as well as a patient's predominant current defense level using the Defensive Functioning Scale.

Coping Styles

Although defense mechanisms in DSM-IV-TR are said to include coping styles, the literature on coping discusses styles not included in the DSM list. *Coping* refers to specific thoughts and behaviors that a person uses to manage the internal and external demands of situations appraised as stressful (Folkman and Moskowitz 2004; Lazarus and Folkman 1984; Pearlin and Schooler 1978). Coping involves cognitive, behavioral, and emotional responses and may or may not be consistent across stressful situations or functional roles. Two major broad styles of coping are problem-focused coping and emotion-focused coping. *Problem-focused coping* refers to efforts to resolve a threatening problem or diminish its impact by taking direct action. *Emotion-focused coping* refers to efforts to reduce the negative emotions aroused in response to a threat by changing the way the threat is attended to or interpreted. Meaning-focused and social coping are other observed coping strategies. Coping has traditionally been assessed by retrospective self-report measures (e.g., the Coping Responses Inventory [Moos 1993], the Ways of Coping Questionnaire [Folkman and Lazarus 1988], and the COPE Inventory [Carver et al. 1989])—and more recently by ecological momentary assessment (real-time) techniques (Stone et al. 1998); but the major types of coping, such as problem solving, seeking support, distancing and distracting, accepting responsibility, positive reappraisal, or self-blame, can also be assessed by clinical interview.

Cognitive Schemas

Cognitive therapists want to characterize patients with personality disorders according to patients' dysfunctional cognitive schemas (core beliefs by which they process information) or their automatic thoughts, interpersonal strategies, and cognitive distortions. Again, particular personality disorders tend to have particular core beliefs. For example, patients with BPD frequently have beliefs such as "I am needy and weak" or "I am helpless if left on my own," whereas patients with OCPD believe "It is important to do a perfect job on everything" or "People should do things my way" (Beck et al. 2004). In contrast to beliefs, which map onto personality disorders specifically, *schemas* are broader themes regarding the self and relationships with others and can cut across personality disorder categories. For example, a schema of "impaired limits" can encompass the entitlement of narcissistic personality disorder as well as the lack of self-control of ASPD or BPD (Young and Klosko 2005).

Objective Behaviors Versus Inferential Traits

Another difficulty in diagnosing personality disorders stems from the degree of inference and judgment necessary to make many of the diagnoses. Numerous critics have noted that it is easy to disagree about symptoms such as affective instability, self-dramatization, shallow emotional expression, exaggerated fears, or feelings of inadequacy—all symptoms of DSM-IV-TR personality disorders. Only the antisocial criteria, among the personality disorders, have historically yielded acceptable levels of reliability, and those criteria have emphasized overtly criminal and delinquent acts.

These observations led several investigators to attempt to determine sets of behaviors that might serve to identify types of personality disorder. Although any one behavior might not be sufficient to indicate a particular personality trait, multiple behavioral indicators considered together would increase confidence in recognizing the trait.

Behaviors that typify a particular personality style have been referred to as *prototypical*. Livesley (1986) developed a set of prototypical behaviors for the DSM-III (American Psychiatric Association 1980) personality disorders and compared them with prototypical traits. He found that highly prototypical behaviors could be derived from corresponding traits. For example, with regard to the concepts of social awkwardness and withdrawal of the schizoid personality disorder, Livesley found that behaviors such as "does not speak unless spoken to," "does not initiate social contacts," and "rarely reveals self to others" were uniformly rated as highly prototypical. Corresponding to the overly dramatic and emotional traits of the histrionic personality disorder were behaviors such as "expressed feelings in an exaggerated way," "considered a minor problem catastrophic," and "flirted with several members of the opposite sex." Behaviors such as "has routine schedules and is upset by deviations," "overreacted to criticism," and "spent considerable time on the minutest details" corresponded to the controlled, perfectionist traits of OCPD.

DSM-IV-TR makes strides in translating the characteristic traits of the personality disorders into explicit behaviors. The criteria for each personality disorder begin with the definition of the overall style or set of traits, followed by a listing of ways this might be expressed. In some instances, for example, for dependent personality disorder, the criteria are quite behavioral. For dependent personality disorder, a pervasive and excessive need to be taken care of that leads to submissive and clinging behavior and fears of separation is indicated by such items as "has difficulty making everyday decisions without an excessive amount of advice and reassurance from others" and "needs others to assume responsibility for most major areas of his or her life" (American Psychiatric Association 2000, p. 725). For other disorders, such as OCPD, an example of the behavior is given along with the trait. For OCPD, perfectionism is indicated by the following criterion: "shows perfectionism that interferes with task completion (e.g., is unable to complete a project because his or her own overly strict standards are not met)" (American Psychiatric Association 2000, p. 729).

COMORBIDITY

Since the introduction of a multiaxial system for recording diagnoses in DSM-III, which provided for the diagnosis of personality disorders on an axis (II) separate from the majority of other mental disorders, it has become apparent that most patients with personality disorders also meet criteria for other disorders. Rates have ranged from about two-thirds to almost 100% (Dolan-Sewell et al. 2001). The co-occurrence of Axis I and Axis II disorders has often been referred to as *comorbidity*, although our current understanding of the fundamental nature of most mental disorders is insufficient to justify the use of the term according to its formal definition, which requires that a comorbid disorder be "distinct" from the index disease or condition (Feinstein 1970). The DSM system, with its tendency to "split" as opposed to "lump" psychopathology via its many and expanding lists of disorders, encourages the diagnosis of multiple putative disorders to describe a patient's psychopathology and virtually ensures that patients will receive more than one diagnosis. In addition to the co-occurrence of personality disorders with Axis I disorders, it is also common for patients to receive more than one personality disorder diagnosis to fully describe their personality problems (Lilienfeld et al. 1994; Oldham et al. 1992). In the sections that follow, major patterns of personality disorder "comorbidity" will be described.

Co-Occurrence of Personality Disorders and Axis I Disorders

There are a number of explanations for the high rates of co-occurrence of personality disorders and Axis I disorders (Lyons et al. 1997). Co-occurring disorders may share a common etiology and be different phenotypic expressions of a common causal factor or factors. They may also be linked by etiology or pathological mechanism, but one disorder may be a milder version of the other on a spectrum of severity of pathology or impairment. One disorder may precede and increase the risk for the occurrence of another disorder, making a person more "vulnerable" to developing the second disorder. A second disorder may arise after a first as a complication or residual phenomenon or "scar." People with certain personality disorders and related Axis I disorders may share common psychobiological substrates that regulate cognitive or affective processes or impulse control. The Axis I disorders may be the direct symptomatic expression of dysfunctions in these systems, whereas personality disorders may reflect coping mechanisms and more general personality predispositions arising from the same systems (Siever and Davis 1991). This more comprehensive model of disorder co-occurrence integrates aspects of the common cause, spectrum, and vulnerability hypotheses.

Axis I/Axis II co-occurrence may be viewed from the perspectives of the course of a person's lifetime or the current presenting illness. Lifetime rates will obviously be higher. Patients with personality disorders who are seeking treatment also tend to have elevated rates of Axis I disorder co-occurrence, because the development or exacerbation of an Axis I disorder is often the reason a personality disorder patient comes for clinical attention (Shea 1997). For disorder co-occurrence to be significant from a scientific perspective, rates must be elevated above those expected by chance, based on the rates of occurrence of the individual disorders in a given clinical setting or population. From a treatment perspective, any co-occurrence may be significant.

The personality disorders of Cluster A—paranoid, schizoid, and schizotypal—are linked by theory and phenomenology to Axis I psychotic disorders such as delusional disorder, schizophreniform disorder, or schizophrenia. Few studies have actually documented these associations, however, possibly because of problems in being able to differentiate between clinical presentations of attenuated and full-blown psychotic symptoms that warrant two diagnoses instead of just one. Oldham et al. (1995) found elevated odds of a current psychotic disorder in patients with Cluster A personality disorders but also found elevated odds for Clusters B and C personality disorders as well, suggesting less disorder specificity than might be expected.

In contrast, Cluster B personality disorders, especially BPD, which is linked by theory and phenomenology to Axis I mood and impulse control disorders, have repeatedly been shown to have high rates of co-occurring MDD and other mood disorders, substance use disorders, and bulimia nervosa (Oldham et al. 1995; Skodol et al. 1993, 1999; Zanarini et al. 1989, 1998). Taking into account co-occurrence expected by chance alone, however, neither Oldham et al. (1995) nor McGlashan et al. (2000) substantiated the relationship between BPD and MDD. In addition, several studies have shown significantly elevated rates of anxiety disorders, including panic disorder and posttraumatic stress disorder, in patients with BPD (McGlashan et al. 2000; Skodol et al. 1995). ASPD

is most strongly associated with substance use disorders in clinical and general population samples (Compton et al. 2007; Grant et al. 2004; Hasin et al. 2007; Kessler et al. 1997; Morgenstern et al. 1997; see also Chapter 19, "Substance Abuse"). This association supports an underlying dimension of impulsivity or externalization (acting-out and being at odds with mainstream goals and values) shared by these disorders (Krueger et al. 1998, 2002, 2007).

Cluster C personality disorders, especially avoidant and dependent personality disorders, are linked by theory and phenomenology to anxiety disorders (Tyrer et al. 1997). Several studies have demonstrated high rates of co-occurrence of avoidant personality disorder with MDD, agoraphobia, social phobia, and obsessive-compulsive disorder (Herbert et al. 1992; Oldham et al. 1995; Skodol et al. 1995). The co-occurrence rates between avoidant personality disorder and social phobia (particularly the generalized type) have been so high in some studies that investigators have argued that they are the same disorder. Several studies have indicated that dependent personality disorder co-occurs with a wide variety of Axis I disorders, consistent with the notion of excessive dependency as a nonspecific maladaptive behavior pattern that may result from coping with other chronic mental disorders (Skodol et al. 1996). OCPD may be specifically linked to obsessive-compulsive disorder; however, an association between them has only inconsistently been found.

Following the co-occurrence of Axis I and Axis II disorders is more than an intellectual exercise. The presence of an Axis I disorder in a patient with a personality disorder may suggest a more specific treatment approach, either with pharmacological agents, psychotherapy, or self-help groups (as in the case of substance use disorders), that will favorably affect outcome in these patients. Conversely, the presence of personality disorder in a patient with an Axis I disorder often indicates greater and more widespread levels of impairment (Jackson and Burgess 2002; Skodol et al.

2002), more chronicity (Grilo et al. 2005; Hart et al. 2001), and an overall poorer response to treatment requiring more intensive and prolonged care (Reich and Vasile 1993; Shea et al. 1992). Twenty years later, co-occurring Axis I and Axis II disorders present a higher risk for negative prognoses than do disorders on either axis alone (Crawford et al. 2008).

Co-Occurrence of Personality Disorders With Other Personality Disorders

When thorough assessments of the full range of Axis II disorders are conducted, as in research studies employing semistructured interviews, approximately half of patients receive more than one personality disorder diagnosis. Patterns of co-occurrence of personality disorders generally follow the DSM cluster structure (i.e, schizotypal personality disorder occurs more frequently with paranoid and schizoid personality disorders than with personality disorders outside Cluster A). These patterns are consistent with factor-analytic studies that support the clustering of personality disorders in DSM (Kass et al. 1985; Sanislow et al. 2002). Some personality disorders, however, particularly those in Cluster C, show associations with personality disorders from other clusters. Dependent personality disorder commonly occurs in patients with BPD, which makes clinical sense because patients with BPD can display regressive, clinging, and dependent behavior in interpersonal relationships. Some personality disorders rarely co-occur. OCPD and ASPD would be an exceedingly rare combination, because the careful planning and work orientation of OCPD are the antithesis of the impulsivity and irresponsibility of ASPD.

Elevated rates of personality disorder co-occurrence raise questions about the appropriate application of DSM-IV-TR categories to phenomenology that rarely appears to have discrete boundaries. Although DSM-IV-TR clearly stipulates that for many patients, personality disturbance would frequently meet criteria for more than one disorder, clinicians have found the practice of diagnosing multiple disorders conceptually difficult and therefore seldom attempt such diagnoses.

Prior to DSM-III-R (American Psychiatric Association 1987), part of the problem had been that most of the personality disorders were defined as classical categories (Cantor et al. 1980)—that is, ones in which all members clearly share certain identifying features. Classical categories imply a clear demarcation between members and nonmembers, but natural phenomena rarely fit neatly into such categories.

CATEGORICAL VERSUS DIMENSIONAL ASSESSMENTS OF PERSONALITY

Traditionally, in much of the psychological literature, personality has been described and measured along certain dimensions (Frances 1982). Dimensions of personality frequently are continuous with opposite traits at either end of a spectrum, such as dominant-submissive or hostile-friendly. People can then vary in the extent to which each of the traits describes them. Dimensional models of personality diagnosis appear to be more flexible and specific than categorical models when the phenomenology lacks clear-cut boundaries between normal and abnormal and between different constellations of maladaptive traits, as seems true of personality disturbance (Widiger et al. 1987). Scaled rating systems have been devised to transform Axis II disorders into dimensions (Kass et al. 1985; Oldham and Skodol 2000), but they are not representative of dimensional approaches currently in wide use. Dimensional models of personality disorders are being seriously considered for DSM-V (see Chapter 20, "Future Directions: Toward DSM-V."

Some personality disorder researchers advocate a prototype matching approach to the diagnosis of personality disorders rather than the current DSM procedure, which continues to involve making present/absent judgments about individual criteria (Shedler and Westen 2004; Westen et al. 2006). They would replace the diagnostic criteria sets with descriptions of various personality disorder prototypes in paragraph form and ask clinicians to rate the degree of similarity between the prototypes and the patient undergoing evaluation. They argue that a prototype matching approach allows the clinician to consider individual criteria in the context of the whole personality disorder description, such that no single criterion can "make or break" the diagnosis. They also argue that a prototype matching approach is closer to the way clinicians make personality disorder diagnoses in actual practice.

CONCLUSION

Although considerable dissatisfaction has been expressed over the DSM approach to these disorders and a major overhaul has been recommended by many researchers and clinicians in the field (Clark et al. 1997; Shedler and Westen 2004; Widiger 1991, 1993), the DSM approach remains the official standard for diagnosing personality disorder psychopathology. Work on DSM-V has recently begun, but its publication is not anticipated until at least 2012. Therefore, even if a dimensional approach to personality disorders were to replace the categorical approach in DSM-V, these changes would not be implemented for several years.

REFERENCES

Adler DA, Drake RE, Teague GB: Clinicians' practices in personality assessment: does gender influence the use of DSM-III Axis II? Compr Psychiatry 31:125–133, 1990

Alarcon RD: Cross-cultural issues, in American Psychiatric Publishing Textbook of Personality Disorders. Edited by Oldham JM, Skodol AE, Bender DS. Washington, DC, American Psychiatric Publishing, 2005, pp 561–578

American Psychiatric Association: Diagnostic and Statistical Manual of Mental Disorders, 3rd Edition. Washington, DC, American Psychiatric Association, 1980

American Psychiatric Association: Diagnostic and Statistical Manual of Mental Disorders, 3rd Edition, Revised. Washington, DC, American Psychiatric Association, 1987

American Psychiatric Association: Diagnostic and Statistical Manual of Mental Disorders, 4th Edition, Text Revision. Washington, DC, American Psychiatric Association, 2000

Andreoli A, Gressot G, Aapro N, et al: Personality disorders as a predictor of outcome. J Personal Disord 3:307–321, 1989

Beck AT, Freeman A, Davis DD, et al: Cognitive Therapy of Personality Disorders, 2nd Edition. New York, Guilford, 2003

Bender DS, Skodol AE: Borderline personality as a self-other representational disturbance. J Personal Disord 21:500–517, 2007

Benjamin LS: Interpersonal Diagnosis and Treatment of Personality Disorders, 2nd Edition. New York, Guilford, 1996

Bernstein DP, Cohen P, Skodol AE, et al: Childhood antecedents of adolescent personality disorders. Am J Psychiatry 153:907–913, 1996

Blashfield RK, Herkov MJ: Investigating clinician adherence to diagnosis by criteria: a replication of Morey and Ochoa (1989). J Personal Disord 10:219–228, 1996

Bond MP, Vaillant JS: An empirical study of the relationship between diagnosis and defense style. Arch Gen Psychiatry 43:285–288, 1986

Cantor N, Smith EE, French RS, et al: Psychiatric diagnosis as prototype categorization. J Abnorm Psychol 89:181–193, 1980

Carver CS, Scheier MF, Weintraub JK: Assessing coping strategies: a theoretically based approach. J Pers Soc Psychol 56:267–283, 1989

Casey PR, Tyrer P: Personality disorder and psychiatric illness in general practice. Br J Psychiatry 156:261–265, 1990

Clark LA, Livesley WJ, Morey L: Special feature: personality disorder assessment: the challenge of construct validity. J Personal Disord 11:205–231, 1997

Compton WM, Thomas YF, Stinson FS, et al: Prevalence, correlates, disability, and comorbidity of DSM-IV drug abuse and dependence in the United States: results from the National Epidemiologic Survey on Alcohol and Related Conditions. Arch Gen Psychiatry 64:566–576, 2007

Crawford TN, Cohen P, First MB, et al: Comorbid Axis I and Axis II disorders in early adolescence: outcomes 20 years later. Arch Gen Psychiatry 65:641–648, 2008

Dolan-Sewell RT, Krueger RF, Shea MT: Co-occurrence with syndrome disorders, in Handbook of Personality Disorders: Theory, Research, and Treatment. Edited by Livesley WJ. New York, Guilford, 2001, pp 84–104

Drake RE, Vaillant GE: A validity study of Axis II of DSM-III. Am J Psychiatry 142:553–558, 1985

Feinstein AR: The pre-therapeutic classification of comorbidity in chronic disease. J Chronic Dis 23:455–468, 1970

First M, Gibbon M, Spitzer RL, et al: User's Guide for the Structured Clinical Interview for DSM-IV Axis II Personality Disorders. Washington, DC, American Psychiatric Press, 1997

Folkman S, Lazarus RS: The Ways of Coping Questionnaire. Palo Alto, CA, Consulting Psychologists Press, 1988

Folkman S, Moskowitz JT: Coping: pitfalls and promise. Ann Rev Psychol 55:745–774, 2004

Frances A: Categorical and dimensional systems of personality diagnosis: a comparison. Compr Psychiatry 23:516–527, 1982

Grant BF, Stinson FS, Dawson DA, et al: Co-occurrence of 12-month alcohol and drug use disorders and personality disorders in the United States: results from the National Epidemiologic Survey on Alcohol and Related Conditions. Arch Gen Psychiatry 61:361–368, 2004

Grilo CM, Sanislow CA, Gunderson JG, et al: Two-year stability and change of schizotypal, borderline, avoidant, and obsessive-compulsive personality disorders. J Consult Clin Psychol 72:767–775, 2004

Grilo CM, Sanislow CA, Shea MT: Two-year prospective naturalistic study of remission from major depressive disorder as a function of personality disorder comorbidity. J Consult Clin Psychol 73:78–85, 2005

Gunderson JG: Disturbed relationships as a phenotype for borderline personality disorder. Am J Psychiatry 164:1637–1640, 2007

Hart AB, Craighead WE, Craighead LW: Predicting recurrence of major depressive disorder in young adults: a prospective study. J Abnorm Psychol 110:633–643, 2001

Hasin DS, Stinson FS, Ogburn E, et al: Prevalence, correlates, disability, and comorbidity of DSM-IV alcohol abuse and dependence in the United States: results from the National Epidemiologic Survey on Alcohol and Related Conditions. Arch Gen Psychiatry 64:830–842, 2007

Herbert JD, Hope DA, Bellack AS: Validity of the distinction between generalized social phobia and avoidant personality disorder. J Abnorm Psychol 101:332–339, 1992

Herkov MJ, Blashfield RK: Clinicians' diagnoses of personality disorder: evidence of a hierarchical structure. J Pers Assess 65:313–321, 1995

Hill J, Pilkonis P, Morse J, et al. Social domain dysfunction and disorganization in borderline personality disorder. Psychol Med 38:135–146, 2008

Hyler SE: Personality Diagnostic Questionnaire—4 (PDQ-4). New York, New York State Psychiatric Institute, 1994

Hyler SE, Skodol AE, Kellman D, et al: Validity of the Personality Diagnostic Questionnaire: comparison with two structured interviews. Am J Psychiatry 147:1043–1048, 1990

Hyler SE, Skodol AE, Oldham JM, et al: Validity of the Personality Diagnostic Questionnaire–Revised (PDQ-R): a replication in an outpatient sample. Compr Psychiatry 33:73–77, 1992

Jackson HJ, Burgess PM: Personality disorders in the community: results from the Australian National Survey of Mental Health and Well-Being, part II. Relationships between personality disorder, Axis I mental disorders, and physical conditions with disability and health consultations. Soc Psychiatry Psychiatr Epidemiol 37:251–260, 2002

Johnson JG, Cohen P, Skodol AE, et al: Personality disorders in adolescence and risk of major mental disorders and suicidality during adulthood. Arch Gen Psychiatry 56:805–811, 1999

Johnson JG, Cohen P, Kasen S, et al: Age-related change in personality disorder trait levels between early adolescence and adulthood: a community-based longitudinal investigation. Acta Psychiatr Scand 102:265–275, 2000

Karasu TB, Skodol AE: Fourth axis for DSM-III: psychodynamic evaluation. Am J Psychiatry 137:607–610, 1980

Kasen S, Cohen P, Skodol AE, et al: Influence of child and adolescent psychiatric disorders on young adult personality disorder. Am J Psychiatry 156:1529–1535, 1999

Kasen S, Cohen P, Skodol AE, et al: Childhood depression and adult personality disorder: alternative pathways of continuity. Arch Gen Psychiatry 58:231–236, 2001

Kass F, Skodol AE, Charles E, et al: Scaled ratings of DSM-III personality disorders. Am J Psychiatry 142:627–630, 1985

Kessler RC, Crum RM, Warner LA, et al: Lifetime co-occurrence of DSM-III-R alcohol abuse and dependence with other psychiatric disorders in the National Comorbidity Survey. Arch Gen Psychiatry 54:313–321, 1997

Kiesler DJ: Contemporary Interpersonal Theory and Research: Personality, Psychopathology, and Psychotherapy. New York, Wiley, 1996

Klein DN: Patients' versus informants' reports of personality disorders in predicting 7½-year outcome in outpatients with depressive disorders. Psychol Assess 15: 216–222, 2003

Klonsky ED, Oltmanns TF, Turkheimer E: Informant-reports of personality disorder: relation to self-reports and future directions. Clin Psychol Sci Pract 9:300–311, 2002

Kobak KA, Skodol AE, Bender DS: Diagnostic measures for adults, in Handbook of Psychiatric Measures, 2nd Edition. Edited by Rush AJ, First MB, Blacker D. Washington, DC, American Psychiatric Publishing, 2008, pp 35–60

Krueger RF, Caspi A, Moffitt TE, et al: The structure and stability of common mental disorders (DSM-III-R): a longitudinal-epidemiological study. J Abnorm Psychol 106:216–227, 1998

Krueger RF, Hicks BM, Patrick CJ, et al: Etiologic connections among substance dependence, antisocial behavior, and personality: modeling the externalizing spectrum. J Abnorm Psychol 111:411–424, 2002

Krueger RF, Markon KE, Patrick CJ, et al: Linking antisocial behavior, substance use, and personality: an integrative quantitative model of the adult externalizing spectrum. J Abnorm Psychol 116:645–666, 2007

Lazarus RS, Folkman S: Stress, Appraisal, and Coping. New York, Springer, 1984

Lenzenweger MF: Stability and change in personality disorder features: the Longitudinal Study of Personality Disorders. Arch Gen Psychiatry 56:1009–1015, 1999

Lewinsohn PM, Rohde P, Seeley JR, et al: Axis II psychopathology as a function of Axis I disorder in childhood and adolescents. J Am Acad Child Adolesc Psychiatry 36:1752–1759, 1997

Lilienfeld SO, Waldman ID, Israel AC: A critical examination of the use of the term "comorbidity" in psychopathology research. Clin Psychol Sci Pract 1:71–83, 1994

Livesley WJ: Trait and behavioral prototypes of personality disorder. Am J Psychiatry 143:728–732, 1986

Loranger AW: International Personality Disorder Examination (IPDE). Odessa, FL, Psychological Assessment Resources, 1999

Lyons MJ, Tyrer P, Gunderson J, et al: Special feature: heuristic models of comorbidity of Axis I and Axis II disorders. J Personal Disord 11:260–269, 1997

McDermut W, Zimmerman M: Personality disorders, personality traits, and defense mechanisms, in Handbook of Psychiatric Measures, 2nd Edition. Edited by Rush AJ, First MB, Blacker D. American Psychiatric Publishing, 2008, pp 687–729

McGlashan TH, Grilo CM, Skodol AE, et al: The Collaborative Longitudinal Personality Disorders Study: Axis I/II and II/II diagnostic co-occurrence. Acta Psychiatr Scand 102:256–264, 2000

McGlashan TH, Grilo CM, Sanislow CA, et al: Two-year prevalence and stability of individual DSM-IV criteria for schizotypal, borderline, avoidant and obsessive-compulsive personality disorders: toward a hybrid model of Axis II disorders. Am J Psychiatry 162:883–889, 2005

Millon T, Millon C, Davis R: MCMI-III Manual, 2nd Edition. Minneapolis, MN, National Computer Systems, 1997

Moos RH: Coping Responses Inventory. Odessa, FL, Psychological Assessment Resources, 1993

Morey LC, Ochoa ES: An investigation of adherence to diagnostic criteria. J Personal Disord 3:180–192, 1989

Morey LC, Alexander GM, Boggs C: Gender, in American Psychiatric Publishing Textbook of Personality Disorders. Edited by Oldham JM, Skodol AE, Bender DS. Washington, DC, American Psychiatric Publishing, 2005, pp 541–559

Morgenstern J, Langenbucher J, Labouvie E, et al: The comorbidity of alcoholism and personality disorders in a clinical population: prevalence rates and relation to alcohol typology variables. J Abnorm Psychol 106:74–84, 1997

Noyes R Jr, Reich J, Christiansen J, et al: Outcome of panic disorder: relationship to diagnostic subtypes and comorbidity. Arch Gen Psychiatry 47:809–818, 1990

Oldham JM, Skodol AE: Charting the future of Axis II. J Personal Disord 14:17–29, 2000

Oldham JM, Skodol AE, Kellman HD, et al: Diagnosis of DSM-III-R personality disorders by two structured interviews: patterns of comorbidity. Am J Psychiatry 149:213–220, 1992

Oldham JM, Skodol AE, Kellman HD, et al: Comorbidity of Axis I and Axis II disorders. Am J Psychiatry 152:571–578, 1995

Pearlin LI, Schooler C: The structure of coping. J Health Soc Behav 19:2–21, 1978

Perry JC, Bond M: Defensive functioning, in American Psychiatric Publishing Textbook of Personality Disorders. Edited by Oldham JM, Skodol AE, Bender DS. Washington, DC, American Psychiatric Publishing, 2005, pp 523–540

Perry JC, Cooper SH: An empirical study of defense mechanisms, I: clinical interview and life vignette ratings. Arch Gen Psychiatry 46:444–452, 1989

Pfohl B, Stangl D, Zimmerman M: The implications of DSM-III personality disorders with major depression. J Affect Disord 7:309–318, 1984

Pfohl B, Blum N, Zimmerman M: Structured Interview for DSM-IV Personality. Washington, DC, American Psychiatric Press, 1997

Pope HG Jr, Jonas JM, Hudson JI, et al: The validity of DSM-III borderline personality disorder:

a phenomenologic, family history, treatment response, and long-term follow-up study. Arch Gen Psychiatry 40:23–30, 1983

Reich J, Vasile RG: Effect of personality disorders on the treatment outcome of Axis I conditions: an update. J Nerv Ment Dis 181:475–484, 1993

Reich J, Yates W, Nduaguba M: Prevalence of DSM-III personality disorders in the community. Soc Psychiatry Psychiatr Epidemiol 24:12–16, 1989

Rey JM, Morris-Yates A, Singh M, et al: Continuities between psychiatric disorders in adolescents and personality disorders in young adults. Am J Psychiatry 152:895–900, 1995

Roberts BW, Caspi A, Moffitt TE: Work experiences and personality development in young adulthood. J Pers Soc Psychol 84:582–593, 2003

Sanislow CA, Morey LC, Grilo CM, et al: Confirmatory factor analysis of DSM-IV borderline, schizotypal, avoidant, and obsessive-compulsive personality disorders: findings from the Collaborative Longitudinal Personality Study. Acta Psychiatr Scand 105:28–36, 2002

Seivewright H, Tyrer P, Johnson T: Persistent social dysfunction in anxious and depressed patients with personality disorder. Acta Psychiatr Scand 109:104–109, 2004

Shea MT: Assessment of change in personality disorders, in Measuring Changes in Mood, Anxiety, and Personality Disorders: Toward a Core Battery. Edited by Strupp HH, Horowitz LM, Lambert MJ. Washington, DC, American Psychological Association, 1997, pp 389–400

Shea MT, Pilkonis PA, Beckham E, et al: Personality disorder and treatment outcome in the NIMH Treatment of Depression Collaborative Research Program. Am J Psychiatry 147:711–718, 1990

Shea MT, Widiger TA, Klein MH: Comorbidity of personality disorders and depression: implications for treatment. J Consult Clin Psychol 60:857–868, 1992

Shedler J, Westen D: Refining personality disorder diagnosis: integrating science and practice. Am J Psychiatry 161:1350–1365, 2004

Siever LJ, Davis KL: A psychobiological perspective on the personality disorders. Am J Psychiatry 148:1647–1658, 1991

Skodol AE: Problems in Differential Diagnosis: From DSM-III to DSM-III-R in Clinical Practice. Washington, DC, American Psychiatric Press, 1989

Skodol AE, Gunderson JG: Personality disorders, in The American Psychiatric Publishing Textbook of Psychiatry, 5th Edition. Edited by Hales RE, Yudofsky SC, Gabbard GO. Washington, DC, American Psychiatric Punblishing, 2008, pp 829–851

Skodol AE, Williams JBW, Spitzer RL, et al: Identifying common errors in the use of DSM-III through diagnostic supervision. Hosp Community Psychiatry 35:251–255, 1984

Skodol AE, Rosnick L, Kellman D, et al: Validating structured DSM-III-R personality disorder assessments with longitudinal data. Am J Psychiatry 145:1297–1299, 1988

Skodol AE, Oldham JM, Rosnick L, et al: Diagnosis of DSM-III-R personality disorders: a comparison of two structured interviews. Int J Methods Psychiatr Res 1:13–26, 1991

Skodol AE, Oldham JM, Hyler SE, et al: Comorbidity of DSM-III-R eating disorders and personality disorders. Int J Eating Disorders 14:403–416, 1993

Skodol AE, Oldham JM, Hyler SE, et al: Patterns of anxiety and personality disorder comorbidity. J Psychiatr Res 29:361–374, 1995

Skodol AE, Gallaher PE, Oldham JM: Excessive dependency and depression: is the relationship specific? J Nerv Ment Dis 184:165–171, 1996

Skodol AE, Oldham JM, Gallaher PE: Axis II comorbidity of substance use disorders among patients referred for treatment of personality disorders. Am J Psychiatry 156:733–738, 1999

Skodol AE, Gunderson JG, McGlashan TH, et al: Functional impairment in patients with schizotypal, borderline, avoidant, or obsessive-compulsive personality disorder. Am J Psychiatry 159:276–283, 2002

Skodol AE, Pagano MP, Bender DS, et al: Stability of functional impairment in patients with schizotypal, borderline, avoidant, or obsessive-compulsive personality disorder over two years. Psychol Med 35:443–451, 2005

Soloff PH, Ulrich RF: Diagnostic interview for borderline patients: a replication study. Arch Gen Psychiatry 38:686–692, 1981

Somwaru DP, Ben-Porath YS: Development and reliability of MMPI-2 based personality disorder scales. Paper presented at the 30th annual Workshop and Symposium on Recent Developments in the Use of the MMPI-2 and MMPI-A, St. Petersburg, FL, April, 1995

Stone AA, Schwartz JE, Neale JM, et al: A comparison of coping assessed by ecological momentary assessment and retrospective recall. J Pers Soc Psychol 74:1670–1680, 1998

Torgersen S: Genetic and nosological aspects of schizotypal and borderline personality disorders: a twin study. Arch Gen Psychiatry 41:546–554, 1984

Turner SM, Beidel DC, Borden JW, et al: Social phobia: Axis I and II correlates. J Abnorm Psychol 100:102–106, 1991

Tyrer P, Gunderson J, Lyons MJ, et al: Special feature: extent of comorbidity between mental state and personality disorders. J Personal Disord 11:242–259, 1997

Vaillant GE, Bond M, Vaillant CO: An empirically validated hierarchy of defense mechanisms. Arch Gen Psychiatry 43:786–794, 1986

Verheul R, Widiger TA: A meta-analysis of the prevalence and usage of personality disorder not otherwise specified (PDNOS). J Personal Disord 18:309–319, 2004

Westen D: Divergences between clinical and research methods for assessing personality disorders: implications for research and the evolution of Axis II. Am J Psychiatry 154:895–903, 1997

Westen DS, Shedler J, Bradley R: A prototype approach to personality disorder diagnosis. Am J Psychiatry 163:846–856, 2006

Widiger TA: Personality disorder dimensional models proposed for DSM-V. J Personal Disord 5:386–398, 1991

Widiger TA: The DSM-III-R categorical personality disorder diagnoses: a critique and an alternative. Psychol Inq 4:75–90, 1993

Widiger TA: Sex biases in the diagnosis of personality disorders. J Personal Disord 12:95–118, 1998

Widiger TA: Personality disorders, in Handbook of Assessment and Treatment Planning for Psychological Disorders. Edited by Antony MM, Barlow DH. New York, Guilford, 2002, pp 453–480

Widiger TA, Coker LA: Assessing personality disorders, in Clinical Personality Assessment: Practical Approaches, 2nd Edition. Edited by Butcher JN. New York, Oxford University Press, 2002, pp 407–434

Widiger TA, Sanderson CJ: Assessing personality disorders, in Clinical Personality Assessment: Practical Approaches. Edited by Butcher JN. New York, Oxford University Press, 1995, pp 380–394

Widiger TA, Trull TJ, Hurt SW, et al: A multidimensional scaling of the DSM-III personality disorders. Arch Gen Psychiatry 44:557–563, 1987

Widiger TA, Mangine S, Corbitt EM, et al: Personality Disorder Interview–IV: A Semistructured Interview for the Assessment of Personality

Disorders. Odessa, FL, Psychological Assessment Resources, 1995

Young J, Klosko J: Schema therapy, in American Psychiatric Publishing Textbook of Personality Disorders. Edited by Oldham JM, Skodol AE, Bender DS. Washington, DC, American Psychiatric Publishing, 2005, pp 289–306

Zanarini MC, Gunderson JG, Frankenburg FR: Axis I phenomenology of borderline personality disorder. Compr Psychiatry 30:149–156, 1989

Zanarini MC, Frankenburg FR, Sickel AE, et al: Diagnostic Interview for DSM-IV Personality Disorders. Belmont, MA, McLean Hospital, 1996

Zanarini MC, Frankenburg FR, Dubo ED, et al: Axis I comorbidity of borderline personality disorder. Am J Psychiatry 155:1733–1739, 1998

Zanarini MC, Frankenburg FR, Hennen J, et al: Prediction of the 10-year course of borderline personality disorder. Am J Psychiatry 163:827–832, 2006

Zanarini MC, Frankenburg FR, Reich DB, et al: The subsyndromal phenomenology of borderline personality disorder: a 10-year follow-up study. Am J Psychiatry 164:929–935, 2007

Zimmerman M: Diagnosing personality disorders: a review of issues and research methods. Arch Gen Psychiatry 51:225–245, 1994

Zimmerman M, Coryell W: DSM-III personality disorder diagnoses in a nonpatient sample: demographic correlates and comorbidity. Arch Gen Psychiatry 46:682–689, 1989

Zimmerman M, Mattia JI: Differences between clinical and research practices in diagnosing borderline personality disorder. Am J Psychiatry 156:1570–1574, 1999

Zimmerman M, Pfohl B, Stangl D, et al: Assessment of DSM-III personality disorders: the importance of interviewing an informant. J Clin Psychiatry 47:261–263, 1986

Zimmerman M, Pfohl B, Coryell W, et al: Diagnosing personality disorder in depressed patients: a comparison of patient and informant interviews. Arch Gen Psychiatry 45:733–737, 1988

Zoccolillo M, Pickles A, Quinton D, et al: The outcome of conduct disorder: implications for defining adult personality disorder and conduct disorder. Psychol Med 22:971–986, 1992

4

Course and Outcome

Carlos M. Grilo, Ph.D.
Thomas H. McGlashan, M.D.

The diagnostic construct of personality disorder has evolved considerably over the past few decades (see Skodol 1997 for a detailed ontogeny of the DSM system; and see Chapter 1, "Personality Disorders: Recent History and the DSM System," for a historical overview). Substantial changes have occurred in both the number and types of specific personality disorder diagnoses over time, as well as in the "admixture of criteria" (Sanislow and Mc-Glashan 1998) representing possible manifestations of personality disorders (e.g., DSM-IV-TR [American Psychiatric Association 2000] specifies that the "enduring pattern" can be manifested by problems in at least two of the following areas: cognition, affectivity, interpersonal functioning, or impulse control). One central tenet—that a personality disorder reflects a persistent, pervasive, enduring, and stable pattern—has not changed. The concept of stability is salient in both major classifica-

tion systems, DSM-IV-TR and ICD-10 (World Health Organization 1992), although the two systems differ somewhat in their classification and definitions for personality disorders and thus demonstrate only moderate convergence for some diagnoses (Ottosson et al. 2002). The extent of stability of personality disorders remains uncertain (Shea and Yen 2003; Tyrer and Simonsen 2003). This chapter provides an overview of the course and outcome of personality disorders and synthesizes the empirical literature on the stability of personality disorders.

STABILITY AS THE CENTRAL TENET OF PERSONALITY DISORDERS

The concept of stability has remained a central tenet of personality disorders throughout the various editions of DSM, dating back to the first edition (American Psychiatric Association 1952). In what some experts have referred to as a "bold step" (Tyrer and Simonsen 2003), personality disorders were placed on a separate axis (Axis II) of the multiaxial DSM-III (American Psychiatric Association 1980). DSM-III stated that the separation to Axis II was intended, in part, to encourage clinicians to assess "the possible presence of disorders that are frequently overlooked when attention is directed to the usually more florid Axis I disorder." Conceptually, this separation reflected the putative stability of personality disorders relative to the episodically unstable course of Axis I psychiatric disorders (Grilo et al. 1998; Skodol 1997).

FIRST- AND SECOND-GENERATION RESEARCH STUDIES ON STABILITY

First, we provide a brief review of the empirical literature through the end of the twentieth century. This period can be thought of as including the first generation (mostly clinical-descriptive accounts) and the second generation (the emerging findings based on attempts at greater standardization of diagnoses and assessment methods) of research efforts on personality disorders. Second, we provide a brief overview of methodological problems and conceptual gaps that characterize this literature and that must be considered when interpreting ongoing research and designing future studies. Third, we summarize emerging findings from ongoing longitudinal studies that have shed light on a number of key issues about the course of personality disorders.

OVERVIEW OF THE LITERATURE THROUGH 1999

A number of previous reviews have been published addressing aspects of the course and outcome of personality disorders (Grilo and McGlashan 1999; Grilo et al. 1998; Mc-

David and Pilkonis 1996; Perry 1993; Ruegg and Frances 1995; Stone 1993; Zimmerman 1994). These reviews, although varied, have agreed on the pervasiveness of methodological problems that characterize much of the literature and thereby preclude any firm conclusions regarding the nature of the stability of personality disorders. The reviews, however, have also generally agreed that available research raises questions regarding many aspects of the construct validity of personality disorders (Zimmerman 1994), including their hypothesized high degree of stability (Grilo and McGlashan 1999).

The few early (pre-DSM-III era) studies of the course of personality disorders reported findings that borderline (Carpenter and Gunderson 1977; Grinker et al. 1968) and antisocial (Maddocks 1970; Robbins et al. 1977) personality disorders were highly stable. Carpenter and Gunderson (1977), for example, reported that the impairment in functioning observed for borderline personality disorder (BPD) was comparable with that observed for patients with schizophrenia over a 5-year period. As previously noted (Grilo et al. 1998), the dominant clinical approach to assessing personality disorder diagnoses based partly on treatment refractoriness naturally raises the question of whether these findings simply reflect a tautology.

The separation of personality disorders to Axis II in DSM-III contributed to increased research attention to these clinical problems (Blashfield and McElroy 1987). The development and utilization of a number of structured and standardized approaches to clinical interviewing and diagnosis during the 1980s represented notable advances (Zimmerman 1994). The greater attention paid to defining the criteria required for diagnosis in the classification systems and by researchers during the development of standardized interviews greatly facilitated research efforts in this field.

In our previous reviews of the DSM-III and DSM-III-R (American Psychiatric Association 1987) studies, we concluded that the available research suggested that "personality disorders demonstrate only moderate stability and that, although personality disorders are generally associated with negative outcomes, they can improve over time and can benefit from specific treatments" (Grilo and McGlashan 1999, p. 157). In our 1998 review (Grilo et al. 1998), we noted that the 20 selected studies of DSM-III-R criteria generally found low to moderate stability of any personality disorder over relatively short follow-up periods (6 to 24 months). For example, the major studies that employed diagnostic interviews reported kappa coefficients for the presence of any personality disorder of 0.32 (Johnson et al. 1997), 0.40 (Ferro et al. 1998), 0.50 (Loranger et al. 1994), and 0.55 (Loranger et al. 1991). Especially noteworthy is that the stability coefficients for specific personality disorder diagnoses (in the few cases in which they could be calculated given the sample sizes) were generally lower. In addition, follow-up studies of adolescents diagnosed with personality disorders also reported modest stability; for example, Mattanah et al. (1995) reported a 50% rate of stability for any personality disorder at 2-year follow-up. More recently, Grilo et al. (2001) also found modest stability in dimensional personality disorder scores in this adolescent follow-up study. Squires-Wheeler et al. (1992), as part of the New York State high-risk offspring study, reported low stability for schizotypal personality disorder and features, although the stability was higher for the offspring of patients with schizophrenia than for those with mood disorders or control subjects.

Subsequently, we (Grilo and McGlashan 1999) reviewed nine reports of longitudinal findings for personality disorder diagnoses published in 1997 and 1998. In terms of specific diagnoses, the studies generally reported moderate stability (kappa approximately 0.5) for BPD and antisocial personality disorder (ASPD). These reports, like most of the previous literature, had small sample sizes and infrequently followed more than one personality disorder.

CONCEPTUAL AND METHODOLOGICAL QUESTIONS ABOUT COURSE

Previous reviews of personality disorders have raised many methodological problems. Common limitations highlighted include small sample sizes; concerns about nonstandardized assessments, interrater reliability, blindness to baseline characteristics, and narrow assessments; failure to consider alternative (e.g., dimensional) models of personality disorder; reliance on only two assessments typically over short follow-up periods; insufficient attention to the nature and effects of co-occurring Axis I and Axis II diagnoses; and inattention to treatment effects. Diagnoses other than ASPD and BPD have received little attention. Particularly striking is the absence of "relevant" comparison or control groups in the longitudinal literature. We comment briefly on a few of these issues.

Reliability

Reliability of assessments represents a central issue for any study of course and outcome. The creation of standardized instruments for collecting data was a major development of the 1980s (Loranger et al. 1991; Zimmerman 1994). Such instruments, however, were less-than-perfect assessment methods and have been criticized for a variety of reasons (Westen 1997; Westen and Shedler 1999). It is critical to keep in mind that interrater reliability and test–retest reliability represent the limits (or ceiling) for estimating the stability of a construct.

Previous reviews (Grilo and McGlashan 1999; Zanarini et al. 2000; Zimmerman 1994) of reliabilities for Axis II diagnostic interviews have generally reported median interrater reliabilities of roughly 0.70 and short-interval, test–retest reliabilities of 0.50 for diagnoses. These reliabilities compare favorably with those generally reported for diagnostic instruments for Axis I psychiatric disorders. Both interrater and test–retest reliability coefficients tend to be higher for dimensional scores than for categorical diagnoses of personality disorders. Another finding of note is that even when experts administer diagnostic interviews, the degree of convergence or agreement produced by two different interviews administered only 1 week apart is limited (Oldham et al. 1992).

Reliability and "Change"

Test–retest reliability is also relevant for addressing, in part, the well-known problem of "regression to the mean" in repeated measures studies (Nesselroade et al. 1980). It has been argued that the multiwave or repeated measures approach lessens the effects of regression to the mean (Lenzenweger 1999). This argument may be true in terms of the obvious decreases in severity with time (i.e., very symptomatic participants meeting eligibility at study entry are likely to show some improvement because, by definition, they are already reporting high levels of symptoms). However, other effects need to be considered whenever assessments are repeated within a study. As cogently noted by Shea and Yen (2003), repeated measures studies of both Axis II (Loranger et al. 1991) and Axis I (Robins 1985) disorders have found hints that participants systematically report or endorse fewer problems during repeated interviews to reduce interview time. For example, Loranger et al. (1991), in his test–retest study of the Personality Disorder Examination interview (Loranger 1988) conducted between 1 and 26 weeks after baseline, documented significant decreases in personality disorder criteria for all but two of the DSM-III-R diagnoses. Recall that the Personality Disorder Examination, which requires skilled and trained research clinicians, has a required minimum duration stipulation of 5 years for determining persistence and pervasiveness of the criteria being assessed. Thus, the magnitude of changes observed during such a short period of time, which was shown to be unrelated to "state-trait effects," reflects some combination of the following: regression to the mean, error in either or both the baseline and repeated assessments, and overreporting by patients at hospital admission and underreporting during retest at discharge (Loranger et al. 1991; Shea and Yen 2003). These phenomena were discussed further by Gunderson et al. (2000).

Categorical Versus Dimensional Approaches

Long-standing debate regarding the conceptual and empirical advantages to dimensional models of personality disorders (Frances 1982; Livesley et al. 1992; Loranger et al. 1994; Widiger 1992) has accompanied the DSM categorical classification system. Overall, longitudinal studies of personality disorder have reported moderate levels of stability for dimensional scores for most personality disorders, with the stability coefficients tending to be higher than for categorical or diagnostic stability (Ferro et al. 1998; Johnson et al. 1997; Klein and Shih 1998; Loranger et al. 1991, 1994).

Comorbidity

Most studies have ascertained participants who meet criteria for multiple Axis I and Axis II diagnoses. This problem of diagnostic overlap, or comorbidity, represents a well-known, long-standing major challenge (Berkson 1946) in working with clinical samples. One expert and critic of DSM (Tyrer 2001), in speaking of the "spectre of comorbidity," noted that "the main reason for abandoning the present classification is summed up in one word, comorbidity. Comorbidity is the nosologist's nightmare; it shouts, 'you have failed'" (p. 82). We suggest, however, that such clinical realities (multiple presenting problems that are especially characteristic of treatment-seeking patients) represent not only potential confounds but also potential opportunities to understand personality and dysfunctions of personality better. Comorbidity begs the question: what are the fundamental personality dimensions and disorders of personality, and how do their courses influence (and conversely, how are their courses affected by) the presence and course of Axis I psychiatric disorders?

Continuity

A related issue pertaining to course concerns "longitudinal comorbidities" (Kendell and Clarkin 1992) or "continuities." An obvious example is that conduct disorder during adolescence is required for the diagnosis of ASPD to be given to adults. This definitional isomorphism is one likely reason for the consistently strong associations between conduct disorder and later ASPD in the literature. This association is, however, more than an artifactual relationship, because longitudinal research has clearly documented that children and adolescents with behavior disorders have substantially elevated risk for antisocial behavior during adulthood (Robins 1966). More generally, studies with diverse recruitment and ascertainment methods reported that disruptive behavior disorders during the adolescent years prospectively predicted personality disorders during young adulthood (Bernstein et al. 1996; Lewinsohn et al. 1997; Myers et al. 1998; Rey et al. 1995). The Yale Psychiatric Institute follow-up study found that personality disorder diagnoses in adolescent inpatients prospectively predicted greater drug use problems but not global functioning (Levy et al. 1999).

The importance of considering comorbidity is underscored in the findings of the longitudinal study by Lewinsohn et al. (1997). They found that the apparent longitudinal continuity noted for disruptive behavioral disorders during adolescence and subsequent ASPD in adulthood was accounted for, in part, by Axis I psychiatric comorbidity. A longitudinal study of young adult men found that personality disorders predicted the subsequent onset of psychiatric disorders during a 2-year follow-up, even after controlling for previous psychiatric history (Johnson et al. 1997).

Comorbidity and Continuity Models

A variation of the comorbidity concept is that certain disorders may be associated with one another in a number of possible ways over time. A variety of models have been proposed for the possible relationships between Axis II and Axis I disorders (Dolan-Sewell et al. 2001; Lyons et al. 1997; Tyrer et al. 1997). These include, for example, the predisposition or vulnerability model, the complication or scar model, the pathoplasty or exacerbation model, and various spectrum models. We emphasize that these models do not necessarily assume categorical entities. Indeed, an especially influential spectrum model proposed by Siever and Davis (1991) posits four psychobiological dimensions to account for Axis II and Axis I psychopathology. The Cloninger et al. (1993) psychobiological model of temperament and character represents another valuable approach that considers dimensions across personality and psychopathology. More broadly, Krueger noted that although most research has focused on pairs of constructs (i.e., Axis II and Axis I associations) (Krueger 1999; Krueger and Tackett 2003), it seems important to examine the "multivariate structure of the personality-psychopathology domain" (Krueger and Tackett 2003, p. 109).

Age (Early Onset)

A related point, stressed by Widiger (2003), is that personality disorders need to be more clearly conceptualized and carefully characterized as having an early onset. However, the validity of personality disorders in adolescents remains controversial (Krueger and Carlson 2001). It can be argued, for example, that determining early onset of personality disorders is impossible because adolescence is a period of profound changes and flux in personality and identity. A critical review of the longitudinal literature on personality traits throughout the life span revealed that personality traits are less stable during childhood and adolescence than they are throughout adulthood (Roberts and DelVecchio 2000). Roberts and DelVecchio's (2000) meta-analysis of data from 152 longitudinal studies of personality traits revealed that rank-order consistency for personality traits increased steadily throughout the life span; test–retest correlations (over 6.7-year time intervals) increased from 0.31 (during childhood) to 0.54 (during college), to 0.64 (age 30 years), to a high of 0.74 (ages 50–70 years).

Nonetheless, if childhood precursors of personality disorders could be identified (as in the case of conduct disorder for ASPD), they could become part of the diagnostic criteria and thus create some degree of longitudinal continuity in the diagnostic system. Myers et al. (1998), for example, found that early onset (before 10 years of age) of conduct disorder problems predicted subsequent ASPD. More generally, temperamental vulnerabilities or precursors to personality disorders have been posited as central in a variety of models of personality disorders (Cloninger et al. 1993; Siever and Davis 1991). Specific temperamental features evident in childhood have been noted to be precursors for diverse personality disorders (Paris 2003; Rettew et al. 2003; Wolff et al. 1991) as well as for differences in interpersonal functioning (Newman et al. 1997) in adulthood. For example, studies have noted early odd and withdrawn patterns for schizotypal personality disorder in adults (Wolff et al. 1991) and shyness for avoidant personality disorder (Rettew et al. 2003). Speaking more generally, although the degree of stability for personality traits is higher throughout adulthood than throughout childhood and adolescence (Roberts and DelVecchio 2000), longitudinal analyses of personality data have revealed that the transition from adolescence to adulthood is characterized by greater personality continuity than change (Roberts et al. 2001).

Age and the Aging Process

Another age issue concerns the aging process itself. Considerable research suggests that personality remains relatively stable thorough adulthood (Heatherton and Weinberger 1994; Roberts and DelVecchio 2000) and is highly stable after age 50 (Roberts and DelVecchio 2000). Little is known, however, about personality disorders in older persons (Abrams et al. 1998). The 12-year follow-up of personality disorders that was part of the Nottingham Study of Neurotic Disorder (Seivewright et al. 2002) documented substantial changes in personality disorder trait scores based on blind administration of a semistructured interview. Seivewright et al. (2002) reported that Cluster B personality disorder diagnoses (ASPD, histrionic) showed significant improvements, whereas Cluster A and Cluster C diagnoses appeared to worsen with age. Although the Seivewright et al. (2002) findings are limited somewhat by the two-point cross-sectional assessment (little is known about the intervening period), Tyrer et al. (1983) previously reported good reliability (weighted kappa of 0.64) for this diagnostic interview over a 3-year test–retest period. These findings echo somewhat the results of the seminal Chestnut Lodge follow-up studies (McGlashan 1986a, 1986b) that suggested distinctions between BPD and schizotypal personality disorders, decreases in impulsivity and interpersonal instability with age, and increased avoidance with age. There are other reports of diminished impulsivity with increasing age in BPD (Paris and Zweig-Frank 2001; Stevenson et al. 2003), although this type of reduction was not observed in a recent prospective analysis of individual BPD criteria (McGlashan et al. 2005).

The reader is referred to Judd and McGlashan (2003) for detailed accounts of four specific cases that elucidate the course and outcome of BPD. These detailed case studies, based on rich clinical material available through the Chestnut Lodge study, demonstrate the considerable heterogeneity in the course of BPD.

Summary and Implications

To resolve these complex issues, complementary research efforts are required, with large samples of both clinical and community populations. It is clear that prospective longitudinal studies with repeated assessments over time are needed to understand the course of personality disorders. Such studies must consider (and cut across) different developmental eras, broad domains of functioning, and multimodal approaches to personality and disorders of personality. These approaches have, in fact, been performed with personality traits (Roberts et al. 2001) and with other forms of psychiatric problems and have yielded invaluable insights. Notable are the contributions of the National Institutes of Health (NIH)–funded multisite efforts on depression (Collaborative Depression Study; Katz et al. 1979) and anxiety (Harvard/Brown Anxiety Research Project; Keller 1991).

REVIEW OF RECENT EMPIRICAL ADVANCES AND UNDERSTANDING OF STABILITY

Of particular relevance for this review are three prospective studies on the longitudinal course of adult personality disorders funded by the NIH during the 1990s. These studies included the Longitudinal Study of Personality Disorders (Lenzenweger 1999), the McLean Study of Adult Development (Zanarini et al. 2003), and the multisite Collaborative Longitudinal Personality Disorders Study (CLPS; Gunderson et al. 2000). The NIH also funded a community-based prospective longitudinal study of personality, psychopathology, and functioning of children/adolescents and their mothers (Children in the Community study; Brook et al. 2002) that began in 1975. These four studies are especially noteworthy in that they, to varying degrees, partly correct for a number of the conceptual and methodological issues noted earlier. These studies utilized multiple and standardized assessment methods, carefully considered training and reliability, and—perhaps most notably—multiwave repeated assessments that are essential for determining longitudinal change. They have employed, to varying degrees, multiple assessment methods and have considered personality and its disorders (personality disorders) as well as Axis I psychiatric disorders. Collectively, these studies have provided valuable insights into the complexities of personality (traits and disorders) and its vicissitudes over time.

Longitudinal Study of Personality Disorders

The Longitudinal Study of Personality Disorders (Lenzenweger 1999; Lenzenweger et al. 1997) assessed 250 participants drawn from Cornell University at three points over a 4-year period. It utilized a semistructured diagnostic interview (International Personality Disorder Examination; Loranger et al. 1994) and a self-report measure (Millon Clinical Multiaxial Inventory—II; Millon 1987) to obtain complementary information on personality. Of the 250 participants, 129 met criteria for at least one personality disorder and 121 did not meet any personality disorder diagnosis. Dimensional scores for the personality disorders were characterized by significant levels of stability on both the interview and self-report measures. Stability coefficients for the total number of personality disorder features ranged from 0.61 to 0.70. Cluster B personality disorders had the highest stability coefficients, and Cluster A personality disorders had the lowest. Personality disorder dimensions showed significant declines over time, and the decline was more rapid for the personality disorder group than for the non–personality disorder group. Axis I psychiatric disorders (diagnosed in 63% of personality disorder subjects and 26% of non–personality disorder subjects) did not significantly influence changes in personality disorder dimensions over time.

The Longitudinal Study of Personality Disorders BPD findings are generally consistent (although the three-point assessment is an important incremental contribution) with those previously reported by Trull et al. (1997, 1998) in a prospective study of BPD features using two different assessment instruments administered to a college student sample assessed twice over a 2-year period.

The Longitudinal Study of Personality Disorders (Lenzenweger 1999), however, is limited by its relatively homogeneous study group of college students, its narrow developmental time frame, and most importantly the insufficient frequency of any personality disorder diagnosis at a categorical (diagnostic) level to allow analysis of a clinical entity. Lenzenweger (1999) noted the need for repeated measures longitudinal data from clinically based personality disorder samples to address the question of the course and stability of dysfunctions of personality.

McLean Study of Adult Development

The McLean Study of Adult Development (Zanarini et al. 2003, 2005) is an ongoing prospective, longitudinal study comparing the course and outcome of hospitalized patients with BPD with those of patients with other personality disorders. It utilizes repeated assessments performed every 2 years (Zanarini et al. 2003) and has reported outcomes through 6 years (Zanarini et al. 2003) and 10 years (Zanarini et al. 2006) of follow-up. Zanarini et al. (2003) assessed personality disorders in 362 inpatients (290 with BPD and 72 with other personality disorders) using two semistructured diagnostic interviews and administered assessments to characterize Axis I psychiatric disorders, psychosocial functioning domains, and treatment utilization. Of the patients diagnosed with BPD, remission was observed for 35% by year 2, 49%

by year 4, and 74% by year 6. Recurrences were rare and were reported for only 6% of those patients who achieved a remission. The authors concluded that "symptomatic improvement is both common and stable, even among the most disturbed borderline patients, and that the symptomatic prognosis for most, but not all, severely ill borderline patients is better than previously recognized" (Zanarini et al. 2003; p. 274). Zanarini et al. (2004) reported that Axis I psychiatric disorders are less common over time in patients with BPD and particularly among those who remit from BPD.

Collaborative Longitudinal Personality Disorders Study

The CLPS (Gunderson et al. 2000; McGlashan et al. 2000; Skodol et al. 2005b) is an ongoing prospective, longitudinal, repeated measures study designed to examine the course and outcome of patients meeting DSM-IV (American Psychiatric Association 1994) criteria for one of four personality disorders: schizotypal, borderline, avoidant, and obsessive-compulsive. The CLPS includes a comparison group of patients with major depressive disorder (MDD) without any personality disorder. This comparison group was selected because of its episodic and fluctuating course (thought to distinguish Axis I from Axis II) and because MDD has been carefully studied in similar longitudinal designs (e.g., Collaborative Depression Study; [Katz et al. 1979; Solomon et al. 1997]). The CLPS has employed multimodal assessments (Gunderson et al. 2000; Zanarini et al. 2000) to prospectively follow and capture different aspects of the fluctuating nature of personality disorders and dimensions (both interviewer-based and self-report representing different conceptual models) (Morey et al. 2007), Axis I psychiatric disorders and symptoms (Grilo et al. 2005, 2007), various domains of psychosocial functioning (Markowitz et al. 2007; Skodol et al. 2005a, 2005d), and treatment utilization (Bender et al. 2007).

To date, the CLPS has reported on different concepts of categorical and dimensional stability of four personality disorders over 12 months (Shea et al. 2002) and 24 months (Grilo et al. 2004) using prospective data obtained for 668 patients recruited from diverse settings at four universities. Based on the traditional test–retest approach, blind repeated administration of a semistructured interview conducted 24 months after baseline revealed "remission" rates (based solely on falling below DSM-IV diagnostic thresholds) ranging from 50% (avoidant personality disorder) to 61% (schizotypal personality disorder). Grilo et al. (2004) applied lifetable survival analyses to prospective data obtained using an assessment methodology modeled after the Collaborative Depression Study (Keller et al. 1982) and the Longitudinal Interval Follow-Up Evaluation (Keller et al. 1987) methodology. These findings are summarized in Figures 4–1 and 4–2.

Figure 4–1 shows the times to remission for the four personality disorder groups and for the MDD comparison group, which were calculated based on parallel definitions of two consecutive months with minimal symptoms (Grilo et al. 2004). As can be seen, the MDD group had a significantly higher remission rate than the personality disorder groups. This study represents the first empirical demonstration of the central tenet that personality disorders are characterized by greater degree of stability than the hypothesized episodic course of Axis I psychiatric disorders (Grilo et al. 1998; Shea and Yen 2003).

The reader is referred to Shea and Yen (2003) for a broader discussion of this issue. These researchers, who have played roles in the CLPS as well as the longitudinal studies of depression (Collaborative Depression Study) and anxiety (Harvard/Brown Anxiety Research Project), provide an overview of the central findings that pertain to the issue of stability as a distinction between Axis II and Axis I diagnoses (Shea and Yen 2003). Briefly, comparison across the studies (which

can be done given the parallel assessment instrumentation) reveals that personality disorders demonstrate greater stability than Axis I mood and anxiety disorders (as hypothesized) but show less diagnostic (categorical) stability than conceptualized. Perhaps noteworthy is that the longitudinal studies for both mood and anxiety disorders documented much greater chronicity (much lower remission rates) than previously known.

Returning to the CLPS findings (Grilo et al. 2004), Figure 4–1 reveals that although personality disorders were more stable than MDD, a substantial number of "remissions" occurred during the 24 months of follow-up. Using the arbitrarily selected 2-month definition (2 months with two or fewer criteria) adopted from the MDD field (Keller et al. 1982; Solomon et al. 1997), remission rates range from 33% (schizotypal personality disorder) to 55% (obsessive-compulsive personality disorder). Figure 4–2 shows the comparable remission rates if a very stringent definition of 12 consecutive months with two or fewer criteria is adopted. As can be seen, the remission rates using the 12-month definition range from 23% (schizotypal personality disorder) to 38% (obsessive-compulsive personality disorder). Grilo et al. (2004) concluded that these four personality disorders show substantial improvements in symptomatology over a 2-year period even when a stringent definition is used.

The CLPS also provided complementary analyses using dimensional approaches for 12-month (Shea et al. 2002) and 24-month (Grilo et al. 2004) follow-ups. Grilo et al. (2004) documented a significant decrease in the mean proportion of criteria met in each of the personality disorder groups over time, which is suggestive of decreased severity. However, when the relative stability of individual differences was examined across the multiwave assessments (baseline and 6-, 12-, and 24-month time points), a high level of consistency was observed as evidenced by

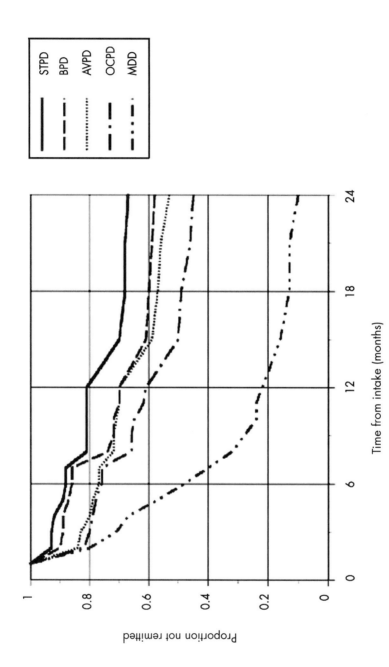

Figure 4–1.   Time to remission for four personality disorder groups and major depressive disorder (MDD) comparison group using a 2-month criterion in Collaborative Longitudinal Personality Study.

AVPD=avoidant personality disorder; BPD=borderline personality disorder; OCPD=obsessive-compulsive personality disorder; STPD=schizotypal personality disorder.

Source.   From Grilo CM, Shea MT, Sanislow CA, et al: "Two-Year Stability and Change in Schizotypal, Borderline, Avoidant, and Obsessive-Compulsive Personality Disorders." *Journal of Consulting and Clinical Psychology* 72:767–775, 2004. Reprinted with permission.

correlation coefficients ranging from 0.53 to 0.67 for proportion of criteria met between baseline and 24 months. Grilo et al. (2004) concluded that patients with personality disorder are consistent in terms of their rank order of personality disorder criteria (i.e., that individual differences in personality disorder features are stable), although they may fluctuate in the severity or number of personality disorder features over time. It is worth noting that the range of the stability coefficients was quite similar to that documented by the Longitudinal Study of Personality Disorders (Lenzenweger 1999) for a nonclinical sample.

In contrast to their symptomatic improvement, however, patients with personality disorders show less significant and more gradual improvement in their functioning, particularly in social relationships (Skodol et al. 2005c). In addition, depressed patients with personality disorders show longer time to remission from MDD (Grilo et al. 2005) and have greater risks for recurrences and for new onsets of MDD (Gunderson et al. 2008). Personality disorders, however, were unrelated to the course of some Axis I psychiatric disorders, such as eating disorders (Grilo et al. 2007). Because personality psychopathology usually begins in adolescence or early adulthood, the potential for delays in occupational and interpersonal development is great—and even after symptomatic improvement, it might take time to overcome deficits and make up the necessary ground to achieve "normal" functioning. Developmental issues for patients with personality disorders are discussed in more detail in Chapter 7, "Developmental Issues."

Several reports from the CLPS are also relevant here given the issue of longitudinal comorbidities and continuities. Shea et al. (2004) examined the time-varying (longitudinal) associations between personality disorders and psychiatric disorders, in part guided by the Siever and Davis (1991) crosscutting psychobiological dimension model. BPD demonstrated significant associations with certain psychiatric disorders (MDD and posttraumatic stress disorder), whereas avoidant personality disorder was significantly associated with two anxiety disorders (social phobia and obsessive-compulsive disorder). While these findings were consistent with predictions based on the Siever and Davis (1991) model, other personality disorders (schizotypal and obsessive-compulsive) did not demonstrate significant longitudinal associations. Gunderson et al. (2004) followed up on the Shea et al. (2004) findings regarding changes in BPD and MDD by performing a more fine-grained analysis of specific changes in the two disorders using 3 years of longitudinal data. Changes (improvements) in BPD severity preceded improvements in MDD but not vice versa (Gunderson et al. 2004).

Another report (Warner et al. 2004) examined whether personality traits are stable in patients with personality disorders and tested the hypothesis that the stability of these personality disorders is due in part to the stability in these traits (Lynam and Widiger 2001). A series of latent longitudinal models tests whether changes in specific traits prospectively predicted changes in relevant personality disorders. Warner et al. (2004) documented significant cross-lagged relationships between changes in specific traits and subsequent (later) changes for schizotypal, borderline, and avoidant personality disorders but not for obsessive-compulsive personality disorder.

McGlashan et al. (2005) examined the individual criteria for schizotypal, borderline, avoidant, and obsessive-compulsive personality disorders and how they changed over a 2-year period. The individual criteria for these four personality disorders showed varied patterns of stability and change over time. Overall, within personality disorders, the relatively fixed (least changeable) criteria were generally more traitlike (and attitudinal), whereas the more fluctuating criteria were generally behavioral (or reactive). McGlashan et al. (2005) posited that perhaps

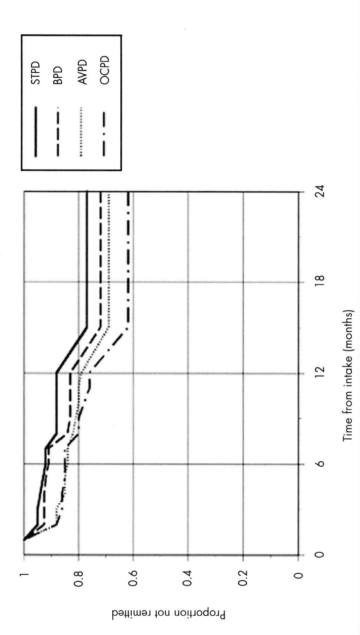

Figure 4–2. Time to remission for four personality disorder groups using a 12-month criterion in Collaborative Longitudinal Personality Study. AVPD=avoidant personality disorder; BPD=borderline personality disorder; OCPD=obsessive-compulsive personality disorder; STPD=schizotypal personality disorder.

Source. From Grilo CM, Shea MT, Sanislow CA, et al: "Two-Year Stability and Change in Schizotypal, Borderline, Avoidant, and Obsessive-Compulsive Personality Disorders." *Journal of Consulting and Clinical Psychology* 72:767–775, 2004. Reprinted with permission.

personality disorders are hybrids of traits and symptomatic behaviors and that it is the interaction of these over time that helps to define the observable diagnostic stability. Collectively, along with the recent CLPS efforts, these findings suggest that personality disorder traits are stable over time and across developmental eras and may generate intra- and interpersonal conflicts that result in behaviors symptomatic of personality disorders (which are less stable over time).

Children in the Community Study

The Children in the Community study (Brook et al. 1995, 2002; Cohen et al. 2005) is an especially impressive longitudinal effort that has already provided a wealth of information about the course of personality and behavioral traits, psychiatric problems, substance abuse, and adversities. It is an ongoing prospective study of nearly 1,000 families with children ages 1–10 years originally recruited in 1975 in New York State using a random sampling procedure. The study has employed repeated multimodal assessments and has followed over 700 participants since childhood and through the development eras of childhood, adolescence, and early adulthood.

This landmark study, which has reported 20-year outcomes (Crawford et al. 2008), has provided data that speak to the critical issues of longitudinal comorbidities and continuities. In a series of papers, the collaborating researchers have documented important findings relevant to the issues raised in this review but especially to the critical issues of continuity of risk and functioning across developmental eras. These include documentation of the validity of certain forms of dramatic-erratic personality disorders in adolescents (Crawford et al. 2001a, 2001b); findings of age-related changes in personality disorder traits, including their moderate levels of stability throughout adolescence and early adulthood (Johnson et al. 2000b); and indications that early forms of behavioral distur-

bances predict personality disorders in adolescents and that personality disorders during adolescence, in addition to demonstrating significant levels of continuity into adulthood, also predict psychiatric disorders, suicidality, and violent and criminal behavior during young adulthood (Crawford et al. 2008; Johnson et al. 2000a, 2000b, 2005). Collectively, these findings support the continuity and persistence of personality disturbances, although their developmental pathways are not yet understood.

CONCLUSION

We have reviewed the literature regarding the course and stability of personality disorders. We once again conclude that personality disorders demonstrate only moderate stability and that they can improve over time. This conclusion is offered with less caution than during our previous reviews (Grilo and McGlashan 1999), given some notable advances in research. We also conclude that when personality disorders are considered dimensionally, the degree of stability is substantial. Emerging work has suggested that personality disorder traits, although deviant, are stable over time and across developmental eras and may generate intra- and interpersonal conflicts that result in personality disorder–symptomatic behaviors (which are less stable over time). Future research in personality disorders is necessary to dissect and understand this trait-state interaction and track its vicissitudes across time and circumstances.

REFERENCES

Abrams RC, Spielman LA, Alexopoulos GS, et al: Personality disorder symptoms and functioning in elderly depressed patients. Am J Geriatr Psychiatry 6:24–30, 1998

American Psychiatric Association: Diagnostic and Statistical Manual of Mental Disorders. Washington, DC, American Psychiatric Association, 1952

American Psychiatric Association: Diagnostic and Statistical Manual of Mental Disorders, 3rd Edition. Washington, DC, American Psychiatric Association, 1980

American Psychiatric Association: Diagnostic and Statistical Manual of Mental Disorders, 3rd Edition, Revised. Washington, DC, American Psychiatric Association, 1987

American Psychiatric Association: Diagnostic and Statistical Manual of Mental Disorders, 4th Edition. Washington, DC, American Psychiatric Association, 1994

American Psychiatric Association: Diagnostic and Statistical Manual of Mental Disorders, 4th Edition, Text Revision. Washington, DC, American Psychiatric Association, 2000

Bender DS, Skodol AE, Dyck IR, et al: Ethnicity and mental health treatment utilization by patients with personality disorders. J Consult Clin Psychol 75:992–999, 2007

Berkson J: Limitations of the application of four-fold table analysis to hospital data. Biometrics Bulletin 2:47–53, 1946

Bernstein DP, Cohen P, Skodol AE, et al: Childhood antecedents of adolescent personality disorders. Am J Psychiatry 153:907–913, 1996

Blashfield RK, McElroy RA: The 1985 journal literature on the personality disorders. Compr Psychiatry 28:536–546, 1987

Brook DW, Brook JS, Zhang C, et al: Drug use and the risk of major depressive disorder, alcohol dependence, and substance use disorders. Arch Gen Psychiatry 59:1039–1044, 2002

Brook JS, Whiteman M, Cohen P, et al: Longitudinally predicting late adolescent and young adult drug use: childhood and adolescent precursors. J Am Acad Child Adolesc Psychiatry 34:1230–1238, 1995

Carpenter WT, Gunderson JG: Five year follow-up comparison of borderline and schizophrenic patients. Compr Psychiatry 18:567–571, 1977

Cloninger CR, Svrakic DM, Przybeck TR: A psychobiological model of temperament and character. Arch Gen Psychiatry 50:975–990, 1993

Cohen P, Crawford TN, Johnson JG, et al: The Children in the Community study of developmental course of personality disorder. J Personal Disord 19:466–486, 2005

Crawford TN, Cohen P, Brook JS: Dramatic-erratic personality disorder symptoms, I: continuity from early adolescence into adulthood. J Personal Disord 15:319–335, 2001a

Crawford TN, Cohen P, Brook JS: Dramatic-erratic personality disorder symptoms, II: develop-mental pathways from early adolescence to adulthood. J Personal Disord 15:336–350, 2001b

Crawford TN, Cohen P, First MB, et al: Comorbid Axis I and Axis II disorders in early adolescence: outcomes 20 years later. Arch Gen Psychiatry 65:641–648, 2008

Dolan-Sewell RT, Krueger RF, Shea MT: Co-occurrence with syndrome disorders, in Handbook of Personality Disorders. Edited by Livesley WJ. New York, Guilford, 2001, pp 84–104

Ferro T, Klein DN, Schwartz JE, et al: 30-month stability of personality disorder diagnoses in depressed outpatients. Am J Psychiatry 155:653–659, 1998

Frances A: Categorical and dimensional systems of personality diagnosis: a comparison. Compr Psychiatry 23:516–527, 1982

Grilo CM, McGlashan TH: Stability and course of personality disorders. Curr Opin Psychiatry 12:157–162, 1999

Grilo CM, McGlashan TH, Oldham JM: Course and stability of personality disorders. J Pract Psychiatry Behav Health 4:61–75, 1998

Grilo CM, Becker DF, Edell WS, et al: Stability and change of personality disorder dimensions in adolescents followed up two years after psychiatric hospitalization. Compr Psychiatry 42:364–368, 2001

Grilo CM, Sanislow CA, Gunderson JG, et al: Two-year stability and change of schizotypal, borderline, avoidant, and obsessive-compulsive personality disorders. J Consult Clin Psychol 72:767–775, 2004

Grilo CM, Sanislow CA, Shea MT, et al: Two-year prospective naturalistic study of remission from major depressive disorder as a function of personality disorder comorbidity. J Consult Clin Psychol 73:78–85, 2005

Grilo CM, Pagano ME, Skodol AE, et al: Natural course of bulimia nervosa and of eating disorder not otherwise specified: 5-year prospective study of remissions, relapses, and the effects of personality disorder psychopathology. J Clin Psychiatry 68:738–746, 2007

Grinker RR, Werble B, Drye RC: The Borderline Syndrome. New York, Basic Books, 1968

Gunderson JG, Shea MT, Skodol AE, et al: The Collaborative Longitudinal Personality Disorders Study, I: development, aims, designs and sample characteristics. J Personal Disord 14:300–315, 2000

Gunderson JG, Morey LC, Stout RL, et al: Major depressive disorder and borderline personality disorder revisited: longitudinal interactions. J Clin Psychiatry 65:1049–1056, 2004

Gunderson JG, Stout RL, Sanislow CA, et al: New episodes and new onsets of major depression in borderline and other personality disorders. J Affect Disord 111:40–45, 20008

Heatherton TF, Weinberger JL (eds): Can Personality Change? Washington, DC, American Psychological Press, 1994

Johnson JG, Williams JBW, Goetz RR, et al: Stability and change in personality disorder symptomatology: findings from a longitudinal study of HIV+ and HIV– men. J Abnorm Psychol 106:154–158, 1997

Johnson JG, Cohen P, Kasen S, et al: Age-related change in personality disorder trait levels between early adolescence and adulthood: a community-based longitudinal investigation. Acta Psychiatr Scand 102:265–275, 2000a

Johnson JG, Cohen P, Smailes E, et al: Adolescent personality disorders associated with violence and criminal behavior during adolescence and early adulthood. Am J Psychiatry 157:1406–1412, 2000b

Johnson JG, First MB, Cohen P, et al: Adverse outcomes associated with personality disorder not otherwise specified in a community sample. Am J Psychiatry 162:926–932, 2005

Judd PH, McGlashan TH: A Developmental Model of Borderline Personality Disorder: Understanding Variations in Course and Outcome. Washington, DC, American Psychiatric Publishing, 2003

Katz MM, Secunda SK, Hirschfeld R, et al: NIMH Clinical Research Branch Collaborative Program on Psychobiology of Depression. Arch Gen Psychiatry 36:765–771, 1979

Keller MB, Shapiro RW, Lavori PW, et al: Recovery in major depressive disorder: analysis with the lifetable and regression models. Arch Gen Psychiatry 39:905–910, 1982

Keller MB, Lavori PW, Friedman B, et al: The Longitudinal Interval Follow-Up Evaluation. Arch Gen Psychiatry 44:540–548, 1987

Keller MB: Social anxiety disorder clinical course and outcome: review of Harvard/Brown Anxiety Research Program (HARP) findings. J Clin Psychiatry 67(suppl):14–19, 2006

Kendell PC, Clarkin JF: Introduction to special section: comorbidity and treatment implications. J Consult Clin Psychol 60:833–834, 1992

Klein DN, Shih JH: Depressive personality: associations with DSM-III-R mood and personality disorders and negative and positive affectivity, 30-month stability, and prediction of course of axis I depressive disorders. J Abnorm Psychol 107:319–327, 1998

Krueger RF: The structure of common mental disorders. Arch Gen Psychiatry 56:921–926, 1999

Krueger RF, Carlson SR: Personality disorders in children and adolescents. Curr Psychiatry Rep 3:46–51, 2001

Krueger RF, Tackett JL: Personality and psychopathology: working toward the bigger picture. J Personal Disord 17:109–128, 2003

Lenzenweger MF: Stability and change in personality disorder features: the Longitudinal Study of Personality Disorders. Arch Gen Psychiatry 56:1009–1015, 1999

Lenzenweger MF, Loranger AW, Korfine L, et al: Detecting personality disorders in a nonclinical population: application of a 2-stage procedure for case identification. Arch Gen Psychiatry 54:110–133, 1997

Levy KN, Becker DF, Grilo CM, et al: Concurrent and predictive validity of the personality disorder diagnosis in adolescent inpatients. Am J Psychiatry 156:1522–1528, 1999

Lewinsohn PM, Rohde P, Seeley JR, et al: Axis II psychopathology as a function of Axis I disorder in childhood and adolescents. J Am Acad Child Adolesc Psychiatry 36:1752–1759, 1997

Livesley WJ, Jackson DN, Schroeder ML: Factorial structure of traits delineating personality disorders in clinical and general population samples. J Abnorm Psychol 101:432–440, 1992

Loranger AW. Personality Disorder Examination (PDE) Manual. Yonkers, NY, DV Communications, 1988

Loranger AW, Lenzenweger MF, Gartner AF, et al: Trait-state artifacts and the diagnosis of personality disorders. Arch Gen Psychiatry 48:720–728, 1991

Loranger AW, Sartorius N, Andreoli A, et al: The International Personality Disorder Examination (IPDE): the World Health Organization/Alcohol, Drug Abuse, and Mental Health Administration International Pilot Study of Personality Disorders. Arch Gen Psychiatry 51:215–224, 1994

Lynam DR, Widiger TA: Using the five-factor model to represent the DSM-IV personality disorders: an expert consensus approach. J Abnorm Psychol 110:401–412, 2001

Lyons MJ, Tyrer P, Gunderson J, et al: Special feature: heuristic models of comorbidity of Axis I and Axis II disorders. J Personal Disord 11:260–269, 1997

Maddocks PD: A five year follow-up of untreated psychopaths. Br J Psychiatry 116:511–515, 1970

Markowitz JC, Skodol AE, Petkova E, et al: Longitudinal effects of personality disorders on psychosocial functioning of patients with major depressive disorder. J Clin Psychiatry 68:186–193, 2007

Mattanah JJ, Becker DF, Levy KN, et al: Diagnostic stability in adolescents followed up 2 years after hospitalization. Am J Psychiatry 152:889–894, 1995

McDavid JD, Pilkonis PA: The stability of personality disorder diagnoses. J Personal Disord 10:1–15, 1996

McGlashan TH: The Chestnut Lodge Follow-Up Study, part III: long-term outcome of borderline personalities. Arch Gen Psychiatry 42:20–30, 1986a

McGlashan TH: The Chestnut Lodge Follow-up Study, part VI: schizotypal personality disorder. Arch Gen Psychiatry 43:329–334, 1986b

McGlashan TH, Grilo CM, Skodol AE, et al: The Collaborative Longitudinal Personality Disorders Study: baseline Axis I/II and II/II diagnostic co-occurrence. Acta Psychiatr Scand 102:256–264, 2000

McGlashan TH, Grilo CM, Sanislow CA, et al: Two-year prevalence and stability of individual DSM-IV criteria for schizotypal, borderline, avoidant, and obsessive-compulsive disorders: toward a hybrid model of Axis II disorders. Am J Psychiatry 162:883–889, 2005

Millon T: Millon Clinical Multiaxial Inventory–III. Minneapolis, MN, National Computer Systems, 1987

Morey LC, Hopwood CJ, Gunderson JG, et al: Comparison of alternative models for personality disorders. Psychol Med 37:983–994, 2007

Myers MG, Stewart DG, Brown SA: Progression from conduct disorder to antisocial personality disorder following treatment for adolescent substance abuse. Am J Psychiatry 155:479–485, 1998

Nesselroade JR, Stigler SM, Baltes PB: Regression toward the mean and the study of change. Psychol Bull 88:622–637, 1980

Newman DL, Caspi A, Moffitt TE, et al: Antecedents of adult interpersonal functioning: effects of individual differences in age three temperament. Dev Psychol 33:206–217, 1997

Oldham JM, Skodol AE, Kellman HD, et al: Diagnosis of DSM-III-R personality disorders by two structured interviews: patterns of comorbidity. Am J Psychiatry 149: 213–220, 1992

Ottosson H, Ekselius L, Grann M, et al: Cross-system concordance of personality disorder diagnoses of DSM-IV and diagnostic criteria for research of ICD-10. J Personal Disord 16:283–292, 2002

Paris J: Personality disorders over time: precursors, course and outcome. J Personal Disord 17:479–488, 2003

Paris J, Zweig-Frank H: A twenty-seven year follow-up of borderline patients. Compr Psychiatry 42:482–487, 2001

Perry JC: Longitudinal studies of personality disorders. J Personal Disord 7 (suppl):63–85, 1993

Rettew DC, Zanarini MC, Yen S, et al: Childhood antecedents of avoidant personality disorder: a retrospective study. J Am Acad Child Adolesc Psychiatry 42:1122–1130, 2003

Rey JM, Morris-Yates A, Singh M, et al: Continuities between psychiatric disorders in adolescents and personality disorders in young adults. Am J Psychiatry 152:895–900, 1995

Robbins E, Gentry KA, Munoz RA, et al: A contrast of the three more common illnesses with the ten less common in a study and 18-month follow-up of 314 psychiatric emergency room patients, III: findings at follow-up. Arch Gen Psychiatry 34:285–291, 1977

Roberts BW, DelVecchio WF: The rank-order consistency of personality traits from childhood to old age: a quantitative review of longitudinal studies. Psychol Bull 126:3–25, 2000

Roberts BW, Caspi A, Moffitt TE: The kids are alright: growth and stability in personality development from adolescence to adulthood. J Pers Soc Psychol 81:670–683, 2001

Robins LN: Deviant Children Grown Up: A Sociological and Psychiatric Study of Sociopathic Personality. Baltimore, MD, Williams & Wilkins, 1966

Robins LN: Epidemiology: reflections on testing the validity of psychiatric interviews. Arch Gen Psychiatry 42:918–924,1985

Ruegg R, Frances A: New research in personality disorders. J Personal Disord 9:1–48, 1995

Sanislow CA, McGlashan TH: Treatment outcome of personality disorders. Can J Psychiatry 43:237–250, 1998

Seivewright H, Tyrer P, Johnson T: Change in personality status in neurotic disorders. Lancet 359:2253–2254, 2002

Shea MT, Yen S: Stability as a distinction between Axis I and Axis II disorders. J Personal Disord 17:373–386, 2003

Shea MT, Stout RL, Gunderson JG, et al: Short-term diagnostic stability of schizotypal, borderline, avoidant, and obsessive-compulsive personality disorders. Am J Psychiatry 159:2036–2041, 2002

Shea MT, Stout RL, Yen S, et al: Associations in the course of personality disorders and Axis I disorders over time. J Abnorm Psychol 113:449–508, 2004

Siever LJ, Davis KL: A psychobiological perspective on the personality disorders. Am J Psychiatry 148:1647–1658, 1991

Skodol AE: Classification, assessment, and differential diagnosis of personality disorders. J Pract Psychiatry Behav Health 3:261–274, 1997

Skodol AE, Grilo CM, Pagano ME, et al: Effects of personality disorders on functioning and well-being in major depressive disorder. J Psychiatr Pract 11:363–368, 2005a

Skodol AE, Gunderson JG, Shea MT, et al: The Collaborative Longitudinal Personality Disorders Study (CLPS): overview and implications. J Personal Disord 19:487–504, 2005b

Skodol AE, Oldham JM, Bender DS, et al: Dimensional representations of DSM-IV personality disorders: relationships to functional impairment. Am J Psychiatry 162:1919–1925, 2005c

Skodol AE, Pagano ME, Bender DS, et al: Stability of functional impairment in patients with schizotypal, borderline, avoidant, or obsessive-compulsive personality disorder over two years. Psychol Med 35:443–451, 2005d

Solomon DA, Keller MB, Leon AC, et al: Recovery from major depression: a 10-year prospective follow-up across multiple episodes. Arch Gen Psychiatry 54:1001–1006, 1997

Squires-Wheeler E, Skodol AE, Erlenmeyer-Kimling L: The assessment of schizotypal features over two points in time. Schizophrenia Res 6:75–85, 1992

Stevenson J, Meares R, Comerford A: Diminished impulsivity in older patients with borderline personality disorder. Am J Psychiatry 160:165–166, 2003

Stone MH: Long-term outcome in personality disorders. Br J Psychiatry 162:299–313, 1993

Trull TJ, Useda JD, Conforti K, et al: Borderline personality disorder features in nonclinical young adults, 2: two-year outcome. J Abnorm Psychol 106:307–314, 1997

Trull TJ, Useda JD, Doan BT, et al: Two-year stability of borderline personality measures. J Personal Disord 12:187–197, 1998

Tyrer P: Personality disorder. Br J Psychiatry 179:81–84, 2001

Tyrer P, Simonsen E: Personality disorder in psychiatric practice. World Psychiatry 2:41–44, 2003

Tyrer P, Strauss J, Cicchetti D: Temporal reliability of personality in psychiatric patients. Psychol Med 13:393–398, 1983

Tyrer P, Gunderson J, Lyons M, et al: Special feature: extent of comorbidity between mental state and personality disorders. J Personal Disord 11:242–259, 1997

Warner MB, Morey LC, Finch JF, et al: The longitudinal relationship of personality traits and disorders. J Abnorm Psychol 113:217–227, 2004

Westen D: Divergences between clinical and research methods for assessing personality disorders: implications for research and the evolution of Axis II. Am J Psychiatry 154:895–903, 1997

Westen D, Shedler J: Revising and assessing Axis II, part II: toward an empirically based and clinically useful classification of personality disorders. Am J Psychiatry 156: 273–285, 1999

Widiger TA: Categorical versus dimensional classification: implications from and for research. J Personal Disord 6:287–300, 1992

Widiger TA: Personality disorder and Axis I psychopathology: the problematic boundary of Axis I and Axis II. J Personal Disord 17:90–108, 2003

Wolff S, Townshend R, McGuire RJ, et al: Schizoid personality in childhood and adult life, II: adult adjustment and the continuity with schizotypal personality disorder. Br J Psychiatry 159:620–629, 1991

World Health Organization: The ICD-10 Classification of Mental and Behavioural Disorders: Clinical Description and Diagnostic Guidelines. Geneva, World Health Organization, 1992

Zanarini MC, Skodol AE, Bender D, et al: The Collaborative Longitudinal Personality Disorders Study: reliability of Axis I and II diagnoses. J Personal Disord 14:291–299, 2000

Zanarini MC, Frankenburg FR, Hennen J, et al: The longitudinal course of borderline psychopathology: 6-year prospective follow-up of the phenomenology of borderline personality disorder. Am J Psychiatry 160:274–283, 2003

Zanarini MC, Frankenburg FR, Hennen J, et al: Axis I comorbidity in patients with borderline personality disorder: 6-year follow-up and prediction of time to remission. Am J Psychiatry 161:2108–2114, 2004

Zanarini MC, Frankenburg FR, Hennen J, et al: The McLean Study of Adult (MSAD): overview and implications of the first six years of prospective follow-up. J Personal Disord 19:505–523, 2005

Zanarini MC, Frankenburg FR, Hennen J, et al: Prediction of the 10-year course of borderline personality disorder. Am J Psychiatry 163:827–832, 2006

Zimmerman M: Diagnosing personality disorders: a review of issues and research methods. Arch Gen Psychiatry 51:225–245, 1994

Part III

Etiology

5

Prevalence, Sociodemographics, and Functional Impairment

Svenn Torgersen, Ph.D.

From clinical work we get an impression of which personality disorders are more common and which are rarer. However, people with some types of personality disorders may be more likely to seek treatment and obtain treatment compared with people with other types of personality disorders. Consequently, if we are interested in how prevalent different personality disorders are in the general population, we have to study representative samples of the general population. Epidemiological research does just that.

Clinical work also gives us ideas about relationships between socioeconomic and sociodemographic factors and personality disorders. However, in a clinical setting we only meet those from an unfavorable environment who have developed a personality disorder. We do not meet those from an unfavorable environment who have *not* developed a disorder. Furthermore, the combination of a specific personality disorder and specific so-

ciodemographic features may increase the likelihood of a particular person to seek treatment. These complexities mean that only population (epidemiological) studies can demonstrate the "true" relationship between personality disorders and socioeconomic and sociodemographic variables, or any other variables such as traumas, disastrous events, upbringing, or partner relationships.

PREVALENCE

We know much about the prevalence of Axis I disorders in the general population (Kringlen et al. 2001). As to personality disorders, however, less is known. Some studies have been performed, but few of them adequately represent the general population (Torgersen et al. 2001). In this chapter I review published studies that are closest to what one might call an epidemiological population study. These individual studies are discussed below (and presented in Table 5–1) in view of different elements of epidemiology, beginning with a discussion of sample selection for each study.

Sample Selection

The sample studied by Zimmerman and Coryell (1989, 1990) included first-degree relatives of normal subjects (23%) and of psychiatric patients (mood disorders and schizophrenia) as well as a smaller group of first-degree relatives of nonpsychotic psychiatric patients. Thus, even if this is a "nonpatient sample," it is not an average population sample. However, the prevalence of mania was not higher than 2%, and the prevalence of schizophrenia was not higher than 1%. Interviews were conducted in person (27%) and by telephone (73%). The Structured Interview for DSM-III Personality Disorders was applied (Stangl et al. 1985). The study took place in Iowa City.

The sample reported on by Black et al. (1993) consisted of 120 relatives of 32 outpatients with obsessive-compulsive disorder and 127 relatives of a comparison group screened for Axis I disorders. Strangely, no difference was found between the prevalence of personality disorders in the two relative groups. More than half of the sample were siblings, a quarter were parents, and the rest were children. A little more than half were women. The mean age was 42 years. More than half were interviewed in person and the rest by telephone.

Maier et al. (1992) conducted one of the few reported studies in which the sample is relatively representative of the general population. Control probands were selected by a marketing company to match patients older than age 20 on sex, age, residential area, and educational level. The participants had to have at least one living first-degree relative who also had agreed to be interviewed. Otherwise, this sample represented the general population of a mixed urban/rural German residential area near Mainz. No screening for medical or psychiatric history was performed. The control probands, their spouses, and first-degree relatives constituted the sample.

The sample studied by Moldin et al. (1994) consisted of parents and their offspring in two control groups used in the New York High Risk Project. One of the groups was recruited from two schools in the New York metropolitan area. The other group came from the pool of a population sampling firm. The subjects were white, English-speaking families screened for psychiatric disorder.

In the study by Klein et al. (1995), the sample comprised relatives of a control group screened for Axis I disorders in Stony Brook, New York. The interviews were partly conducted in person and partly by telephone.

Lenzenweger et al. (1997) examined a sample consisting initially of 1,684 undergraduate students from Cornell University in New York. They were screened by means of a questionnaire; a sample of those expected and those not expected to have a personality disorder was interviewed. The total number of subjects interviewed was 258. In this overview (Table 5–1), I apply the actual numbers. The estimated prevalence for any personality disorder is a little different.

The study by Torgersen et al. (2001) was conducted in Oslo, the capital of Norway. A random sample of names of 3,590 citizens between age 18 and 65 years was selected from the National Register of Oslo. Some had moved out of town, some were impossible to trace, and some were dead. Others refused to participate or postponed the interview beyond the period of the study (18%). Of the original sample, 2,053 (57%) delivered interviews of sufficient quality for the study. All interviews were performed in person. The sampling procedure made it possible to identify all causes of reduction in the sample from the initial to the final sample. There were almost equal numbers of men and women.

The sampling procedure used by Samuels et al. (2002) was very complicated. Initially, a sample of 3,481 adult household residents in Baltimore was studied in the 1980s. About 10 years later, a subsample was selected that included individuals previously evaluated by psychiatrists or those who appeared to have an Axis I diagnosis based on the Diagnostic Interview Schedule. In addition, a random sample was selected. A number of subjects could not be traced, refused, were too ill to participate, or were deceased. The remaining sample consisted of 742 individuals. Their ages varied between 34 and 94 years, and two-thirds were women.

In the study by Grant et al. (2004), a very large sample (N=43,093; the so-called National Epidemiologic Survey on Alcohol and Related Conditions [NESARC]), was interviewed. A measure named Alcohol Use Disorder and Associated Disabilities Interview Schedul–IV (AUDADIS-IV) was applied. Borderline, schizotypal, and narcissistic personality disorders were not included. The results were weighted to represent the U.S. population age 18 years and older.

Crawford et al. (2005) studied prospectively 597 community members from age 14 to 33 years. The reported percentages in Table 5–1 are based on the application of the Structured Clinical Interview for DSM-IV Axis II Personality Disorders (SCID-II) to respondents at age 33 years.

Coid et al. (2006) interviewed 626 individuals age 16–74 years in the United Kingdom. Table 5–1 reports the weighted prevalences (unweighted prevalences for the specific disorders are not stated in the publication). The SCID-II screening questionnaire was applied.

Personality disorders were assessed in the National Comorbidity Survey Replication (NCS-R). A set of the International Personality Disorder Examination (IPDE) screening questions was applied to 5,692 individuals age 18 years or older (Lenzenweger et al. 2007). A subsample of 214 individuals "who screened positive for one or more of our outcome measures on the basis of the IPDE screening questions in the NCS-

R" (p. 554) was interviewed with the complete IPDE.

Results

Table 5–1 presents the prevalences in the published studies discussed above, including all personality disorders. So-called mixed personality disorders, defined by the absence of one criterion for two or more personality disorders and not having the required number of criteria for any disorder, are excluded. The same is the case for personality disorders not otherwise specified (NOS), defined by having 10 or more criteria, but not a sufficient number of criteria obtained for any specific disorder. Unweighted prevalences (rather than weighted prevalences based on questionable weighting procedures) are presented, if possible, because the prevalences among those not reached cannot be known. The qualified, although questionable, guesswork gives one an impression of increased accuracy. A nonweighted rate is transparent and does not claim more than it can stand for.

In almost half of the studies, the prevalence of any disorder is between 7% and 13%. The median prevalence is above 10%. The median prevalence of specific personality disorders is mostly between 1% and 2%.

Obsessive-compulsive personality disorder is the most frequently occurring personality disorder (above 2%). Next come paranoid, avoidant, and passive-aggressive personality disorder (1.7%); then borderline (1.6%), histrionic (1.5%), antisocial (1.1%), and schizoid and schizotypal (0.9%); and finally narcissistic personality disorder (0.5%). The only two studies that included self-defeating and sadistic personality disorder reported an average of 0.4% and 0.1% respectively.

The correlations between the different studies are very low, around 0.17. The only two studies that reflect the average prevalences (calculated by intraclass correlation) are those of Maier et al. (1992) and Torgersen et al. (2001).

Table 5–1.   Prevalences of personality disorders in twelve population studies

	Zimmerman and Coryell 1989	Black et al. 1993	Maier et al. 1992	Moldin et al. 1994	Klein et al. 1995	Lenzenweger et al. 1997	Torgersen et al. 2001	Samuels et al. 2002	Grant et al. 2004	Crawford et al. 2005	Coid et al. 2006	Lenzenweger et al. 2007	Median
Place	Iowa	Iowa	Mainz	NYC	New York	New York	Oslo	Baltimore	USA	New York	UK	USA	
Method	SIDP	SIDP	SCID-II	PDE	PDE	PDE	SIDP-R	IPDE	AUDADIS-IV	SCID-II	SCID-II screening	IPDE	
DSM system	III	III	III-R	III-R	III-R	III-R	III-R	IV	IV	IV	IV	IV	
Personality disorder													
Paranoid	0.9	1.6	1.8	0.0	1.8	0.4	2.2	0.7	4.4	5.1	5.1	2.3	1.7
Schizoid	0.9	0.0	0.4	0.0	0.9	0.4	1.6	0.7	3.1	1.7	1.7	4.9	0.9
Schizotypal	2.9	3.2	0.7	0.7	0.0	0.0	0.6	1.8	—	1.1	1.1	3.3	0.9
Antisocial	3.3	0.8	0.2	2.6	2.6	0.8	0.6	4.5	3.6	1.2	1.2	1.0	1.1
Borderline	1.7	3.2	1.1	2.0	1.8	0.0	0.7	1.2	—	3.9	3.9	1.6	1.6
Histrionic	3.0	3.2	1.3	0.3	1.8	1.9	1.9	0.4	1.8	0.9	0.9	0.0	1.5
Narcissistic	0.0	0.0	0.0	0.0	4.4	1.2	0.8	0.1	—	2.2	2.2	0.0	0.5
Avoidant	1.3	2.0	1.1	0.7	5.7	0.4	5.0	1.4	2.4	6.4	6.4	5.2	1.7
Dependent	1.8	1.6	1.6	1.0	0.4	0.4	1.5	0.3	0.5	0.8	0.8	0.6	0.7
Obsessive-compulsive	2.0	9.3	2.2	0.7	2.6	0.0	1.9	1.2	7.9	4.7	4.7	2.4	2.1
Passive-aggressive	3.3	10.5	1.8	1.7	1.8	0.0	1.6	—	—	—	—	—	1.7
Self-defeating	—	—	—	—	—	0.0	0.8	—	—	—	—	—	0.4
Sadistic	—	—	—	—	—	0.0	0.2	—	—	—	—	—	0.1

Table 5–1.   Prevalences of personality disorders in twelve population studies *(continued)*

	Zimmerman and Coryell 1989	Black et al. 1993	Maier et al. 1992	Moldin et al. 1994	Klein et al. 1995	Lenzenweger et al. 1997	Torgersen et al. 2001	Samuels et al. 2002	Grant et al. 2004	Crawford et al. 2005	Coid et al. 2006	Lenzenweger et al. 2007	Median
Any personality disorder	14.3	22.7	10.0	7.3	14.8	3.9	13.1	10.0		15.7	4.4	10.3	10.3
Number	797	247	452	303	229	258	2,053	742	43,093	597	626	214	

Note.   IPDE=International Personality Disorders Examination; NYC=New York City; PDE=Personality Disorder Examination; SCID-II=Structured Clinical Interview for DSM-IV Axis II Personality Disorders; SIDP=The Structured Interview for DSM-III Personality Disorders; SIDP-R=The Structured Interview for DSM-III-R Personality Disorders.

Dependent and borderline personality disorders display the most stable prevalences from study to study, while narcissistic and passive-aggressive personality disorders vary most from study to study (based on spreading/mean ratio or *t* test). It is noteworthy that these two disorders are not included among the ICD-10 (World Health Organization 1992) or DSM-IV (American Psychiatric Association 1994) personality disorders.

Table 5–2 shows a comparison between the prevalences in a large outpatient clinic in Oslo (Alnæs and Torgersen 1988) and in the general population of that city (Torgersen et al. 2001). The ratio between the prevalence in the clinic and that in the population is calculated separately for women and men and in the total sample. There are relatively small differences in the range of the ratios between women and men, even if the ratios are a little larger for the specific personality disorder among men (not for any personality disorders). Those with dependent, borderline, avoidant, and obsessive-compulsive personality disorder are strongly overrepresented among the patients based on prevalence rates in the general population, whereas those with antisocial, schizoid, and paranoid personality disorder are less common in the clinical compared with the general population. To have a borderline, avoidant, or schizotypal personality disorder implies pain and dysfunction, as I discuss later in the chapter. One may speculate that those who are dependent seek help, whereas obsessive-compulsive patients want to do something with their problems, even if they do not suffer as much. In the other direction, those who are antisocial do not want psychological help and are also refused help. Schizoid individuals keep their distance, whereas paranoid subjects do not believe in any cure.

In conclusion, while the prevalences of the specific personality disorders vary strongly from study to study, the number of published studies makes it possible to draw some conclusions today. At least in the United States and Europe, the prevalences are between 1% and 2%. The validity of the prevalences of those personality disorders that are less frequently occurring is questionable. The prevalence of "any personality disorder" is around 10%. The sum of the percentages for the specific disorders is higher, around 15%, pointing to the fact that around one-third of those with one disorder have one more. (The distribution is skewed with most having only one, some having two, and few having many personality disorders, hence 50% of individuals will not have more than one disorder.) Studies of patients give us a distorted impression of the absolute and relative prevalences of personality disorders, because those with dependent and borderline much more often seek treatment.

SOCIODEMOGRAPHIC CORRELATES

Gender

Gender differences are common among mental disorders. Women more often have mood and anxiety disorders, and men more often have substance-related disorders (Kringlen et al. 2001). For personality disorders, women and men also differ.

With regard to personality disorders, Zimmerman and Coryell (1989) observed a higher prevalence of any personality disorders among males as did Jackson and Burgess (2000) for ICD-10 screening when regression analysis was applied. However, differences between genders were very small, and Torgersen et al. (2001) did not observe any differences.

As to the personality disorder clusters, Samuels et al. (2002) and Torgersen et al. (2001) reported that Cluster A (odd/eccentric) and Cluster B (dramatic/emotional) personality disorders or traits were more common among men. Coid et al. (2006) found the same for Cluster B only.

Among the specific Cluster A disorders, both Torgersen et al. (2001) and Zimmerman and Coryell (1990) found that schizoid per-

Table 5–2. Prevalences of personality disorders in the common population and among outpatients in Oslo, Norway

Personality disorder	Females			Males			Total		
	Torgersen et al. 2001	Alnæs and Torgersen 1988	Ratio (range)	Torgersen et al. 2001	Alnæs and Torgersen 1988	Ratio (range)	Torgersen et al. 2001	Alnæs and Torgersen 1988	Ratio (range)
Paranoid	2.2	3.9	1.8 (9)	2.3	7.6	3.3 (9)	2.2	5.0	2.3 (9)
Schizoid	1.1	0.0	0.0 (10)	2.2	5.4	2.5 (10)	1.6	1.7	1.1 (10)
Schizotypal	0.6	3.9	6.5 (6)	0.5	12.0	24.0 (3)	0.6	6.4	10.7 (4)
Antisocial	0.0	0.0	0.0 (10)	1.3	0.0	0.0 (11)	0.6	0.0	0.0 (11)
Borderline	0.9	17.0	18.9 (2)	0.4	9.8	24.5 (2)	0.7	14.8	21.1 (2)
Histrionic	2.5	15.0	6.0 (7)	1.2	10.9	9.1 (7)	1.9	13.8	7.3 (6)
Narcissistic	0.8	1.9	2.4 (8)	0.9	10.9	12.1 (6)	0.8	4.7	5.9 (8)
Avoidant	5.0	53.4	10.7 (3)	4.9	59.8	12.2 (5)	5.0	55.4	11.1 (3)
Dependent	2.0	47.6	23.8 (1)	0.9	45.7	50.8 (1)	1.5	47.0	31.3 (1)
Obsessive-compulsive	1.3	13.6	10.5 (4)	2.6	33.7	13.0 (4)	1.9	19.8	10.4 (5)
Passive-aggressive	0.9	6.3	7.0 (5)	2.2	18.5	8.4 (8)	1.6	10.1	6.3 (7)
Any personality disorder	12.6	76.7	6.1	13.7	90.2	6.6	13.1	80.9	6.2
Number	1,142	206	—	911	92	—	2,053	298	—

sonality disorder or traits were more common among men. Zimmerman and Coryell (1990) found this also for paranoid traits. Grant et al. (2004), however, observed that women more often had a paranoid personality disorder. Neither Zimmerman and Coryell (1989, 1990) nor Torgersen et al. (2001) observed any gender difference for schizotypal personality disorder. Among the Cluster B personality disorders, antisocial disorder is much more common among men (Torgersen et al. 2001; Zimmerman and Coryell 1989, 1990). Those with histrionic personality disorder or traits appear more often to be women (Torgersen et al. 2001; Zimmerman and Coryell 1990). Narcissistic traits are found more often among men, and there are no statistically significant gender differences for borderline personality disorder or traits (Torgersen et al. 2001; Zimmerman and Coryell 1990).

Among the Cluster C (anxious/fearful) personality disorders, dependent personality disorder is much more common among women (Grant et al. 2004; Torgersen et al. 2001; Zimmerman and Coryell 1989, 1990), and obsessive-compulsive personality disorder or traits are found more often among men (Torgersen et al. 2001; Zimmerman and Coryell 1989, 1990). Zimmerman and Coryell (1989, 1990) and Grant et al. (2004) reported more avoidant personality disorder and traits among women.

Regarding personality disorders "provided for further study" (American Psychiatric Association 2000), Torgersen et al. (2001)—but not Zimmerman and Coryell (1989, 1990)—found that men more often had passive-aggressive personality disorder. Torgersen and colleagues also found that women more often presented with self-defeating traits, and men more often presented with sadistic traits.

The most clear-cut results from the studies are that men tend to be antisocial and women tend to be dependent. These results are perhaps not surprising. However, more surprising is a lack of gender difference for

borderline traits. In patient samples, borderline personality disorder is not more prevalent among women than among men (Alnæs and Torgersen 1988; Fossati et al. 2003; Golomb et al. 1995). In one study of patients, borderline personality disorder was, in fact, more common among men than among women (Carter et al. 1999). In our unsystematic impression of people, we are more likely to "see" borderline features in women than in men. That schizotypal personality disorder does not show any gender bias will more easily be recognized. A trend in the direction of men being more often schizoid, narcissistic, and obsessive-compulsive and women being more often histrionic and avoidant is in accordance with common opinion.

Age

To diagnose a personality disorder in an individual younger than age 18 years, the features must have been present at least 1 year (American Psychiatric Association 2000). At the same time, it is assumed that personality disorders start early in life and are relatively stable. For some personality disorders, especially the dramatic types, it is also assumed that they are typical for young people. On the other hand, the older people are, the longer they have had to develop personality disorders, even though personality disorders may also disappear. Suicide and fatal accidents also may happen more often among those with personality disorders than among other individuals. These facts will influence the rate of specific personality disorders in older age.

What does empirical research show? Zimmerman and Coryell (1989) observed that individuals with personality disorders were younger than those without. Jackson and Burgess (2000) found the same using a short ICD-10 screening instrument (IPDE screener). Torgersen et al. (2001), however, observed the opposite. This can be explained by the high prevalence of introverted and low prevalence of impulsive personality traits in Norway as compared with the United States.

As to the clusters of personality disorders, Torgersen et al. (2001) found that individuals with odd/eccentric personality disorders were older, whereas Samuels et al. (2002), Coid et al. (2006), and Lenzenweger et al. (2007) did not find any age variation. For the dramatic/emotional cluster, Samuels et al. (2002), Coid et al. (2006), and Lenzenweger et al. (2007) found a higher prevalence among the younger subjects, whereas Torgersen et al. (2001) found that the dramatic/emotional trait dimensions decreased with age. As to the anxious/fearful cluster, neither group observed any age trend.

Among the odd/eccentric personality disorders, schizoid personality disorder or traits seem to be associated with being older (Torgersen et al. 2001; Zimmerman and Coryell 1989, 1990). Several studies have found that paranoid personality disorder is unrelated to age (Torgersen et al. 2001; Zimmerman and Coryell 1989, 1990). Zimmerman and Coryell (1989, 1990) observed that those with schizotypal personality disorder were younger, and Torgersen et al. (2001) found that they were older. Grant et al. (2004) found that both schizoid and paranoid personality disorder decreased with age.

Among the dramatic/emotional personality disorders, those with antisocial and borderline personality disorder or traits are younger (Torgersen et al. 2001; Zimmerman and Coryell 1989, 1990), and Zimmerman and Coryell (1990) observed that those with histrionic and narcissistic traits are younger as well. These results were not confirmed by Torgersen et al. (2001). Grant et al. (2004) observed that histrionic and antisocial personality disorders are more prevalent among younger respondents.

Zimmerman and Coryell (1989, 1990) did not find any age trend for any of the fearful disorders, whereas Torgersen et al. (2001) observed that individuals with obsessive-compulsive disorder and avoidant traits are older. No difference was found for dependent personality disorders. Finally, Grant et al. (2004) reported that avoidant, dependent,

and obsessive-compulsive personality disorders are more common in younger age.

Zimmerman and Coryell (1989) found that individuals with passive-aggressive personality disorder are typically of a younger age, and Torgersen et al. (2001) observed that such traits were negatively correlated with age. The latter study also examined self-defeating and sadistic traits and found that sadistic traits were associated with younger age.

To summarize, persons with antisocial, borderline, or histrionic personality disorder seem to be younger. As for other disorders, the studies are conflicting. The reason for the age difference in disorders is that people become less impulsive and overtly aggressive as they age. Agreeableness and conscientiousness increase with age (Srivastava et al. 2003). Cluster B disorders are typically negatively correlated with agreeableness and conscientiousness (Saulsman and Page 2004).

Marital Status

Most of the results concerning marital status are from Zimmerman and Coryell (1989). Some of the data from Torgersen et al. (2001) have been calculated for this chapter to fit the tables in Zimmerman and Coryell (1989) (see Table 5–3). Grant et al. (2004) also provide information.

As illustrated in Table 5–3, subjects with personality disorder have more often been separated or divorced compared with those without a personality disorder, and they are more often divorced at the time of the interview (Zimmerman and Coryell 1989). They are less frequently married (Jackson and Burgess 2000; Zimmerman and Coryell 1989), and they are more often never married (Zimmerman and Coryell 1989). If we include living nonmarried persons with a partner, subjects with personality disorder live more often alone without a partner compared with those without a personality disorder in the general population (Torgersen et al. 2001).

However, as the risk of having a personality disorder is related to gender and age,

Table 5–3.　Marital status and personality disorders, calculated from Torgersen et al. (2001)

Personality disorder	Number	Single (never married) (%)	Married (%)	Separated[a] (%)	Divorced[a] (%)	Widowed (%)	Ever separated[b] (%)	Ever divorced[c] (%)
Paranoid	46	34.8	34.8	6.5	21.7[c]	2.2	15.8	36.7
Schizoid	32	56.3	31.3	0.0	6.3	6.3	20.0	28.6
Schizotypal	12	50.0	33.3	0.0	8.3	8.3	20.0	16.7
Antisocial	12	75.0[d]	8.3[d]	0.0	16.7	0.0	0.0	66.7
Borderline	14	57.1	35.7	7.1	0.0	0.0	20.0	16.7
Histrionic	39	46.2	35.9	0.0	17.9	0.0	0.0	47.6[d]
Narcissistic	17	35.6	52.9	0.0	5.9	5.9	10.0	9.1
Avoidant	102	45.1	36.3	1.0	14.7	2.9	7.5	28.6
Dependent	31	58.1[d]	25.8[d]	3.2	12.9	0.0	11.1	30.8
Obsessive-compulsive	39	41.6	43.6	0.0	10.3	5.1	5.6	21.7
Passive-aggressive	32	35.3	31.3	6.3	9.4	3.1	18.2	31.3
Self-defeating	17	35.3	17.6[d]	0.0	41.2[e]	5.9	25.0	63.6
Sadistic	4	50.0	56.0	0.0	0.0	0.0	0.0	0.0
Eccentric	80	45.6	33.8[d]	3.8	15.0	2.5	13.8	34.1
Dramatic	62	49.3	35.2	1.4	12.7	1.4	8.3	33.3
Fearful	189	45.5	36.5[d]	1.3	14.1	2.6	8.2	28.2
Any personality disorder	269	43.9	36.8[f]	2.2	15.6[d]	1.5	7.9	33.1[f]
No personality disorder	1,784	38.8	46.5	2.4	10.4	1.8	5.1	23.2
Number	**2,053**	693	830	43	185	33	43	253

[a] At the time of interview.
[b] Excluding those who are never married.
[c] Excluding those who are never married and those who are divorced.
[d] X^2 test, $P < 0.05$
[e] X^2 test, $F < 0.001$
[f] X^2 test, $F < 0.01$

the real effect of other sociodemographic variables such as marital status is difficult to determine. Younger people are less often married, and education is related to gender and age. The best way to determine the independent effect of other sociodemographic variables is to apply multivariate methods. However, to apply such methods one needs large samples. Thus multivariate methods have been used in very few studies. In the study of Torgersen et al. (2001), such multivariate analyses have been carried out for living alone versus living with a partner.

Those with eccentric personality disorders have more often been divorced or separated (Coid et al. 2006; Samuels et al. 2002); they are more often divorced when interviewed, and they have seldom been married (Samuels et al. 2002; Table 5–3). Those with dramatic personality disorders are also often unmarried and live more often alone (Torgersen et al. 2001), and they are more often separated or divorced (Coid et al. 2006). Those with fearful personality disorders are also less often married (Samuels et al. 2002) and live more often alone (Torgersen et al. 2001).

When we examine the specific personality disorders, we encounter problems in comparing the different studies. Marital status does not seem to be as important in the Norwegian study, perhaps because many Norwegians live in stable relationships without being married. When we include "living together with a partner" from the study of Torgersen et al. (2001) and consider this life situation as analogous to marriage, we find more similarity between this study and the study by Zimmerman and Coryell (1989). It is important to note that the relationships in the Torgersen et al. study are based on logistic and linear regression analysis, taking into account a number of other sociodemographic variables.

Among the odd/eccentric personality disorders, those with paranoid personality disorder are more often never married (Grant et al. 2004), divorced (Grant et al. 2004; Table 5–3), or living alone (Torgersen et

al. 2001). Those with schizoid personality disorder are more seldom separated (Zimmerman and Coryell 1989), more often never married or separated/divorced/widowed (Grant et al. 2004), and more often living alone (Torgersen et al. 2001). Those with schizotypal personality disorder have more often been separated (Zimmerman and Coryell 1989) and live more often alone (Torgersen et al. 2001).

Among the Cluster B disorders, persons with histrionic personality disorder have more often been separated or divorced (Zimmerman and Coryell 1989). They are also more often not married when interviewed (Zimmerman and Coryell 1989), more often never married or divorced/separated/widowed (Grant et al. 2004), and live more often alone (Torgersen et al. 2001). Those with antisocial personality disorder also more often have been divorced, separated (Zimmerman and Coryell 1989), or never married (Grant et al. 2004; Table 5–3); are less often married when interviewed; and live more often alone (Torgersen et al. 2001). Persons with borderline personality disorder also have more often been separated if married, are more often divorced, and are not married when interviewed (Zimmerman and Coryell 1989). They are more often never married (Zimmerman and Coryell 1989), and live more often alone (Torgersen et al. 2001). Finally, those with narcissistic personality disorder also more often live alone (Torgersen et al. 2001).

Among persons with anxious/fearful personality disorders, those with avoidant personality disorder have more often been separated (Zimmerman and Coryell 1989). They are more often separated/divorced/widowed when interviewed, and more often never married (Grant et al. 2004). Those with dependent personality disorder more often have been separated when interviewed (Zimmerman and Coryell 1989), never married (Grant et al. 2004; Table 5–3), or separated/divorced/widowed (Grant et al. 2004). Those with obsessive-compulsive traits are less often married (Torgersen et al. 2001).

Among the proposed personality disorders, persons with passive-aggressive personality disorder have more often been divorced and are less often married when interviewed (Zimmerman and Coryell 1989) and live more often alone (Torgersen et al. 2001). Those with self-defeating personality disorder have more often been divorced (Zimmerman and Coryell 1989), are more often divorced (Table 5–3) and not married when interviewed (Zimmerman and Coryell 1989), and more often live alone (Torgersen et al. 2001).

In conclusion, those with personality disorders typically live alone, which is most likely specifically for those with self-defeating, borderline, or schizotypal personality disorder. Those with obsessive-compulsive personality disorder may be an exception. Never being married is often observed among those with antisocial and dependent personality disorder. The risk of divorce/separation is high among those with paranoid personality disorder. In cultures where it is more common to live together unmarried, a breakup in the relationship is less easy to record. For whatever reason, living without a partner is very common among those with personality disorders.

Education and Income

Relatively few studies have investigated the relationship between personality disorders and education and income. Torgersen et al. (2001) observed that those with any personality disorder had less education. The same was observed for those with odd/eccentric personality disorders, and those with dramatic/emotional as well as anxious/fearful personality disorder traits. Samuels et al. (2002) and Lenzenweger et al. (2007) confirmed that those with dramatic/emotional personality disorders had less education but not those with odd/eccentric or anxious/fearful personality disorders. Coid et al. (2006), however, found lower education among those with Cluster A disorders.

In applying logistic regression analysis and taking into account a number of other sociodemographic variables, Torgersen et al. (2001) observed that paranoid and avoidant personality disorders and traits and schizoid, schizotypal, antisocial, borderline, dependent, and self-defeating personality traits were related to lower education. Interestingly, those with obsessive-compulsive disorder or traits in fact had higher education. Only histrionic, narcissistic, and passive-aggressive personality disorders or traits were unrelated to education. Grant et al. (2004) found that lower education was related to all the studied personality disorders (paranoid, schizoid, antisocial, histrionic, avoidant, and dependent), with the exception of obsessive-compulsive personality disorder, which was related to higher education (as Torgersen et al. [2001]) found.

Coid et al. (2006) found that Cluster A disorders were related to unemployment and lower social class, Cluster B disorders were related to lower social class, and Cluster C disorders were related to being "economically inactive" but not unemployed. Grant et al. (2004) found that lower income was related to all the studied personality disorders, except obsessive-compulsive personality disorder. Lenzenweger et al. (2007) found that only borderline personality disorder was related to unemployment.

Samuels et al. (2002) also investigated the relationship between income and personality disorders but did not find any association. Jackson and Burgess (2000) did not find any relationship to unemployment. It is important to note that these studies applied multivariate methods, taking into account other sociodemographic variables.

In conclusion, personality disorders, with a few exceptions, are related to lower socioeconomic status and economic problems. This holds true for all of the Cluster A disorders (paranoid, schizoid, and schizotypal) and for at least two Cluster B disorders (antisocial and borderline). It is not true for narcissistic personality disorder, and the socioeconomic status of those with histrionic personality disorder is equivocal. As to Cluster C disorders, avoidant and dependent personality disorders imply poorer socioeconomic status, whereas the opposite is true for obsessive-compulsive personality disorder. For the provisional disorders, there exists only one study (Torgersen et al. 2001) suggesting lower education for those with self-defeating and sadistic, but not passive-aggressive, personality disorders.

Urban Location

The study of Torgersen et al. (2001) showed that those living in the populated center of the city more often had a personality disorder. The same was true for all clusters of personality disorders and all specific disorders except antisocial, sadistic, avoidant, and dependent personality. Grant et al. (2004) found this to be true only for paranoid and avoidant personality disorders, not antisocial, histrionic, schizoid, dependent, or obsessive-compulsive personality disorders. The two studies agree that paranoid personality disorder, but not antisocial and dependent personality disorders, are related to urbanicity. They disagree about schizoid, histrionic, avoidant, and obsessive-compulsive personality disorders, while the rest of the personality disorders are not included in the study.

Given that more people with personality disorders are found in the center than in the outskirts of a city, one may speculate about the reason for this. Quality of life is generally lower in the center of the city (Cramer et al. 2004), and there is a higher rate of symptom disorders in the city or in the center of the city (Kringlen et al. 2001; Lewis and Booth 1992, 1994; Marcelis et al. 1998; Sundquist et al. 2004; van Os et al. 2001). One reason may be that the concentrated urban life creates stress leading to personality disorders. Another reason may be that individuals with personality problems drift to the center, where they can lead an anonymous life. A third explanation may be that less social control simply

makes it easier to express the less socially acceptable aspects of one's personality. We used to think that excessive social control creates mental problems. Perhaps social control hinders the development of accentuated eccentric, narcissistic, and impulsive personality styles.

QUALITY OF LIFE AND DYSFUNCTION

Central to the definition of personality disorder are the interpersonal problems, reduced well-being, and dysfunction that personality disorders imply. In the sample studied by Torgersen et al. (2001), quality of life was assessed by interview and included the following aspects: subjective well-being, self-realization, relation to friends, social support, negative life events, relation to family of origin, and neighborhood quality (Cramer et al. 2003, 2006, 2007). All aspects were integrated in a global quality-of-life index.

Personality disorders turned out to be more strongly related to quality of life than Axis I mental disorders, somatic health, and any other socioeconomic, demographic, or life situation variable. Among the specific personality disorders, avoidant personality disorder was most strongly related to quality of life, controlling for all the aforementioned variables. Next came schizotypal, then paranoid, schizoid, borderline, dependent, antisocial personality disorders, and narcissistic and self-defeating personality disorders to a lesser degree. Histrionic, obsessive-compulsive, and passive-aggressive personality disorders were unrelated to quality of life. Some may be surprised that borderline personality disorder was not more strongly related to reduced quality of life. The reason for this is that the disorder is related to a number of other variables that are related to quality of life. Hence, the variables become weaker in a multiple regression analysis.

A dysfunction index was created by combining quality of life (reversed); the answer to the Structured Interview for DSM-III Personality Disorders–Revised question "do you feel that the way you usually deal with people and handle situations causes you problems?"; the number of lifetime Axis I diagnoses; and any incidence of seeking treatment with varying degrees of seriousness, from private psychologist and psychiatrist—via outpatient and inpatient clinics—to psychiatric hospitals. The dysfunction index was related to personality disorder much as the global quality-of-life index was. The only differences found in comparing results derived from the dysfunction index with those from the global quality-of-life index were that those persons with borderline, dependent, or self-defeating personality disorder appeared more dysfunctional, and those persons with antisocial personality disorder appeared less dysfunctional. The reason for the differences is mainly that those with borderline, histrionic, dependent, and self-defeating personality disorders are more likely to seek treatment and those with antisocial personality disorders are less likely to seek treatment.

However, the most important result in this study was that for both quality of life and dysfunction, there was a perfect linear dose–response relationship to numbers of criteria fulfilled for all personality disorders together and to the number of criteria fulfilled for any specific personality disorder. Thus, if a person has one criterion fulfilled for one or another personality disorder, the quality of life is lower and dysfunction is higher than among those with no criteria fulfilled. Those with two criteria fulfilled on one or more specific disorders have more problems than those with one, those with three criteria have more problems than those with two, and so on. In other words, when those with zero criteria on all disorders were grouped together—that is, those with a maximum of one criterion on any disorder, those with a maximum of two, and so on—the relationship to global quality of life and dysfunction was perfectly linear (Figures 5–1 and 5–2). This result means that there are no argu-

ments for any specific number of criteria to define a personality disorder if one uses quality of life or dysfunction as validation variables. There is no natural cutoff point.

A high level of dysfunction and disability was also observed among those with schizotypal personality disorder, followed by borderline and avoidant personality disorders, in a large-scale multicenter study (Skodol et al. 2002). It was also observed that those with obsessive-compulsive personality disorder showed much less disability.

In another study, Ullrich et al. (2007), found that obsessive-compulsive personality disorder was not related to poor functioning—in fact, it was quite the opposite. Also histrionic personality disorder was positively related to "status and wealth," while narcissistic and paranoid personality disorders were unrelated to this index as well as to "successful intimate relationships." Taken together, those with schizoid personality disorder scored poorest on these two indexes, followed by antisocial, schizotypal, avoidant, borderline, and dependent personality disorders.

Zimmerman and Coryell (1989) also found a high frequency of psychosexual dysfunction among persons with avoidant personality disorder. Surprisingly, this dysfunction was infrequent among persons with borderline personality disorder, and, not surprisingly, it was also infrequent among those with antisocial personality disorder.

Grant et al. (2004) applied a short form of quality of life assessment, the Short Form Health Survey, Version 2 (SF-12v2; Ware et al. 2002) and found that those with dependent personality disorder had the poorest quality of life, followed by those with avoidant, paranoid, schizoid, or antisocial personality disorders. There was no reduction in quality of life for those with histrionic personality disorder, and a reduction on only one of three scores for those with obsessive-compulsive personality disorder.

Crawford et al. (2005) studied impairment using the Global Assessment of Functioning (GAF) scale. Those with borderline

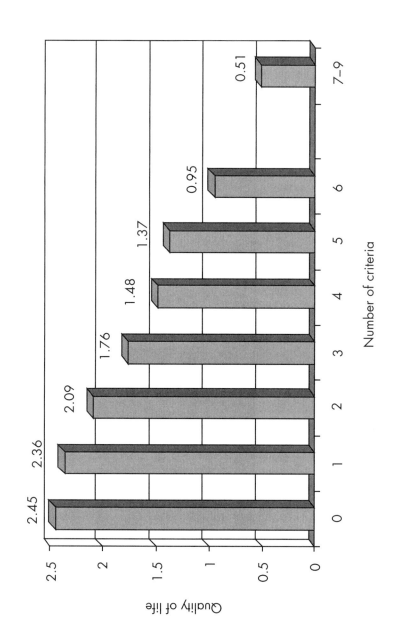

Figure 5–1.   The relationship between maximum number of criteria fulfilled on any personality disorder and quality of life.

As explained in text, the ordinate (quality of life) is a composite of subjective well-being, self-realization, social support, negative life events, and relation to family, friends and neighbors. The mean is set to 2 and the standard deviation is 1.

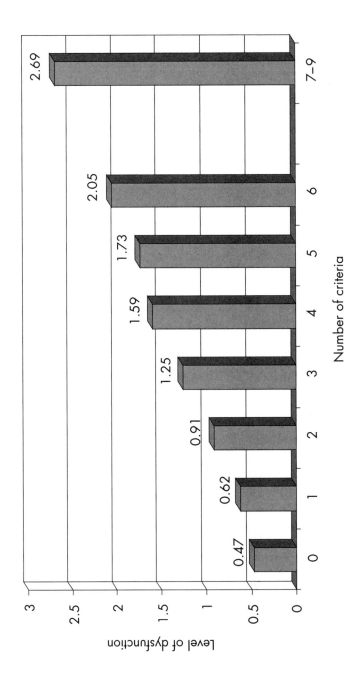

Figure 5–2. The relationship between maximum number of criteria fulfilled on any personality disorder and dysfunction.

As explained in the text, the ordinate (dysfunction) is a composite of life quality (reversed), treatment seeking, the number of lifetime Axis I diagnoses, and the notion that one's behavior causes problems. The mean and standard deviation are 1.

personality disorder had the poorest functioning, followed by avoidant, schizotypal, narcissistic, antisocial, paranoid, histrionic, dependent, and schizoid personality disorders. Only obsessive-compulsive personality disorder had no indication of dysfunction.

In conclusion, all studies taken together show that reduced quality of life and dysfunction are highest among those with avoidant personality disorder, followed closely by those with schizotypal or borderline personality disorders. Those with paranoid, schizoid, dependent, or antisocial personality disorder follow. There are few studies showing impaired quality of life for histrionic, narcissistic, or obsessive-compulsive personality disorder. The same is true for the quality of provisional personality disorders, passive-aggressive, self-defeating, and sadistic personality disorders. However, it should be noted that a problem with many of these studies is a lack of control for other variables correlating with specific personality disorders and quality of life, dysfunction, and impairment.

There is reason to question whether histrionic and obsessive-compulsive personality disorders, in spite of their long histories, deserve a status as personality disorder. Narcissistic personality disorder was not included in ICD-10, which some would view as a wise decision. The provisional disorders "provided for further study" do not appear to deserve an inclusion in the nosology of personality disorders.

In the future, there is reason to believe that we will see more studies of quality of life, dysfunction, impairment, and disability among subjects with personality disorders, either in the general population or in patient samples.

POINT PREVALENCE AND LIFETIME PREVALENCE

Lifetime prevalence for disorders is necessarily higher than point prevalence. If we measure the percentage of the population with a disorder during the last 2 weeks, 1 month, 1 year, 2 years, or 5 years, the percentage will be lower than if we follow a population throughout the whole life span. This obvious fact has long since been established for Axis I mental disorders. The same will hold true for personality disorders, provided the disorders are not there already in early age and stay chronic throughout life. While some theories may suggest this to be the case, empirical research shows that many individuals are free of the personality disorder after a relatively short time (Grilo et al. 2004; Zanarini et al. 2006). At the same time, the 2–5 years point prevalence is much the same over age, as we have seen. The implication is that new cases have to debut in the population replacing those that disappear, even if some few reappear (Ferro et al. 1998; Durbin and Klein 2006). The consequence is that the percentage of the population that will fulfill the criteria for a personality disorder in one or more periods of their life is much higher than 10%. This may be surprising for some, but it is an inevitable consequence of the continuous nature of personality disorders and the application of a threshold number of criteria to define personality disorders. (Some with personality disorders regress toward the population mean and do not any longer show the prescribed number of criteria. Other individuals with too few criteria display an increase and jump over and above the threshold.)

In the future, longitudinal studies will give us valuable insight into the epidemiology of personality disorders.

CONCLUSION

Personality disorders are prevalent: more than 1 in 10 adult individuals has a personality disorder.

The average prevalence of the specific personality disorders is a little above 1%, somewhat higher for obsessive-compulsive, passive-aggressive, avoidant, histrionic, and antisocial personality disorders, and somewhat lower for sadistic, narcissistic, and self-defeating personality disorders. Two of these low-prevalence disorders, sadistic and self-defeating, are only "provided for further study" in DSM-III-R (American Psychiatric Association 1987), and none of the three exists in ICD-10.

Those with dependent, borderline, obsessive-compulsive, avoidant, and schizotypal personality disorders are overrepresented in patient populations, both overall and when gender is controlled for, whereas those with antisocial, schizoid, and paranoid personality disorders are underrepresented.

The highest prevalences of personality disorders in the general population are observed among subjects with lower education living in populated areas, for example in the city center. They often have a history of divorce and separation and are more often living without a partner.

Men have typically a schizoid, antisocial, or obsessive-compulsive personality disorder, whereas women are more inclined toward a dependent or histrionic personality disorder. Antisocial, borderline, and passive-aggressive personality disorders are more often observed among younger persons, whereas older individuals more often have a schizoid personality disorder. It is typical for those with personality disorder (with an exception for obsessive-compulsive personality disorder) to to live alone. In many cases, some are never married (antisocial, dependent), have a history of frequent divorces (borderline), are divorced (paranoid), or not married (histrionic) when interviewed.

Lower education is most typical for those with paranoid and avoidant personality disorders, whereas those with obsessive-compulsive personality disorder in fact have higher education than those without the disorder. Those with paranoid, schizotypal, and passive-aggressive personality disorders are most inclined to live in the city center.

Personality disorders imply dysfunction and reduction in quality of life, including reduced subjective well-being and self-realization, relational problems, lack of social support, and frequent negative life events.

Among the personality disorders, individuals with avoidant, schizotypal, and borderline personality disorders tend to have the most reduced quality of life, dysfunction, and disability, followed by those with paranoid, schizoid, dependent, and antisocial personality disorders. Individuals with obsessive-compulsive, histrionic, narcissistic, passive-aggressive, or sadistic personality disorders tend to have little or no reduction in quality of life, dysfunction, and disability.

There is an even reduction in quality of life and an even increase in dysfunction for each criterion manifested. Thus, there is a continuous relationship between those with no or small personality problems, those with moderate problems, and those with severe problems. No natural cutoff point exists. Any definition of how many criteria are required for a personality disorder is arbitrary. Even so, to have a definition is important for communication. However, a change in criteria will immediately change the prevalence estimates in the society. Consequently, correlations between personality disorders and other variables are more important than prevalence rates. These correlations appear to be independent of how strictly personality disorders are defined.

Because of the continuous nature of personality disorders, their tendency to disappear, and the even distribution of point prevalence over age, new personality disorders have to arise over the life span. Consequently, the likelihood of having a personality disorder once in the lifetime may be surprisingly high.

Epidemiological research has perhaps changed some stereotypic notions about personality disorders. They are more frequent in the general population than we generally believed, especially the introverted personality disorders. Borderline personality disorder is not a "female disorder." Living without a partner is a risk factor for personality disorders, but being unmarried is less a risk factor than many would have believed. Those living in a partnership without being married function well.

Care must be taken to avoid believing that these correlations display one-directional causal relationships. Personality disorders may hinder obtaining higher levels of education and may create socioeconomic difficulties. Problematic personality traits may prevent a person from going into a relationship or may lead to the breaking-up of relationships, rather than having relationship issues and problems causing problematic personality traits.

Personality disorders are not something that a person necessarily has for life. Impulsive and aggressive features may decrease quickly with age, whereas introverted traits increase as people get older.

Perhaps one of the most important aspects of personality disorders is the reduction of quality of life that is implied. However, a low quality of life does not necessarily create a personality disorder; the opposite is just as likely.

REFERENCES

Alnæs R, Torgersen S: DSM-III symptom disorders (Axis I) and personality disorders (Axis II) in an outpatient population. Acta Psychiatr Scand 78:348–355, 1988

American Psychiatric Association: Diagnostic and Statistical Manual of Mental Disorders, 3rd Edition, Revised. Washington, DC, American Psychiatric Association, 1987

American Psychiatric Association: Diagnostic and Statistical Manual of Mental Disorders, 4th Edition. Washington, DC, American Psychiatric Association, 1994

American Psychiatric Association: Diagnostic and Statistical Manual of Mental Disorders, 4th Edition, Text Revision. Washington, DC, American Psychiatric Association, 2000

Black DW, Noyes R Jr, Pfohl B, et al: Personality disorder in obsessive-compulsive volunteers, well comparison subjects, and their first-degree relatives. Am J Psychiatry 150:1226–1232, 1993

Carter JD, Joyce PR, Mulder RT, et al: Gender differences in the frequency of personality disorders in depressed outpatients. J Personal Disord 13:67–74, 1999

Coid J, Yang M, Tyrer P, et al: Prevalences and correlates of personality disorder. Br J Psychiatry 188:423–431, 2006

Cramer V, Torgersen S, Kringlen E: Personality disorders, prevalence, sociodemographic correlations, quality of life, dysfunction, and the question of continuity. Persønlichkeitsstørungen. Theorie und Therapie 7:189–198, 2003

Cramer V, Torgersen S, Kringlen E: Quality of life in a city: the effect of population density. Soc Indic Res 69:103–116, 2004

Cramer V, Torgersen S, Kringlen E: Personality disorders and quality of life. A population study. Compr Psychiatry 47:178–184, 2006

Cramer V, Torgersen S, Kringlen E: Socio-demographic conditions, subjective somatic health, Axis I disorders and personality disorders in the common population: the relationship to quality of life. J Personal Disord 21:552–567, 2007

Crawford TN, Cohen P, Johnson JG, et al: Self-reported personality disorder in the children in the community sample: convergent and prospective validity in late adolescence and adulthood. J Personal Disord 19:30–52, 2005

Durbin EC, Klein DN: Ten-year stability of personality disorders among outpatients with mood disorders. J Abnorm Psychol 115:75–84, 2006

Ferro T, Klein DN, Schwartz JE, et al: Thirty-month stability of personality disorder diagnoses in depressed outpatients. Am J Psychiatry 155:653–659, 1998

Fossati A, Feeney JA, Donati D, et al: Personality disorders and adult attachment dimensions in a mixed psychiatric sample: a multivariate study. J Nerv Ment Dis 191:30–37, 2003

Golomb M, Fava M, Abraham M, et al: Gender differences in personality disorders. Am J Psychiatry 152:579–582, 1995

Grant BF, Hasin DS, Stinson FR, et al: Prevalences, correlates, and disability of personality disorders in the United States: results from the National Epidemiologic Survey on Alcohol and Related Conditions. J Clin Psychiatry 65:948–958, 2004

Grilo CM, Sanislow CA, Gunderson JG, et al: Two-year stability and change of schizotypal, borderline, avoidant, and obsessive-compulsive personality disorders. J Consult Clin Psychol 72:767–775, 2004

Jackson HP, Burgess PM: Personality disorders in the community: a report from the Australian National Survey of Mental Health and Well Being. Soc Psychiatry Psychiatr Epidemiol 35:531–538, 2000

Klein DN, Riso LP, Donaldson SK, et al: Family study of early onset dysthymia: mood and personality disorders in relatives of outpatients with dysthymia and episodic major depressive and normal controls. Arch Gen Psychiatry 52:487–496, 1995

Kringlen E, Torgersen S, Cramer V: A Norwegian psychiatric epidemiological study. Am J Psychiatry 158:1091–1098, 2001

Lenzenweger MF, Loranger AW, Korfine L, et al: Detecting personality disorders in a nonclinical population: application of a 2-stage procedure for case identification. Arch Gen Psychiatry 54:345–351, 1997

Lenzenweger MF, Lane MC, Loranger AW, et al: DSM-IV personality disorders in the national comorbidity survey replication. Biol Psychiatry 62:553–564, 2007

Lewis G, Booth M: Regional differences in mental health in Great Britain. J Epidemiol Community Health 46:608–611, 1992

Lewis G, Booth M: Are cities bad for your mental health? Psychol Med 24:913–915, 1994

Maier W, Lichtermann D, Klingler T, et al: Prevalences of personality disorders (DSM-III-R) in the community. J Personal Disord 6:187–196, 1992

Marcelis M, Navarro-Mateu F, Murray R: Urbanization and psychosis: a study of 1942–1978 birth cohorts in the Netherlands. Psychol Med 28:1197–1203, 1998

Moldin SO, Rice JP, Erlenmeyer-Kimling L, et al: Latent structure of DSM-III-R Axis II psychopathology in a normal sample. J Abnorm Psychol 103:259–266, 1994

Samuels J, Eaton WW, Bienvenu OJ III, et al: Prevalences and correlates of personality disorders in a community sample. Br J Psychiatry 180:536–542, 2002

Saulsman LM, Page AC: The five-factor model and personality disorders empirical literature: a meta-analytic review. Clin Psychol Rev 23:1055–1085, 2004

Skodol AE, Gunderson JG, McGlashan TH, et al: Functional impairment in patients with schizotypal, borderline, avoidant, or obsessive-compulsive personality disorder. Am J Psychiatry 159:276–283, 2002

Srivastava S, John OP, Gosling SD, et al: Development of personality in early and middle adulthood: set like plaster or persistent change? Journal of Personal Social Psychology 84:1041–1053, 2003

Stangl D, Pfohl B, Zimmerman M, et al: A structured interview for the DSM-III personality disorders. Arch Gen Psychiatry 42:591–596, 1985

Sundquist K, Frank G, Sundquist J: Urbanisation and incidence of psychosis and depression. Br J Psychiatry 184:293–298, 2004

Torgersen S, Kringlen E, Cramer V: The prevalence of personality disorders in a community sample. Arch Gen Psychiatry 58:590–596, 2001

Ullrich S, Farrington DP, Coid JW: Dimensions of DSM-IV personality disorders and life-success. J Personal Disord 21:657–663, 2007

van Os J, Hanssen M, Bijl RV, et al: Prevalence of psychotic disorder and community level of psychotic symptoms: an urban-rural comparison. Arch Gen Psychiatry 58:663–668, 2001

Ware JE, Kosinski M, Turner-Bowker DM, et al: How to Score Version 2 of the SF-12 Health Survey. Lincoln, RI, Quality Metric, 2002

World Health Organization: The ICD-10 Classification of Mental and Behavioural Disorders: Clinical Description and Diagnostic Guidelines. Geneva, World Health Organization, 1992

Zanarini MC, Frankenburg FR, Hennen J, et al: Prediction of the 10-years course of borderline personality disorder. Am J Psychiatry 163:827–832, 2006

Zimmerman M, Coryell W: DSM-III personality disorder diagnoses in a nonpatient sample: demographic correlates and comorbidity. Arch Gen Psychiatry 46:682–689, 1989

Zimmerman M, Coryell WH: Diagnosing personality disorders in the community: a comparison of self-report and interview measures. Arch Gen Psychiatry 47:527–531, 1990

6

Neurobiology

Emil F. Coccaro, M.D.
Larry J. Siever, M.D.

The study of personality disorders involves the study of both disordered character and disordered temperament. *Character* relates to how we see and operate in our world and is based on how we develop and what we are taught about how to go through life. *Temperament*, in contrast, relates to our innate tendency to behave and to react to any of a variety of challenges presented by other people and our environment. Although both aspects of personality may be studied empirically, the study of temperament is uniquely suited to biological study because temperament has known genetic and neurobiological correlates, both of which are linked to critical processes involving cognition, emotion, and behavior.

The neurobiology of temperament, as it appears in personality disorders, can be studied in a variety of ways, including those that involve behavioral genetics, neuropsychopharmacology, molecular genetics, psychophysiology, and neuroimaging. Behavioral-genetic study informs us about the degree to which personality (or temperamental) traits are under genetic influence. This work largely involves studies of families and twins and is designed to document familial, if not genetic, components to behavior. Previous work defining the genetic underpinnings of temperament has been critical to our current understanding that temperament is inherently biological in nature. Neuropsychopharmacological study informs us about the nature of brain chemistry and how the regulation of any of a variety of brain neurotransmitters influences temperament. Work in this area has led to the understanding that brain serotonin, for example, is critical in modulating impulsive aggressive behavior in individuals with personality disorder. Consequently, work in neuropsychopharmacology leads to work in molecular genetics whereby the presence of a specific copy of a specific gene (e.g., for a component of the brain serotonin system) influences a temperamental trait. For example, individuals carrying a specific gene for the serotonin transporter may be more anxious than other individuals who do not carry this gene. Finally, work in psychophysiology and neuroimaging brings investigative work up to a level that integrates genes, neuropsychopharmacology, and networks of neural transmission. In this methodology, both brain structure and brain function are examined regarding their contribution to the expression of various temperamental traits. In some groups of patients with personality disorder, neuroimaging has revealed differences in the size and function of specific structures.

Ultimately, the study of the neurobiology of personality disorders is conducted to lead to a more comprehensive understanding of the biological substrates of personality disorder so that better treatments may be discovered and existing treatments may be improved. Uncovering the biological substrate for a specific temperamental trait naturally leads to treatment strategies aimed at this specific substrate. The best example of this approach is the use of serotonin uptake inhibitors in the treatment of impulsive aggression in individuals with personality disorders. Curiously, work in this area revealed the likely presence of two treatment response groups: one responsive to serotonin uptake inhibitors, the other responsive to mood stabilizers.

In this chapter, we discuss the various aspects of the neurobiology of personality disorder on a cluster-by-cluster basis. We have chosen this organization because the prototypical personality disorders of interest tend to break out into one of the three personality disorder clusters. Despite this type of organization, we should note that research has clearly shown the relevance of a dimensional approach to the study of personality. Each section begins with a brief summary of the phenomenology characteristic of each personality disorder cluster and follows with a summary of data relevant to behavioral genetics, neuropsychopharmacology (and molecular genetics where relevant), and neuropsychology and neuroimaging. Each of the first two sections ends with a brief vignette il-

lustrating some of the points made about the psychobiology of prototypical patients with selected personality disorders.

CLUSTER A PERSONALITY DISORDERS

The Cluster A personality disorders include schizotypal, paranoid, and schizoid personality disorder. The criteria of these disorders capture shared characteristics of social isolation, detachment, suspiciousness, and in the case of schizotypal personality disorder, psychotic-like cognitive/perceptional distortion. Schizotypal personality was formulated in part on the clinical profile observed in relatives of schizophrenic probands, whereas the other two were defined more in a clinical tradition. A high degree of overlap exists between schizotypal and paranoid personality disorder, whereas schizoid personality disorder is not frequently diagnosed in the clinical setting and may represent a milder version of the Cluster A personality disorders. These disorders can be perceived as consisting of a dimension of social deficits (no friends, detached affect) and cognitive impairment, and in the case of schizotypal personality disorder, a psychotic-like dimension. Because of its relationship to schizophrenia and its more common prevalence in clinical populations, most of the neurobiological research on this cluster has focused on schizotypal personality disorder and is summarized here in relation to these dimensions.

Behavioral Genetics

Schizotypal personality disorder is found more frequently in the relatives of schizophrenic probands than in the relatives of control subjects, and this association is grounded in genetics rather than shared familial environment as suggested by adoptive and twin studies (Siever 1991). The genetics of paranoid personality disorder are less well understood, but it has a high overlap with schizotypal personality disorder, and its presence may be greater in families of patients with schizophrenia or delusional disorder (Webb and Levinson 1993). Schizoid personality disorder has received little or no genetic study but is more common in the relatives of patients with schizophrenia (Kalus et al. 1993).

Neuropsychopharmacology: Dopamine System

The dopamine system has been extensively studied in patients with schizophrenia and particularly associated with the psychotic symptoms of this disorder, consistent with the antipsychotic effects of the neuroleptics, which act as dopamine antagonists. Accordingly, given the phenomenological and genetic relationships between schizophrenia and schizotypal personality disorder, the dopaminergic system has been the primary neurotransmitter system studied in schizotypal personality disorder.

Neurochemistry

Plasma homovanillic acid (HVA), a major metabolite of dopamine, has been found to be elevated in clinically selected patients with schizotypal personality disorder, and this elevation is significantly correlated with psychotic-like criteria for this disorder, such that statistical correction for the presence of psychotic-like symptoms abolishes the difference between groups (Siever et al. 1991). An identical configuration of results is found with respect to cerebrospinal fluid (CSF) HVA (Siever et al. 1993). On the other hand, among relatives of patients with schizophrenia, who are generally characterized more by the social and cognitive deficit-like symptoms of schizotypal personality disorder, plasma HVA is lower in subjects with schizotypal personality disorder than control subjects (Amin et al. 1999). In these studies, plasma HVA was negatively correlated with the negative or deficit-like symptoms of

schizotypal personality disorder. Interestingly, however, when the negative symptoms were entered as a covariant, the positive relationship with psychotic-like symptoms in plasma HVA emerged (Amin et al. 1997). Reduced plasma HVA concentrations have been associated with impairment in tests of frontally mediated executive function such as the Wisconsin Card Sort Test (Siever et al. 1991). Thus, these results suggest that dopaminergic activity may be relatively increased or decreased depending on the predominance of psychotic-like versus deficit-like symptoms, respectively. This distinction is consistent with formulations that increased dopaminergic activity, particularly in striatum, is associated with psychotic-like symptoms and that decreased dopaminergic activity, particularly in prefrontal regions, is especially associated with deficit-like symptoms (Siever and Davis 2004).

Acute Pharmacological Interventions

Amphetamine, which stimulates the release of the monoamines, particularly dopamine and norepinephrine, has been shown to improve the cognitive performance of schizotypal personality disorder subjects on tests of executive function, working memory, and to a lesser extent, sustained attention and verbal learning (Kirrane et al. 2000; Siegel et al. 1996). These improvements are more consistent than those observed in schizophrenic subjects given amphetamine and are not accompanied by the behavioral worsening— that is, increased psychotic symptoms— found after amphetamine administration in schizophrenic patients. Indeed, the deficit-like symptoms of schizotypal personality disorder tend to improve following amphetamine administration (Laruelle et al. 2002; Siegel et al. 1996). These results suggest that agents that enhance catecholamines, including dopamine, may have beneficial effects on cognition, presumably through stimulation of D_1 receptors in prefrontal cortex.

Similarly, the administration of a glucopyruvic stressor, 2-deoxyglucose, which activates stress-sensitive subcortical systems such as the dopamine system and the hypothalamic-pituitary-adrenal (HPA) axis, results in greater stress-related (i.e., plasma cortisol and HVA) responses in patients with schizophrenia than in control subjects. In contrast, patients with schizotypal personality disorder show normal (plasma HVA) or even reduced (cortisol) activation compared with control subjects, suggesting that patients with schizotypal personality disorder have better-buffered subcortical stress-responsive systems than patients with schizophrenia. Consequently, it is possible that this buffer provides a protective factor against psychosis in patients with schizotypal personality disorder (Siever and Davis 2004).

Longer-term pharmacological interventions have been evaluated in individuals with schizotypal personality disorder to determine their effects on cognitive function. Studies of guanfacine, an α_2-adrenergic agonist, and pergolide, a D_1/D_2 agonist, suggest improvement in cognitive function, particularly working memory, with these catecholaminergic interventions, consistent with the facilitatory effects of the catecholamines on cognitive function and prefrontal cortex (McClure et al. 2007). Cognitive function may also improve with risperidone (Koenigsberg et al. 2003), possibly due to the effects that 5-hydroxytryptamine (serotonin) type 2 receptor (5-HT$_2$) blockade has on facilitating dopaminergic activity in frontal lobe. Antipsychotic effects have been documented in a number of clinical trials of atypical and typical neuroleptics in individuals with schizotypal personality disorder (Hymowitz et al. 1986; Schulz et al. 2003).

DNA Polymorphisms

Catechol-*O*-methyltransferase (COMT) plays a critical role in inactivation of dopamine in the frontal lobe, where the dopamine transporter is not the primary mode of inactivation of dopamine. Recently, a single nucleotide polymorphism in the COMT gene has been discovered. With this polymor-

phism, the allele for the COMT gene codes for the amino acid valine (Val), as opposed to methionine (Met), in the COMT enzyme. The substitution of Val for Met leads to a COMT enzyme that has far more activity than a *COMT* enzyme coded by the MET allele. Thus, individuals with VAL alleles should have increased activity of COMT compared with those with the MET allele. Because increased COMT activity is associated with increased destruction of catecholamines, individuals with VAL alleles should have less central dopamine activity than those with MET alleles. Consistent with this idea, cognitive impairment, particularly evident in dopamine-dependent working memory, has been associated with the presence of the *VAL* allele in patients with schizophrenia (Weinberger et al. 2001) as well as their healthy siblings and control subjects (Goldberg et al. 2003). Studies in patients with schizotypal personality disorder also suggest an association between cognitive impairment and the VAL allele, consistent with the role of reduced dopaminergic activity hypothesized to contribute to the cognitive dysfunction in the schizophrenia spectrum disorders such as schizotypal personality disorder (Minzenberg et al. 2006).

Cognitive Function and Psychophysiology

Although cognitive dysfunction may exist in subtle forms in a variety of personality disorders, the most consistent and robust changes are found in people with Cluster A personality disorders, more specifically schizotypal personality disorder. Patients with schizotypal personality disorder show attenuated patterns of cognitive impairment similar to those of patients with schizophrenia but somewhat more specific. For example, overall intelligence may not be impaired (Mitropoulou et al. 2002; Trestman et al. 1995), whereas specific disturbances in sustained attention, in verbal learning, and particularly in working memory have been reported in patients with schizotypal personality disorder compared with patients with other non-schizophrenia-related personality disorders, the latter of whom are generally not impaired in these indices, and with normal control subjects (Mitropoulou et al. 2002, 2005). Although patients with schizophrenia showed deviations from normal control subjects on the order of two standard deviations, patients with schizotypal personality disorder have more on the order of one standard deviation below the mean or less (Mitropoulou et al. 2002, 2005). The deficits in working memory and attention may contribute to the impaired rapport and misreading of verbal and facial cues in patients with schizotypal personality disorder, who often clinically complain that they have a hard time focusing on others, which detracts from their ability to engage. Indeed, performances on working memory tasks have been reported to be correlated with interpersonal impairment and account for the other cognitive impairments in schizotypal personality disorder (Mitropoulou et al. 2005; Siever et al. 2002).

A variety of psychophysiological endophenotypes that may reflect genetic substrates to the schizophrenia spectrum disorders have been found to be abnormal in patients with schizotypal personality disorder as well as in patients with chronic schizophrenia. Many of these psychophysiological abnormalities have also been found in relatives of patients with schizophrenia, who may have mild schizophrenia-spectrum symptoms or may even appear to be clinically healthy, raising the possibility that these abnormalities reflect an underlying genetic susceptibility to the schizophrenia spectrum that is variably expressed. Although a detailed review of psychophysiological abnormalities is beyond the scope of this chapter, abnormalities in eye movement, visual processing, and inhibition of startle response are among the most consistently replicated. Thus, individuals with schizotypal personality disorder showed impaired smooth-pursuit eye movement, antisaccade generation, and velocity discrimination. Furthermore, they show less capacity for inhibition on a prepulse inhibition paradigm and P_{50}-evoked potential paradigm (Cadenhead 2002). The latter finding is of particular interest because it has been linked to a specific allele of the nicotinic receptor in families of patients with schizophrenia. Backward masking, reflecting early visual processing, has also been reported to be abnormal in patients with schizotypal personality disorder and schizophrenia (Siever and Davis 2004; see Braff and Freedman [2002] for an overview of these psychophysiological abnormalities).

Neuroimaging

Structural Imaging

Patients with schizotypal personality disorders show ventricular enlargement and reduced volumes of several brain regions, as do patients with schizophrenia. In studies of patients with schizotypal personality disorder, ventricular volume is increased, although studies of relatives of patients with schizotypal personality disorder are mixed (Shihabuddin et al. 1996; Siever 1995). Temporal volume reductions in patients with schizotypal personality disorder appear to be comparable with those observed in schizophrenic patients and occur in both superior temporal gyrus and other temporal regions. However, some data suggest that frontal volumes are relatively preserved, especially frontal pole (Brodmann area 10 [BA10]), suggesting that greater frontal capacity may serve as a buffer against the severe cognitive and social deterioration we see in schizophrenia (Hazlett et al. 2008). Whereas striatal volumes of patients with schizophrenia are enlarged secondary (in large part) to neuroleptic medications, the striatal volumes (including putamen [Shihabuddin et al. 2001] and caudate [Levitt et al. 2002]) of patients with schizotypal personality disorder are reduced in comparison with normal control subjects and unmedicated patients with schizophrenia. Reduced striatal volumes are consistent with the possibility of reduced dopaminergic activity, which may be protective against the emergence of psychosis.

Functional Imaging

Both positron emission tomography (PET) and single photon emission computed tomography (SPECT) functional imaging studies suggest that patients with schizotypal personality disorder do not activate regions such as dorsolateral prefrontal cortex in response to an executive function or learning task to the same degree as control subjects, but do so to a greater degree than do patients with schizophrenia. However, patients with schizotypal personality disorder are able to activate other compensatory regions, including the anterior pole of frontal cortex (BA 10), which is believed to be a high-level executive region (Buchsbaum et al. 2002). A recent functional magnetic resonance imaging (fMRI) study (Koenigsberg et al. 2005) using a visuospatial working-memory task also showed increased activation in patients with schizotypal personality disorder in BA 10, but lesser activation in dorsolateral prefrontal cortex than in normal control subjects. Thus, patients with schizotypal personality disorder may have compensatory mechanisms available to them that patients with schizophrenia do not have in the face of diminished capacity to use dorsolateral prefrontal cortex. The compensatory mechanisms may involve using higher executive regions than are required for normal individuals.

An IBZM SPECT study measuring dopamine released by displacement of [^{11}C] iodine-methoxybenzamide (IBZM) demonstrated that subjects with schizotypal personality disorder released significantly more dopamine in response to amphetamine administration than did normal control subjects but less than did acute schizophrenic patients (Siever et al. 2002). These results are consistent with functional imaging studies suggesting increased activation of ventral striatum, which is normally inhibited by dopamine, in unmedicated schizotypal patients compared with control subjects and unmedicated schizophrenic patients as well as the reduced plasma HVA responses to 2-deoxyglucose and striatal volumes noted earlier in these studies, suggesting dopaminergic activity that is better buffered than that of schizophrenic patients.

Case Example

Mr. B is a 56-year-old, common-law married male, employed in his extended family's business, whose current complaint is that "people at work are accusing me of saying things that I am not saying." Mr. B has been seen by the psychiatry service for more than 20 years, after he was admitted to medicine for complaints of back pain. He was transferred to psychiatry because he "couldn't stand up." He was first psychiatrically hospitalized when he was in the Navy for an episode of "going crazy" after a dispute with his captain. He had symptoms of depersonalization, irritability, and difficulty getting along with his peers. Six years after his tour in the Navy, he saw a therapist but would have vivid dreams that were disturbing to both the therapist and himself, at which point Mr. B states his therapy ended. He has had paranoid ideation, thinking that people at work are against him, although this suspiciousness and ideation are responsive to reality testing, as are his ideas of reference. He has prolonged periods of anhedonia and demoralization but, other than insomnia at times, does not have extensive vegetative symptoms of depression. He has experienced episodes of depersonalization described as looking down at himself. He complains of low self-esteem but denies worthlessness, hopelessness, or helplessness. Mr. B notes that he was always a loner and had no close friends since the fifth grade. He went to college just before he went to Vietnam. He smokes one pack of cigarettes per day, does not use recreational drugs, and drinks up to three drinks per night, although he goes for periods without drinking significantly.

Mr. B underwent a research evaluation in the Mood and Personality Disorders Program. Research diagnostic evaluation revealed the presence of a schizotypal personality disorder with traits of paranoid and narcissistic personality disorder; he was also found to meet DSM-IV-TR (American Psychiatric Association 2000) criteria for alcohol abuse (past). Neurobiological evaluation uncovered a number of abnormalities. First, he displayed modestly impaired eye-movement accuracy (3.38 on a 1=best to 5=worst scale) and mild cognitive impairment. His dopaminergic indices were high, with a plasma HVA level of 14.5 ng/mL (mean for normal subjects is 7.4 ± 1.8 ng/mL) and a CSF HVA level of 38.0 ng/mL (mean for normal control subjects = 24.1 ± 6 ng/mL). In addition, Mr. B showed hypofrontality on a PET scan during a verbal memory task. Finally, he showed modest improvement following administration of amphetamine. Since evaluation, Mr. B has been treated with low-dose neuroleptic medication that helps him control multiple symptoms, including an olfactory hallucination-like experience of the smell of "cordite," a feeling that others are staring at him, a feeling of being detached or "separated by a bubble" from other people, a lack of any close friends other than a common-law wife, feelings in the past that his wife might be "following around," and a feeling in the past that he has seen future events.

Summary

These studies suggest that patients with schizotypal personality disorder have at least a profile of cognitive impairment and structural brain abnormalities, particularly in temporal cortex, similar to that found in patients with schizophrenia, but a combination of better prefrontal reserves and more subdued dopaminergic activity subcortically protects them from the emergence of psychosis. Their more subtle cognitive impairments are reflected in their eccentricity and interpersonal disengagement but do not reach the threshold of overt psychosis. For these reasons, they present more in the context of their disturbed interpersonal style and coping mechanisms rather than in the context of overt psychosis as in schizophrenia. However, this disorder provides an example of a spectrum that in its more extreme forms manifests as an Axis I disorder (schizophrenia) but in milder forms as an Axis II disorder. There are few biological data regarding paranoid personality disorder when it is not comorbid with schizotypal personality disorder.

CLUSTER B PERSONALITY DISORDERS

The Cluster B personality disorders include antisocial, borderline, histrionic, and narcissistic personality disorders. Individuals with these disorders present with varied degrees of impulsivity, aggression, and emotional dysregulation. As in other clusters, there is a high degree of overlap among the disorders in Cluster B, particularly between antisocial personality disorder (ASPD) and borderline personality disorder (BPD). ASPD and BPD are the best studied of the cluster, due to clear and reliable criteria for the former and the high prevalence of the latter in clinical populations.

Behavioral Genetics

Twin studies suggest that the genetic influence underlying personality disorders is at least as high as that of personality traits that underlie the various personality disorders. In a relatively small twin study (Torgersen et al. 2000) that may tend to overestimate the underlying genetic influence of any of a variety of personality disorders, the heritability for Cluster B personality disorders was 0.60. The heritabilities of the specific Cluster B disorders in this study were 0.79 for narcissistic personality disorder, 0.69 for BPD, and 0.67 for histrionic personality disorder. The best-fitting models did not include shared familial environment effects, although such effects may influence the development of BPD. Adoption studies of ASPD confirm a strong genetic, although a less strong environmental, influence for this disorder (Cadoret et al. 1985). Although adoption studies of other Cluster B personality disorders have not been conducted, the results of family history studies suggest a complex pattern of familial aggregation in which traits related to impulsive aggressiveness and mood dysregulation, rather than BPD itself, are transmitted in families (Silverman et al. 1991).

Neuropsychopharmacology

The 5-HT system has been extensively studied in individuals with personality disorder in general and in particular as an inverse correlate of impulsive aggressive behavior. Other neurotransmitters and/or modulators have also been studied in this regard, but to a much lesser degree.

Serotonin

There is a clear and consistent role for 5-HT in the regulation of aggression and/or impulsivity, particularly in individuals with personality disorder. Most data suggest an inverse relationship between any of a variety of measures of 5-HT levels and levels of aggression or impulsivity. Although some studies suggest a primary relationship with impulsivity, most studies report a 5-HT relationship more consistent with the construct of "impulsive aggression."

Neurochemical studies. Inverse relationships between human aggression and measures of central 5-HT function have been reported since 1979, when Brown and colleagues reported an inverse relationship between CSF levels of the main central 5-HT metabolite, 5-hydroxyindoleacetic acid (5-HIAA), and life history of actual aggressive behavior in males with a variety of DSM-II (American Psychiatric Association 1968) personality

disorder diagnoses (Brown et al. 1979). This finding was extended (Brown et al. 1982) to include a trivariate relationship between history of aggression, suicide attempts, and reduced CSF 5-HIAA, whereby history of aggression and suicide attempts were correlated directly with each other and inversely with CSF 5-HIAA. Later work with violent offenders (Linnoila et al. 1983) found reduced CSF 5-HIAA in impulsive, but not nonimpulsive, violent offenders with a variety of DSM-II personality disorder diagnoses, suggesting that impulsive aggression was the form most associated with reduced CSF 5-HIAA concentration. Although these findings have been replicated, an inverse relationship between CSF 5-HIAA and aggression has not been reported in samples of individuals with personality disorder without a prominent history of criminal activity (Coccaro et al. 1997a, 1997b; Gardner et al. 1990; Simeon et al. 1992). It is likely that CSF 5-HIAA, being a relatively insensitive index of 5-HT activity, is most reduced in the most severely aggressive individuals and that it is difficult to detect this relationship in less severely aggressive individuals.

Acute pharmacological interventions. There are a variety of 5-HT acute pharmacological challenge studies that have been performed in individuals with personality disorder in the context of the study of aggression. Typically, hormonal (e.g., prolactin) responses to the 5-HT selective agents are reported to correlate inversely with various measures of aggression and impulsivity (Coccaro et al. 1989, 1997a, 1997b; Dolan et al. 2001; Moss et al. 1990; O'Keane et al. 1992; Paris et al. 2004; Siever and Trestman 1993). Pharmacological challenge studies using putatively receptor-selective 5-HT agents also seem to support the hypothesis of an inverse relationship between 5-HT and measures of aggression and suggest a role for at least the 5-HT_{1A} receptor in particular (Cleare and Bond 2000; Coccaro et al. 1990, 1995; Hansenne et al. 2002). A more complex picture in regard to central 5-HT_{1A} receptors has been suggested by the observation of reduced 5-HT_{1A} receptor–mediated responses in females with BPD with a history of sustained child abuse (Rinne et al. 2000). Because childhood abuse has been linked to impulsive aggression in later adolescence and adulthood (Crick and Dodge 1996), it remains to be determined whether the relationships between 5-HT and aggression are linked to this environmental/developmental variable. Although behavioral responses to 5-HT stimulation in individuals with personality disorder have not received much attention, at least one study reported a significant reduction in anger in 12 patients with BPD after administration of the mixed 5-HT agonist m-chlorophenylpiperazine (m-CPP) but not placebo (Hollander et al. 1994); a reduction in fear was also observed in the males with BPD.

Platelet receptor markers. Despite considerable platelet receptor work in other psychiatric populations, relatively little research in this area has been published on subjects with personality disorder. Inverse correlations between the number of platelet ^{3}H-imipramine (5-HT transporter) binding sites and self-mutilation and impulsivity have been reported in individuals with personality disorder but not in patients without a history of self-mutilation (Simeon et al. 1992). Similarly, an inverse correlation between the number of platelet ^{3}H-paroxetine (5-HT transporter) binding sites (Coccaro et al. 1996), the quantity of platelet serotonin (Goveas et al. 2004), and life history of aggression has been reported in persons with personality disorder.

DNA polymorphism studies. Work in this area began with an examination of DNA polymorphisms in the gene for tryptophan hydroxylase (TPH). TPH is the rate-limiting step for the synthesis of serotonin, and it was thought that polymorphisms in TPH would lead to TPH enzymes of different activities. Although this *TPH* polymorphism was not found to have a clear functional consequence regarding serotonin synthesis, the presence of the L allele (L referred to the "lower band"

on the genotyping gel) was found to have some association with clinically relevant variables. For example, impulsive violent offenders (nearly all with a personality disorder) with at least one copy of the L TPH allele have been reported to have significantly lower CSF 5-HIAA compared with impulsive violent offenders with the UU genotype (U referred to the "upper band" on the genotyping gel) in at least one study (Nielson et al. 1994). This finding did not generalize to nonimpulsive violent offenders (many of whom also had a personality disorder) or to normal control subjects and was not replicated in a later study by the same authors (Nielson et al. 1998).

The presence of the L allele was associated with an increased risk of suicidal behavior in all violent offenders in this and in a later study by these authors (Nielson et al. 1994, 1998). New et al. (1998) have also reported that the self-reported tendency toward aggression varies as a function of *TPH* genotype whereby subjects with the LL genotype had higher aggression scores than those with the UU genotype. Curiously, however, the reverse finding was reported by Manuck et al. (1999) in a sample of healthy volunteers from the community: higher aggression scores were associated with the presence of the U allele.

These disparate findings may be due to critical differences in the subject samples. As such, the relationship between the TPH allele and 5-HT function may be dependent on the TPH allele's relationship with some other gene depending on the subject sample. Lappalainen et al. (1998) reported an association between "antisocial alcoholism" (i.e., alcoholism with ASPD or intermittent explosive disorder) and the C allele for the 5-HT_{1D} beta-receptor polymorphism. Because the 5-HT_{1D} beta receptor is a critical receptor involved in the regulation of 5-HT release on neuronal impulse, this finding could be highly relevant to the understanding of ASPD comorbid with alcoholism. Alleles of the 5–HTT transporter, 5-HT_{2A}, and *TPH2* have been found to be associated with BPD or its traits (Ni et al. 2006a, 2006b, 2007; Siever et al. 2006).

Catecholamines

Compared with serotonin, far fewer data have been published regarding the role of other neurotransmitters and behavioral dimensions of relevance to the Cluster B personality disorders.

Neurochemical studies. A positive correlation between CSF 3-methoxy-4-hydroxy-phenylclycol (MHPG, the major metabolite of norepinephrine) concentrations and life history of aggression has been reported in males with personality disorder, although further analysis revealed that CSF 5-HIAA concentration accounted for most (80%) of the variance in aggression scores. Similarly, one study reported a small positive correlation between plasma norepinephrine and self-reported impulsivity in males with personality disorder (Siever and Trestman 1993). In contrast, at least one study (Virkkunen et al. 1987) reported a significant reduction in CSF MHPG concentration in males who have committed violent offenses. Finally, Coccaro et al. (2003) reported an inverse relationship between plasma-free MHPG and life history of aggression in males with personality disorder. Compared with patients with nonborderline personality disorders, patients with BPD had lower plasma free MHPG compared with the nonborderline control subjects; a finding that disappeared after differences in aggression scores were accounted for.

Evidence for the role of dopamine in aggression in individuals with personality disorder is limited and contradictory. Although some studies demonstrate no relationship between CSF HVA concentration and aggression (Brown et al. 1979; Virkkunen et al. 1987), other studies demonstrate an inverse relationship between these variables (Linnoila et al. 1983; Virkkunen et al. 1989). Given the consistent observation of a strong correlation between CSF 5-HIAA and CSF HVA

concentrations, it is possible that findings with CSF HVA may be related to similar findings with CSF 5-HIAA concentration. If so, a specific assessment of CSF HVA may not be made unless the effect of CSF 5-HIAA concentration is accounted for, a statistical adjustment that has not been made in published studies to date.

Acute pharmacological interventions. Early studies of the acute administration of amphetamine in patients with BPD demonstrated a greater behavioral sensitivity to amphetamine challenge among the patients with personality disorder than among control subjects (Schulz et al. 1985). Replication studies found that global worsening in psychopathology after amphetamine was typical of patients with both borderline and schizotypal personality disorder, whereas global improvement was typical of borderline subjects without comorbid schizotypal personality disorder (Schulz et al. 1988). This finding suggests important biological differences among patients with BPD as a function of comorbid schizotypy (perhaps because of preexisting dopaminergic hyperactivity in mesolimbic dopamine circuits). In other studies of amphetamine challenge relevant to Cluster B personality disorder, a direct relationship with affective lability has been noted in healthy volunteers, suggesting that increases in norepinephrine and/or dopamine may play a role in the moment-to-moment dysregulation of affect seen in patients with BPD (Kavoussi et al. 1993).

Limited data are available regarding the study of norepinephrine receptor–mediated responses related to the features of Cluster B personality disorder. One study reported a positive correlation between the growth hormone response to the α_2 norepinephrine agonist clonidine and self-reported "irritability" (a correlate of aggression) in a small sample of males with personality disorder and healthy volunteers (Coccaro et al. 1991). A more recent study of females with BPD, however, reported no difference in growth hormone responses to clonidine (Paris et al. 2004).

DNA polymorphism studies. The presence of the low-functioning monoamine oxidase A (MAO-A) allele in young men combined with a history of childhood maltreatment has recently been shown to be associated with an increased risk of aggressive and criminal offending (e.g., antisocial) behavior (Caspi et al. 2002). This specific MAO-A allele is associated with reduced catabolism of catecholamines (and serotonin) and accordingly with higher levels of these neurotransmitters that may be associated with aggressive behavior. These data suggest that although the presence of this allele may be important in increasing the risk of antisocial behavior, the co-occurrence of childhood maltreatment in vulnerable individuals is also needed to meaningfully increase the risk of antisocial behavior.

Acetylcholine and Other Neurotransmitters/Neuromodulators

Studies of acetylcholine function in personality disorder have been limited to two studies. In the first (Steinberg et al. 1997), patients with BPD reported greater self-rated depression scores in response to the cholinomimetic agent physostigmine than did patients with nonborderline personality disorders or healthy volunteer control subjects. Peak physostigmine-induced depression scores correlated positively with the number of "affective instability," but not with the number of "impulsive aggression," borderline personality traits. This finding suggests that the trait of affective lability in patients with BPD may be mediated in part by a heightened sensitivity to acetylcholine. In the second study (Paris et al. 2004), however, no differences in hormonal responses to a different cholinomimetic agent, pyridostigmine, were seen between females with BPD and control subjects. These divergent findings suggest the possibility that the cholinergic receptors mediating behavioral and hormonal responses to cholinergic agents in these subjects may be very different by virtue of brain location.

Other neurotransmitters or neuromodulators that may play a role in Cluster B–related features include vasopressin, which may have a direct relationship with aggression (Coccaro et al. 1998); substances related to limbic HPA axis functioning (corticotropin releasing factor, adrenocorticotropic hormone, cortisol), which may have varied relationships regarding aggressive behavior dependent on social context and stress (Rinne et al. 2002); testosterone, which is variably correlated with aggression, particularly in violent offenders with ASPD (Virkkunen et al. 1994); and cholesterol and fatty acids, which may play a role in both aggression (both: Atmaca et al. 2002; New et al. 1999) and mood regulation (fatty acids: Zanarini and Frankenburg 2003).

Neuroimaging

Structural Imaging

Reduced prefrontal gray matter (e.g., by 11%) has been associated with autonomic deficits in individuals with ASPD characterized by aggressive behaviors (Raine et al. 2000). Conversely, increases in corpus callosum white matter volume and length have been described in similar subjects (Raine et al. 2003), where larger callosal volumes were also associated with affective/interpersonal deficit, low autonomic stress reactivity, and spatial ability. Given the complex role these structures play in mediating cognitive and affective processes, these findings may represent anatomical correlates of the complex behaviors seen in ASPD. A confounding role for alcoholism in these matters must always be addressed, however, because it also has been shown that volume changes may be correlated with duration of alcoholism (Laakso et al. 2002).

Similar structural imaging studies of females with BPD report reductions in the volume of subcortical structures such as the amygdala (Rusch et al. 2003; Schmahl et al. 2003; Tebartz van Elst et al. 2003; but see New et al. 2007) and hippocampus (Schmahl et al.

2003; Tebartz van Elst et al. 2003). Studies also report reductions in the volumes of both orbitofrontal and anterior cingulate (Hazlett et al. 2005; Tebartz van Elst et al. 2003). Given the role these structures are thought to play in emotional information processing, it is tempting to speculate that these structures represent anatomical correlates of the emotional dysregulation (including impulsive aggression) seen in patients with BPD.

Functional Imaging (PET and SPECT)

Whereas structural imaging yields only a static picture of the brain, SPECT or PET scanning can yield functional information related to cerebral blood flow or cerebral glucose metabolism, respectively. For example, SPECT studies have demonstrated reduced perfusion in prefrontal cortex as well as focal abnormalities in left temporal lobe and increased activity in anteromedial frontal cortex in limbic system in aggressive individuals with ASPD and alcoholism (Amen et al. 1996). A more recent study using SPECT reported significant correlations between reduced cerebral blood flow in frontal and temporal brain regions and the "disturbed interpersonal attitude" factor from the Psychopathy Checklist—Revised (Soderstrom et al. 2002). In homicide offenders (many of whom presumably had ASPD), a bilateral diminution of glucose metabolism has been reported in both medial frontal cortex and at a trend level in orbital frontal cortex (Raine et al. 1994). In a study of patients with a variety of personality disorders, an inverse relationship was found between life history of aggressive impulsive behavior and regional glucose metabolism in orbital frontal cortex and right temporal lobe (Goyer et al. 1994). Patients meeting criteria for BPD had decreased metabolism in frontal regions corresponding to BA 46 and BA 6 and increased metabolism in superior and inferior frontal gyrus (BA 9 and BA 45; Goyer et al. 1994). More-recent PET studies in females with BPD reported hypometabolism in both fron-

tal and prefrontal regions as well as in the hippocampus and cuneus (Juengling et al. 2003), supporting previous structural studies that demonstrated reductions in the volumes of these brain areas. Although most of these PET studies were performed in the resting condition, one PET study in females with BPD showed that the replay of abandonment scripts prior to PET scan was associated with greater increases in activity in dorsolateral prefrontal cortex (bilaterally) and in cuneus, but with reductions in activity in the right anterior cingulate (Schmahl et al. 2003). Given that several of these structures have been shown to be smaller in these subjects compared with control subjects, the increased activity in these regions after the abandonment task is quite notable.

PET studies may also be performed after the administration of neurotransmitter-specific agents so that the activity of brain regions in response to activation of specific receptors by these agents can be assessed. To date, at least four studies of patients with personality disorder have been performed in this way. Two utilized the indirect 5-HT agonist fenfluramine, one utilized the more direct postsynaptic 5-HT agonist m-CPP, and one examined the trapping of a ^{11}C analogue of tryptophan. In the first fenfluramine study, patients with prominent histories of impulsive aggression and BPD demonstrated blunted responses of glucose metabolism in orbital frontal, ventral medial frontal, and cingulate cortex compared with normal subjects (Siever et al. 1999). A similar result was reported in the second fenfluramine study, in which patients with BPD displayed reduced glucose metabolism (relative to placebo) compared with control subjects in right medial and orbital frontal cortex, left middle and superior temporal gyri, left parietal lobe, and left caudate (Soloff et al. 2000). In the PET study involving m-CPP, patients with prominent histories of impulsive aggression and personality disorder were found to have reduced activation of the anterior cingulate and increased activation of the posterior cingulate compared with control subjects, as well as a relative amygdala-prefrontal disconnection (New et al. 2002, 2007). Given the role of the anterior cingulate in emotional information processing, it is noteworthy that this area is underactivated by 5-HT stimulation. In the PET study examining the unilateral trapping of a ^{11}C analogue of tryptophan, evidence for a reduction in 5-HT synthesis was present in the corticostriatal (e.g., medial frontal, anterior cingulate, superior temporal gyri, and corpus striatum) brain areas of subjects with BPD (Leyton et al. 2001). Reduction in 5-HT synthesis in these regions was reported to correlate with a laboratory measure of behavioral disinhibition. Reduced transporter binding has also been reported in patients with impulsive aggressive personality disorder (Frankle et al. 2005), and increased 5–HT_{2A} receptor binding has been reported in currently aggressive subjects (Siever et al. 2006).

Functional Imaging (fMRI)

Unlike PET or SPECT, fMRI does not require the injection of a radiolabeled agent. Instead, fMRI assesses changes in cerebral blood flow using changes in the blood oxygenation level–dependent (BOLD) signal in the magnetic resonance imaging scanner. This offers a much greater spatial and temporal resolution compared with either PET or SPECT and allows a finer assessment of the activation and deactivation of discrete regions of the brain in response to specific stimuli. To date, at least three studies using fMRI in patients with personality disorder have been published. In one study using fMRI, males with (psychopathic) ASPD activated preselected frontal and temporal regions of interest less than did control subjects during trials of negatively charged emotional words (Kiehl et al. 2001), suggesting an important deficit in emotional information processing. In a similar fMRI study in females with BPD, the study group demonstrated greater activation of the amygdala bilaterally (as well as activation of selected frontal regions) while viewing emotionally aversive images (e.g., crying children) than did control subjects (Herpertz et al. 2001). Another fMRI study in females with BPD reported a generally similar finding (left amygdala as opposed to bilateral activation) using emotional faces (Donegan et al. 2003). Other recent studies from the two separate laboratories of the authors suggest a) increased activation in amygdala, and reduced activation in orbitomedial prefrontal cortex, to anger faces in impulsively aggressive subjects with personality disorders (none of whom was psychopathic; Coccaro et al. 2007) and b) increased superior temporal cortex, rather than middle temporal cortex, BOLD responses, suggesting increased reflexive processing and increased amygdala, fusiform, and occipital visual area activation to emotional provocation (Koenigsberg et al. 2007). Given the clear differences in known emotional information processing between psychopathic antisocial subjects on the one hand and borderline subjects on the other, these data suggest the brain sites of these differences.

Case Example

Mr. C is a 29-year-old, married male computer technician referred for treatment of his impulsive aggressive outbursts in the context of a threatened separation from his wife of 4 years. Mr. C reports impulsive aggressive outbursts since his mid-teens. These outbursts typically involve screaming, shouting, and throwing things around; he has only occasionally physically hit anyone. However, these aggressive outbursts occur several times a month and usually several times a week, particularly when Mr. C is "held up" in traffic. Most recently, he has been having serious marital difficulty, and his wife is now threatening to leave him if he does not get help for his anger problem. He reports that his relationship with his wife is often "stormy," with frequent fighting that sometimes goes on for hours. Sometimes in the aftermath of these fights Mr. C runs off and gets exceedingly drunk and drives recklessly around town while high. At other times, he reports, he beats his head so hard against a wall that his forehead bleeds (once he needed stitches). Still, at other times he frantically pleads with his wife not to leave him; once he took an overdose of aspirin, in front of his wife, to get her to stay with him. Mr. C reports a history of alcohol abuse in his late teens and early twenties and a history of gambling to excess up until 1 year prior to evaluation.

Mr. C underwent a research evaluation in the Mood and Personality Disorders Program. Diagnostic evaluation revealed the presence of BPD with traits of histrionic, narcissistic, and obsessive-compulsive personality disorder. He was also found to meet DSM-IV-TR criteria for two episodes of major depression in the past and for alcohol abuse (past) and pathological gambling (past). He underwent a variety of research-related studies including *d*-fenfluramine (d-FEN) challenge and was found to have a blunted, but not absent, prolactin response to d-FEN (2.3 ng/mL compared with 6.3 ± 3.4 ng/mL for healthy male control subjects); his CSF 5-HIAA level was not abnormal (23.9 ng/mL compared with 20.0 ± 4.9 ng/mL for healthy male control subjects). The modest magnitude of his prolactin response to d-FEN suggests a limited degree of central serotonin system dysfunction.

Mr. C entered a treatment trial of fluoxetine and experienced a reduction in overt aggressive behavior over a period of several weeks. Over this time his relationship with his wife somewhat improved, and he is now in dialectical behavioral therapy to work on other aspects of his interpersonal difficulties with others in his life.

Summary

The studies discussed in this section suggest that patients with Cluster B personality disorder have dysfunction in a variety of neurobiological areas that may underlie their clinical presentation. Dysfunction can occur in multiple monoaminergic systems (e.g., serotonin,

norepinephrine, vasopressin for impulsivity and aggression, possibly acetylcholine for mood reactivity) and in brain structures related to behavioral inhibition and emotional information processing (e.g., orbitofrontal cortex, amygdala). Although patients with BPD are often the most extreme in these features and in related biological dysfunction, specific biological dysfunction related to specific traits (e.g., serotonin dysfunction with impulsive aggression) can be seen in patients with other, nonborderline personality disorders. As such, it is doubtful that any assessment of specific neurobiological function will be specific to patients with BPD.

CLUSTER C

The Cluster C personality disorders include avoidant, dependent, and obsessive-compulsive personality disorders. Individuals with these disorders present with varied degrees of anxiety sometimes expressed as "rigidity," particularly in the case of obsessive-compulsive personality disorder. Of the three disorders, avoidant personality disorder is most like generalized social phobia in Axis I, and a great degree of comorbidity occurs between the two diagnoses (Dahl 1996). As in other personality disorder clusters, there is overlap among the disorders in this cluster and with those in other personality disorder clusters, particularly Cluster B. To date, there has been much less empirical neurobiological research with patients in Cluster C.

Behavioral Genetics

As with the Cluster B personality disorders, twin studies suggest substantial genetic influence for each of the Cluster C personality disorders (Torgersen et al. 2000). Heritability for Cluster C personality disorders as a group was estimated at 0.62; heritabilities for each disorder in the study were 0.78 for obsessive-compulsive, 0.57 for dependent, and 0.28 for avoidant personality disorder. The best-fitting models did not include shared familial environment effects, although a model consisting only of shared familial and unique environmental effects could not be definitively ruled out for dependent personality disorders. Family studies suggest a familial association between social anxiety disorder and avoidant personality disorder (Schneier et al. 2002). Avoidant, dependent, and anxious cluster personality disorders show significant familiarity (Reich 1989), and both avoidant and independent personality traits are found in relatives of patients with panic disorder (Reich 1991).

Neuropsychopharmacology

There has been little biological study of the Cluster C personality disorders. However, low dopamine metabolites in CSF have been identified in patients with social anxiety disorder (Johnson et al. 1994), which overlaps to a great extent with avoidant personality disorder, whereas nonselective monoamine oxidase inhibitors (which increase dopamine transmission) or dopaminergic antidepressants improve social anxiety (Schneier et al. 2002). Imaging studies are also consistent with this finding, with low dopamine transporter binding demonstrated in generalized social anxiety disorder (Tiihonen et al. 1997) and lower D_2 receptor binding in a SPECT study of generalized social anxiety disorder (Schneier et al. 2000). In addition, three PET studies support a relationship of reduced D_2 binding associated with detachment, which correlates with social avoidance consistent with that observed both in patients with Cluster C personality disorders and in patients with schizoid personality disorder (Schneier et al. 2000). Genetic studies of these types of behaviors have been found in association with the dopamine transporter gene *DAT1* (Blum et al. 1997). These studies cumulatively suggest low dopaminergic activity in social anxiety disorder and likely in avoidant personality disorder as well.

In the serotonergic system, on the other hand, patients with social anxiety have in-

creased cortisol responses to serotonergic agents (Tancer et al. 1999), and social anxiety disorders respond to selective serotonin reuptake inhibitors that re-regulate serotonergic activity (Schneier et al. 2003). Shyness (related to avoidant traits) has been associated with the serotonin transporter reporter region L allele but not to COMT, MAO-A, or DRD4 alleles. Growth hormone regulation has also been associated with social anxiety (Schneier et al. 2002).

Neuropsychological and Psychophysiological Correlates

Increased amygdala activation in fMRI has been shown in social phobia in one study (Schneier et al. 1999) as well as in recognition bias for recall of disapproving faces in another (Foa et al. 2000). However, skin conductance and heart rate change and startle response during viewing of slides with emotionally charged themes did not distinguish patients with avoidant personality disorder from control subjects (Herpertz et al. 2000). Psychophysiological studies have not been extensively undertaken in the other Cluster C personality disorders.

Summary

Genetic and neurobiological research has been limited in patients with Cluster C personality disorders, but reductions in dopaminergic activity and increases in serotonergic activity are hinted at in the data available.

FUTURE DIRECTIONS

Research in the psychobiology of personality disorder has advanced much since the 1980s. Although there is clear evidence of a number of biogenetic correlates of personality disorder traits, future efforts need to be directed along a variety of lines to increase our understanding of how alterations in brain function lead to the development and manifestation of these traits. Such lines of investigation may be aimed at 1) how genetic and environmental influences interact with neurotransmitter function to lead to specific traits; 2) how neurotransmitter function interacts with the regulation of cognitive and emotional function across distributed neural networks to lead to specific traits; and 3) how understanding brain function at these levels can enable us to devise more effective ways to treat personality disorder traits both pharmacologically and psychotherapeutically.

REFERENCES

Amen DG, Stubblefield M, Carmicheal B: Brain SPECT findings and aggressiveness. Ann Clin Psychiatry 3:129–137, 1996

American Psychiatric Association: Diagnostic and Statistical Manual of Mental Disorders, 2nd Edition. Washington, DC, American Psychiatric Association, 1968

American Psychiatric Association: Diagnostic and Statistical Manual of Mental Disorders, 4th Edition, Text Revision. Washington, DC, American Psychiatric Association, 2000

Amin F, Coccaro EF, Mitropoulou V, et al: Plasma HVA in schizotypal personality disorder, in Plasma Homovanillic Acid Studies in Schizophrenia: Implications for Presynaptic Dopamine Dysfunction. Edited by Friedhoff AJ, Amin F. Washington, DC, American Psychiatric Press, 1997, pp 133–149

Amin F, Silverman JM, Siever LJ, et al: Genetic antecedents of dopamine dysfunction in schizophrenia. Biol Psychiatry 45:1143–1150, 1999

Atmaca M, Kuloglu M, Tezcan E, et al: Serum cholesterol and leptin levels in patients with borderline personality disorder. Neuropsychobiology 45:167–171, 2002

Blum K, Braverman ER, Wu S: Association of polymorphisms of dopamine D2 receptor (DRD2), and dopamine transporter (DAT1) genes with schizoid/avoidant behaviors (SAB). Mol Psychiatry 2:239–246, 1997

Braff DL, Freedman R: Endophenotypes in studies of the genetics of schizophrenia, in Neuropsychopharmacology: The Fifth Generation of Progress. Edited by Davis KL, Charney D, Coyle JT, et al. Philadelphia, PA, Lippincott Williams & Wilkins, 2002, pp 703–716

Brown GL, Goodwin FK, Ballenger JC, et al: Aggression in humans correlates with cerebrospinal fluid amine metabolites. Psychiatry Res 1:131–139, 1979

Brown GL, Ebert MH, Goyer PF, et al: Aggression, suicide, and serotonin: relationships to CSF amine metabolites. Am J Psychiatry 139:741–746, 1982

Buchsbaum MS, Nenadic I, Hazlett EA, et al: Differential metabolic rates in prefrontal and temporal Brodmann areas in schizophrenia and schizotypal personality disorder. Schizophr Res 54:141–150, 2002

Cadenhead KS: Vulnerability markers in the schizophrenia spectrum: implications for phenomenology, genetics, and the identification of the schizophrenia prodrome. Psychiatr Clin North Am 25:837–853, 2002

Cadoret RJ, O'Gorman TW, Troughton E, et al: Alcoholism and antisocial personality: interrelationships, genetic and environmental factors. Arch Gen Psychiatry 42:161–167, 1985

Caspi A, McClay J, Moffitt TE, et al: Role of genotype in the cycle of violence in maltreated children. Science 297:851–854, 2002

Cleare AJ, Bond AJ: Ipsapirone challenge in aggressive men shows an inverse correlation between 5-HT1A receptor function and aggression. Psychopharmacology 148:344–349, 2000

Coccaro EF, Siever LJ, Klar HM, et al: Serotonergic studies in patients with affective and personality disorder: correlates with suicidal and impulsive aggressive behavior. Arch Gen Psychiatry 46:587–599, 1989

Coccaro EF, Gabriel S, Siever LJ: Buspirone challenge: preliminary evidence for a role for 5-HT-1A receptors in impulsive aggressive behavior in humans. Psychopharmacol Bull 26:393–405, 1990

Coccaro EF, Lawrence T, Trestman R, et al: Growth hormone responses to intravenous clonidine challenge correlates with behavioral irritability in psychiatric patients and in healthy volunteers. Psychiatry Res 39:129–139, 1991

Coccaro EF, Kavoussi RJ, Hauger RL: Physiologic responses to d-fenfluramine and ipsapirone challenge correlate with indices of aggression in males with personality disorder. Int Clin Psychopharmacol 10:177–180, 1995

Coccaro EF, Kavoussi RJ, Sheline YI, et al: Impulsive aggression in personality disorder: correlates with 3H-paroxetine binding in the platelet. Arch Gen Psychiatry 53:531–536, 1996

Coccaro EF, Kavoussi RJ, Cooper TB, et al: Central serotonin and aggression: inverse relationship with prolactin response to d-fenfluramine, but not with CSF 5-HIAA concentration in human subjects. Am J Psychiatry 154:1430–1435, 1997a

Coccaro EF, Kavoussi RJ, Trestman RL, et al: Serotonin function in personality and mood disorder:

intercorrelations among central indices and aggressiveness. Psychiatry Res 73:1–14, 1997b

Coccaro EF, Kavoussi RK, Hauger RL, et al: Cerebrospinal fluid vasopressin: correlates with aggression and serotonin function in personality disordered subjects. Arch Gen Psychiatry 55:708–714, 1998

Coccaro EF, Lee R, McCloskey M: Norepinephrine function in personality disorder: plasma free MHPG correlates inversely with life history of aggression. CNS Spectr 8:731–736, 2003

Coccaro EF, McCloskey MS, Fitzgerald DA, et al: Amygdala and orbitofrontal reactivity to social threat in individuals with impulsive aggression. Biol Psychiatry 62:168–178, 2007

Crick NR, Dodge KA: Social information-processing mechanisms in reactive and proactive aggression. Child Dev 67:993–1002, 1996

Dahl AA: The relationship between social phobia and avoidant personality disorder: workshop report 3. Int Clin Psychopharmacol 11(suppl 3):109–112, 1996

Dolan M, Anderson IM, Deakin JF: Relationship between 5-HT function and impulsivity and aggression in male offenders with personality disorders. Br J Psychiatry 178:352–359, 2001

Donegan NH, Sanislow CA, Blumberg HP, et al: Amygdala hyperreactivity in borderline personality disorder: implications for emotional dysregulation. Biol Psychiatry 54:1284–1293, 2003

Foa EB, Gilboa-Schechtman E, Amir N: Memory bias in generalized social phobia: remembering negative emotional expressions. J Anxiety Disord 14:501–519, 2000

Frankle WG, Lombardo I, New AS, et al: Brain serotonin transporters distribution in subjects with impulsive aggressvity: a positron emission study with [11C] McN5652. Am J Psychiatry 162:915–923, 2005

Gardner DL, Lucas PB, Cowdry RW: CSF metabolites in borderline personality disorder compared with normal controls. Biol Psychiatry 28:247-54, 1990

Goldberg TE, Egan MF, Gscheidle T, et al: Executive subprocesses in working memory: relationship to catechol-*O*-methyltransferase Val158Met genotype and schizophrenia. Arch Gen Psychiatry 60:889–896, 2003

Goveas JS, Csernansky JG, Coccaro EF: Platelet serotonin content correlates inversely with life history of aggression in personality-disordered subjects. Psychiatry Res 126:23–32, 2004

Goyer PF, Andreason PJ, Semple WE, et al: Positron-emission tomography and personality disorders. Neuropsychopharmacology 10:21–28, 1994

Hansenne M, Pitchot W, Pinto E, et al: 5-HT1A dysfunction in borderline personality disorder. Psychol Med 32:935–941, 2002

Hazlett EA, New AS, Newmark R, et al: Reduced anterior and posterior cingulated gray matter in borderline personality disorder. Biol Psychiatry 58:614–623, 2005

Hazlett EA, Buchsbaum MS, Haznedar MM, et al: Cortical gray and white matter volume in unmedicated schizotypal and schizophrenia patients. Schizophr Res 101:111–123, 2008

Herpertz SC, Schwenger UB, Kunert HJ, et al: Emotional responses in patients with borderline as compared with avoidant personality disorder. J Personal Disord 14: 339–351, 2000

Herpertz SC, Dietrich TM, Wenning B, et al: Evidence of abnormal amygdala functioning in borderline personality disorder: a functional MRI study. Biol Psychiatry 50: 292–298, 2001

Hollander E, Stein D, DeCaria CM, et al: Serotonergic sensitivity in borderline personality disorder: preliminary findings. Am J Psychiatry 151:277–280, 1994

Hymowitz P, Frances A, Jacobsberg LB, et al: Neuroleptic treatment of schizotypal personality disorders. Compr Psychiatry 27:267–271, 1986

Johnson MR, Lydiard RB, Zealberg JJ: Plasma and CFS levels in panic patients with comorbid social phobia. Biol Psychiatry 36:426–427, 1994

Juengling FD, Schmahl C, Hesslinger B, et al: Positron emission tomography in female patients with borderline personality disorder. J Psychiatr Res 37:109–115, 2003

Kalus O, Bernstein DP, Siever LJ: Schizoid personality disorder: a review of its current status. J Personal Disord 7: 43–52, 1993

Kavoussi RJ, Coccaro EF: The amphetamine challenge test correlates with affective lability in healthy volunteers. Psychiatry Res 48:219–228, 1993

Kiehl K, Smith AM, Hare RD, et al: Limbic abnormalities in affective processing by criminal psychopaths as revealed by functional magnetic resonance imaging. Biol Psychiatry 50:677–684, 2001

Kirrane RM, Mitropoulou V, Nunn M, et al: Effects of amphetamine on visuospatial working memory performance in schizophrenia spectrum personality disorder. Neuropsychopharmacology 22:14–18, 2000

Koenigsberg HW, Reynolds D, Goodman M, et al: Risperidone in the treatment of schizotypal personality disorder. J Clin Psychiatry 64:628–634, 2003

Koenigsberg HW, Buchsbaum MS, Buchsbaum BR, et al: Fuctional MRI of visuospatial working memory in schizotypal personality disorder: a region-of-interest analysis. Psychol Med 35:1019–1030, 2005

Koenigsberg HW, Prohovnik I, Lee H, et al: Neural correlates of the processing of negative and positive social scenes in borderline personality disorder. Biol Psychiatry 61:8S, 1045, 2007

Laakso MP, Gunning-Dixon F, Vaurio O, et al: Prefrontal volumes in habitually violent subjects with antisocial personality disorder and type 2 alcoholism. Psychiatry Res 114:95–102, 2002

Lappalainen J, Long JC, Eggert M, et al: Linkage of antisocial alcoholism to the serotonin 5-HT1B receptor gene in two populations. Arch Gen Psychiatry 55:989–994, 1998

Laruelle M, Kegeles L, Zea-Pance Y, et al: Amphetamine-induced dopamine release in patients with schizotypal personality disorders studies by SPECT and [123] IBZM. Neuroimage 16:S61, 2002

Levitt JJ, McCarley RW, Dickey CC, et al: MRI study of caudate nucleus volume and its cognitive correlates in neuroleptic-naive patients with schizotypal personality disorder. Am J Psychiatry 159:1190–1197, 2002

Leyton M, Okazawa H, Diksic M, et al: Brain regional alpha-[11C]methyl-L-tryptophan trapping in impulsive subjects with borderline personality disorder. Am J Psychiatry 158:775–782, 2001

Linnoila M, Virkkunen M, Scheinin M, et al: Low cerebrospinal fluid 5-hydroxyindolacetic acid concentration differentiates impulsive from nonimpulsive violent behavior. Life Sci 33:2609–2614, 1983

Manuck SB, Flory JD, Ferrell RE, et al: Aggression and anger-related traits associated with a polymorphism of the tryptophan hydroxylase gene. Biol Psychiatry 45:603–614, 1999

McClure MM, Barch DM, Romero MJ, et al: The effects of guanfacine on context processing abnormalities in schizotypal personality disorder. Biol Psychiatry 61:1157–1160, 2007

Minzenberg MJ, Xu K, Mitropoulou V, et al: Catechol-O-methyltransferase Val 158 Met genotype variation is associated with prefrontal dependent task performance in schizotypal personality disorder patients and comparison groups. Psychiatr Genet 16:117–124, 2006

Mitropoulou V, Harvey PD, Maldari LA, et al: Neuropsychological performance in schizotypal personality disorder: evidence regarding diagnostic specificity. Biol Psychiatry 52:1175–1182, 2002

Mitropoulou V, Harvey PD, Zegarelli G, et al: Neuropsychological performance in schizotypal personality disorder: importance of working memory. Am J Psychiatry 162:1896–1903, 2005

Moss HB, Yao JK, Panzak GL: Serotonergic responsivity and behavioral dimensions in antisocial personality disorder with substance abuse. Biol Psychiatry 28:325–338, 1990

New AS, Gelernter J, Yovell Y, et al: Tryptophan hydroxylase genotype is associated with impulsive aggression measures. Am J Med Genet 81:13–17, 1998

New AS, Sevin EM, Mitropoulou V, et al: Serum cholesterol and impulsivity in personality disorders. Psychiatry Res 85:145–150, 1999

New AS, Hazlett EA, Buchsbaum MS, et al: Blunted prefrontal cortical ^{18}fluorodeoxyglucose positron emission tomography response to *meta*-chlorophenylpiperazine in impulsive aggression. Arch Gen Psychiatry 59:621–629, 2002

New AS, Hazlett EA, Buchsbaum MS, et al: Amygdala-prefrontal disconnection in borderline personality disorder. Neuropsychopharmacology 32:1629–1640, 2007.

Ni X, Bismil R, Chan K, et al: Serotonin 2A receptor gene is associated with personality traits, but not to disorder, in patients with borderline personality disorder. Neurosci Lett 408:214–219, 2006a

Ni X, Chan K, Bulgin N, et al: Association between serotonin transporter gene and borderline personality disorder. J Psychiatr Res 40:448–453, 2006b

Ni X, Sicard T, Bulgin N, et al: Monoamine oxidase a gene is associated with borderline personality disorder. Psychiatr Genet 17:153–157, 2007

Nielsen DA, Goldman D, Virkkunen M, et al: Suicidality and 5-hydroxyindoleacetic acid concentration associated with a tryptophan hydroxylase polymorphism. Arch Gen Psychiatry 51:34–38, 1994

Nielsen DA, Virkkunen M, Lappalainen J, et al: A tryptophan hydroxylase gene marker for suicidality and alcoholism. Arch Gen Psychiatry 55:593–602, 1998

O'Keane V, Moloney E, O'Neill H, et al: Blunted prolactin responses to d-fenfluramine in sociopathy: Evidence for subsensitivity of central serotonergic function. Br J Psychiatry 160:643–646, 1992

Paris J, Zweig-Frank H, Kin NM, et al: Neurobiological correlates of diagnosis and underlying traits in patients with borderline personality disorder compared with normal controls. Psychiatry Res 121:239–252, 2004

Raine A, Buchsbaum M, Stanley J, et al: Selective reductions in prefrontal glucose metabolism in murderers. Biol Psychiatry 36:365–373, 1994

Raine A, Lencz T, Bihrle S, et al: Reduced prefrontal gray matter volume and reduced autonomic activity in antisocial personality disorder. Arch Gen Psychiatry 57:119–127, 2000

Raine A, Lencz T, Taylor K, et al: Corpus callosum abnormalities in psychopathic antisocial individuals. Arch Gen Psychiatry 60:1134–1142, 2003

Reich JH: Familiality of DSM-III dramatic and anxious personality clusters. J Nerv Ment Dis 177:96–100, 1989

Reich JH: Avoidant and dependent personality traits in relatives of patients with panic disorder, patients with dependent personality disorder, and normal controls. Psychiatry Res 39:89–98, 1991

Rinne T, Westenberg HG, den Boer JA, et al: Serotonergic blunting to *meta*-chlorophenylpiperazine (m-CPP) highly correlates with sustained childhood abuse in impulsive and autoaggressive female borderline patients. Biol Psychiatry 47:548–556, 2000

Rinne T, de Kloet ER, Wouters L, et al: Hyperresponsiveness of hypothalamic-pituitary-adrenal axis to combined dexamethasone/corticotropin-releasing hormone challenge in female borderline personality disorder subjects with a history of sustained childhood abuse. Biol Psychiatry 52:1102–1112, 2002

Rusch N, van Elst LT, Ludaescher P, et al: A voxel-based morphometric MRI study in female patients with borderline personality disorder. Neuroimage 20:385–392, 2003

Schmahl CG, Vermetten E, Elzinga BM, et al: Magnetic resonance imaging of hippocampal and amygdala volume in women with childhood abuse and borderline personality disorder. Psychiatry Res 122:193–198, 2003

Schneier F, Weiss U, Kessler C: Subcortical correlates of differential classical conditioning of aversive emotional reactions in social phobia. Biol Psychiatry 45:863–871, 1999

Schneier FR, Liebowitz MR, Abi-Dargham A: Low dopamine D2 receptor binding potential in social phobia. Am J Psychiatry 157:457–459, 2000

Schneier FR, Blanco C, Smita XA, et al: The social anxiety spectrum. Psychiatr Clin North Am 25:757–774, 2002

Schneier FR, Blanco C, Campeas R, et al: Citalopram treatment of social anxiety disorder with comorbid major depression. Depress Anxiety 17:191–196, 2003

Schulz SC, Schulz PM, Dommisse C, et al: Amphetamine response in borderline patients. Psychiatry Res 15:97–108, 1985

Schulz SC, Cornelius J, Schulz PM, et al: The amphetamine challenge test in patients with borderline personality disorder. Am J Psychiatry 145:809–814, 1988

Schulz SC, Thomson R, Brecher M: The efficacy of quetiapine vs. haloperidol and placebo: a meta-analytic study of efficacy. Schizophr Res 62:1–12, 2003

Shihabuddin L, Silverman JM, Buchsbaum MS, et al: Ventricular enlargement associated with linkage marker for schizophrenia-related disorders in one pedigree. Mol Psychiatry 1:215–222, 1996

Shihabuddin L, Buchsbaum MS, Hazlett EA, et al: Striatal size and relative glucose metabolic rate in schizotypal personality disorder and schizophrenia. Arch Gen Psychiatry 58:877–884, 2001

Siegel BV, Trestman RL, O'Flaithbheartaigh SO, et al: D-amphetamine challenge effects on Wisconsin Card Sort Test performance in schizotypal personality disorder. Schizophr Res 20:29–32, 1996

Siever LJ: The biology of the boundaries of schizophrenia, in Advances in Neuropsychiatry and Psychopharmacology, Vol 1: Schizophrenia Research. Edited by Tamminga CA, Schulz SC. New York, Raven, 1991, pp 181–191

Siever LJ: Brain structure/function and the dopamine system in schizotypal personality disorder, in Schizotypal Personality. Edited by Raine A, Lencz T, Mednick F. New York, Cambridge University Press, 1995, pp 272–286

Siever LJ, Davis KL: The pathophysiology of the schizophrenic disorders: perspective from the spectrum. Am J Psychiatry 161:398–413, 2004

Siever LJ, Trestman RL: The serotonin system and aggressive personality disorder. Int Clin Psychopharmacol 8 (suppl 2):33–39, 1993

Siever LJ, Amin F, Coccaro EF, et al: Plasma homovanillic acid in schizotypal personality disorder patients and controls. Am J Psychiatry 148:1246–1248, 1991

Siever LJ, Amin F, Coccaro EF, et al: CSF homovanillic acid in schizotypal personality disorder. Am J Psychiatry 150:149–151, 1993

Siever LJ, Buchsbaum M, New A, et al: D,L-fenfluramine response in impulsive personality disorder assessed with [18]-fluorodeoxyglucose positron emission tomography. Neuropsychopharmacology 20:413–423, 1999

Siever LJ, Koenigsberg HW, Harvey P, et al: Cognitive and brain function in schizotypal personality disorder. Schizophr Res 54:157–167, 2002

Siever LJ, Frankle WG, Ducci F, et al: The serotonin transporter binding and genotypes in impulsive personality disorders. Abstract, The Society of Biological Psychiatry 61st Annual Scientific Convention & Program, 2006

Silverman JM, Pinkham L, Horvath TB, et al: Affective and impulsive personality disorder traits in the relatives of patients with borderline personality disorder. Am J Psychiatry 148:1378–1385, 1991

Simeon D, Stanley B, Frances A, et al: Self-mutilation in personality disorders: psychological and biological correlates. Am J Psychiatry 149:221–226, 1992

Soderstrom H, Hultin L, Tullberg M, et al: Reduced frontotemporal perfusion in psychopathic personality. Psychiatry Res 114:81–94, 2002

Soloff PH, Meltzer CC, Greer PJ, et al: A fenfluramine-activated FDG-PET study of borderline personality disorder. Biol Psychiatry 47:540–547, 2000

Steinberg BJ, Trestman R, Mitropoulou V, et al: Depressive response to physostigmine challenge in borderline personality disorder patients. Neuropsychopharmacology 17:264–273, 1997

Tancer ME, Mailman RB, Stein MB, et al: Subcortical correlates of differential classical conditioning of aversive emotional reactions in social phobia. Biol Psychiatry 45:863–871, 1999

Tebartz van Elst L, Hesslinger B, Thiel T, et al: Frontolimbic brain abnormalities in patients with borderline personality disorder: a volumetric magnetic resonance imaging study. Biol Psychiatry 54:163–171, 2003

Tiihonen J, Kuikka J, Bergstrom K: DA reuptake site densities in patients with social phobia. Am J Psychiatry 154:239–242, 1997

Torgersen S, Lygren S, Oien PA, et al: A twin study of personality disorders. Compr Psychiatry 41:416–425, 2000

Trestman RL, Keefe RSE, Harvey PD, et al: Cognitive function and biological correlates of cognitive performance in schizotypal personality disorder. Psychiatry Res 59:127–136, 1995

Virkkunen M, Nuutila A, Goodwin FK, et al: Cerebrospinal fluid monoamine metabolite levels in male arsonists. Arch Gen Psychiatry 44:241–247, 1987

Virkkunen M, DeJong J, Bartko J, et al: Relationship of psychobiological variables to recidivism in violent offenders and impulsive fire setters. Arch Gen Psychiatry 46: 600–603, 1989

Virkkunen M, Rawlings R, Tokola R: CSF biochemistries, glucose metabolism, and diurnal activity rhythms in alcoholic, violent offenders, fire setters, and healthy volunteers. Arch Gen Psychiatry 51:20–27, 1994

Webb CT, Levinson DF: Schizotypal and paranoid personality disorder in the relatives of patients with schizophrenia and affective disorders: a review. Schizophr Res 11:81–92, 1993

Weinberger DR, Egan MF, Bertolino A, et al: Prefrontal neurons and the genetics of schizophrenia. Biol Psychiatry 50:825–844, 2001

Zanarini MC, Frankenburg FR: Omega-3 fatty acid treatment of women with borderline personality disorder: a double-blind, placebo-controlled pilot study. Am J Psychiatry 160:167–169, 2003

7

Developmental Issues

Patricia Cohen, Ph.D.
Thomas Crawford, Ph.D.

Aside from well-documented developmental links between early conduct disorder and antisocial personality disorder (ASPD), there are large gaps in our knowledge about childhood antecedents of other DSM-IV-TR personality disorders (American Psychiatric Association 2000; Widiger and Sankis 2000). In this chapter we discuss how developmental processes and selected risk factors lead to the emergence and persistence of personality disorders in young people. We highlight changes in how children and adolescents construct mental representations of themselves and other people and then consider how distortions in this developmental process manifest in personality disorder. We outline what we have learned about early trajectories of personality disorders and discuss how clinicians and researchers can evaluate the normative and clinical significance of symptoms in children and adolescents. Fi-

nally, we address problems in assessing these disorders in young people based on the limited number of measurement instruments currently available.

ETIOLOGICAL AND DEVELOPMENTAL FACTORS

In an early paper on the "borderline-child-to-be," Pine (1986) identified three key factors in his developmental model of borderline personality disorder (BPD) in young people. First, he hypothesized how early abuse or trauma overwhelms the child, especially when the trauma is ongoing or experienced from a variety of sources. Second, childhood trauma may interfere with the development of how trust, personal attachments, anxiety, aggression, and self-esteem are experienced and expressed. Third, young people may fasten onto immature defenses almost as though these defenses were survival techniques for desperate situations. More recent empirical research points to other factors that contribute to the emergence and persistence of personality disorders over time, including genetic effects (Coolidge et al. 2001; Jang 2005) and co-occurring Axis I disorders (Crawford et al. 2001b, 2008; Kasen et al. 2007).

When individual risk factors occur in isolation, they often may be offset by normative maturational factors in social or cognitive domains. Conduct disorder in childhood, for instance, does not usually lead to ASPD in adulthood. When risk factors occur in combination, however, they may overwhelm the young person's ability to cope, thus leading immature defenses to become inflexible and maladaptive over time. On the other hand, even a child who has experienced a significant trauma may be protected from lasting damage to personality functioning if he or she is securely attached to parents who can buffer the impact of the trauma. If traumatized children are anxiously attached to parents instead, thus reducing the protective effects, they may be at greater risk for lasting personality dysfunction (Alexander 1992; Bleiberg 2001; Levy 2005). Because genetic, interpersonal, and early trauma risk factors are all addressed elsewhere (see Cloninger 2005 and Jang 2005; see in this volume Chapter 8, "Childhood Experiences and the Development of Maladaptive and Adaptive Personality Traits," and Chapter 11, "Mentalization-Based Treatment of Borderline Personality Disorder"), we focus here on disturbances in how children perceive themselves and the people around them and how developmental changes in cognitive ability may play a role in the formation of personality disorders. In this context we draw on the theoretical literature on attachment in infancy and childhood (e.g., Cassidy and Shaver 2008; Fonagy et al. 2003) and identity development in adolescence (Erikson 1968) and seek to bridge the two using Harter's (1998) work on development of self-representation.

Early Working Models of Self and Other

Attachment theory (Bowlby 1969, 1973) focuses on developmental experiences reflecting secure and insecure relationships between infants and caregivers and emphasizes how young people come to perceive themselves and others (Lyddon and Alford 2007). A secure attachment typically occurs when the caregiver has been available and sensitive to the needs of the infant or toddler, especially in times of distress. Young children can better manage negative emotions, such as anger or fear, within a secure relationship because these feelings have been associated with soothing and effective responses by the caregiver (Sroufe 1996). By providing this external form of affect regulation, caregivers prevent infants from being overwhelmed and help them gradually develop the ability to regulate their own affect (Mikulincer et al. 2003). When caregivers are inconsistent or rejecting, infants and toddlers instead may underregulate their own affect or restrict it excessively.

As hypothesized in attachment theory, very basic mental representations of self and others are thought to emerge during infancy through affective experiences that characterize the child–caregiver relationship. These preverbal experiences are labeled "internal working models" and broadly reflect whether infants expect caregivers to be available or helpful when needed. Young children may also internalize a basic sense of whether they are worthy of love and whether other people can be trusted to provide love and emotional support. Individuals who have predominantly negative self-representations usually have anxious attachment styles, and those who have predominantly negative representations of others tend to have avoidant attachment styles. Avoidant attachment is thought to stem from cool, rejecting, and distant treatment by attachment figures, and anxious attachment is traced to inconsistent and unpredictable treatment by early attachment figures (Ainsworth et al. 1978; Roth-bard and Shaver 1994).

As a guide to behavior, internal working models influence whether young children seek to regulate affective distress by approaching or by avoiding attachment figures, or even by alternating between these opposing strategies for managing negative emotions. With growth in cognitive capacity, these basic mental representations of self and other ("schemas") are subject to elaboration, refinement, and increasing differentiation from affective experiences that occur in close relationships. Nevertheless, these schemas appear to have a remarkably enduring impact on interpersonal strategies used to regulate emotional distress (e.g., Waters et al. 2000). Developmental changes often reflect heterotypic continuity in how attachment styles are expressed in different relationships across developmental stages. That is, a negative self-schema may generate anxious preoccupation with changing attachment figures—a primary caregiver in early childhood, a peer group in adolescence, a romantic partner in adulthood—but nevertheless reflect the same basic difficulty regulating affect across the different kinds of relationships.

Although distorted working models accompanying insecure attachment are not pathological by themselves, they may nevertheless contribute to the formation of Axis II psychopathology, especially when combined with other risks or biological vulnerability. Markedly negative representations of others, for instance, may explain higher levels of distrust and suspiciousness in avoidant preadolescents when compared with more securely attached age peers. From this developmental starting point, a variety of pathways leading to pathological and nonpathological outcomes may depend on heritable and environmental risk factors that also influence how personality unfolds. A negative working model of others, reinforced by a hostile and secretive family environment and combined with a biological vulnerability to Cluster A disturbances, may foster a developmental

trajectory leading toward paranoid or schizotypal disturbances in adolescence and adulthood. In the absence of biological vulnerability, negative schemas regarding others and corresponding behaviors may gradually be modified as young people learn that their family is not typical of the broader social environment. Normal maturation processes thus may reduce the likelihood that early Cluster A disturbances persist over time.

Early maltreatment by caregivers may produce a serious disturbance called disorganized attachment (Solomon and George 1999; van Ijzendoorn and Bakermans-Kranenburg 2003). Abused infants and children often experience sharp conflicts when approaching caregivers for comfort and support when they also expect maltreatment from them—thus provoking unstable fluctuations between conflicting attachment strategies and behavior. Furthermore, children may fear the loss of the caregivers they depend on, thus limiting their ability to experience or express any age-appropriate anger or aggression toward that person. This phenomenon probably pertains most to the development of the marked instability in interpersonal relationships associated with borderline psychopathology (Fonagy et al. 2000; Levy 2005; Westen et al. 2006).

Developmental Changes in How the Self and Others Are Perceived

Harter (1998) described how cognitive development in infancy, childhood, and adolescence leads to changes in how young people experience their sense of self. Harter characterized the *self* as a cognitive structure around which behavior is organized, thus anchoring it squarely within the larger framework of personality. As a product of the interaction of biological and social forces, the self undergoes progressive change throughout development. Despite these changes, the self provides a sense of continuity and a source for scripts to organize behavior, thereby creating a foundation for later identity.

Harter emphasized how self-representation often reflects self-evaluation, a process of comparing oneself with other people or with an ideal self, which evolves over time as new cognitive abilities emerge during development. Self-evaluation may be filled with inflated self-worth at one end of the spectrum or laden with self-contempt at the other, and both ends of the spectrum may play an early role in the formation of personality disorders. Even at these extremes, cognitive development may nevertheless allow gradual movement toward a more accurate self-representation with a balanced integration of positive and negative attributes. Although not addressed in self-perception literature, per se, changes in cognitive development probably influence how others are perceived in an analogous manner.

One aspect of the cognitive development of the self can be seen in how children describe themselves at different ages. At early ages children usually describe themselves by their physical characteristics, typical behaviors, or material possessions. Self-perception thus lacks much coherence or integration and self-representation is organized instead around all-or-none thinking (all good or all bad). Because negative and positive characteristics are polar opposites, the child cannot recognize that a single person can have both. Given their inability to distinguish real and ideal selves, young children typically have unrealistically positive self-perceptions that often shade into childhood grandiosity. Older children can admit to negative characteristics in one domain while retaining a positive self-representation in another. Vacillation between positive and negative self-image in early adolescence is gradually replaced by a more integrated sense of self and a greater awareness of the importance of the context to behavior. Early grandiosity thus subsides as young people gain the ability to integrate conflicting self-perceptions into a coherent whole in adolescence and early adulthood.

Inaccurate but age-appropriate self-perceptions in young children thus may resemble later symptoms of narcissistic personality disorder. If unrealistically positive self-representations become inflexible and persist over time, they may limit the young person's ability to abandon immature self-representations as their cognitive resources and perceptual skills increase during the course of normal development. When serving defensive functions against childhood adversity, early grandiosity may persist and harden into personality disorder symptoms. Furthermore, grandiosity may be pathological when asserted aggressively as a way to prevent "all good" self-representations from shifting and suddenly becoming "all bad." This defensive style may lead young people with narcissistic disturbances to have dismissing or derogatory perceptions of others. In BPD, young people may lack sufficient internal defenses to prevent self-representations from alternating frequently between the extremes of all good and all bad. Their perception of others similarly alternates between extremes of idealization and devaluation, thus constituting the clinical phenomenon called "splitting." Although they remain unstable, these mental images of self and others are frequently marked by self-contempt and attributions of malevolence in others (Bender and Skodol 2007)

Among severely abused children, negative self-perceptions may predominate over positive self-images and lead those children to feel profoundly unworthy and unlovable (Fischer and Ayoub 1994). In abusive family environments, caregivers typically reinforce negative evaluations of the child that are then incorporated into the child's self-representations. As a result, there may be little foundation for any cognitive structure of self that would allow the child to develop and integrate both positive and negative self-evaluations. Furthermore, negative self-evaluations may become automatic (Beck et al 2004; Siegler 1991) in ways that make them even more resistant to change.

Formal operational thinking, including logical and abstract reasoning abilities, normally emerges in adolescence (Keating 1990). Dramatic increases in differentiation between self and other also occur during adolescence (Bowlby 1973) and thus increase young people's ability to view themselves as distinct from caregivers. Because differentiation facilitates greater autonomy, dependence on parental attachment figures normally declines during adolescence as young people identify more with peer groups intead. At present we know little about how peer relationships influence personality maturation during adolescence, but this important social factor may reinforce self-perceptions that are more internally based and less centered around the parent–child relationship. Although elevated dependency might not necessarily be pathological in early adolescence, it may become a symptom of dependent personality disorder if it persists past late adolescence and into early adulthood.

The advent of formal operational thinking provides adolescents with a greater capacity to evaluate and compare their relationships with different attachment figures, not just with one another but also against hypothetical ideals. The adolescent's ability to consider attachment relationships in the abstract may bring with it recognition that parents are deficient in some ways (Kobak and Cole 1994), perhaps provoking a dismissive rejection of the parents or angry preoccupation with their shortcomings. Gains in adolescent insight into parent–child relationships will ideally lead to greater openness, objectivity, and flexibility as young people reevaluate attachment relationships and attain a more realistic and integrated perception of parents. This developmental process may reduce dismissing behaviors or dramatic outbursts of anger that might appear earlier in adolescence to be symptoms of narcissism or histrionic personality disorder. If parents respond to these adolescent behaviors in maladaptive ways based on their own interpersonal disturbances, they may not facilitate the resolution of parent–child conflicts and may instead reinforce narcissistic and histrionic tenden-

cies past developmental stages when they normally decline. Linehan (1993) emphasized how invalidating responses from parents can contribute substantially to the formation of BPD, and Bezirganian et al. (1993) have documented that kind of relationship empirically.

Self-Understanding, Self-Direction, and Identity

Erikson (1968) argued that once young people gain greater awareness of themselves and more accurate perceptions of others, they often experience a normative crisis of identity during adolescence and early adulthood. This identity crisis is one of eight age-specific normative crises that occur in human development from infancy through old age. According to Erikson, a crisis is a turning point when development must move in one direction or another. In adolescence, young people either move toward consolidating a secure and stable sense of self or they experience diffuse identities that provide limited direction or sense of continuity over time. When the developmental crisis of identity is successfully resolved, it normally leads to increased integration of personality. When an identity crisis goes unresolved, it may result in potentially pathological delays in maturation instead.

Identity consolidation during adolescence primarily entails establishing a clear sense of self and finding a place in the community. *Identity* is broadly defined in Erikson's theory to encompass self-esteem, satisfaction with personal and occupational goals, and confidence in coping skills. Group membership and sexual identity represent other important domains in a young person's identity. Identity diffusion, on the other hand, is typically expressed in the inability to select clear occupational goals or the adoption of roles deviating from conventional social norms. Erikson notes that identity diffusion may at times include delinquent behavior or psychotic-like symptoms but cautions that these disturbances are often transient during adolescence. Any significant disturbances in social and emotional development may act to distort or interfere with normative identity consolidation, perhaps thereby contributing to the persistence of early personality disorder symptoms that otherwise might resolve through normal maturational processes.

As defined by Erikson, identity diffusion shares many characteristics with Axis II symptoms (Cloninger et al. 1993; Kernberg 1975; Taylor and Goritsas 1994). Indeed, identity disturbances are explicitly included in diagnostic criteria for BPD. Identity disturbances are strongly implied in the suggestibility to other people's influence in histrionic personality disorder, idealized but unrealistic self-perceptions in narcissistic personality disorder, marked worry about other people's criticism in avoidant personality disorder, and difficulties in making everyday decisions in dependent personality disorder. Moreover, identity diffusion and personality disorder symptoms share similar developmental trajectories: both decline with age during adolescence and early adulthood (Johnson et al. 2000a; Meeus et al. 1999).

Distinctions between normal identity diffusion and more enduring personality disorder symptoms in adolescence may be difficult to make in clinical evaluations. Erikson noted that it is normal for young people to "try on" different identities during adolescence and later abandon them when they fail to fit comfortably with their sense of identity. For instance, early attempts to express sexuality may manifest in provocative dress during adolescence without necessarily being a symptom of histrionic personality disorder (Crawford and Cohen 2007). After trying out that overt expression of sexuality, young people may subsequently opt for less provocative attire that corresponds more with their internal sense of self. On the other hand, if provocative dressing co-occurs with poorly regulated affect and maladaptive preoccupation with interpersonal relationships, it may signal a more lasting disturbance of personality.

Despite the broad overlap between personality disorder symptoms and Erikson's construct of identity diffusion, relatively little research has investigated the association between the two. It thus remains unclear whether identity disturbances contribute to the emergence of personality disorders in adolescence and later persistence into adulthood or if personality disorder symptoms delay the consolidation of identity. Consistent with Erikson's epigenetic theory of development, Cluster B symptoms do appear to interfere with the formation of lasting and committed romantic relationships that represent the key developmental task of early adulthood (Crawford et al. 2004). Identity consolidation may occur at a critical stage in the development of personality disorders because it coincides with a period when parental influence declines and youths increasingly assert their independence. As young people gradually separate from the family, the identity they choose plays that much greater a role in defining their personality. If adolescents are unable to clearly differentiate themselves from their parents or to resolve any ongoing disturbances in their relationship, they are likely to carry internalized versions of those difficulties with them in how they perceive themselves and others, perhaps even recapitulating those disturbances in new relationships in adulthood. In other words, if identity remains poorly differentiated as young people separate from their family, any corresponding interpersonal disturbances may become self-perpetuating during adulthood.

PERSONALITY MATURATION AND AXIS II PSYCHOPATHOLOGY

Personality traits reflect a complex adaptive system to internal and environmental conditions, including changes in affective and cognitive structures during development (Caspi 1998; Caspi et al. 2005). Specific affects, behaviors, and cognitions that are age appropriate or normative at one stage of personality development may reflect immaturity or psychopathology at subsequent ages. As young people gain emotional and cognitive skills, they usually abandon immature ways of experiencing and interacting with the world around them. On the other hand, when young people continue to experience affects, behaviors, or cognitions that their peers have outgrown, they may encounter interpersonal difficulties that in some cases accumulate over time. Interpersonal difficulties may be traced to various deficits in the development of affect regulation during infancy, the formation of conscience during early childhood, the establishment of age-appropriate impulse control in childhood and adolescence, or the consolidation of identity in late adolescence and early adulthood. Although deficits or delays in emotional development do not necessarily signify Axis II pathology, they may indicate that an individual is on a deviant pathway with increased risk for further maladaptive behavior. Persistence on a deviant pathway is related to increasing difficulty in returning to a more normal developmental trajectory. Maturational change remains possible, but given the organizational function of personality, developmental change will be constrained by the individual's previous history. (For a further discussion of developmental considerations, see Bleiberg 2001; Cohen 2008; De Clercq and De Fruyt 2007; Freeman and Reinecke 2007; Geiger and Crick 2001; and Kernberg et al. 2000.)

Emotional and Behavioral Problems and Personality Disorder Symptoms

Children and adolescents appear to outgrow many problem behaviors that are reflected in current symptom criteria for personality disorder diagnoses. For instance, parent reports on the Child Behavior Checklist (CBCL; Achenbach 1991) show a significant linear decline in withdrawn behavior from age 4 to age 18 (Bongers et al. 2003). Withdrawn behavior pertains not just to Cluster A personality disorders (paranoid, schizoid, and schizotypal personality disorders) but also to avoidant personality disorder. Parent reports on individual CBCL items associated with Cluster B personality disorders (borderline, histrionic, and narcissistic personality disorders and conduct disorder that precedes ASPD) similarly indicate declines in bragging, showing off, demanding attention, getting into fights, lying, cheating, having a hot temper, crying a lot, feeling excessive dependence, having problems with peers, and experiencing jealousy (Achenbach 1991). Despite broad normative reductions in emotional and behavioral problems, parents report average increases in some childhood and adolescent symptoms such as being suspicious, secretive, and obsessively preoccupied with certain thoughts. Furthermore, age changes in symptoms in normative samples do not necessarily follow the same trajectories as children and adolescents brought in for clinical evaluation or treatment (Achenbach 1991). Parents may take normative age changes into account when assessing the well-being of their children and thus become concerned only when the expected normative decline does not appear, at least for some problems.

It may be useful to put these changes in symptom levels in the context of changes in the prevalence of Axis I symptoms and disorders over childhood and adolescence. Disruptive behavior shows a standard inverted U-shaped prevalence distribution in a wide range of studies (see Moffitt 2007 for a review), with large increases from childhood to adolescence and a sharp drop in young adulthood. Based on parent reports, there are different curvilinear trajectories for mean levels of anxious and depressive symptoms for boys and girls over the full age range from age 4 to 18 years, with higher rates of problems for boys in childhood followed by an adolescent decline (Bongers et al. 2003). For girls these problems increase until the transitional stage of puberty and then level off. Using teachers as informants in a large national epidemiological study, McDermott

(1996) found means on every symptom cluster changing with age between ages 5 and 17 years, often quite differently for males and females.

Normal and Abnormal Personality Traits

Many researchers view personality disorder symptoms as extreme variants of personality traits that are continuously distributed in the population (Costa and Widiger 2002; Livesley and Jang 2000). We currently have only partial information on developmental changes in trait levels and no information in childhood because of problems in conceptualizing and measuring personality before adolescence (Shiner and Caspi 2003).

Perhaps the most complete information available on age changes is based on the five-factor model (FFM) and its component facets that attempt to measure variation in the full normative range of personality. These broad dimensions and more narrowly defined facets have also been proposed as a way of understanding and potentially measuring personality disorder (Costa and Widiger 2002). The dimension labeled neuroticism is especially pertinent because it is hypothesized to reflect many of the criteria for personality disorder. Age changes in self-reported scores on the NEO Personality Inventory—Revised (NEO-PI-R; Costa and McCrae 1992) were evaluated in a longitudinal sample of gifted children between age 12 and 16 years and in a much larger cross-sectional sample of Flemish adolescents between age 14 and 18 years (McCrae et al. 2002). Most age changes were very small and did not follow previously established adult trajectories that show a gradual decline in neuroticism from the college years to age 30 years (e.g., McCrae et al. 1999). When evaluated in younger adolescent samples, neuroticism showed an elevation in girls up to about age 14 years and stability thereafter, and there were no significant age changes in boys. Within each broader factor of the FFM, individual facet–age correlations were sometimes different in direction in this study, with some neuroticism facets increasing with age, some stable over the age span, and some declining.

Although knowledge of normative age changes in personality disorder symptoms is limited, the available data clearly show that nearly every Axis II disorder has a gradual linear decrease in average symptom levels between ages 10 and 35. When tracked across 20 years in approximately 800 youths in the Children in the Community random sample (Cohen et al. 2005; Crawford et al. 2005), mean personality disorder symptoms were highest in early adolescence (Johnson et al. 2000a) and steadily declined with age well into adulthood (Crawford et al. 2006). Since mean levels are higher in early adolescence, more youths are likely to meet fixed diagnostic criteria that do not take changing age norms into account, thereby possibly increasing the rate of false-positive diagnoses during adolescence. These data suggest that age-specific norms may be desirable for an assessment instrument in this age range. However, they also make clear that the problem of changing normative symptom levels is not limited to childhood and adolescence. Despite changes in symptom level norms, adolescent psychiatric disorders warrant clinical attention even in developmental periods when they are most prevalent.

On the whole, normative data do not show any clear congruence between average age changes in normal personality dimensions measured on the NEO-PI-R and normative changes observed using personality disorder measures based on combined youth and parent reports or parent-reported measures of clinically relevant emotional and behavior symptoms. Some of the discrepancy may reflect how the NEO-PI-R assesses personality traits in the normal range and may be limited by ceiling effects at the extreme range of functioning assessed by personality disorder measures or the CBCL. Once again, the direction of age-related changes in symptoms in normative community samples may not always correspond to age-related change in symptoms in children from clinical populations.

CHANGE AND STABILITY IN CHILDHOOD

Given our knowledge that the prevalence of particular behaviors changes with age, what can be said about the correlational or rank-order stability of personality or its temperamental precursors over childhood and adolescence? In particular, to what extent may we expect that the same individuals who manifest the most extreme personality problems at one age will be among those who do so at another age?

Temperament

Temperament is often regarded as an early precursor to personality (Shiner 2005) that reflects basic biological differences in childhood characteristics such as activity level, fearful withdrawal, ability to be soothed, responsiveness to stimuli, and affective intensity. Temperament is typically measured by observational ratings or maternal report. Cloninger and his colleagues have developed a measure assessing temperament dimensions in preschool children that are posited to be related to later personality disorder (Constantino et al. 2002). Mervielde et al. (2005) and De Clercq et al. (2006) have also conceptualized and developed measures to track continuities between childhood temperament, personality, and personality pathology.

In general, temperament shows significant but low stability in early childhood (Rothbart and Bates 1998) for reasons that may be intrinsic to the developmental process. For example, there may be effects specific to maturational levels due to genetic or other constitutional influences. The impact of contextual factors may vary at different maturational levels. Constitutional–environ-

mental interactions also may be an important source of variation in early childhood, when strong behavioral habits have not yet become firmly established. There may be more error in observation-based measures of temperament in infants and preschool children than in older children due to their greater reactivity to fatigue, hunger, and other temporary influences. Increased measurement error thus may contribute to lower stability estimates in younger children.

An additional problem has been an absence of consensus on how to define the major temperament dimensions, an issue that has only recently begun to be resolved. Some dimensions of temperament and the measures devised to assess them have been theoretically derived (Rothbart et al. 2001; Tellegen 1985), including predicted relationships with specific personality disorders (Cloninger 1987; Cloninger et al. 1993). However, theoretically derived dimension names sometimes do not clearly correspond to the content of items. Despite an array of unique construct-derived names, certain dimensions of temperament can be viewed in the frame of the FFM (Shiner and Caspi 2003). This frame has the advantage of uniting the personality and temperament literatures but does only partial justice to the original conceptions of the important individual differences in early childhood such as executive control and emotional reactivity. Research linking temperament measured in early childhood to later personality disorder is only beginning to appear (Constantino et al. 2002).

Personality Dimensions

There is clear evidence that, on average, a personality dimension assessed by a self-report instrument will show lower correlation over equivalent time for younger persons than for older persons (Roberts and DelVecchio 2000). Because instability in personality dimensions continues throughout life, correlations measuring stability reach a maximum at about age 50 years. Stabilities for symptom measures of personality disorder are very likely to show a similar pattern. Although we have no preadolescent data, correlations measuring stability are moderate in adolescence (Crawford et al. 2001a), and it is not clear that they increase from adolescence into young adulthood (Johnson et al. 2000a). General stability may not be the issue if disorders are outcomes of gene–environment interactions, so that it is expected that there may be lower stability on extreme scores than over the full range of relevant dimensions (DiLalla et al. 2000).

Axis II diagnoses, on the other hand, tend to be much less stable in clinical and community samples of adolescents (Bernstein et al. 1993; Mattanah et al. 1995). Axis II diagnoses in adults similarly tend to be unstable even in clinical samples (Shea et al. 2002; Zanarini et al. 2003). This instability is likely to be a consequence not only of the generally poorer measurement quality of dichotomized continuous measures (MacCallum et al. 2002) but also of somewhat arbitrary decisions about diagnostic cut-points. Despite the relative instability of categorically defined diagnoses, there is increasing evidence of long-term impairment and poor prognosis associated with adolescent personality disorder or a high level of personality disorder symptoms independent of Axis I disorders or symptoms (Chen et al. 2006a, 2006b; Crawford et al. 2008; Johnson et al. 1999, 2000b; Kasen et al. 1999, 2007; Lofgren et al. 1991; Rey et al. 1997; Skodol et al. 2007; Winograd et al. 2008). We are thus accumulating evidence that the criteria for adult disorders may be useful indicators of Axis II pathology even in young samples and not necessarily less predictive at times when they are more normative (also see Cohen et al. 2007; Ehrensaft et al. 2006; Kasen et al. 2001).

Comorbidity With Axis I Disorders

Axis II disorders in adolescence frequently co-occur with Axis I disorders (Cohen et al. 2005). Of adolescents diagnosed with Cluster A disorders in a community sample, 35% had disruptive disorders, 25% had anxiety disorders, and 20% had depressive disorders (Kasen et al. 1999). A full 47% of those with Cluster B disorders had a comorbid disruptive behavior disorder, 38% had an anxiety disorder, and 28% had a depressive disorder. Over half (51%) of those with Cluster C diagnoses had an anxiety disorder, 34% had a disruptive behavior disorder, and 23% had a depressive disorder.

Co-occurrence of Axis I and Axis II disorders is important because of its impact on prognosis. When adolescent Cluster A disorders co-occurred with disruptive behavior disorders, the risk for a subsequent Cluster A diagnosis in early adulthood was 24.6 times higher than the risk for adolescents with no psychiatric disorder (Kasen et al. 1999). By comparison, the risk for Cluster A disorders in early adulthood was only 2.76 times higher when Cluster A disorders in adolescence were diagnosed without any disruptive behavior disorder. Similarly, the risk for Cluster B diagnoses in early adulthood was 19 times higher when earlier Cluster B disorders co-occurred with major depression, but only 3.83 times higher when these personality disorders occurred without major depression.

Recent research shows that the effects of comorbid Axis I and Axis II disorders continue well beyond early adulthood. Compared with adolescents with no psychiatric disorder, adolescents with diagnoses on both axes had an almost nine-fold increase in risk for psychiatric disorders 20 years later, when assessed at mean age 33 years (Crawford et al. 2008). Adolescents with co-occurring Axis I and II disorders also were more likely to have been in treatment or take psychotropic drugs when subsequently assessed as adults (Kasen et al. 2007). Impairment and lower functioning were still evident 20 years later among adolescents with Axis II diagnoses alone, but prognosis was consistently worse for academic, occupational, interpersonal, and psychiatric functioning when Axis I and

Axis II disorders co-occurred in adolescence (Crawford et al. 2008). Given effects that persisted across two decades, it is important for clinicians to evaluate and treat adolescent personality disorders, especially when they co-occur with Axis I disorders.

Case Examples

Given what we know about developmental trajectories of personality disorder symptoms in adolescents, it appears unwise to make categorical diagnoses during initial clinical assessment except perhaps in extreme cases. Nevertheless, it is meaningful to consider youths at risk for subsequent personality disorder based on how they present for treatment and based on collateral risk factors in close family members, as illustrated by the following vignette.

> A 15-year-old boy from an intact family was brought for individual psychotherapy to address uncontrolled anger, a pervasive hatred toward age peers, and oppositional and self-defeating behavior (e.g., threatening to drop out of high school). His self-image reflected grandiosity or self-contempt depending on different social contexts, and he tended to be avoidant and dismissive of others. During treatment it became evident that one parent tried to cope with excessive anxiety by becoming overinvolved in the patient's long-term plans in ways that provoked stubborn and oppositional behavior. The other parent had recurrent depressive episodes, an explosive and unpredictable temper, identity diffusion, and a dismissive interpersonal style.
>
> On initial evaluation, this 15-year-old youth appeared at increased risk for lasting BPD based on persistent symptoms of uncontrolled anger, marked antipathy for others, and poorly integrated representations of self and others. The long-term risk may be compounded by the presence of parental anxiety and mood disturbances, especially as they are woven into parent–child relationships. Personality disturbances thus ap-

peared to be reinforced by defensive reactions to one parent's overinvolvement and also by identification with the other parent's angry and dismissive interpersonal style. Despite poor social adjustment with peers, this youth nevertheless reported having a positive relationship with his parents. Given this protective factor and an absence of key risk factors such as childhood trauma, his personality disorder symptoms may well subside over time as he gains maturity. Treatment in this case focused on assisting the youth to regulate angry affect more adaptively and to articulate how peers upset him so much. Treatment also helped the parents to become more aware of how their own anxiety and mood disturbances contributed to maladaptive parent–child interactions in ways that inhibited the youth's gradual movement toward independent adult functioning.

Just as maturational factors appear to confound the assessment of personality disorders in adolescents, they may also obscure the presence of personality disorder in adults who have outgrown some earlier manifestations of the disorder. Knowledge of normative trajectories of personality disorder thus can inform the assessment and treatment of personality disturbances in adult patients whose symptoms fall short of current diagnostic criteria:

> A 42-year-old woman presented for treatment with complaints of loneliness and an enduring inability to establish a stable romantic relationship. She recalled adolescence and early adulthood as periods characterized by labile mood, frequent abandonment fears, volatile and unpredictable romantic relationships, reactive anger toward parents and peers, and a series of suicidal gestures. During childhood she witnessed violent conflicts between mother and father before they divorced and experienced significant emotional neglect afterward. When presenting for treatment, this patient denied any mood lability or suicidal ideation and

functioned well at work. However, she experienced abandonment fears, reactive anger, and mood lability whenever she became involved in new romantic relationships, thereby prompting a general avoidance of close relationships and reinforcing unwanted feelings of loneliness.

Even allowing for inaccuracies that distort retrospective clinical reports, this patient undoubtedly met full criteria for BPD during adolescence and early adulthood. Although her symptoms have since fallen below diagnostic threshold, either due to maturational factors or the effects of prior individual psychotherapies, she nevertheless continues to experience significant borderline psychopathology in ways that become painfully apparent whenever new romantic attachments evoke long-standing abandonment fears she otherwise seeks to avoid. Treatment in this case focused on clarifying and then reducing abandonment fears and addressing how her reactive anger undermined the stability of her romantic relationships. Treatment also addressed the disorganizing effects of childhood trauma and neglect.

WHAT IS THE BEST MEASUREMENT STRATEGY FOR ASSESSING EARLY PERSONALITY DISORDERS?

Three overall issues pose problems for the assessment of personality disorders in children and adolescents. First, DSM-IV-TR does not take into account normative developmental changes in the prevalence of certain problems and the consequent possibility that certain diagnostic criteria should not be seen as abnormal behavior at some ages. Second, there is a shortage of appropriate and validated diagnostic instruments for children and adolescents and unresolved questions about the best measurement strategy. Third, aspects of personality are less stable in childhood and adolescence, thus raising concern that early

diagnosis of personality disorders might lead to premature labeling.

CHOICE OF INFORMANT

In clinical assessment of adults the patient is usually the primary informant, although the corroboration and independent perspectives of knowledgeable sources such as family members are welcome and often useful. Research measures designed for use with adults in clinical or other samples generally are confined to self-report. In the child mental health field, there is still little consensus about which informants should be considered primary and which should be seen as auxiliary at different points in childhood development. It is often assumed that the primary caretaker should be the principal informant for preschool children. As such, instruments measuring temperament, personality, and psychopathology in children younger than age 9 or 10 years are most often based on information supplied by parents—for example, the Children's Behavior Questionnaire (Rothbart et al. 2001), the Personality Inventory for Children (PIC-2; Lachar 1999a), and the CBCL. For young children in preschool or day care, teachers or childcare leaders may provide the best data based on greater familiarity with normative patterns of behavior for the age.

Similarly, parents and teachers are both thought to provide relevant data for older children in elementary school, although agreement on the child's problems is often poor across these informants (Achenbach et al. 1987). Sometime in childhood, at least by age 9 or 10, most children are able to provide data on their own characteristics and problems. For instance, the youth-reported version of the Diagnostic Interview Schedule for Children Version IV (Shaffer et al. 2000) assesses psychopathology in children as young as age 9 years. Similarly, the Personality Inventory for Youth (PIY; Lachar and Gruber 1995) uses self-reports to assess personality in children starting at the same age. Most self-report measures of normal personality, however, are used only with adolescents and adults (Shiner and Caspi 2003).

Agreement between parent and offspring on youth behaviors and problems is often poor (Achenbach et al. 1987). Age changes in prevalence based on youth self-report look different from those based on parent report or teacher report. Agreement between self and informant reports on personality disorder measures for adults is similarly poor (Klonsky et al. 2002). Despite these difficulties, the research field generally agrees that all informants add usefully to the assessment of Axis I disorders in children and adolescents. As a consequence, the preferred strategy is to obtain data from at least two informants and consider any symptomatic report to be valid providing there is evidence of associated impairment. However, evidence indicates that adolescents are better informants about emotions and often acknowledge disruptive or antisocial behaviors that may be unknown to the parent when only a single informant is used. Parents or teachers are thought to be better informants on issues where normative comparisons are relevant.

Where does this leave us when deciding which informants to assess for personality disturbances in children and adolescents? At present we do not know whether diagnostic criteria for Axis II are intrinsically more difficult to assess in youth than most criteria for Axis I. All things considered, it appears prudent to gather data from multiple sources whenever possible when assessing children and adolescents.

CLINICAL MEASURES OF CHILD OR ADOLESCENT PERSONALITY DISORDER

As interest in early Axis II disturbances in young people has grown, a variety of instruments designed to measure normal and abnormal personality in adults have been evaluated for use in adolescent samples. Certain

personality disorder instruments for adults have been specifically adapted to be age appropriate for child or adolescent respondents. Among self- and parent-reported instruments, Axis II scales are typically combined with various measures of Axis I disturbances and thus facilitate the assessment of co-occurrence between these psychiatric constructs.

Structured Clinical Interviews

Of the structured interviews designed to assess DSM-defined personality disorders in adults, the Personality Disorder Examination (Loranger 1988) has been most thoroughly evaluated and appears to be a valid measure of Axis II disturbance in adolescents. Nevertheless, more work is needed to identify age-related differences in adolescent and adult manifestations of personality disorders. In a longitudinal comparison of adolescent and adult inpatient samples, personality disorders assessed with the Personality Disorder Examination were less stable over a 2-year interval in adolescents than in adults (Mattanah et al. 1995). However, threshold effects often add unreliability to stability estimates of categorically defined personality disorders, thus making comparisons across age groups more difficult to interpret. When assessed as dimensional constructs, stability estimates for personality disorders usually appear higher than when assessed as categorical constructs.

Self-Report Instruments

Although self-report instruments are easier and more cost-efficient to administer than structured interviews, questions are raised about whether respondents have sufficient self-awareness or willingness to acknowledge Axis II symptoms that might stigmatize them. Given problems in setting reliable thresholds, the available instruments for children and adolescents tend to assess Axis II symptoms using continuous scales instead of making formal diagnoses.

The Millon Adolescent Clinical Inventory (MACI) is a well-known instrument modeled on the Millon Clinical Multiaxial Inventory designed for adults (see Davis et al. 1999). Intended for adolescents as young as age 13, the MACI uses 160 self-report items to measure personality disorder constructs congruent with DSM-defined personality disorders but also reflecting Millon's (1990) theory of personality. The MACI thus measures 12 personality styles labeled Introversive, Inhibited, Doleful, Submissive, Dramatizing, Egotistic, Unruly, Forceful, Conforming, Oppositional, Self-Demeaning, and Borderline Tendency. Computer-generated scores on the MACI make adjustments for age and gender differences in Axis II disturbances based on norms from separate samples of normal and disturbed adolescents. Standardized scores are further adjusted to take estimated base rates of psychopathology into account even though the prevalence of Axis II disturbances in adolescents has yet to be established. These built-in adjustments are not readily transparent and effectively preclude their use for investigating the population prevalence of adolescent Axis II disturbances or for assessing developmental change.

Parallel Parent- and Youth-Reported Instruments

The PIC-2 and PIY were both originally modeled on the Minnesota Multiphasic Personality Inventory and thus do not correspond directly to DSM-IV (American Psychiatric Association 1994) Axis II disorders. The parent-reported PIC-2 uses 275 forced-choice items to measure constructs labeled Cognitive Impairment, Impulsivity and Distractibility, Delinquency, Family Dysfunction, Reality Distortion, Somatic Concern, Psychological Discomfort, Social Withdrawal, and Social Skills Deficits. The youth-reported PIY uses 270 forced-choice items to measure the same constructs. As suggested by the labels, the PIY and PIC-2 measure constructs that probably tap a mixture of Axis I and Axis II

disturbances. Despite substantial similarity on the PIY and PIC-2, youth and parent informants show moderate agreement (median correlation=0.43, range 0.28–0.53) (Lachar 1999b). These concordance rates appear better than the 0.25 correlation between youth and parent reports for comparable age groups on the CBCL (Achenbach et al. 1987).

Additional Instruments for DSM-IV/DSM-IV-TR Personality Disorders

The Adolescent Psychopathology Scale (Reynolds 1998) is a self-report measure designed for adolescents age 12–19 years. It measures five of the 10 DSM-IV personality disorders (borderline, avoidant, obsessive-compulsive, paranoid, and schizotypal personality disorders) along with conduct disorder as the childhood precursor of ASPD. The Coolidge Personality and Neuropsychological Inventory for Children (CPNI; Coolidge 1998) assesses DSM-IV Axis II disorders in children and adolescents from age 5–17 years by parent report. The CPNI assesses symptoms of all DSM-IV personality disorders as well as conduct disorder symptoms. The Shedler-Westen Assessment Procedure–200 for Adolescents (SWAP-200-A; Westen et al. 2003, 2005) is a Q-sort instrument designed for use by skilled clinical observers to assess Axis II pathology in adolescent patients they see in treatment. Q-sort is a method by which items are arrayed by the clinician from most descriptive of the adolescent to least descriptive of the adolescent. This measure was adapted from the Shedler-Westen Assessment Procedure–200, a Q-sort designed for adults that has shown evidence of validity, reliability, and utility in taxonomic research with adult samples (e.g., Shedler and Westen 1998). At present none of the available instruments has demonstrated clear superiority in clinical and research applications, and there are limited validity data available for newly developed scales measuring DSM-IV and DSM-IV-TR personality disorders.

CONCLUSION

Since the late 1980s, there has been accumulating evidence that clinically meaningful personality disorders occur in adolescents. Adolescent personality disorders are associated with emotional distress and psychosocial impairment in community samples (Bernstein et al. 1993, 1996; Golombek et al. 1987; Lewinsohn et al. 1997; Marton et al. 1987; Rogosch and Cicchetti 2005; Stein et al. 1987) and clinical samples in inpatient and outpatient settings (Becker and Grilo 2006; Brent et al. 1994; Grilo et al. 1996; Pinto et al. 1996; Westen et al. 2003). When adolescent and adult personality disorders are compared, many similarities can be observed. Just as adult personality disorders are associated with co-occurring Axis I disturbances (Bienvenu and Stein 2003; Skodol 2005), so have adolescent personality disorders (Becker et al. 2000; Crawford et al. 2001a, 2008). However, more work is needed on age-related differences in adolescent and adult manifestations of personality disorders.

Although elevated personality disorder scores in adolescence represent a risk for later psychiatric and psychosocial disturbances, early personality disorder symptoms are likely to decline over time. Caution is warranted in evaluating the clinical significance of symptoms during adolescence. Yet, there is almost universal agreement that prevention of mental disorders is best accomplished at a very young age and in collaboration with parents, particularly when other risk factors are also present. Therefore, children with elevated symptoms or their precursors are prime targets for secondary prevention—that is, prevention of further developmental delays or elevation to frank disorder. Regardless of how childhood and adolescent personality disorders are defined—either as an early version of adult disorder or an early indicator of elevated risk of adult disorder—it appears appropriate to consider interventions to alleviate Axis II disturbances when they manifest in young people.

REFERENCES

Achenbach TM: Manual for the Child Behavior Checklist, Ages 4–18 and 1991 Profile. Burlington, VT, University of Vermont, Department of Psychiatry, 1991

Achenbach TM, McConaughy SH, Howell CT: Child/adolescent behavioral and emotional problems: implications of cross-informant correlations for situational specificity. Psychol Bull 101:213–232, 1987

Ainsworth MDS, Blehar MC, Waters E, et al: Patterns of Attachment: A Psychological Study of the Strange Situation. Hillsdale, NJ, Erlbaum, 1978

Alexander PC: Application of attachment theory to the study of sexual abuse. J Consult Clin Psychol 60:185–195, 1992

American Psychiatric Association: Diagnostic and Statistical Manual of Mental Disorders, 4th Edition. Washington, DC, American Psychiatric Association, 1994

American Psychiatric Association: Diagnostic and Statistical Manual of Mental Disorders, 4th Edition, Text Revision. Washington, DC, American Psychiatric Association, 2000

Beck AT, Freeman A, Davis DD, et al: Cognitive Therapy of Personality Disorders, 2nd Edition. New York, Guilford Press, 2004

Becker DF, Grilo CM: Validation studies of the borderline personality disorder construct in adolescents. Adolesc Psychiatry 29:217–235, 2006

Becker DF, Grilo CM, Edell WS, et al: Comorbidity of borderline personality disorder with other personality disorders in hospitalized adolescents and adults. Am J Psychiatry 157:2011–2016, 2000

Bender DS, Skodol AE: Borderline personality as self-other representational disturbance. J Personal Disord 21:500–517, 2007

Bernstein DP, Cohen P, Velez CN, et al: Prevalence and stability of the DSM-III-R personality disorders in a community-based survey of adolescents. Am J Psychiatry 150:1237–1243, 1993

Bernstein DP, Cohen P, Skodol A, et al: Childhood antecedents of adolescent personality disorders. Am J Psychiatry 153:907–913, 1996

Bezirganian S, Cohen P, Brook JS: The impact of mother-child interaction on the development of borderline personality disorder. Am J Psychiatry 150:1836–1842, 1993

Bienvenu OJ, Stein MB: Personality and anxiety disorders: a review. J Personal Disord 17:139–151, 2003

Bleiberg E: Treating Personality Disorders in Children and Adolescents: A Relational Approach. New York, Guilford, 2001

Bongers IL, Kool IIM, van der Ende J, et al: The normative development of child and adolescent problem behavior. J Abnorm Psychol 112:179–192, 2003

Bowlby J: Attachment and Loss, Vol 1: Attachment. New York, Basic Books, 1969

Bowlby J: Attachment and Loss, Vol 2: Separation. New York, Basic Books, 1973

Brent DA, Johnson B, Perper J, et al: Personality disorder, personality traits, impulsive violence and completed suicide in adolescents. J Am Acad Child Adolesc Psychiatry 33:1080–1086, 1994

Caspi A: Personality development across the life course, in Handbook of Child Psychology, Vol 3: Social, Emotional, and Personality Development, 5th Edition. Edited by Damon W, Eisenberg N. New York, Wiley, 1998, pp 311–388

Caspi A, Roberts BW, Shiner RL: Personality development: stability and Change. Ann Rev Psychology 56: 453–484, 2005

Cassidy J, Shaver PR: Handbook of Attachment: Theory, Research, and Clinical Applications, 2nd Edition. New York, Guilford, 2008

Chen H, Cohen P, Kasen S, et al: Adolescent Axis I and personality disorders predict quality of life during young adulthood. J Adolesc Health 39:14–19, 2006a

Chen H, Cohen P, Kasen S, et al: Impact of adolescent mental disorders and physical illnesses on quality of life 17 years later. Arch Pediatr Adolesc Med 160:93–99, 2006b

Cloninger CR: A systematic method for clinical description and classification of personality variants: a proposal. Arch Gen Psychiatry 44:573–588, 1987

Cloninger CR: Genetics, in The American Psychiatric Publishing Textbook of Personality Disorders. Edited by Oldham JM, Skodol AE, Bender D. Washington, DC, American Psychiatric Publishing, 2005, pp 143–154

Cloninger CR, Svrakic DM, Przybeck TR: A psychobiological model of temperament and character. Arch Gen Psychiatry 50:975–990, 1993

Cohen P: Child development and personality disorder. Psychiatr Clin North Am 31:477–493, vii, 2008

Cohen P, Crawford TN, Johnson JG, et al: The Children in the Community Study of developmental course of personality disorder. J Personal Disord 19:466–486, 2005

Cohen P, Chen H, Crawford TN, et al: Personality disorders in early adolescence and the development of later substance use disorders in the general population. Drug and Alcohol Addiction 88S:S71–S84, 2007

Constantino JN, Cloninger CR, Clarke AR, et al: Application of the seven-factor model of personality to early childhood. Psychiatr Res 109:229–244, 2002

Coolidge FL: Coolidge Personality and Neuropsychological Inventory for Children Manual: CPNI. Colorado Springs, CO, FL Coolidge, 1998

Coolidge FL, Thede LL, Jang KL: Heritability of personality disorders in childhood: a preliminary investigation. J Personal Disord 15:33–40, 2001

Costa PT Jr, McCrae RR: Revised NEO Personality Inventory (NEO-PI-R) and NEO Five-Factor Inventory (NEO-FFI) Professional Manual. Odessa, FL, Psychological Assessment Resources, 1992

Costa PT Jr, Widiger TA (eds): Personality Disorders and the Five-Factor Model of Personality, 2nd Edition. Washington, DC, American Psychological Association, 2002

Crawford TN, Cohen P: Histrionic personality disorder, in Personality Disorders in Children and Adolescents. Edited by Freeman A, Reinecke M. New York, John Wiley & Sons, 2007, pp 495–532

Crawford TN, Cohen P, Brook JS: Dramatic erratic personality disorder symptoms, I: continuity from early adolescence into adulthood. J Personal Disord 15:319–335, 2001a

Crawford TN, Cohen P, Brook JS: Dramatic erratic personality disorder symptoms, II: developmental pathways from early adolescence to adulthood. J Personal Disord 15:336–350, 2001b

Crawford TN, Cohen P, Johnson JG, et al: The course and psychosocial correlates of personality disorder symptoms in adolescence: Erikson's developmental theory revisited. J Youth Adolesc 33:373–387, 2004

Crawford TN, Cohen P, Johnson JG, et al: Self-reported personality disorder in the Children in the Community sample: convergent validity and prospective validity in late adolescence and adulthood. J Personal Disord 19:30–52, 2005

Crawford TN, Shaver PR, Cohen P et al: Self-reported attachment, interpersonal aggression, and personality disorder in a prospective community sample of adolescents and adults. J Personal Disord 20:331–353, 2006

Crawford TN, Cohen P, First MB, et al: Comorbid Axis I and Axis II disorders in early adolescence: outcomes 20 years later. Arch Gen Psychiatry 65:641–648, 2008

Davis RD, Woodward M, Goncalves A, et al: Treatment planning and outcome in adults: the Millon Clinical Multiaxial Inventory-III, in The Use of Psychological Testing for Treatment Planning and Outcomes Assessment, 2nd Edition. Edited by Maruish ME. Mahwah, NJ, Erlbaum, 1999, pp 1051–1081

De Clercq B, De Fruyt: Childhood antecedents of personality disorder. Curr Opin Psychiatry 20:57–61, 2007

De Clercq B, De Fruyt F, Van Leeuwen K, et al: The structure of maladaptive personality traits in childhood: a step toward an integrative developmental perspective for DSM-V. J Abnorm Psychol 115:639–657 2006

DiLalla DL, Gottesman II, Carey G: Madness beyond the threshold? Associations between personality and psychopathology, in Temperament and Personality Development Across the Life Span. Edited by Molfese VJ, Molfese DL. Mahwah, NJ, Erlbaum, 2000, pp 177–210

Ehrensaft M, Cohen P, Johnson JG: Development of personality disorder symptoms and the risk for partner violence. J Abnormal Psychol 115:474–483, 2006

Erikson EH: Identity: Youth and Crisis. New York, WW Norton, 1968

Fischer KW, Ayoub C: Affective splitting and dissociation in normal and maltreated children: developmental pathways for self in relationships, in Disorders and Dysfunctions of the Self: Rochester Symposium on Developmental Psychopathology, Vol 5. Edited by Cicchetti D, Toth SL. New York, Plenum Press, 1994, pp 149–222

Fonagy P, Target M, Gergely G: Attachment and borderline personality disorder: a theory and some evidence. Psychiatr Clin North Am 23:103–122, 2000

Fonagy P, Target M, Gergely G, et al: The developmental roots of borderline personality disorder in early attachment relationships: a theory and some evidence. Psychoanalytic Inquiry 23:412–459, 2003

Freeman A, Reinecke M (eds): Personality Disorders in Children and Adolescents. New York, John Wiley & Sons, 2007

Geiger TC, Crick NR: A developmental psychopathology perspective on vulnerability to personality disorders, in Vulnerability to Psychopathology. Edited by Ingram RE, Price JM. New York, Guilford, 2001, pp 57–102

Golombek H, Marton P, Stein B, et al: Personality functioning status during early and middle adolescence. Adolesc Psychiatry 14:365–377, 1987

Grilo CM, Becker DF, Fehon DC, et al: Gender differences in personality disorders in psychiatrically hospitalized adolescents. Am J Psychiatry 153:1089–1091, 1996

Harter S: The development of self-representations, in Handbook of Child Psychology, Vol 3: Social, Emotional, and Personality Development, 5th Edition. Edited by Damon W, Eisenberg N. New York, Wiley, 1998, pp 553–617

Jang KL: The Behavioral Genetics of Psychopathology: A Clinical Guide. Mahwah, NJ, Erlbaum, 2005

Johnson JG, Cohen P, Skodol AE, et al: Personality disorders in adolescence and risk of major mental disorders and suicidality during adulthood. Arch Gen Psychiatry 56: 805–811, 1999

Johnson JG, Cohen P, Kasen S, et al: Age-related change in personality disorder trait levels between early adolescence and adulthood: a community-based longitudinal investigation. Acta Psychiatr Scand 102:265–275, 2000a

Johnson JG, Cohen P, Smailes E, et al: Adolescent personality disorders associated with violence and criminal behavior during adolescence and early adulthood. Am J Psychiatry 157:1406–1412, 2000b

Kasen S, Cohen P, Skodol AE, et al: Influence of child and adolescent psychiatric disorders on young adult personality disorder. Am J Psychiatry 156:1529–1535, 1999

Kasen S, Cohen P, Skodol AE, et al: Childhood depression and adult personality disorder: alternative pathways of continuity. Arch Gen Psychiatry 58:231–236, 2001

Kasen S, Cohen P, Skodol AE, et al: Comorbid personality disorder and treatment use in a community sample of youths: a 20-year follow-up. Acta Psychiatr Scand 115:56–65, 2007

Keating D: Adolescent thinking, in At the Threshold: The Developing Adolescent. Edited by Feldman SS, Elliott G. Cambridge, MA, Harvard University Press, 1990, pp 54–90

Kernberg OF: Borderline Conditions and Pathological Narcissism. Northvale, NJ, Jason Aronson, 1975

Kernberg PF, Weiner AS, Bardenstein KK: Personality Disorders in Children and Adolescents. New York, Basic Books, 2000

Klonsky ED, Oltmanns TF, Turkheirmer E: Informant reports of personality disorders: relation to self-reports and future research directions. Clinical Psychology: Science and Practice 9:300–311, 2002

Kobak R, Cole C: Attachment and metamonitoring: implications for adolescent autonomy and psychopathology, in Rochester Symposium on Development and Psychopathology, Vol 5: Disorders of the Self. Edited by Cicchetti D. Rochester, NY, University of Rochester Press, 1994, pp 267–297

Lachar D: Personality Inventory for Children-2 (PIC-2) Manual. Los Angeles, CA, Western Psychological Services, 1999a

Lachar D: Personality Inventory for Children, 2nd Edition (PIC-2), Personality Inventory for Youth (PIY), and Student Behavior Survey (SBS), in The Use of Psychological Testing for

Treatment Planning and Outcomes Assessment, 2nd Edition. Edited by Maruish ME. Mahwah, NJ, Lawrence Erlbaum Associates, 1999b, pp 399–427

Lachar D, Gruber CP: Personality Inventory for Youth (PIY) Manual. Los Angeles, CA, Western Psychological Services, 1995

Levy KN: The implications of attachment theory and research for understanding borderline personality disorder. Developmental Psychopathology 17:959–986, 2005

Lewinsohn PM, Rohde P, Seeley JR, et al: Axis II psychopathology as a function of Axis I disorders in childhood and adolescence. J Am Acad Child Adolesc Psychiatry 36:1752–1759, 1997

Linehan MM: Cognitive Behavioral Treatment of Borderline Personality Disorder. New York, Guilford, 1993

Livesley WJ, Jang KL: Toward an empirically based classification of personality disorder. J Person Disord 14:137–151, 2000

Lofgren DP, Bemporad J, King J, et al: A follow-up study of so-called borderline children. Am J Psychiatry 148:1541–1547, 1991

Loranger AW: Personality Disorder Examination (PDE) Manual. Yonkers, NY, DV Communications, 1988

Lyddon WJ, Alford DJ: Personality disorders: a cognitive behavioral perspective, in Personality Disorders in Children and Adolescents. Edited by Freeman A, Reinecke M. New York, John Wiley & Sons, 2007, pp 99–130

MacCallum RC, Zhang S, Preacher KJ, et al: On the practice of dichotomization of quantitative variables. Psychol Methods 7:41–63, 2002

Marton P, Golombek H, Stein B, et al: Behavior disturbance and changes in personality dysfunction from early to middle adolescence. Adolesc Psychiatry 14:394–406, 1987

Mattanah JJF, Becker DF, Levy KN, et al: Diagnostic stability in adolescents followed 2 years after hospitalization. Am J Psychiatry 152:889–894, 1995

McCrae RR, Costa PT, de Lima MP, et al: Age differences in personality across the adult life span: parallels in five cultures. Dev Psychol 35:466–477, 1999

McCrae RR, Costa PT, Terracciano A, et al: Personality trait development from age 12 to age 18: longitudinal, cross-sectional, and cross-cultural analyses. J Pers Soc Psychol 83:1456–1468, 2002

McDermott PA: A nationwide study of developmental and gender prevalence for psychopathology in childhood and adolescence. J Abnorm Child Psychol 24:53–66, 1996

Meeus W, Iedema J, Helsen M, et al: Patterns of adolescent identity development: review of

literature and longitudinal analysis. Dev Rev 19:419–461, 1999

Mervielde I, De Clercq B, De Fruyt F, et al: Temperament, personality, and developmental psychopathology as childhood antecedents of personality disorders. J Person Disord 19:171–201, 2005

Mikulincer M, Shaver PR, Pereg D: Attachment theory and affect regulation: the dynamics, development, and cognitive consequences of attachment-related strategies. Motiv Emot 2:77–102, 2003

Millon T: Toward a New Personology: An Evolutionary Model. New York, Wiley, 1990

Moffitt TE: A review of research on the taxonomy of life-course persistent versus adolescence-limited antisocial behavior, in The Cambridge Handbook of Violent Behavior and Aggression. Edited by Flannery DJ, Vazsonyi AT, Waldman ID. New York, Cambridge University Press, 2007, pp 49–74

Pine F: On the development of the "borderline-child-to-be." Am J Orthopsychiatry 56:450–457, 1986

Pinto A, Grapentine WL, Francis G, et al: Borderline personality disorder in adolescents: affective and cognitive features. J Am Acad Child Adolesc Psychiatry 35:1338–1343, 1996

Rey JM, Singh M, Morris-Yates A, et al: Referred adolescents as young adults: the relationship between psychosocial functioning and personality disorder. Aust N Z J Psychiatry 31:219–226, 1997

Reynolds WM: Adolescent Psychopathology Scale. Odessa, FL, Psychological Assessment Resources, 1998

Roberts BW, DelVecchio WF: The rank-order consistency of personality traits from childhood to old age: a quantitative review of longitudinal studies. Psychol Bull 126:3–25, 2000

Rogosch FA, Cicchetti D: Child maltreatment, attention networks, and potential precursors to borderline personality disorder. Dev Psychopathol 17:1071–1089, 2005

Rothbard JC, Shaver PR: Continuity of attachment across the life span, in Attachment in Adults: Clinical and Developmental Perspectives. Edited by Sperling MB, Berman WH. New York, Guilford, 1994, pp 31–71

Rothbart MK, Bates JE: Temperament, in Handbook of Child Psychology, Vol 3: Social, Emotional, and Personality Development, 5th Edition. Edited by Damon M, Eisenberg N. New York, Wiley, 1998, pp 105–176

Rothbart MK, Ahadi SA, Hershey KL, et al: Investigations of temperament at three to seven years: the Children's Behavior Questionnaire. Child Dev 72:1394–1408, 2001

Shaffer D, Fisher P, Lucas CP, et al: NIMH Diagnostic Interview Schedule for Children Version IV (NIMH DISC-IV): description, differences from previous versions, and reliability of some common diagnoses. J Am Acad Child Adolesc Psychiatry 39:28–38, 2000

Shea MT, Stout R, Gunderson J, et al: Short-term diagnostic stability of schizotypal, borderline, avoidant, and obsessive-compulsive personality disorders. Am J Psychiatry 159:2036–2041, 2002

Shedler J, Westen D: Refining the measurement of Axis II: a Q-sort procedure for assessing personality pathology. Assessment 5:335–355, 1998

Shiner R: A developmental perspective on personality disorders: lessons from research on normal personality development in childhood and adolescence. J Personal Disord 19:202–210, 2005

Shiner R, Caspi A: Personality differences in childhood and adolescence: measurement, development, and consequences. J Child Psychol Psychiatry 44:2–32, 2003

Siegler RS: Children's Thinking, 2nd Edition. Englewood Cliffs, NJ, Prentice Hall, 1991

Skodol AE: Manifestations, clinical diagnosis, and comorbidity, in The American Psychiatric Publishing Textbook of Personality Disorders. Edited by Oldham JM, Skodol AE, Bender D. Washington, DC, American Psychiatric Publishing, 2005, pp 57–87

Skodol AE, Johnson JG, Cohen P, et al: Personality disorder and impaired functioning from adolescence to adulthood. Br J Psychiatry 190:415–420, 2007

Solomon J, George C: Attachment Disorganization. New York, Guilford, 1999

Sroufe LA: Emotional Development: The Organization of Emotional Life in the Early Years. New York, Cambridge University Press, 1996

Stein B, Golombek H, Marton P, et al: Personality functioning and change in clinical presentation from early to middle adolescence. Adolesc Psychiatry 14:378–393, 1987

Taylor S, Goritsas E: Dimensions of identity diffusion. J Personal Disord 8:229–239, 1994

Tellegen A: Structure of mood and personality and their relevance to assessing anxiety, with an emphasis on self-report, in Anxiety and the Anxiety Disorders. Edited by Tuma AH, Maser JD. Hillsdale, NJ, Erlbaum, 1985, pp 681–706

van Ijzendoorn MH, Bakermans-Kranenburg MJ: Attachment disorders and disorganized attachment: similar and different. Attach Hum Dev 5:313–320, 2003

Waters E, Merrick S, Treboux D, et al: Attachment security in infancy and early adulthood: a longitudinal study. Child Dev 71:684–689, 2000

Westen D, Shedler J, Glass S, et al: Personality diagnoses in adolescence: DSM-IV Axis II diagnoses and an empirically derived alternative. Am J Psychiatry 160:952–966, 2003

Westen D, Dutra L, Shedler J: Assessing adolescent personality pathology. Br J Psychiatry 186:227–238, 2005

Westen D, Nakash O, Thomas C, et al: Clinical assessment of attachment patterns and personality disorder in adolescents and adults. J Consult Clin Psychol 74:1065–1085, 2006

Widiger TA, Sankis L: Adult psychopathology: issues and controversies. Ann Rev Psychol 51:377–404, 2000

Winograd G, Cohen P, Chen H: Adolescent borderline symptoms in the community: prognosis for functioning over 20 years. J Child Psychol Psychiatry 49:933–941, 2008

Zanarini MC, Frankenburg FR, Hennen J, et al: The longitudinal course of borderline psychopathology: 6-year prospective follow-up of the phenomenology of borderline personality disorder. Am J Psychiatry 160:274–283, 2003

8

Childhood Experiences and Development of Maladaptive and Adaptive Personality Traits

Jeffrey G. Johnson, Ph.D.
Elizabeth Bromley, M.D.
Pamela G. McGeoch, M.A.

During the past century, clinical experience and research have provided considerable support for the hypothesis that interpersonal experiences during childhood and adolescence play an important role in personality development (e.g., Erikson 1963). Childhood adversities such as maladaptive parenting and childhood abuse and neglect may be likely to have an adverse impact on personality development because they interfere with or alter the trajectory of normative socialization processes during childhood and adolescence (Cohen 1999; Johnson et al. 2001a). Positive experiences during childhood and adolescence, such as parental warmth and support, may be likely to promote the development of adaptive traits such as trust, altruism, and optimism, due to social learning processes and development of a secure attachment style during childhood (e.g., Erikson 1963; Sroufe et al. 1999). This chapter presents a summary of research findings that are currently available regarding the role that childhood experiences may play in the development of maladaptive and adaptive personality traits. We begin by summarizing the evidence that is currently available from retrospective and prospective studies regarding the hypothesized association between childhood adversities and personality disorders. The association of childhood abuse and neglect with risk for the development of personality disorders is examined in particular depth because this association is of considerable interest to clinicians and because comparatively little information is available regarding other adversities that may contribute to the development of maladaptive traits. The chapter concludes with an examination of the available evidence regarding the association of positive childhood experiences with the development of adaptive traits.

CHILDHOOD ADVERSITIES ASSOCIATED WITH DEVELOPMENT OF PERSONALITY DISORDERS

A large body of research has provided findings that are indirectly consistent with the hypothesis that some types of childhood adversities may contribute to the development of maladaptive personality traits and personality disorders. Retrospective studies, the majority of which have been conducted with clinical samples, have demonstrated that individuals with personality disorders tend to be more likely than individuals without personality disorders to report a history of childhood maltreatment and other traumatic childhood experiences. These findings have also been of interest because they have provided evidence of specificity, indicating that patients with personality disorders are particularly likely to report having experienced specific types of childhood abuse or neglect. However, retrospective studies cannot rule out the alternative hypotheses that the association of childhood adversities with maladaptive personality traits is attributable to recall bias or to preexisting childhood traits that may contribute to the onset of some types of childhood adversities (Maughan and Rutter 1997; Paris 1997).

Both of these alternative hypotheses have presented significant challenges to researchers in this field. Although there have been

findings supporting the validity of retrospective reports of childhood adversities (e.g., Bifulco et al. 1997; Robins et al. 1985), and although retrospective studies have promoted the formulation of developmental hypotheses, it is nevertheless problematic to make strong causal inferences based on retrospective data. In addition, a number of studies have supported the hypothesis that genetic and prenatal factors may play an important role in the development of behavioral and emotional problems that may become evident during childhood (Livesley et al. 1993; Neugebauer et al. 1999; Thomas and Chess 1984). Furthermore, research has indicated that maladaptive childhood traits may have an adverse influence on parenting behavior, potentially increasing risk for childhood maltreatment (Kendler 1996). Such findings have contributed to skepticism about the hypothesis that childhood adversities play an important role in the development of maladaptive personality traits and personality disorders.

However, in recent years, investigations utilizing a number of different research paradigms have provided new and compelling evidence in support of the hypothesis that childhood experiences have an important influence on personality development. Research has indicated that maladaptive personality traits are likely to be caused by the interaction of genetic and environmental risk factors (Caspi et al. 2002), including maternal behavior, health, and environmental characteristics affecting prenatal development (Neugebauer et al. 1999). Epidemiological studies and co-twin analyses that have controlled for genetic factors have indicated that childhood abuse is likely to be causally related to an increased risk for a broad spectrum of psychiatric symptoms (Kendler et al. 2000). Neurobiological studies have provided considerable evidence suggesting that childhood maltreatment may cause persistent deficits in brain activity associated with a wide range of psychiatric symptoms (Teicher et al. 2003). Prospective longitudinal studies and investigations that obtained evidence of childhood maltreatment from official records have supported the hypothesis that childhood abuse and neglect may contribute to increased risk for the development of personality disorders. (Drake et al. 1988; Guzder et al. 1996; Johnson et al. 1999a, 2000, 2001a, 2001b; Luntz and Widom 1994). The findings of these studies and those that have provided relevant retrospective data are described in greater detail below.

Childhood Physical Abuse

Research conducted with clinical, forensic, and epidemiological samples has indicated that indices of childhood physical abuse may be associated with antisocial, borderline, and other personality disorder traits. Patients with antisocial personality disorder (ASPD) have been found to be more likely than patients with other psychiatric disorders to report a history of physical abuse during childhood (e.g., Bierer et al. 2003; Bradley et al. 2005; Norden et al. 1995; see also Bernstein et al. 1998). Confirmatory findings have indicated that individuals identified as having experienced childhood physical abuse are likely to have problems with aggressive, criminal, or antisocial behavior (Pollock et. al. 1990; Widom 1989). Patients with borderline personality disorder (BPD) have also been found to be likely to report a history of physical abuse during childhood (e.g., Brown and Anderson 1991; Goldman et al. 1992). Other studies have yielded findings indicating that paranoid, schizoid, and schizotypal traits were associated with reports of childhood physical abuse in clinical samples (Bernstein et al. 1998; Bierer et al. 2003; Yen et al. 2002).

Data from the Children in the Community study (CICS; for detailed information about the study methodology, please see http://nyspi.org/childcom), a community-based longitudinal study, indicated that documented physical abuse was associated with elevated antisocial, borderline, dependent, depressive, passive-aggressive, and schizoid personality disorder traits after parental education and parental psychopathology were controlled statistically (Johnson et al. 1999a). Antisocial and depressive personality disorder traits remained significantly associated with documented physical abuse after other personality disorder traits were controlled statistically. Evidence of physical abuse, obtained from either official records or retrospective self-reports, was associated with elevated antisocial, borderline, passive-aggressive, and schizotypal personality disorder traits after controlling for parental education, parental psychopathology, sexual abuse, and neglect (Johnson et al. 1999a).

In summary, prospective epidemiological studies and retrospective clinical studies have provided considerable evidence in support of the hypothesis that childhood physical abuse may contribute to the onset of ASPD, independent of the effects of other types of childhood maltreatment. Epidemiological studies that relied on prospective and retrospective data and retrospective clinical findings have suggested that childhood physical abuse may be associated with elevated risk for the development of borderline and schizotypal personality disorders after other kinds of childhood maltreatment are accounted for. In addition, prospective or retrospective studies have provided evidence suggesting that childhood physical abuse may be associated with the development of depressive, paranoid, passive-aggressive, and schizoid personality disorder traits.

Childhood Sexual Abuse

Many studies have provided evidence indicating that patients with personality disorders are significantly more likely than patients without personality disorders to report a history of sexual abuse. Patients with BPD are more likely than other patients to report a history of childhood sexual abuse (Brown and Anderson 1991; Laporte and Guttman 1996; Westen et al. 1990). Evidence also has suggested that patients with BPD may tend to have experienced chronic (as opposed to episodic) sexual abuse during childhood (Weaver and Clum 1993). Systematic studies have suggested that other personality disorders may also be associated with a history of reported sexual abuse. Norden et al. (1995) found that reports of childhood sexual abuse were associated with borderline, histrionic, narcissistic, and schizotypal personality disorders. Bierer et al. (2003) reported that childhood sexual abuse was associated with paranoid personality disorder in a sample of psychiatric outpatients. Shea et al. (1999) obtained convergent findings from both inpatient and outpatient samples indicating that reported childhood sexual abuse in both samples was associated with elevated avoidant, paranoid, and schizotypal personality disorder symptom levels. Ruggiero et al. (1999) found that military veterans who reported severe childhood sexual abuse had higher antisocial, avoidant, passive-aggressive, schizoid, and schizotypal personality disorder symptom levels than did men who reported minimal childhood maltreatment. Reports of childhood sexual abuse have also been found to be associated with depressive symptoms and interpersonal difficulties (Browne and Finkelhor 1986).

Community-based research findings have indicated that documented sexual abuse was associated with elevated BPD traits after parental education and parental psychopathology were controlled statistically (Johnson et al. 1999a). Evidence of sexual abuse, obtained from either official records or retrospective self-reports, was associated with elevated borderline, depressive, and histrionic personality disorder traits after controlling for parental education, parental psychopathology, physical abuse, and neglect (Johnson et al. 1999a).

In summary, prospective epidemiological studies and retrospective clinical studies have provided considerable support for the hypothesis that childhood sexual abuse may contribute to the onset of BPD, independent of the effects of other types of childhood maltreatment. Epidemiological studies that relied on prospective and retrospective data and retrospective clinical findings have suggested that childhood sexual abuse may be associated with elevated risk for the development of histrionic and depressive personality disorder traits after other kinds of childhood maltreatment are accounted for. In addition, prospective or retrospective studies have provided evidence suggesting that childhood sexual abuse may be associated with the development of antisocial, avoidant, narcissistic, paranoid, passive-aggressive, schizoid, and schizotypal personality disorder traits.

Childhood Emotional Abuse

Research has suggested that emotional abuse (including verbal abuse, humiliation, and other psychological maltreatment) may contribute, independently, to the development of personality disorder traits during childhood and adolescence. Childhood emotional abuse may increase risk for the development of personality disorders in part by increasing the likelihood that youths will experience maladaptive thoughts and feelings, such as excessive guilt, resentment, social anxiety, shame, and mistrust of others during their most critical years of psychosocial development. Severe childhood verbal abuse may leave deeper scars than other types of abuse, because children tend to internalize verbally abusive statements and to self-inflict these abusive thoughts throughout their lives (Ney 1987).

Clinical studies have indicated that many patients with BPD and other personality disorders report a history of childhood verbal abuse (Laporte and Guttman 1996; Oldham et al. 1996; Zanarini et al. 1997). Childhood emotional abuse and intolerant, shaming parental behavior have been found to be associated with avoidant personality traits among psychiatric patients (Grilo and Masheb 2002; Stravynski et al. 1989). Bierer et al. (2003) reported that childhood emotional abuse was associated with paranoid personality disorder in a sample of psychiatric outpatients. Bernstein et al. (1998) reported that Cluster B and C personality disorders were significantly associated with retrospective reports of childhood emotional abuse. When sexual and physical abuse have been statistically controlled, emotional abuse has also been found to be independently associated with depressive personality traits, including poor self-esteem and suicidality (Briere and Runtz 1990; Mullen et al. 1996).

Longitudinal research has indicated that verbal abuse during childhood, assessed in a series of maternal interviews, was associated with increased risk for borderline, narcissistic, obsessive-compulsive, and paranoid personality disorders and with elevated borderline, narcissistic, paranoid, schizoid, and schizotypal personality disorder symptom levels during adolescence and early adulthood (Johnson et al. 2001b). These findings were obtained after behavioral and emotional problems during childhood, physical abuse, sexual abuse, neglect, physical punishment, parental education, parental psychopathology, and co-occurring psychiatric disorders were controlled statistically. Such findings have suggested that childhood verbal abuse may contribute to the development of some types of personality disorders, independent of the effects of other types of childhood maltreatment.

When the available data from prospective epidemiological studies and retrospective clinical studies are considered together, considerable evidence supports the hypothesis that childhood emotional abuse may contribute to the onset of BPD, independent of the effects of other types of childhood maltreatment. In addition, prospective or retrospective studies have provided evidence suggesting that childhood emotional abuse may be associated with the development of avoidant, depressive, narcissistic, obsessive-compulsive, paranoid, schizoid, and schizotypal personality disorder traits.

Childhood Neglect

The association of childhood neglect with the development of personality disorders has been investigated less extensively than the corresponding associations regarding childhood sexual and physical abuse. Nevertheless, the available evidence suggests that childhood neglect may contribute as or more strongly than physical and sexual abuse to the development of personality disorder symptoms and other maladaptive personality traits (Gauthier et al. 1996; Johnson et al. 1999a). Many patients with personality disorders report a history of childhood neglect (Oldham et al. 1996), and reports of a lack of parental affection during childhood have been found in clinical samples to be associated with antisocial, avoidant, borderline, dependent, paranoid, and schizoid personality disorder symptoms (Arbel and Stravynski 1991; Carter et al. 1999; Norden et al. 1995). Reports of severe childhood neglect have been found to be associated with elevated avoidant, schizoid, and schizotypal personality disorder symptom levels among military veterans (Ruggiero et al. 1999). Childhood neglect has also been found to be associated with a wide range of other maladaptive personality traits, including antisocial or avoidant behavior, attachment difficulties, hostility, paranoia, and self-destructive behavior (Dubo et al. 1997; Gauthier et al. 1996; Robins 1966; Sroufe et al. 1999).

Longitudinal research has suggested that childhood neglect may increase risk for the development of personality disorders. Evidence of childhood neglect (i.e., lack of parental affection and supervision during early adolescence) has been found to be associated with risk for dependent and passive-aggressive personality disorders during adulthood (Drake et al. 1988). CICS findings indicated that documented childhood neglect was associated with elevated antisocial, avoidant, borderline, dependent, narcissistic, paranoid, passive-aggressive, and schizotypal personality disorder traits after parental education and parental psychopathology were controlled statistically (Johnson et al. 1999a). Antisocial, avoidant, borderline, narcissistic, and passive-aggressive personality disorder traits remained significantly associated with documented neglect after other personality disorder traits were controlled statistically. Evidence of childhood neglect, obtained from either official records or retrospective self-reports, was associated with elevated antisocial, avoidant, borderline, dependent, narcissistic, passive-aggressive, and schizotypal personality disorder traits after controlling for parental education, parental psychopathology, sexual abuse, and neglect (Johnson et al. 1999a).

In recent years, research has suggested that specific types of childhood neglect may be differentially associated with specific types of personality disorder traits. Patients with BPD have been found to be more likely than patients with other personality disorders to report a history of childhood emotional, physical, and supervision neglect (Zanarini et al. 1997). Patients with antisocial, avoidant, dependent, and paranoid personality disorders have been found to be more likely than other patients to report a history of childhood emotional neglect (Carter et al. 1999). Patients with elevated schizoid personality disorder symptom levels have been found to be particularly likely to report a history of childhood emotional neglect (Bernstein et al. 1998). Dubo et al. (1997) found that symptoms of self-mutilation and suicidality were associated with retrospective reports of childhood emotional neglect among patients with BPD. Johnson et al. (2000) reported that childhood emotional neglect was independently associated with increased risk for avoidant personality disorder and elevated paranoid personality disorder symptom levels, physical neglect was independently associated with elevated schizotypal symptom levels, and supervision neglect was independently associated with elevated borderline, paranoid, and passive-aggressive personality disorder symptom levels. In addition,

emotional, physical, and supervision neglect were independently associated with elevated overall personality disorder symptom levels and overall risk for personality disorders during adolescence or early adulthood after other types of childhood maltreatment were accounted for (Johnson et al. 2000). These findings suggest that specific types of childhood neglect may contribute in unique ways, in combination with other childhood adversities, to the development of different types of personality disorder symptoms.

In summary, prospective epidemiological studies and retrospective clinical studies have provided considerable evidence in support of the hypothesis that childhood neglect may contribute to the onset of avoidant, borderline, passive-aggressive, and schizotypal personality disorders, independent of the effects of other types of childhood maltreatment. In addition, epidemiological studies that relied on prospective and retrospective data and retrospective clinical findings have suggested that childhood neglect may be associated with risk for ASPD after other kinds of childhood maltreatment are accounted for. Furthermore, prospective or retrospective studies have provided evidence suggesting that childhood neglect may be associated with the development of dependent, narcissistic, paranoid, and schizoid personality disorder traits.

Prospective epidemiological studies have suggested that specific types of childhood neglect may be differentially associated with elevated risk for specific types of personality disorder symptoms.

Case Example

Ms. D was a 19-year-old psychiatric outpatient diagnosed with depressive, obsessive-compulsive, and borderline personality disorder symptoms and severe narcissistic personality disorder symptoms. During psychotherapy sessions, she reported that she had been molested and sexually abused by an older half-brother from age 4 years until early adolescence, when she became aware of the meaning of sexual activity. The sexual abuse began with episodic molestation but became more severe from age 7 onward, occurring during lengthy periods of time when she and her half-brother were left alone and unsupervised by her parents. Ms. D tried to tell her mother about the sexual abuse—she wrote a suicide note that her mother found—but her mother did not put an end to her half-brother's behavior.

Ms. D also reported that her father frequently relied on harsh physical punishment to discipline her, for example, using a belt to whip her when she received poor grades in school. At times, this punishment was so severe that it resulted in bruises or lacerations, including an open gash in her leg, indicative of physical abuse. Ms. D also reported that her father abused her emotionally, calling her names like "stupid," "lazy," and a "whore." In addition, she reported that her mother was emotionally and physically abusive, although this abuse was not as severe as that perpetrated by her father.

Ms. D frequently witnessed physical violence between her parents, who were often verbally or physically combative. Her father often drank heavily and had a number of extramarital affairs. Ms. D informed her mother about one of her father's indiscretions, and her mother became so enraged that she shot Ms. D's father. There was abundant evidence indicating that Ms. D's history of maltreatment and problematic parenting contributed to the development and persistence of her depressive, obsessive-compulsive, borderline, and narcissistic personality disorder traits, which were associated with considerable impairment and distress.

Case Example

Ms. E was a 22-year-old psychiatric inpatient with severe BPD, dependent personality disorder traits, and posttraumatic stress disorder, with a history of dissociative symptoms, severe insomnia, depressed mood, and psychotic episodes. Ms. E reported that she had been emotionally abused and "scapegoated" by her mother throughout her childhood. For example, she reported that her mother frequently forced her to wait until the other family members had finished their meals before allowing her to eat. She also reported that her mother made her spend substantially more of her time than her siblings doing housework and other chores. Ms. E reported that her mother often humiliated her by doing things such as making her wear boys' clothing to school, and that her mother punished her severely for any appearance of sexual behavior. In addition, Ms. E reported that her mother neglected her emotionally and that her mother rarely, if ever, was affectionate, nurturing, or supportive toward her.

Ms. E reported that she was forced to leave the family home at age 17 and soon afterward became homeless. She became involved in an abusive relationship with a man who beat and raped her repeatedly. She ran away from him and asked her mother to take her in, but her mother told her, "You chose your bed. Now you can lie in it." Ms. E went to a homeless shelter, where she was beaten by some other young women on the day she arrived. During her stay at the shelter, Ms. E began receiving psychiatric treatment for the first time. However, her sense of well-being was frequently threatened while she lived there, and she reported that she constantly felt endangered during that time. She reported that on one occasion she was raped by a stranger while at the shelter. Prior to her initial hospitalization, Ms. E reported having cut her wrists on several occasions when she found the adversities of life in the homeless shelter to be overwhelming. She received several years of treatment that enabled her to recover sufficiently to be able to live semi-independently. However, many of her symptoms were so severe and unremitting that she was eventually classified as chronically disabled.

CLINICAL IMPLICATIONS OF RESEARCH ON CHILDHOOD MALTREATMENT AND RISK FOR PERSONALITY DISORDER

It may be possible to prevent the onset of chronic personality disorders among some youths by providing high-risk parents with services that assist them in developing more adaptive parenting behaviors. Research has indicated that it is possible to reduce the likelihood that children will develop psychiatric disorders by helping parents to learn more effective child-rearing techniques (Redmond et al. 1999). In addition, because treatment of parental disorders may help to reduce the likelihood of childhood maltreatment and problematic parenting, it may be possible to decrease offspring risk for personality disorders by improving the recognition and treatment of psychiatric disorders among parents in the community (Chilcoat et al. 1996).

OTHER CHILDHOOD ADVERSITIES ASSOCIATED WITH THE DEVELOPMENT OF PERSONALITY DISORDERS

Although childhood abuse and neglect are likely to play a particularly important role in the development of personality disorder symptoms, a number of studies have indicated that problematic parenting (e.g., parenting behavior that, although problematic, is not sufficiently severe to be classified as "abuse" or "neglect") is likely to be associated with the development of maladaptive personality traits and personality disorders (see Chapter 7, "Developmental Issues"). Research has indicated that a lack of parental affection during childhood, low family communication and expressiveness, a lack of parental time with the child, and harsh, controlling parenting behavior are associated with elevated personality disorder traits among adolescent nonpatients and adult psychiatric patients (Baker et al. 1996; Head et al. 1991; Johnson et al. 1997, 2006; Parker et al. 1999; Stravynski et al. 1989). Retrospective reports of a lack of parental affection during childhood by patients with personality disorders have been found, in a patient sample, to be associated with ASPD and schizoid person-

ality disorder symptoms, and paternal overprotection was associated with schizoid personality disorder symptoms (Norden et al. 1995). Community-based longitudinal research has also indicated that a wide range of problematic parenting behaviors may be associated with risk for personality disorders (Drake et al. 1988; Johnson et al. 2001a, 2006). In addition, research has indicated that a number of other childhood adversities including parental death, parental separation or divorce, socioeconomic adversities, traumatic life events, and victimization (e.g., assault, bullying) may be associated with elevated risk for personality disorders (Coid 1999; Johnson et al. 1999b, 2006; Zanarini and Frankenburg 1997).

PROTECTIVE FACTORS ASSOCIATED WITH THE DEVELOPMENT OF ADAPTIVE TRAITS

Research has identified a wide variety of experiences, relationships, and community resources that may promote the development of adaptive personality traits, such as hardiness or resiliency during childhood and adolescence. Familial warmth, extrafamilial support, and other facilitative environmental characteristics have been found to be associated with the development of adaptive traits. These traits, in turn, are likely to play an important mediating role in determining whether individuals are able to adapt effectively to adversities during adulthood (Garmezy 1985; Shiner 2000; Werner and Smith 1982).

Familial Protective Factors

A wide range of parenting behaviors (e.g., affection, communication, time spent with children) and characteristics of the family and home environment play an important role in healthy child development (Johnson et al. 2001a; see also Chapter 7, "Developmental Issues"). Parental empathy, support, and warmth have been found to help children and adolescents cope effectively with many types of adversities (Cowen et al. 1997; Jaffee et al. 2007; Luthar and Zigler 1991; Wyman et al. 1991). Research has also indicated that children who develop a close, strong, and mutually respectful relationship with their parents tend to be particularly resilient and to have adaptive coping skills (Kobak and Sceery 1988). Furthermore, strong and supportive relationships with parents and family members tend to be associated with healthy interpersonal functioning during adulthood and successful adaptation to adult responsibilities (Werner and Smith 1982; see also Chapter 7, "Developmental Issues"). Young adults who perceive their family as warm and supportive tend to be relatively confident and adaptable and to have high self-esteem, whereas those who perceive their parents as authoritarian tend to be more uncertain about themselves and the future (Strage 1998).

It is important to note that a variety of parenting styles may lead to positive outcomes (Baldwin et al. 1990) and that the child-rearing behavior of the parent is determined, in part, by the disposition or temperament of the child (Cohen 1999; Kendler 1996). For example, youths with externalizing behavior problems may need extra parental supervision, and youths with internalizing problems may be in particular need of parental warmth and support. However, research has indicated that most youths benefit from having responsible, nurturing, supportive parents who gradually encourage them to function in an increasingly autonomous manner as they mature (Cowen et al. 1997; Luthar and Zigler 1991; Rikhye et al. 2008; Strage 1998; Wyman et al. 1991).

Extrafamilial Protective Factors

Many different types of community and neighborhood resources may help to promote healthy personality development during childhood and adolescence. Supportive community organizations that help young people to develop ethics and values; mentors such as teachers, godparents, and adult role models; and confidants in the form of highly functioning and supportive peers may facilitate the development of adaptive personality traits (Werner 1989). The presence of a mentor during adolescence has been found to be associated with improved academic achievement, attitudes about school, insight, relationships with parents and peers, and self-esteem, and with reductions in aggressive behavior and psychoactive substance use (Wolkow and Ferguson 2001; Zimmerman et al. 2002).

Participation in community activities and organizations may also have a variety of beneficial consequences. Community involvement may help to provide a sense of purpose, to increase the availability of social support, and to foster resiliency (Vaillant 1977). Youths who have a strong sense of membership in and identification with the community may adapt more effectively to stressful life events (Heath et al. 1999). Extracurricular activities, such as participation in athletic activities, arts and crafts, hobbies, musical ensembles, and organized recreational activities may also promote healthy adaptation to adversity (Bell and Suggs 1998). Thus, communities and schools that provide young people with a wide range of opportunities to engage in such activities may help to promote healthy personality development during childhood and adolescence.

ADAPTIVE PERSONALITY TRAITS

The research findings cited earlier are consistent with Erik Erikson's (1963) hypothesis that personality development during childhood and adolescence is determined, in large measure, by the child's upbringing, chronic adversities, and other important interpersonal experiences. Although each child begins life with behavioral tendencies that are influenced by genetic and prenatal factors

(Livesley et al. 1993; Neugebauer et al. 1999; Thomas and Chess 1984), life experiences appear to play a critical role in determining how these temperamental characteristics are expressed (Caspi et al. 2002; Cohen 1999; Wilson et al. 2006). Research has also supported Erikson's hypothesis that children who grow up in a supportive environment are more likely to develop character strengths such as trust in others, autonomy, industriousness, and self-esteem (see Chapter 7, "Developmental Issues"). These and other personality traits have been found to promote the development of strong, supportive relationships with others to decrease risk for the development of psychiatric disorders (Bromley et al. 2006) and to facilitate adaptation to adversities later in life (Garmezy 1985; Rutter 1987; Shiner 2000; Werner and Smith 1982).

Resiliency

Research has identified personality traits, such as optimism and productivity, that tend to be associated with an adaptive, resilient response to stress (Pengilly and Dowd 2000; Rutter 1987). The development of resiliency may stem in part from experiences that teach individuals how to cope effectively with difficulties, thereby "inoculating" them so that they are able to deal with future adversities more effectively (Rutter 1987). Adaptive traits referred to as "ego resiliency" (confident optimism, insight and warmth, productive activity, and skilled expressiveness) have been found to be associated with positive outcomes, such as the ability to arouse liking and acceptance by others (Block and Gjerde 1990; Klohnen 1996; Klohnen et al. 1996).

Hardiness

Kobasa (1979) identified a similar set of adaptive traits as being indicative of hardiness. Individuals with a high level of hardiness tend to view stressful events as being potentially meaningful and interesting, to view themselves as capable of changing the events and circumstances in their lives, and to believe that planning and preparation can mitigate or prevent future problems (Kobasa 1979). In addition, hardy individuals have been found to view changing circumstances as opportunities for growth (Pengilly and Dowd 2000; Werner 1989, 1992).

Self-Efficacy

Children and adults who believe that they are in control of their lives tend to remain well in the face of adversity. Longitudinal research has indicated that children with high self-efficacy scores who experienced a high level of family stress were more likely than other children to have positive outcomes, such as being competent and caring (Werner 1989, 1992). Similarly, self-mastery and an internal locus of control have also been found to be associated with positive outcomes (Wyman et al. 1991). Longitudinal research has indicated that successful peer and school adaptation are particularly evident among children who work enthusiastically, creatively, and persistently and who strive to achieve high standards (Shiner 2000).

Pro-Social Traits

Pro-social traits, including communication skills, confidence, empathy, perceptiveness, and warmth, appear to play an important role in the development of adaptive functioning during childhood and adolescence (Shiner 2000). Resilient youths tend to interact with and reach out to others, rather than withdrawing, in both adverse and normal circumstances. Longitudinal research has shown that adolescents with pro-social tendencies tend to have better long-term psychosocial outcomes (Shiner 2000). This may be attributable in part to the familial and extrafamilial support that may be made particularly abundant to individuals with pro-social personality traits (Garmezy 1985).

Other Adaptive Traits

Conscientiousness, impulse control, integrity, and persistence have been found to be associated with the development of resiliency during adolescence (Funder and Block 1989; Klohnen et al. 1996; Luthar and Zigler 1991; Rutter 1990; Shiner 2000). The ability to respond to humor and to share it with others has been found to promote positive outcomes (Klohnen et al. 1996; Luthar and Zigler 1991; Vaillant 1977). Humor is viewed as an adaptive defense or coping style by psychoanalytic theorists, as are altruism, suppression (i.e., the conscious postponement of attention to disturbing circumstances), anticipation (i.e., consciously planning how to cope with stressful circumstances), self-regulation (Gardner et al. 2008; Martel et al. 2007), and sublimation (Vaillant 1977).

Case Example

Ms. F was a 31-year-old woman with metastatic adenocarcinoma. At the time of her diagnosis, she was living with her boyfriend and working as a painter with some commercial success. She had graduated from a prestigious university and attended graduate art school. The oncologist described Ms. F as a "real fighter, all the way through the chemotherapy and surgery." She learned what she could about the illness and treatment. Ms. F brought small, bright paintings for the nurses and patients every week. She came to the hospital each week with a variety of close friends and loved ones. Her parents were helpful with the treatment arrangements.

When seen by the psychiatrist, Ms. F's boyfriend, mother, and father were sitting around her bed. Flowers and small paintings were on the bedside table. Ms. F, bald and thin, smiled weakly. She said that at the time of her diagnosis, "my career was really taking off, and my boyfriend and I were engaged. It was such a shock, but I had no choice but to learn what I could from the horror." She described how she coped. She grew closer to her father and learned more about his illness experience. She took a long-wished-for trip to Italy to visit her high school art teacher. She committed herself to finishing her work on a large painting exhibit with a friend, saying "I just knew my work and my community would keep me upbeat and give my days hope." Referring to how she coped with a friend's death as a teen, she said she learned at the time that "I had the strength to find some meaning in hardship." Ms. F was also able to explore her anger, sense of loss, and sorrow for those she would leave behind.

Ms. F's story illustrates how community, activity, self-efficacy, parents, and loved ones are called on in times of profound stress. She not only coped with the difficulties of cancer treatment but also found generative ways to help others. The love and encouragement that she received from her parents and mentors, her insight into her own feelings, her perseverance, and her ability to rally others around her were important aspects of her successful coping.

CLINICAL IMPLICATIONS OF RESEARCH ON PROTECTIVE FACTORS AND ADAPTIVE PERSONALITY TRAITS

The present literature review supports the recommendation to assess protective factors and personality strengths as well as symptoms and maladaptive traits. Assessing protective factors and adaptive personality traits may increase the effectiveness of a clinical intervention, in part, by making it clear to the patient that the clinician is interested in developing a well-rounded understanding of the patient's strengths and weaknesses, thereby fostering the development of a strong therapeutic alliance. Moreover, recent evidence suggests that patients with some interpersonal problems who can cite positive developmental experiences may have a better prognosis than those patients who cannot

(Skodol et al. 2007). In addition, there are many ways that clinicians and other professionals who work with young people can help to promote the development of adaptive personality traits during childhood and adolescence. Some examples include promoting extracurricular activities, encouraging youths to take on age-appropriate challenges and responsibilities, facilitating the development of appropriate relationships with suitable adult mentors, and assisting the youth and family in taking advantage of community resources and in participating actively in the life of the community. Furthermore, it may be important to assist parents in improving their child-rearing skills, developing a closer and more supportive relationship with their children, and encouraging parents to minimize reliance on disciplinary methods that have been found to be problematic if utilized too frequently (e.g., harshly controlling, punishing, or shaming offspring; see Redmond et al. 1999).

REFERENCES

Arbel N, Stravynski A: A retrospective study of separation in the development of adult avoidant personality disorder. Acta Psychiatr Scand 83:174–178, 1991

Baker JD, Capron EW, Azorlosa J: Family environment characteristics of persons with histrionic and dependent personality disorders. J Personal Disord 10:82–87, 1996

Baldwin AL, Baldwin C, Cole RE: Stress-resistant families and stress-resistant children, in Risk and Protective Factors in the Development of Psychopathology. Edited by Rolf J, Masten AS, Cicchetti D, et al. Cambridge, England, Cambridge University Press, 1990, pp 257–280

Bell CC, Suggs H: Using sports to strengthen resiliency in children: training heart. Child Adolesc Psychiatr Clin N Am 7:859–865, 1998

Bernstein DP, Stein JA, Handelsman L: Predicting personality pathology among adult patients with substance use disorders: effects of childhood maltreatment. Addict Behav 23:855–868, 1998

Bierer LM, Yehuda R, Schmeidler J, et al: Abuse and neglect in childhood: relationship to personality disorder diagnoses. CNS Spectrums 8:737–754, 2003

Bifulco A, Brown GW, Lillie A, et al. Memories of childhood neglect and abuse: corroboration in a series of sisters. J Child Psychol Psychiatry 38:365–374, 1997

Block J, Gjerde PF: Depressive symptoms in late adolescence: a longitudinal perspective on personality antecedents, in Risk and Protective Factors in the Development of Psychopathology. Edited by Rolf J, Masten AS, Cicchetti D, et al. Cambridge, England, Cambridge University Press, 1990, pp 334–360

Bradley R, Jenei J, Westen D: Etiology of borderline personality disorder: disentangling the contributions of intercorrelated antecedents. J Nerv Ment Dis 193:24–31, 2005

Briere J, Runtz M: Differential adult symptomatology associated with three types of child abuse histories. Child Abuse Neglect 14:357–364, 1990

Bromley E, Johnson JG, Cohen P: Personality strengths in adolescence and decreased risk of developing mental health problems in early adulthood. Compr Psychiatry 47:315–324, 2006

Brown GR, Anderson B: Psychiatric morbidity in adult inpatients with childhood histories of sexual and physical abuse. Am J Psychiatry 148:55–61, 1991

Browne A, Finkelhor D: Impact of child sexual abuse: a review of the research. Psychol Bull 99:66–77, 1986

Carter JD, Joyce PR, Mulder RT, et al: Early deficient parenting in depressed outpatients is associated with personality dysfunction and not with depression subtypes. J Affect Disord 54:29–37, 1999

Caspi A, McClay J, Moffitt TE, et al: Role of genotype in the cycle of violence in maltreated children. Science 297:851–854, 2002

Chilcoat HD, Breslau N, Anthony JC: Potential barriers to parent monitoring: social disadvantage, marital status, and maternal psychiatric disorder. J Am Acad Child Adolesc Psychiatry 35:1673–1682, 1996

Cohen P: Personality development in childhood: old and new findings, in Personality and Psychopathology. Edited by Cloninger CR. Washington, DC, American Psychiatric Press, 1999, pp 101–127

Coid JW: Aetiological risk factors for personality disorders. Br J Psychiatry 174:530–538, 1999

Cowen EL, Wyman PA, Work WC, et al: Follow-up study of young stress-affected and stress-resilient urban children. Dev Psychopathol 9:565–577, 1997

Drake RE, Adler DA, Vaillant GE: Antecedents of personality disorders in a community sample of men. J Personal Disord 2:60–68, 1988

Dubo ED, Zanarini MC, Lewis RE, et al: Childhood antecedents of self-destructiveness in borderline personality disorder. Can J Psychiatry 42:63–69, 1997

Erikson EH: Childhood and Society, 2nd Edition. New York, WW Norton, 1963

Funder DC, Block J: The role of ego-control, ego-resiliency, and IQ in delay of gratification in adolescence. J Pers Soc Psychol 57:1041–1050, 1989

Gardner TW, Dishion TJ, Connell AM: Adolescent self-regulation as resilience: resistance to antisocial behavior within the deviant peer context. J Abnorm Child Psychol 36:273–284, 2008

Garmezy N: Stress-resistant children: the search for protective factors, in Recent Research in Developmental Psychopathology. Edited by Stevenson JE. Oxford, England, Pergamon Press, 1985, pp 213–233

Gauthier L, Stollak G, Messé L, et al: Recall of childhood neglect and physical abuse as differential predictors of current psychological functioning. Child Abuse Neglect 20:549–559, 1996

Goldman SJ, D'Angelo EJ, DeMaso DR, et al: Physical and sexual abuse histories among children with borderline personality disorder. Am J Psychiatry 149:1723–1726, 1992

Grilo C, Masheb RM: Childhood maltreatment and personality disorders in adult patients with binge eating disorder. Acta Psychiatr Scand 106:183–188, 2002

Guzder J, Paris J, Zelkowitz P, et al: Risk factors for borderline pathology in children. J Am Acad Child Adolesc Psychiatry 35:26–33, 1996

Head SB, Baker JD, Williamson DA: Family environment characteristics and dependent personality disorder. J Personal Disord 5:256–263, 1991

Heath AC, Madden PA, Grant JD, et al: Resiliency factors protecting against teenage alcohol use and smoking: influences of religion, religious involvement and values, and ethnicity in the Missouri Adolescent Female Twin Study. Twin Res 2:145–155, 1999

Jaffee SR, Caspi A, Moffitt TE, et al: Individual, family, and neighborhood factors distinguish resilient from non-resilient maltreated children: a cumulative stressors model. Child Abuse Negl 31:231–253, 2007

Johnson JG, Quigley JF, Sherman MF: Adolescent personality disorder symptoms mediate the relationship between perceived parental behavior and Axis I symptomatology. J Personal Disord 11:381–390, 1997

Johnson JG, Cohen P, Brown J, et al: Childhood maltreatment increases risk for personality disorders during early adulthood. Arch Gen Psychiatry 56:600–606, 1999a

Johnson JG, Cohen P, Dohrenwend BP, et al: A longitudinal investigation of social causation and social selection processes involved in the association between socioeconomic status and psychiatric disorders. J Abnorm Psychol 108:490–499, 1999b

Johnson JG, Smailes EM, Cohen P, et al: Associations between four types of childhood neglect and personality disorder symptoms during adolescence and early adulthood: findings of a community-based longitudinal study. J Personal Disord 14:171–187, 2000

Johnson JG, Cohen P, Kasen S, et al: Association of maladaptive parental behavior with psychiatric disorder among parents and their offspring. Arch Gen Psychiatry 58: 453–460, 2001a

Johnson JG, Cohen P, Smailes EM, et al: Childhood verbal abuse and risk for personality disorders during adolescence and early adulthood. Compr Psychiatry 42:16–23, 2001b

Johnson JG, Cohen P, Chen H, et al: Parenting behaviors associated with risk for offspring personality disorder during adulthood. Arch Gen Psychiatry 63:597–587, 2006

Kendler KS: Parenting: a genetic-epidemiologic perspective. Am J Psychiatry 153:11–20, 1996

Kendler KS, Bulik CM, Silberg J, et al: Childhood sexual abuse and adult psychiatric and substance use disorders in women: an epidemiological and co-twin control analysis. Arch Gen Psychiatry 57:953–959, 2000

Klohnen EC: Conceptual analysis and measurement of the construct of ego-resiliency. J Pers Soc Psychol 70:1067–1079, 1996

Klohnen EC, Vandewater EA, Young A: Negotiating the middle years: ego-resiliency and successful midlife adjustment in women. Psychol Aging 11:431–442, 1996

Kobak RR, Sceery A: Attachment in late adolescence: working models, affect regulation, and representations of self and others. Child Dev 59:135–146, 1988

Kobasa SC: Stressful life events, personality and health: an inquiry into hardiness. J Pers Soc Psychol 37:1–11, 1979

Laporte L, Guttman H: Traumatic childhood experiences as risk factors for borderline and other personality disorders. J Personal Disord 10:247–259, 1996

Livesley WJ, Jang KL, Jackson DN, et al: Genetic and environmental contributions to dimensions of personality disorder. Am J Psychiatry 150:1826–1831, 1993

Luntz BK, Widom CS: Antisocial personality disorder in abused and neglected children grown up. Am J Psychiatry 151:670–674, 1994

Luthar SS, Zigler E: Vulnerability and competence: a review of research on resilience in childhood. Am J Orthopsychiatry 61:6–22, 1991

Martel MM, Nigg JT, Wong MM, et al: Childhood and adolescent resiliency, regulation, and executive functioning in relation to adolescent problems and competence in a high-risk sample. Dev Psychopathol 19:541–563, 2007

Maughan B, Rutter M: Retrospective reporting of childhood adversity: issues in assessing long-term recall. J Personal Disord 11:19–33, 1997

Mullen PE, Martin JL, Anderson JC, et al: The long-term impact of the physical, emotional and sexual abuse of children: a community study. Child Abuse Neglect 20:7–21, 1996

Neugebauer R, Hoek HW, Susser E: Prenatal exposure to wartime famine and development of antisocial personality disorder in early adulthood. JAMA 282:455–462, 1999

Ney PG: Does verbal abuse leave deeper scars: a study of children and their parents. Can J Psychiatry 32:371–378, 1987

Norden KA, Klein DN, Donaldson SK, et al: Reports of the early home environment in DSM-III-R personality disorders. J Personal Disord 9:213–223, 1995

Oldham JM, Skodol AE, Gallaher PE, et al: Relationship of borderline symptoms to histories of abuse and neglect: a pilot study. Psychiatr Q 67:287–295, 1996

Paris J: Childhood trauma as an etiological factor in the personality disorders. J Personal Disord 11:34–49, 1997

Parker G, Roy K, Wilhelm K, et al: An exploration of links between early parenting experiences and personality disorder type and disordered personality functioning. J Personal Disord 13:361–374, 1999

Pengilly JW, Dowd ET: Hardiness and social support as moderators of stress. J Clin Psychol 56:813–820, 2000

Pollock VE, Briere J, Schneider L, et al: Childhood antecedents of antisocial behavior: parental alcoholism and physical abusiveness. Am J Psychiatry 147:1290–1293, 1990

Redmond C, Spoth R, Shin C, et al: Modeling long-term parent outcomes of two universal family focused preventive interventions: one-year follow-up results. J Consult Clin Psychol 67:975–984, 1999

Rikhye K, Tyrka AR, Kelly MM, et al: Interplay between childhood maltreatment, parental bonding, and gender effects: impact on quality of life. Child Abuse Negl 32:19–34, 2008

Robins LN: Deviant Children Grow Up: A Sociological and Psychiatric Study of Sociopathic Personality. Baltimore, MD, Williams & Wilkins, 1966

Robins LN, Schoenberg SP, Holmes SJ, et al: Early home environment and retrospective recall: a test for concordance between siblings with and without psychiatric disorders. Am J Orthopsychiatry 55:27–41, 1985

Ruggiero J, Bernstein DP, Handelsman L: Traumatic stress in childhood and later personality disorders: a retrospective study of male patients with substance dependence. Psychiatr Ann 29:713–721, 1999

Rutter M: Psychosocial resiliency and protective mechanisms. Am J Orthopsychiatry 57:316–329, 1987

Rutter M: Psychosocial resilience and protective mechanisms, in Risk and Protective Factors in the Development of Psychopathology. Edited by Rolf J, Masten AS, Cicchetti D, et al. Cambridge, England, Cambridge University Press, 1990, pp 181–214

Shea MT, Zlotnick C, Weisberg RB: Commonality and specificity of personality disorder profiles in subjects with trauma histories. J Personal Disord 13:199–210, 1999

Shiner RL: Linking childhood personality with adaptation: evidence for continuity and change across time into late adolescence. J Pers Soc Psychol 78:310–325, 2000

Skodol AE, Bender DS, Pagano ME, et al: Positive childhood experiences: resilience and recovery from personality disorder in early adulthood. J Clin Psychiatry 68:1102–1108, 2007

Sroufe LA, Carlson EA, Levy AK, et al: Implications of attachment theory for developmental psychopathology. Dev Psychopathol 11:1–13, 1999

Strage AA: Family context variables and the development of self-regulation in college students. Adolescence 33:17–31, 1998

Stravynski A, Elie R, Franche RL: Perception of early parenting by patients diagnosed with avoidant personality disorder: a test of the overprotection hypothesis. Acta Psychiatr Scand 80:415–420, 1989

Teicher MH, Andersen SL, Polcari A, et al: The neurobiological consequences of early stress and childhood maltreatment. Neurosci Biobehav Rev 27:33–44, 2003

Thomas A, Chess S: Genesis and evolution of behavioral disorders: from infancy to early adult life. Am J Orthopsychiatry 141:1–9, 1984

Vaillant GE: Adaptation to Life. Cambridge, MA, Harvard University Press, 1977

Weaver TL, Clum GA: Early family environments and traumatic experiences associated with borderline personality disorder. J Consult Clin Psychol 61:1068–1075, 1993

Werner EE: High-risk children in young adulthood: a longitudinal study from birth to 32 years. Am J Orthopsychiatry 59:72–81, 1989

Werner EE: The children of Kauai: resiliency and recovery in adolescence and adulthood. J Adolesc Health 13:262–268, 1992

Werner EE, Smith RS: Vulnerable But Invincible: A Study of Resilient Children. New York, McGraw-Hill, 1982

Westen D, Ludolph P, Misle B, et al: Physical and sexual abuse in adolescent girls with borderline personality disorder. Am J Orthopsychiatry 60:55–66, 1990

Widom CS: The cycle of violence. Science 244:160–166, 1989

Wilson RS, Krueger KR, Arnold SE, et al: Childhood adversity and psychosocial adjustment in old age. Am J Geriatr Psychiatry 14:307–315, 2006

Wolkow KE, Ferguson HB: Community factors in the development of resiliency: considerations and future directions. Community Ment Health J 37:489–498, 2001

Wyman PA, Cowen EL, Work WC, et al: Developmental and family milieu correlates of resiliency in urban children who have experienced major life stress. Am J Community Psychol 19:405–426, 1991

Yen S, Shea MT, Battle CL, et al: Traumatic exposure and posttraumatic stress disorder in borderline, schizotypal, avoidant, and obsessive-compulsive personality disorders: findings from the Collaborative Longitudinal Personality Disorders Study. J Nerv Ment Dis 190:510–518, 2002

Zanarini MC, Frankenburg FR: Pathways to the development of borderline personality disorder. J Personal Disord 11:93–104, 1997

Zanarini MC, Williams AA, Lewis RE, et al: Reported pathological childhood experiences associated with the development of borderline personality disorder. Am J Psychiatry 154:1101–1106, 1997

Zimmerman MA, Bingenheimer JB, Notaro PC: Natural mentors and adolescent resiliency: a study with urban youth. Am J Community Psychol 30:221–243, 2002

Part IV

Treatment

9

Levels of Care in Treatment

John G. Gunderson, M.D.
Kim L. Gratz, Ph.D.
Edmund C. Neuhaus, Ph.D.
George W. Smith, M.S.W.

In this chapter, we describe the indications, goals, structures, and empirical evidence related to the use of four different and decreasingly intensive levels of care: IV—hospital; III—partial hospital/day treatment; II—intensive outpatient; and I—outpatient. Although we are concerned primarily with the roles these levels of care play in treating personality disorders, we recognize that patients who have a personality disorder often will be placed in levels of care due to a treatment primarily directed at comorbid Axis I conditions. For example, major depression has a comorbidity of about 50% with Cluster B and C disorders (Dolan-Sewell et al. 2001), anxiety disorders have a comorbidity of about 25% with Cluster C disorders (Dyck et al. 2001), and substance abuse is associated with a comorbid Cluster B disorder more than 50% of the time (Oldham et al. 1995).

The presence of a comorbid personality disorder often complicates the treatment of an Axis I disorder (Tyrer et al. 1997); for example, the patient with avoidant personality disorder may not attend group sessions; the patient with borderline personality disorder (BPD) may refuse family contacts; the patient with histrionic personality disorder may express sensitivity to the side effects of medications, and so on. In such ways, personality disorders may diminish the prognosis for the treatment of Axis I disorders.

DEFINITIONS

Treatments can be organized according to the four different levels of care (see Table 9–1). Those personality disorders associated with the most severe crises and highest levels of

Table 9–1.   Levels of care

IV	Hospital; 24 hours/day with option of locked doors and seclusion
III	Partial hospital/day treatment; 2–8 hours/day, 3–5 days/week, 6–30 hours/week; usually heavily involving group therapies
II	Intensive outpatient; 3–10 hours/week of specifically prescribed, scheduled, and integrated therapies
I	Outpatient; 1–3 hours/week of scheduled therapies

dysfunction are more apt to require higher levels of care. The four levels of care are hierarchical in terms of containment, intensity, structure, and costs per day, and they are inversely related to usual length of stay.

GENERAL PRINCIPLES GOVERNING LEVELS OF CARE

The least restrictive level of care possible is usually best—this maximizes and requires use of one's personal strengths, increases the likelihood of being able to apply new capabilities and skills to community settings (i.e., generalization), and decreases the likelihood of regressive aspects of treatment (e.g., reinforcement of dysfunctional behavior).

Availability of all levels is clinically desirable (most treatment settings include only IV and I) and possibly cost beneficial (Quaytman and Scharfstein 1997). The availability of levels II and III decreases use of hospitalizations, decreases dropouts, and increases social rehabilitation interventions.

With each decrease in level of care, the treatments become more specific for different types of personality disorders.

EVIDENTIARY BASE

Several meta-analytic reports have affirmed the value of psychotherapy, which really includes all psychosocial therapies, for personality disorders (Leichsenring and Leibing 2003; Perry and Bond 2000). The extant re-

search involving specified levels of care is shown in Table 9–2. Many of these studies have examined personality disorders in general, and these studies vary in the extent to which they control for or examine the specific impact of particular personality disorders or a personality disorder cluster on treatment efficacy. Most research examining treatment for specific personality disorders involves BPD and antisocial personality disorder (ASPD), with a growing number of studies examining the effectiveness of treatments at different levels of care on Cluster C disorders—in particular, avoidant personality disorder. Cluster A disorders have received the least systematic attention from researchers. Furthermore, empirical support for the comparative efficacy of different levels of care is rare.

OVERALL THEORY FOR USE OF DIFFERENT LEVELS OF CARE

The intended goals for therapeutic change are often classified within four domains: subjective distress, maladaptive behaviors, interpersonal, and intrapsychic (i.e., psychological). These domains are identified in the sequence in which change can be expected (Gabbard et al. 2002; Gunderson and Gabbard 1999; Howard et al. 1986; Kopta et al. 1994; Lanktree and Briere 1995) as well as a sequence that generally should be prioritized in treatment planning. Table 9–3 indicates the relative capacity for the different levels of care to effect

Table 9–2. Studies on level of care for personality disorders

	Hospital	Partial hospital	Intensive outpatient	Outpatient
All personality disorders	Dolan et al. 1992, 1997	Karterud et al. 1992, 2003 Mehlum et al. 1991 Vaglum et al. 1990 Wilberg et al. 1998b, 1999	NA	NA
Cluster A	NA	NA	NA	NA
Cluster B	NA	NA	NA	NA
BPD	Barley et al. 1993 Bohus et al. 2000, 2004 Silk et al. 1994	Bateman and Fonagy 1999, 2001, 2008 McQuillan et al. 2005	Linehan et al. 1991, 1993, 1994, 2006	Blum et al. 2002, 2008 Brown et al. 2004 Davidson et al. 2006 Giesen-Bloo et al. 2006 Gratz and Gunderson 2006 Munroe-Blum and Marziali 1995 Stevenson and Meares 1992 Wilberg et al. 1998a
ASPD	Cacciola et al. 1995 Gabbard and Coyne 1987 Harris et al. 1994) Hildebrand et al. 2004 Messina et al. 1999, 2002 Ogloff et al. 1990 Reiss et al. 1999 Rice et al. 1992 Richards et al. 2003	Cacciola et al. 1995	NA	Brooner et al. 1998 Compton et al. 1998 Messina et al. 2003
Clusters B and C	NA	Krawitz 1997	NA	Hoglend 1993 Winston et al. 1994
Cluster C	Gude and Vaglum 2001	NA	NA	Hardy et al. 1995
AVPD	NA	NA	NA	Alden 1989

Note. ASPD=antisocial personality disorder; AVPD=avoidant personality disorder; BPD=borderline personality disorder; NA=not available.
Source. Search engine used: PsycINFO.

Table 9–3.   Goals and their relationship to levels of care

	Distress	Behavioral	Interpersonal	Intrapsychic
Hospital	++	+	−	−
Partial hospital	++	++	+	−
Intensive outpatient	+	++	++	+
Outpatient	+	+	++	++

Note.   Effectiveness: ++=strong; +=possible; −=unlikely.

change in these four domains. Of course, this profile is tied to the expected lengths of stay.

Another way to classify goals is by the priority they should be assigned in planning treatment interventions (Gunderson 2001). Here, for example, goals include crisis management, behavioral stabilization, social rehabilitation, and psychological growth (Table 9–4). These goals naturally map onto those in Table 9–3 and vary in the extent to which they can and should be addressed within each level of care. For example, crises are often managed by hospitalizations because of the hospital's role in providing containment, asylum from stress, and the potential for rapid medication changes that offer immediate symptom relief. Behavioral stabilization and social rehabilitation are achieved through corrective social learning experiences, as well as the continued opportunities for the acquisition and generalization of coping skills that are central to partial hospital (level III) and intensive outpatient (level II) programs. Psychological growth change requires longer-term and often repetitive learning experiences available only in stable longer-term settings—that is, in level I outpatient care.

Case Example

Ms. G, a 26-year-old, single white woman, was referred from another state for treatment of personality disorder not otherwise specified with borderline, schizotypal, and avoidant features. With an excellent high school grade point average, she had been accepted into a very competitive college. However, her completion of college was repeatedly delayed due to angry conflicts with peers and teachers usually followed by self-endangering behaviors of variable seriousness. For the past several years, she has been living at home doing minimal work.

On arrival, Ms. G was angry at her parents for bringing her but desperate about needing help. She refused to enter the residential program, insisting that she wasn't that "sick." When advised it would provide a way to develop peer relationships, she angrily denied the need for that and claimed she could make friends whenever she wanted. Her parents' effort to correct that claim only made her resistance to entering the partial hospital more resolute. She nonetheless reiterated that she was desperate to receive an intensive outpatient program (IOP, level II) that had been unavailable at home.

A clinical decision needed to be made: either accept Ms. G in an IOP (level II) as she insisted or not (under which circumstances she claimed returning home was not an option, and she would go to the streets of Boston).

At her parents' urging, Ms. G was accepted into an IOP and quickly found residence with someone she met there. She got attached to her individual therapist but became preoccupied with her roommate, who had her own problems. After 6 months, the therapist and group therapy leaders in the IOP concluded that Ms. G was making no progress—that she had insufficient social supports or structure to use treatment for other than crisis management. The therapist felt that to insist on residential care would be experienced as rejection and might precipitate suicidal danger.

Ms. G's case illustrates several common and difficult problems involved in selecting or changing a level of care. One is making a concession on level of care to accommodate a patient's insistence. Making a concession is sometimes necessary but is best done with the proviso that the patient agrees to accept your recommendations if he or she has not achieved some reasonable progress in some agreed-upon time (e.g., has not achieved a job, has not attended therapies regularly, has not established a social support system, or has not diminished high-risk activities). A second problem illustrated by this case is that once treatments are under way, it can be very difficult to change them without breaking the relational alliance with the patient and/or precipitating a potentially dangerous flight. In Ms. G's case, the IOP team called for a consultation. Use of outside consultants to oversee changes helps depersonalize what often looms as a very difficult confrontation. To do this required time-consuming communications by the treaters. It is more easily done within hospitals. How to make such confrontations (advising patients of information that they do not want to hear) and how to impose limits (prohibiting behavior[s] that a patient wishes to continue) without patients becoming self-destructive or leaving treatment is not easy (see Gunderson 2001 for discussion).

LEVELS OF CARE

What follows is an elaboration of indications, goals, and structures for each of the four levels of care (see Table 9–4). Where available, relevant empirical evidence is noted.

Level IV: Hospital

Given that hospitalizations are almost always 2–14 days in duration in practice, the following discussion is geared to those lengths of stay. Still, research that has been done on hospitalizations of longer durations (e.g., 2–3 months) suggests that they can be useful in ways that are not feasible in 2–14 days. That research is described at the end of this section.

Potential risks associated with inpatient hospitalization include reinforcement of maladaptive behaviors (e.g., parasuicidal, attention seeking, control struggles) and/or passive problem solving. Clinicians should consider these issues for the particular patient. Nonetheless, the role of hospitalization should be appreciated, because personality disorder patients treated in community-oriented treatments (level I or II) with an aggressive emphasis on keeping patients out of the hospital have worse outcomes than patients for whom hospitals were used as needed (Tyrer and Simmonds 2003).

Indications

Hospitalization may be clinically indicated during acute crises and in response to increasingly severe behavioral dysfunction, especially with regard to suicidal behaviors and violence toward others. Perhaps also worth noting is that hospitalization may be used as an asylum to permit patients with personality disorders to leave abusive or otherwise harmful situations or relationships. Hospitalizations can also enable patients to leave treatments that were not helpful but that they would otherwise have had difficulty leaving.

Many people with personality disorders enter hospitals because of comorbid psychiatric disorders to which the personality disorder may predispose them. Indeed, more than half of psychiatrically hospitalized patients have a personality disorder, with the most common types being borderline, avoidant, and dependent personality disorders (Loranger 1990). Attention to and consideration of the personality disorder may affect treatment efficacy for the Axis I disorders and should influence treatment decisions.

Given that BPD is the predominant personality disorder found in inpatient hospital services (constituting about 15% of hospitalizations; Koenigsberg et al. 1985; Loranger

Table 9–4.   Levels of care: modalities, goals, duration, and therapeutic processes

Level	Modalities	Goals and procedures	Duration	Therapeutic processes

IV. Hospital	Medication
	Milieu
	Group
	Case management
		Crisis management
		  Decrease distress
		  Decrease suicide risk
		
		Assessments
		  Neurological evaluations
		  Psychological evaluations
		
		Plan/change treatment
		  Develop treatment plan
		  Identify primary therapist
		  Initiate medication changes
		  Expert consultation
			2–14 days
			24 hours/day
				Containment
				Support

III. Partial hospital	Milieu
	Group
	Case management
	Family
	Individual
		Skills training
		  Stabilize daily living skills
		  Structure daily activities
		  Identify maladaptive patterns
		
		Behavioral stabilization
		  Decrease impulsive behavior
		  Increase coping skills
		
		Social rehabilitation
		  Improve social functioning
		  Vocational rehabilitation
		  Community reentry
			1–2 weeks
			6–20 hours/week
			
			3–12 weeks
			6–10 hours/week
			
			16+ weeks
				Structure
				Support
				Involvement

Table 9–4. Levels of care: modalities, goals, duration, and therapeutic processes

Level	Modalities	Goals and procedures	Duration	Therapeutic processes
II. Intensive outpatient	Group Family Individual	Social (behavioral) adaptation Vocational Behavioral Affective Interpersonal	3–18 months 3–10 hours/week	Support Involvement
I. Outpatient	Individual Group	Psychological growth Interpersonal Intrapsychic	12–36 months 1–3 hours/week	Involvement Validation

1990; Widiger and Weissman 1991), it is worth noting a common clinical situation for which hospitalizations should be used with caution. Hospitalization should rarely be used in response to self-injurious behavior without suicidal intent. Furthermore, although inpatient stays may be warranted for BPD patients who are acutely suicidal, such hospitalizations may not decrease the likelihood of future suicide attempts (Van der Sande et al. 1997).

Despite the widespread belief that hospitalization is generally contraindicated for patients with ASPD, research on the effectiveness of inpatient therapeutic community drug treatment programs and inpatient substance abuse programs suggests that ASPD patients may respond positively to certain types of inpatient programs (Cacciola et al. 1995; Messina et al. 1999, 2002). Of course, the generalizability of these results to other, less specialized inpatient hospital programs is indeterminable. With regard to contraindications to hospitalization, Gabbard and Coyne (1987) noted that negative responses to hospitalization are likely for ASPD patients with a history of felony arrests or convictions; a history of repeated lying, aliases, and conning; an unresolved legal situation at admission; forced hospitalization as an alternative to incarceration; and a history of violence toward others. Moreover, research suggests that psychiatric hospitalization is relatively contraindicated for those ASPD patients (approximately 25%–65%; see Widiger and Corbitt 1996) who are psychopathic (i.e., display a lack of remorse, lack of empathy, and shallow affect; Harris et al. 1994; Hart and Hare 1997; Hildebrand et al. 2004; Reiss et al. 1999; Richards et al. 2003; see also Salekin 2002). In contrast, there is evidence to suggest that ASPD patients without psychopathy may respond positively to forensic hospitals with therapeutic community programs (Rice et al. 1992) and that the presence of comorbid anxiety and/or depression may also be associated with a positive response to hospitalization among ASPD patients (see Gabbard and Coyne 1987).

Although level IV care is rarely indicated for Cluster C personality disorders, it is worth noting that hospitalization may offer useful exposures for patients with avoidant personality disorder. For instance, hospitalization may expose avoidant patients to typically avoided social situations (e.g., seeing others in distress) or internal experiences (e.g., feeling helpless or anxious). Although hospitalization may result in initial improvements in symptoms for these patients, however, research suggests that patients with pure Cluster C personality disorders (especially avoidant personality disorder) may be at greater risk for relapsing after discharge than patients with Cluster B personality disorders (see Gude and Vaglum 2001).

Goals: Crisis Management, Assessments, and Planning and Implementing Treatment Changes

Following are the major goals of hospitalizations and the usual time required for meeting them:

- Crisis management (2–6 days): Hospitalization can diminish acute suicidal or violent dangers.
- Extensive neurological or psychological evaluations (2–6 days): These evaluations are more easily coordinated, and may only be feasible, in hospital settings.
- Development of a treatment plan and personnel (3–14 days): Such plans usually require arranging for continuity through appropriate step-downs and assessing the suitability of new therapy personnel. An essential part of these processes is to identify the primary clinician who will be responsible for the patient's treatment. For primary clinicians, an essential first step is to define roles and goals—that is, establish a "contractual alliance"—and to contract with the patient about participation in aftercare services.
- Changes in prior therapies (3–14 days): These changes are often indicated, but

they may require expert consultation and the introduction of new therapists. If the changes are considered undesirable by the patient, working through resistance may be possible only in the hospital, where the options for flight from the proposed changes are reduced.

- Hospitalizations may allow therapists to review prior impasses or establish a clearer framework for their ongoing work. For many patients with personality disorder, hospitalization serves as an environment to initiate medication changes and evaluate medication benefits.

Structures

A businesslike, practical, supportive, and task-oriented atmosphere and orientation is useful. Harmful is a milieu that encourages long one-to-one talks or the development of personal relationships with staff or other patients. Community meetings or group therapies that emphasize cohesion or bonding among patients are relatively contraindicated. Care should be taken not to reinforce maladaptive behaviors or increasingly intense/severe expressions of distress and suicidality. Furthermore, emphasizing the short-term nature of the treatment, retaining a focus on impending discharge, and making aftercare plans for less-restrictive levels of care may be useful strategies for preventing lengthy or contraindicated hospitalizations (see Bohus et al. 2000; Silk et al. 1994). Given that it is easy for staff to feel trapped by escalating suicidal ideation as patients approach discharge, a consultant can help alleviate unrealistic liability fears.

In regard to staffing, a case manager should be assigned and should keep the patient oriented toward the problems preceding the hospitalization that the patient will need to cope with on discharge. A primary task of the case manager is to bring in relatives or other significant people to help understand precipitating events and diminish the likelihood of their recurrence after discharge, to receive psychoeducation about the personality disorder, and to coordinate aftercare plans.

The psychiatrist should oversee medications and involve the patient in any changes. As important, the psychiatrist should caution patients about the relatively modest benefits they can expect. In addition, the psychiatrist should evaluate coexisting Axis I disorders and give them appropriate priority in aftercare planning. For example, comorbid substance or alcohol abuse almost always should be assigned high priority in aftercare, and coexisting depression may not respond well to medications (Gunderson et al. 2004; Koenigsberg et al. 1999; Kool et al. 2003; Shea et al. 1987; Soloff 1998) and may require further monitoring at a less-restrictive level of care.

Longer-Term Hospitalizations: Empirical Lessons

Longer-term hospitalizations may address additional goals. Dolan et al. (1997) found that long-term (i.e., average of 7 months) therapeutic community inpatient treatment was associated with decreased borderline psychopathology. Furthermore, hospitalizations of 2–3 months may result in behavioral stabilization (a goal usually reached in level III and generally not addressed in the 2–10 day hospitalizations described above). Dialectical behavior therapy (DBT)–based inpatient programs in particular may be more effective in fulfilling this goal than other inpatient programs with equally long stays (see Barley et al. 1993; Bohus et al. 2004). The advantages shown for such programs are presumably due to the emphasis on skills training (in particular, distress tolerance skills), behavioral analyses of problem behaviors (with the goal of identifying precipitants and consequences of problem behaviors so as to determine appropriate interventions), and the use of contingency strategies, potentially minimizing unintended reinforcement of maladaptive behaviors (Barley et al. 1993; Bohus et al. 2000, 2004). Moreover, the milieu can be used to practice, and begin to generalize, the skills being learned.

These studies of 2- to 3-month hospitalizations can be used to inform the development of hospital programs with shorter lengths of stay. For instance, Silk et al. (1994) developed a DBT-based inpatient treatment for BPD with an average length of stay of 10–17 days. In assessing patients' perceptions of improvement at the time of discharge, they found that patients in the DBT-based program (compared with patients assigned to a non-DBT discussion group) felt that the lessons they learned would help them to better handle difficult or painful situations. Although the same level of change found with longer-term hospital stays would not be expected with short-term hospitalizations, a similar structure can be utilized with beneficial results.

Level III: Partial Hospital/Day Treatment

The literature presents a diverse picture of partial hospital treatments for personality disorders, varying extensively with regard to treatment duration (i.e., length of stay) and treatment intensity (i.e., hours per week). These programs offer more structure, containment, and intensive treatment than outpatient care while providing the opportunity for behavioral stabilization—and for skills building and generalization—that are not usually available in typical short-term inpatient settings. Our discussion of partial hospital treatment is oriented toward the levels of duration and intensity—that is, the shorter-term partial hospital programs (2–4 weeks in duration) that are usually available in the current health care system. A discussion of the lessons that can be learned from the longer-term partial programs that have been the primary recipients of empirical attention can be found at the end of this section.

Indications

For some patients with a personality disorder, partial hospital programs offer an optimal level of care. They can diminish the likelihood of substance/alcohol abuse relapses or suicide attempts (although they do not have enough monitoring or containment to prevent these behaviors). Moreover, partial hospital programs may be indicated for patients who lack either the social supports or vocational options to make community living viable. Whether as an alternative to or step-down from hospitalization, partial hospital programs are needed for personality disorder patients with marked social or behavioral impairment. Karterud et al. (2003) operationalized the need for partial hospitalization by suggesting that it was indicated for patients with Global Assessment of Functioning scores below 50. Partial hospital programs can assess the types of, and reasons for, social disability and introduce rehabilitative efforts. This level of care can also be used to introduce or stabilize new treatments when close supervision and evaluations are needed.

As with level IV, BPD is the personality disorder most likely to use level III. Although patients with ASPD are also socially impaired, there is some evidence to suggest that they may be likely to drop out of partial hospital programs (Karterud et al. 2003; Wilberg et al. 1998b). However, given evidence of a positive response to level III therapeutic community drug treatment programs among ASPD patients (Cacciola et al. 1995), it is possible that certain specialized programs may be effective in the treatment of ASPD patients. Patients with schizotypal personality disorder are unlikely to be helped by partial hospital programs (see Karterud et al. 1992; Vaglum et al. 1990). Surprisingly, however, patients with paranoid personality disorder treated in an 18-week day treatment program evidenced significant improvements in global functioning, symptom severity, and interpersonal functioning—improvements comparable with those seen among patients with other personality disorders (Wilberg et al. 1998b).

Goals: Skills Training, Stabilization, and Social Rehabilitation

A pragmatic and theoretically grounded approach conceptualizes treatment in stages, each of which has its own goals and interventions. Stages are organized with respect to their duration and intensity as well as to the changes that can reasonably be expected to occur within a given time frame. Based on clinical experience, a high-intensity "front-loaded" treatment is optimal initially, followed by treatment at a titrated intensity over several months. Given that most programs can offer only short-term treatment (what we refer to here as stage 1 of treatment), this titration is particularly relevant. One partial hospitalization program that emphasizes stage 1 targets found that patients can improve in the brief time frame of 1–2 weeks (Neuhaus 2006; Neuhaus et al. 2007). The following are goals for each stage:

Stage 1 (1–2 Weeks)

- Develop a therapeutic alliance and the patient attaches to treatment: This process is assisted by defining goals and establishing an initial treatment contract that gets reviewed and refined over time.
- Psychoeducation: This helps patients frame goals and understand treatment options, and enlists family support.
- Stabilize or teach daily living skills (eating, sleeping, hygiene): The need for this goal varies, as does the optimal approach to achieving it. Most patients need consistent monitoring and education about the importance of eating and sleeping in regular patterns. Sleep medications may prove useful for patients who have trouble falling asleep because of fearfulness.
- Schedule and structure time and activities: This assists with the management and planning of daily activities, promotes self-care routines (e.g., sleep, hygiene, good eating habits), and aids in overall stress management.
- Begin to identify typical patterns (e.g., interpersonal conflicts, loneliness) that lead to maladaptive behaviors: Although maladaptive patterns cannot be expected to change in stage 1, it is often useful to introduce basic behavioral strategies at this point, including chain analyses and impulse control skills.

Stage 2 (3–8 Weeks)

- Stabilize behavior: This goal involves attaining better impulse control, resulting in a decrease in the frequency and severity of impulsive and self-destructive behaviors (e.g., self-harm, suicide attempts, substance use). This stabilization is often a nonspecific effect of asylum, structure, and support.
- Initiate vocational rehabilitation: This goal is not easily accomplished and typically gets overlooked due to the fact that patients with a personality disorder rarely seek vocational rehabilitation. Young or inexperienced staff are unlikely to give this goal adequate value and importance. Program administrators or staff involved with families are more apt to determine whether it is addressed.
- Reevaluate the treatment contract on the basis of the extent to which patients are working collaboratively and responsibly in treatment: In stage 2 treatment, after patients have achieved more competency with regard to coping skills (e.g., better impulse control, improved anxiety management), a greater emphasis is placed on interpersonal relationships.

Structures

Partial hospital and day treatment programs rely heavily on group therapy and the positive effects of a therapeutic milieu. Such structure must be actively constructed, proactively maintained, and updated as needed. With a 1- or 2-week length of stay, patients do not have the luxury of time to "settle in" to treatment. Clear and concise information (e.g., description of the program and treatment philosophy, expectations of patients, roles of treatment team members) provided upon entry can diminish a patient's anxiety and facilitate immediate involvement in treatment. Handouts with daily schedules and brief descriptions of groups may further orient patients and promote memory of what to expect. The structure of the partial hospital program may become a template for structuring their lives outside the program.

As with hospitals, a case manager responsible for implementing the treatment and monitoring progress should be assigned. This person should work directly with the patient, treatment team members both within and outside of the program, and family members. To be an effective case manager with personality disorder patients requires clinical savvy to set limits, confront when necessary (e.g., when patients are missing groups), and stay connected with a patient despite being vilified as not understanding or caring. An effective case manager must also be willing and able to negotiate with treatment team members outside of the program (e.g., the patient's outpatient therapist). In short-term treatment the case manager may be invaluable to the family system in providing information, support, and the framework of an overall treatment plan (e.g., anticipating the issues involved in less intensive levels of care).

Given the potential for treatment noncompliance at this level of care (patients may have difficulty attending treatment when feeling bad), the structure of the program should include provisions for addressing noncompliance through program expectations, policies, and an explicit emphasis on therapy-interfering behaviors. Noncompliance is best addressed by the case manager and then followed up in groups. It is useful to utilize a combination of validation, confronting, limit setting (e.g., patients cannot stay in the program unless attendance improves), and the teaching of coping skills to facilitate improved attendance despite emotional distress.

High-intensity, short-term treatment at this level of care should be front-loaded with skills training and psychoeducation to promote stabilization and safety. It is essential to select and prioritize elemental skills that are feasible for patients to learn quickly. This bottom-up approach draws heavily from cognitive-behavioral therapy (CBT) principles and simplifies the treatment program for patients (Levendusky et al. 1994; Neuhaus 2006). As an extension of cognitive-be-havioral treatment, an intensive DBT approach has also been shown to be effective in treating borderline patients in a 3- to 4-week time frame (McQuillan et al. 2005). Notably, even the psychoanalytic partial hospital program developed by Bateman and Fonagy (2004) is heavily cognitive-behavioral; especially in early phases. As such, a core constellation of groups within stage 1 treatment may include treatment contracting, community meeting (for addressing therapy-interfering behaviors), personality disorder psychoeducation (with information about the influence of Axis I disorders), basic behavioral skills groups (including behavioral scheduling, impulse control, distress tolerance, and anxiety management), self-assessment groups that teach patients how to identify maladaptive behavioral patterns (including the emotional and cognitive precipitants of maladaptive behaviors), and rudimentary interpersonal groups (e.g., assertiveness training, interpersonal effectiveness, and the impact of personality styles on relationships).

Groups during stage 2 of treatment may follow the framework of stage 1, although with greater depth and further opportunities for patients to practice skills and achieve some competency in their use. At this stage of treatment, as patients begin to feel like part of the milieu, there is a natural progression to focus more explicitly on the patient's interpersonal relationships. This stage may see an intensification of treatment relationships and attachments, which offers challenges to patients and treatment providers alike. Any honeymoon phase would likely be over by this stage of treatment, necessitating that the frustrations, disappointments, and realities of treatment be addressed. For effective treatment to continue, the therapeutic alliance must be strong enough to endure these obstacles.

Longer-Term Partial Hospital/Day Treatment Programs: Empirical Lessons

Research on longer-term partial hospital and day treatment programs suggests that they may provide the opportunity for behavioral stabilization (including decreased parasuicidal behavior) and symptom improvement and, unlike shorter-term programs, can also positively affect social and interpersonal functioning. Bateman and Fonagy (1999) found that BPD patients treated in a partial hospital program organized around a mentalization-based model of treatment (Bateman and Fonagy 2004), compared with BPD patients in standard outpatient care, evidenced significantly fewer suicide attempts after 6 months, significant reductions in depression and anxiety after approximately 9 months, and significantly fewer acts of self-harm after 12 months. Moreover, partial hospital program patients not only maintained their gains but reported further improvements at follow-up (Bateman and Fonagy 2001, 2008).

Global symptom severity of patients with Cluster B and C disorders has been shown to decrease significantly after approximately 4 months of level III treatment (Karterud et al. 1992; Krawitz 1997; Vaglum et al. 1990; Wilberg et al. 1998b). These same improvements may also be found for patients with paranoid personality disorder (Wilberg et al. 1998b). Research also suggests that patients with Cluster C personality disorders may experience improvements in social functioning after 4 months (Karterud et al. 1992; Vaglum et al. 1990). For patients with BPD, on the other hand, significant improvements in social adjustment and interpersonal functioning may require up to 18 months of treatment (Bateman and Fonagy 1999).

Moreover, even in these longer-term partial hospital/day treatment programs, vocational rehabilitation is difficult to achieve. Following a 4-month day treatment program, unemployment rates of patients with Cluster B and C disorders did not change during the 2-year follow-up period despite other significant improvements in global functioning and symptom severity (Krawitz 1997). Similarly, in another study, patients with personality disorder (primarily borderline, avoidant, and paranoid) treated in a variety of day treatment programs (ranging from 18–41 weeks and

from 8–16 hours/week) did not evidence any improvements in work functioning at 1-year follow-up (Karterud et al. 2003).

Finally, although it is often assumed that more treatment (i.e., greater intensity) will result in greater improvements, research suggests that when it comes to the day treatment of patients with BPD, "less is more." Karterud et al. (2003) found that lower-intensity (i.e., 8–10 hours per week) partial hospital treatment was more effective (i.e., fewer dropouts and greater improvements in global functioning and symptom severity) for patients with BPD than high-intensity treatments (approximately 16 hours per week). This finding is consistent with the level of intensity found to be effective in Bateman and Fonagy's (1999, 2001, 2008) randomized controlled trial.

Level II: Intensive Outpatient Program

When described as a level of care, an IOP differs from an intensive schedule of individual psychotherapy. For purposes of this review, we define IOP as an integration of two or more modalities in which efforts are coordinated and patients receive 3–10 hours of services per week. Thus, at its higher end, IOPs overlap with low-intensity partial hospital programs. When patients need fewer than 3 hours of service per week and/or the services do not need to regularly coordinate their efforts, the treatment becomes level I. IOP or level II care is of particular value for BPD patients (Gunderson 2001; Smith et al. 2001). Although Linehan's (1993) DBT treatment has been identified as an outpatient service, it involves both individual and group therapy provided by collaborating clinicians at a level of 3.5 hours per week— thus, it could be classified as an IOP.

Indications

IOPs are indicated for personality disorder patients whose problems with living in the community are not acutely self-endangering but are sufficiently severe that only daily, or otherwise unusually intensive, care can bring about changes. IOPs can provide a gradual transition from higher levels of care (i.e., inpatient and partial hospital programs). Because patients often experience this transition as happening too quickly or before they are ready, treatment modalities at this level of care should recognize and validate patients' subjective distress while simultaneously encouraging the use of their personal strengths and skills.

Case Example

Ms. H, a 38-year-old, single white woman with BPD and posttraumatic stress disorder (PTSD), was hospitalized for increased PTSD symptoms and reckless behavior following a serious accident in which her son was injured. Previous hospitalizations had lasted weeks longer than anticipated and were followed by 2–3 months in partial hospital without obvious benefit. On the inpatient unit, the patient was disappointed not to have the case manager and psychiatrist she had worked with in the past and also was eager to go home to spend Christmas with her son. Her therapist was leaving for vacation and seemed worried about the patient returning to outpatient care in her absence. The patient and therapist negotiated with the leaders of the IOP groups about how she could use the groups to manage emotional distress and to monitor any reckless behavior. The patient was discharged to an IOP, resumed her functioning as a mother, and survived her therapist's absence.

This vignette illustrates both the value of an IOP as a step-down from hospital (level IV) care and the ways it can assist during crises (in this case, the absence of a therapist) while in outpatient (level I) care.

Goals: Social (Behavioral) Adaptation

- Vocational (4–12 weeks): Enlist in needed vocational training or develop skills and initiative required to obtain work.

- Behavioral (4–12 months). Improve abilities to control impulsive behaviors and out-of-control (i.e., ineffective) expressions of feelings. Improve ability to engage in goal-directed, valued behaviors.
- Affective (6–52 weeks): Recognize feeling states in self and others and learn to associate them with behaviors (what Fonagy [1991] has termed *mentalization*). This recognition is especially important for the feelings of fear and anger in avoidant personality disorder and BPD, respectively. Increase emotional acceptance.
- Interpersonal (6 months–2 years): Recognize dependent needs as part of self and others. This goal initially involves recognition of such needs; becoming comfortable with them follows (Gunderson et al. 1993). Increase interpersonal effectiveness.

Structures

In addition to individual psychotherapy, IOPs offer complementary groups that meet three to five times per week and promote the resumption of functional capacities within the community. Groups are best offered in the morning or late afternoon to allow time in the patients' schedules to pursue nonclinical activities such as work or volunteering. Offering several different types of groups, each with a different format and function, will help patients meet the various goals of this level of care.

For instance, daily self-assessment groups can provide a structured format for each patient, in turn, to discuss the transition, identify maladaptive behaviors and/or interpersonal difficulties, and obtain support. Daily groups, by virtue of their frequency, enable patients to become familiar with the details of each others' lives, contributing to their sense of being heard and understood. The format of these groups also enables group members to hold each other accountable for managing maladaptive behaviors and interpersonal problems. DBT or CBT skills groups in an IOP provide patients with the opportunity to further develop and refine skills learned in more intensive levels of care (e.g., skills to control impulses, regulate emotions, tolerate distress, and improve their capacity to negotiate relationships).

These groups are more rigorous than supportive groups (such as self-assessment ones) and require a serious commitment to homework assignments and behavioral change. Interpersonal groups are process-oriented psychotherapy groups that have a longer-term focus. These groups encourage patients to examine how they relate to others, both within the group and in their lives. Conflicts between members are expected to be frequent and may reflect ambivalence about dependency needs and competitiveness for attention. Mentalization groups—derived from mentalization-based treatment—are designed to help members develop more awareness of the mental states of other persons and to consider how that awareness affects their own mental state (Bateman and Fonagy 2006).

The nature and function of these groups provide useful information as to how best to incorporate them within the structure of the IOP. Whereas self-assessment groups may be invaluable during the initial period of transition, lasting as little as a few weeks, interpersonal and DBT/CBT skills groups have a longer-term focus and may be expected to continue after the patient leaves the IOP for outpatient care (level I), thereby assisting in this new transition.

Finally, it is essential that the groups of the IOP be coordinated and integrated with the overall goals of the patient's treatment. When a patient's primary clinician works outside the IOP setting, the responsibility for coordination and implementation of the treatment plan can be handicapped. Regular communication between the patient's psychotherapist and group leaders, as well as among the group leaders themselves, is critical. For instance, Linehan's (1993) DBT includes a weekly 2-hour consultation team meeting, considered to be one of the necessary components of the treatment.

Level I: Outpatient

Level I is the level of care in which most of the treatment for personality disorders occurs. In a previous generation, psychoanalytic therapies were considered the treatment of choice for all personality disorders, even though the literature mainly consisted of negative accounts about the resistances encountered. Some of the problems traditionally encountered in outpatient care can be addressed by utilizing higher levels of care—especially IOPs. Other problems were due to applying psychoanalysis to patients who needed more structure, more of a here-and-now focus, and more support. To some extent, psychoanalytic theory has been modified to address these problems, acknowledging the importance of the "real relationships" and putting insight into perspective. Moreover, outpatient treatments for personality disorders have diversified to include a much stronger place for CBTs and medications.

Indications

There are no specific indications or contraindications for outpatient care. There are generic issues; because outpatient care requires conscious willful effort, such care is limited de facto to those who seek it and who can be sufficiently reliable to attend scheduled sessions. Beyond these considerations, some patients primarily seek support or direction, and their motivation to work on changing their personality may not be present. The absence of this motivation may be a relative contraindication for outpatient treatment.

Research on the effectiveness of outpatient treatments for personality disorders has focused primarily on relatively high-functioning clients. For instance, Winston et al. (1994) required that clients with a personality disorder have no suicidal behavior, no history of destructive impulse control problems, no use of psychotropic medications in the past year, and the presence of one close interpersonal relationship; Alden (1989) excluded participants who had ever been hospitalized for psychiatric difficulties, and most of the participants were employed or in school; in Hoglend's (1993) study, most participants were employed and none had severe acting-out behaviors. Because we do not know what fraction of the personality disorder patients in outpatient services meet these requirements, the generalizability of this research is unclear. What may be concluded is that the results will not apply to patients with severe social dysfunction.

Goals: Interpersonal and Intrapsychic Growth

Goals for level I are often the same as those identified for an IOP. Indeed, because most treatments for patients with a personality disorder are delivered in this nonintensive outpatient level of care, the goals identified for an IOP are usually initiated in level I. However, in outpatient care, achieving these goals is more apt to involve active selection and motivation by the particular patient.

An important discontinuity with the IOP is that outpatient care is rarely directed at vocational rehabilitative needs; this may be especially true for psychodynamic individual therapies. CBT- or DBT-based approaches may be more likely to accommodate this lack of vocational rehabilitation through role playing and problem-solving issues related to applying for school or work. Still, because outpatient therapies depend on what patients identify as goals, and because vocational rehabilitation is rarely a reason for which patients with a personality disorder seek therapy, this arena is often neglected.

- Enhance social involvement: Improve level of, and satisfaction from, social and recreational activities (as demonstrated by Winston et al. 1994).
- Improve impulse control: Although often begun at higher levels of care, impulse control can also occur in, or be strengthened by, outpatient care.
- Work on changes in interpersonal relatedness and intrapsychic structure: These are

the primary targets of psychodynamic (and psychoanalytic) psychotherapies. Although the attention given to diagnoses is often limited and idiosyncratic, there is a body of evidence relevant to their effectiveness with personality disorders (see Gunderson and Gabbard 1999). The results published by Knight (1941) indicated that psychoanalytic psychotherapies are more effective for "neurosis" (63%) and character disorders (57%) than for psychosis (25%). A review of available literature suggests that such therapy is particularly likely to help patients with obsessive-compulsive, narcissistic, and dependent personality disorders (Gunderson 2003).

The effectiveness of psychodynamic psychotherapy for BPD has received the most attention. Although a study conducted at McLean Hospital found that it was rare for a patient with BPD to remain in long-term treatment and get dramatically better (Waldinger and Gunderson 1989), such cases could be identified and the processes of change seemed to occur in a predictable sequence (Gunderson et al. 1993). Moreover, three studies with larger samples of BPD patients have added credibility to the claim that long-term psychodynamic psychotherapy can be effective for patients with BPD and have significant cost offsets (Hoke LA: "Longitudinal Patterns of Behaviors in Borderline Personality Disorder," Doctoral dissertation, Boston University, 1989; Howard et al. 1986; Stevenson and Meares 1992). Of particular note, the psychoanalytic psychotherapy offered in the Stevenson and Meares (1992) study (a 1-year manualized treatment conducted by trainees) was followed by continued improvement. However, it is important to note that these studies do not show that the psychoanalytic components distinguish effective psychotherapy, nor do they indicate to what extent the favorable outcomes can be generalized to the larger universe of BPD patients.

Structures

Individual psychotherapy assumes the central role in most outpatient treatments for personality disorders. Still, split treatments (i.e., adding a suitable second modality to accompany the individual psychotherapy) have advantages (Gunderson 2001; see also Chapter 17, "Collaborative Treatment"). At this level of care, the split treatment may involve medications (e.g., for schizotypal, borderline, or avoidant personality disorders; see Chapter 14, "Somatic Treatments"). The second modality could also include a social rehabilitative component, including a CBT group (Blum et al. 2002, 2008; Gratz and Gunderson 2006), an interpersonal therapy group (Marziali and Munroe-Blum 1995; Munroe-Blum and Marziali 1995), a self-help group (e.g., Alcoholics Anonymous, Narcotics Anonymous; see Chapter 19, "Substance Abuse"), and/or some continuation of family involvement. These therapies are often indicated for dependent, borderline, histrionic, avoidant, or schizoid personality disorders. Moreover, a meta-analysis of treatment studies on psychopathy suggests that the augmentation of individual psychotherapy with group or family therapy may enhance its effectiveness (see Salekin 2002).

Case Example

Mr. I was a 34-year-old man who sought help because he wanted to reconcile with his wife, who had kicked him out. He was "obsessed" with his wife and claimed he did not understand why she had rejected him. She had refused couples therapy, saying that Mr. I needed to change himself. Prior efforts to assuage his agitation and insomnia with medications had proven helpful—but he now "needs to change himself," although he could offer no ideas about what he wanted to change. In the ensuing sessions, Mr. I described a very disturbed childhood with a punitive mother.

He became quite devoted to the therapist, a woman, and began calling her frequently for what to her seemed trivial reasons. He was deeply hurt by her ef-

forts to interpret his calls or to set limits on them, and she eventually sought consultation. The consultant suggested an interpersonal group therapy be added. In the group, his anxieties about rejection were seen as unrealistic, and the maladaptive nature of his intrusive wishes for reassurance were confronted. The patient resisted, but after starting the group, his behavior in therapy changed dramatically. He was able to clearly see his reactions to his therapist (and wife) as transference phenomena.

Impasses in individual psychotherapy with patients with a personality disorder often derive from the fact that such patients are often unaware of how they create problems for others and then can feel unjustifiably criticized by therapists who point this out. In many cases, this obstacle can be overcome by the addition of a second modality. In this case, the group therapy diminished the transference and provided a source of feedback to Mr. I that was less personalized.

Some evidence suggests that patients with a personality disorder may require longer-term treatments to reach normative levels of functioning or to maintain treatment gains. Alden (1989) found that although three different behaviorally based treatments for avoidant personality disorder resulted in greater improvements than a waiting list control group, the patients remained significantly more symptomatic than normative samples. Similarly, in a study of the long-term outcomes of patients with and without personality disorders treated with outpatient dynamic psychotherapy, Hoglend (1993) found that for the patients with personality disorders, the number of sessions in treatment was significantly related to acquired insight (i.e., new emotional self-understanding) and to overall personality change at 2- and 4-year follow-up.

Conclusion

Because personality disorders are defined by enduring social maladaptations, they are intrinsically tied to social contingencies. To bring about change, good treatments across all levels of care must embody coherent and repetitive interventions with a primary initial focus on the here and now.

The interventions offered by any level of care will only be effective if patients develop an alliance with treaters. For patients with personality disorders, forming an alliance will be complicated by the obstacles created by their personalities, for example, avoidance, deceit, or attention seeking. This chapter emphasized that establishing an alliance begins with establishing agreed-upon goals, selecting the level of care appropriate to (i.e., best able to fulfill) these goals, and clarifying what is expected of patients. These activities establish a contractual alliance. This form of alliance may be sufficient for hospitals but is also a necessary prerequisite for all other levels of care. The relational alliance (i.e., an alliance based on liking or trusting the treaters) also is necessary. Such alliances usually develop from supportive attention, and in some cases respectful listening may be all that is required. When such an alliance is not formed with clinicians, progress is unlikely. Beyond this relational alliance, the value of many specific forms of intervention depends on what has been termed the *working alliance*—that is, an alliance that is needed for collaborative work toward the patient's goals (e.g., acquiring new skills and capabilities). Although such a mutual task orientation is often assumed when contractual alliances are made, for patients with personality disorders, a working alliance can be hard to achieve. Clinicians working at all levels of care need to be vigilant about whether personality disorder patients are working with the therapist for purposes of changing themselves (i.e., their identity or self).

Earlier in this review, we noted a relationship between the four levels of care and the domains of psychopathology that patients are best able to change. Table 9–3 reflects this progression as it relates to goals. Another way to understand the distinctive effectiveness of the four levels of care is via a hierarchy of therapeutic processes (Gunderson 1978, 2001). Viewed through this lens, the levels of care move from most to least containment, with an attendant increase in reliance on internal controls and self-agency. There is also a progressive decrease in the level of structure across the levels of care, such that the organization of time and activities imposed by the treatment setting is reduced at each step down. Even within the least-structured treatment setting—that is, outpatient psychotherapies—there is a hierarchy in which more directive and active interventions give way to lesser ones as patients progress. Support in the form of reassurance, advice, and expressions of concern are important elements of all levels of care. Because support often bonds people, it becomes an essential element for interpersonal attachments. Such attachments may be a negative factor in the highest levels of care because they can form a resistance to leaving, but they become more important, like the relational alliance noted earlier, as patients move into longer-term settings.

Winnicott (1965) identified a "holding environment" as a social context that is a necessary prerequisite for the development of an internal sense of safety and security. Everyone requires a feeling of being securely contained, but the degree to which this feeling depends on external factors varies. Although Winnicott originally conceptualized the holding environment as a function served by mothers early in development, it has been transformed into a term that is used to describe a function offered by therapies. As one moves through the levels of care, the "holding" action depends progressively less on imposed constraints and structures and more on internal resources. This shift has implications for the levels of care that may be most appropriate for specific personality disorders.

Although the role of hospitalization tends to be limited for the treatment of personality disorders, many patients with personality disorders use hospitalizations to treat comorbid conditions or crises. Hospitalizations may be most useful for those patients whose sense of self is most disorganized or unstable (BPD) or whose unintegrated behaviors pose a danger to self or others (e.g., BPD and nonpsychopathic ASPD). Such patients may need more containment and structure to feel "held." Partial hospital (day treatment) care (level III) is used primarily for stabilizing mental states and initiating longer-term therapies within the 2 weeks usually allotted by the modern managed care environment. However, there is good evidence that longer-term stays can add substantial benefits. The limited durations of stay available in partial hospitals have helped create the need for a relatively new level of care, IOPs (level II). This level of care may be needed for at least 1 year and requires theoretically and structurally integrated individual and group components. These programs have been demonstrated to be useful for BPD, but in principle they should be just as applicable to any personality disorder with severe social functioning handicaps (e.g., schizoid, avoidant, dependent, and antisocial personality disorders). Ironically, this level of care, arguably the most useful for dysfunctional personality disorders, is the least available in the present health care system. Outpatient care is the primary setting for the treatment of most personality disorders. Here, long-term individual psychotherapy by itself is thought to be the treatment of choice for patients with narcissistic, histrionic, and obsessive-compulsive personality disorders. Although it is thought that significant personality change may be possible in outpatient care, availability of this treatment is largely dependent on private pay and thus is frequently inaccessible.

There is very little research relevant to systems of health care services for personality disorders. What little there is supports the value of graduated step-down levels of care. Not surprisingly, the two personality disorders for which higher levels of care are most needed and that have the most public health significance, BPD and ASPD, have generated the most research attention (see Table 9–2).

This research has generally shown that BPD can be responsive to well-structured programs at all levels of institutional services. The results for ASPD are more complicated. Specialized programs at inpatient, partial hospital, and outpatient levels of care have been shown to be useful for nonpsychopathic ASPD patients. Although the higher levels of care are generally contraindicated for psychopathic ASPD patients, the aforementioned meta-analysis of treatments for psychopathy suggests that long-term, intensive individual psychotherapy may have positive results for this population (see Salekin 2002). However, the extent to which these research findings generalize to standard practices in outpatient settings is unclear, given the potential for problems related to treatment retention and compliance at this level of care.

Because research suggests that well-structured and theoretically consistent programs are more useful for patients with a personality disorder than programs that are not, these qualities should become standards for care. More attention should now be given to whether programs with different theoretical models (e.g., dynamic vs. cognitive-behavioral) have different effects. Research should also look at the relative cost-effectiveness of different treatments using follow-up data, and to the extent indicated, reimbursement policies should be changed accordingly. Another area that would benefit from research attention is how well the therapeutic alliance (and what type of alliance) predicts patients' subsequent benefits from treatment. Furthermore, increased research attention should focus on the intensive outpatient level of care (level II), a relatively new level that seems particularly promising for BPD patients. Finally, given the apparent differences in effective treatments for psychopathic and nonpsychopathic ASPD, research should continue to distinguish between these two groups when examining treatments for ASPD as well as begin to identify the extent to which the positive results found for specialized drug treatment programs (at all levels of care) are generalizable to other treatment programs for ASPD patients.

This chapter provides an overview of the structures and goals of different levels of care as well as their relative appropriateness for the treatment of different personality disorders. Attention to and consideration of personality disorder diagnosis will aid clinicians in determining the levels of care likely to be most effective and clinically indicated and should be used to inform treatment decisions. In particular, preliminary evidence suggests the value of using graduated, step-down levels of care, although more research is needed to determine the specific structure and timeline most likely to be effective within such a step-down system.

REFERENCES

Alden L: Short-term structured treatment for avoidant personality disorder. J Consult Clin Psychol 57:756–764, 1989

Barley WD, Buie SE, Peterson EW, et al: Development of an inpatient cognitive-behavioral treatment program for borderline personality disorder. J Personal Disord 7: 232–240, 1993

Bateman A, Fonagy P: Effectiveness of partial hospitalization in the treatment of borderline personality disorder: a randomized controlled trial. Am J Psychiatry 156:1563–1569, 1999

Bateman A, Fonagy P: Treatment of borderline personality disorder with psychoanalytically oriented partial hospitalization: an 18-month follow-up. Am J Psychiatry 158:36–42, 2001

Bateman A, Fonagy P: Psychotherapy for Borderline Personality Disorder: Mentalization-Based Treatment. New York, Oxford University Press, 2004

Bateman A, Fonagy P: Mentalization-Based Treatment for Borderline Personality Disorder: A Practical Guide. Oxford, England, Oxford University Press, 2006

Bateman A, Fonagy P: Eight-year follow-up of patients treated for borderline personality disorder: mentalization-based treatment versus treatment as usual. Am J Psychiatry 165:631–638, 2008

Blum N, Pfohl B, St. John D, et al: STEPPS: a cognitive-behavioral systems-based group treatment for outpatients with borderline personality disorder. A preliminary report. Compr Psychiatry 43:301–310, 2002

Blum N, St. John D, Pfohl B, et al: Systems Training for Emotional Predictability and Problem Solving (STEPPS) for outpatients with borderline personality disorder: a randomized controlled trial and 1-year follow-up. Am J Psychiatry 165:468–478, 2008

Bohus M, Haaf B, Stiglmayr C, et al: Evaluation of inpatient dialectical behavior therapy for borderline personality disorder: a prospective study. Behav Res Ther 38:875–887, 2000

Bohus M, Haaf B, Simms T, et al: Effectiveness of inpatient dialectical behavioral therapy for borderline personality disorder: a controlled trial. Behav Res Therapy 4:487–499, 2004

Brooner RK, Kidorf M, King VL, et al: Preliminary evidence of good treatment response in antisocial drug abusers. Drug Alcohol Depend 49:249–260, 1998

Brown GK, Newman CF, Charlesworth SE, et al: An open clinical trial of cognitive behavior therapy for borderline personality disorder. J Personal Disord 18:257–271, 2004

Cacciola JS, Alterman AI, Rutherford MJ, et al: Treatment response of antisocial substance abusers. J Nerv Ment Dis 183:166–171, 1995

Compton WM, Cottler LB, Spitznagel EL, et al: Cocaine users with antisocial personality improve HIV risk behaviors as much as those without antisocial personality. Drug Alcohol Depend 49:239–247, 1998

Davidson K, Norrie J, Tyrer P, et al: The effectiveness of cognitive behavior therapy for borderline personality disorder: results from the Borderline Personality Disorder Study of Cognitive Therapy (BOSCOT) trial. J Personal Disord 20:450–465, 2006

Dolan BM, Evans C, Wilson J: Therapeutic community treatment for personality disordered adults: changes in neurotic symptomatology on follow-up. Int J Soc Psychiatry 38:243–250, 1992

Dolan B, Warren F, Norton K: Change in borderline symptoms one year after therapeutic community treatment for severe personality disorder. Br J Psychiatry 171:274–279, 1997

Dolan-Sewell RT, Krueger RF, Shea MT: Co-occurrence with syndrome disorders, in Handbook of Personality Disorders: Theory, Research and Treatment. Edited by Livesley WJ. New York, Guilford, 2001, pp 84–104

Dyck IR, Phillips KA, Warshaw MG, et al: Patterns of personality pathology in patients with generalized anxiety disorders, panic disorder with and without agoraphobia, and social phobia. J Personal Disord 15:60–71, 2001

Fonagy P: Thinking about thinking: some clinical and theoretical considerations in the treatment of a borderline patient. Int J Psychoanal 72:1–18, 1991

Gabbard GO, Coyne L: Predictors of response of antisocial patients to hospital treatment. Hosp Community Psychiatry 38:1181–1185, 1987

Gabbard GO, Gunderson JG, Fonagy P: The place of psychoanalytic treatments within psychiatry. Arch Gen Psychiatry 59:505–510, 2002

Giesen-Bloo J, van Dyck R, Spinhoven P, et al: Outpatient psychotherapy for borderline personality disorder: randomized trial of schema-focused therapy vs. transference-focused therapy. Arch Gen Psychiatry 6:649–658, 2006

Gratz KL, Gunderson JG: Preliminary data on an acceptance-based emotional regulation group intervention for deliberate self-harm among women with borderline personality disorder. Behav Ther 37:25–35, 2006

Gude T, Vaglum P: One-year follow-up of patients with Cluster C personality disorders: a prospective study comparing patients with "pure" and "comorbid" conditions within Cluster C, and "pure" C with "pure" Cluster A or B conditions. J Personal Disord 15:216–228, 2001

Gunderson JG: Defining the therapeutic processes in psychiatric milieus. Psychiatry 41:327–335, 1978

Gunderson JG: Borderline Personality Disorder: A Clinical Guide. Washington, DC, American Psychiatric Press, 2001

Gunderson JG: Treatment of personality disorders: an overview. Paper presented at the annual meeting of the American Psychiatric Association, San Francisco, CA, May 2003

Gunderson JG, Gabbard GO: Making the case for psychoanalytic therapies in the current psychiatric world. J Am Psychoanal Assoc 47:679–703, 1999

Gunderson JG, Waldinger R, Sabo A: Stages of change in dynamic psychotherapy with borderline patients: clinical and research implications. J Psychother Pract Res 2:64–72, 1993

Gunderson JG, Morey LC, Stout RL, et al: Major depressive disorder and borderline personality disorder revisited: longitudinal interactions. J Clin Psychiatry 65:1049–1056, 2004

Hardy GE, Barkham M, Shapiro DA, et al: Impact of Cluster C personality disorders on outcome of contrasting brief psychotherapies for depression. J Consult Clin Psychol 63:997–1004, 1995

Harris GT, Rice ME, Cormier CA: Psychopaths: is a therapeutic community therapeutic? Therapeutic Communities 15:283–299, 1994

Hart SD, Hare RD: Psychopathy: assessment and association with criminal conduct, in Handbook of Antisocial Behavior. Edited by Stoff DM, Breiling J, Maser JD. New York, Wiley, 1997, pp 22–35

Hildebrand M, de Ruiter C, Nijman H: PCL-R psychopathy predicts disruptive behavior among offenders in a Dutch forensic psychiatric hospital. J Interpers Violence 19:13–29, 2004

Hoglend P: Personality disorders and long-term outcome after brief dynamic psychotherapy. J Personal Disord 7:168–181, 1993

Howard KI, Kopta SM, Krause MS, et al: The dose-response relationship in psychotherapy. Am Psychol 41:159–164, 1986

Karterud S, Vaglum S, Friis S, et al: Day hospital therapeutic community treatment for patients with personality disorders: an empirical evaluation of the containment function. J Nerv Ment Dis 180:238–243, 1992

Karterud S, Pederson G, Bjordal E, et al: Day treatment of patients with personality disorders: experiences from a Norwegian treatment research network. J Personal Disord 17:243–262, 2003

Knight R: Evaluation of the results of psychoanalytic therapy. Am J Psychiatry 98:434–446, 1941

Koenigsberg HW, Kaplan RD, Gilmore MM, et al: The relationship between syndrome and personality disorder in DSM-III: experience with 2,464 patients. Am J Psychiatry 142:207–212, 1985

Koenigsberg HW, Anwunah I, New AS, et al: Relationship between depression and borderline personality disorder. Depress Anxiety 10:158–167, 1999

Kool S, Dekker J, Duijsens IJ, et al: Efficacy of combined therapy and pharmacotherapy for depressed patients with or without personality disorders. Harv Rev Psychiatry 11:133–141, 2003

Kopta SM, Howard KI, Lowry JL, et al: Patterns of symptomatic recovery in psychotherapy. J Clin Consult Psychol 62:1009–1016, 1994

Krawitz R: A prospective psychotherapy outcome study. Aust N Z J Psychiatry 31:465–473, 1997

Lanktree CB, Briere J: Outcome of therapy for sexual abused children: a repeated measures study. Child Abuse Negl 19:1145–1155, 1995

Leichsenring F, Leibing E: The effectiveness of psychodynamic therapy in the treatment of personality disorders: a meta-analysis. Am J Psychiatry 160:1223–1232, 2003

Levendusky PG, Willis BS, Ghinassi FA: The therapeutic contracting program: a comprehensive continuum of care model. Psychiatr Q 65:189–207, 1994

Linehan MM: Cognitive-Behavioral Treatment of Borderline Personality Disorder. New York, Guilford, 1993

Linehan MM, Armstrong HE, Suarez A, et al: Cognitive-behavioral treatment of chronically parasuicidal borderline patients. Arch Gen Psychiatry 48:1060–1064, 1991

Linehan MM, Heard HL, Armstrong HE: Naturalistic follow-up of a behavioral treatment for chronically parasuicidal borderline patients. Arch Gen Psychiatry 50: 971–974, 1993

Linehan M, Tutek DA, Heard HL, et al: Interpersonal outcome of cognitive behavioral treatment for chronically suicidal borderline patients. Am J Psychiatry 151:1771–1776, 1994

Linehan MM, Comtois KA, Murray AM, et al: Two-year randomized controlled trial and follow-up of dialectical behavior therapy vs. therapy by experts for suicidal behaviors and borderline personality disorder. Arch Gen Psychiatry 7:757–766, 2006

Loranger AW: The impact of DSM-III on diagnostic practice in a university hospital. Arch Gen Psychiatry 47:672–675, 1990

Marziali E, Munroe-Blum H: An interpersonal approach to group psychotherapy with borderline personality disorder. J Personal Disord 9:179–189, 1995

McQuillan A, Nicastro R, Guenot F, et al: Intensive dialectical behavior therapy for outpatients with borderline personality disorder who are in crisis. Psychiatr Serv 56: 193–197, 2005

Mehlum L, Friis S, Irion T, et al: Personality disorders 2–5 years after treatment: a prospective follow-up study. Acta Psychiatr Scand 84:72–77, 1991

Messina NP, Wish ED, Nemes S: Therapeutic community treatment for substance abusers with antisocial personality disorder. J Subst Abuse Treat 17:121–128, 1999

Messina NP, Wish ED, Hoffman JA, et al: Antisocial personality disorder and therapeutic community treatment outcomes. Am J Drug Alcohol Abuse 28:197–212, 2002

Messina N, Farabee D, Rawson R: Treatment responsivity of cocaine-dependent patients with antisocial personality disorder to cognitive-behavioral and contingency management interventions. J Consult Clin Psychol 71:320–329, 2003

Munroe-Blum H, Marziali E: A controlled trial of short-term group treatment for borderline personality disorder. J Personal Disord 9:190–198, 1995

Neuhaus EC: Fixed values and a flexible partial hospital program model. Harv Rev Psychiatry 14:1–14, 2006

Neuhaus EC, Christopher M, Jacob K, et al: Short-term cognitive behavioral partial hospital treatment: a pilot study. J Psychiatr Pract 13:298–307, 2007

Ogloff JR, Wong S, Greenwood A: Treating criminal psychopaths in a therapeutic community program. Behav Sci Law 8:181–190, 1990

Oldham JM, Skodol AE, Kellman HD, et al: Comorbidity of Axis I and Axis II disorders. Am J Psychiatry 152:571–578, 1995

Perry JC, Bond M: Empirical studies of psychotherapy for personality disorders, in Psychotherapy for Personality Disorders. Edited by Gunderson JG, Gabbard GO (Review of Psychiatry Series, Vol 19; Oldham JM and Riba MB, series eds). Washington, DC, American Psychiatric Press, 2000, pp 1–31

Quaytman M, Scharfstein SS: Treatment for severe borderline personality disorder in 1987 and 1997. Am J Psychiatry 154:1139–1144, 1997

Reiss D, Grubin D, Meux C: Institutional performance of male "psychopaths" in a high-security hospital. Journal of Forensic Psychiatry 10:290–299, 1999

Rice ME, Harris GT, Cormier CA: An evaluation of maximum security therapeutic community for psychopaths and other disordered offenders. Law Hum Behav 16: 399–412, 1992

Richards HJ, Casey JO, Lucente SW: Psychopathy and treatment response in incarcerated female substance abusers. Crim Justice Behav 30:251–276, 2003

Salekin RT: Psychopathy and therapeutic pessimism: clinical lore or clinical reality? Clin Psychol Rev 22:79–112, 2002

Shea MT, Glass DR, Pilkonis PA, et al: Frequency and implications of personality disorders in a sample of depressed inpatients. J Personal Disord 1:27–41, 1987

Silk KR, Eisner W, Allport C, et al: Focused time-limited inpatient treatment of borderline personality disorder. J Personal Disord 8:268–278, 1994

Smith G, Ruis-Sancho A, Gunderson JG: An intensive outpatient program for patients with borderline personality disorder. Psychiatr Serv 52:532–533, 2001

Soloff PH: Algorithm for pharmacological treatment of personality dimensions: symptom-specific treatments for cognitive-perceptual, affective and impulsive-behavioral dysregulation. Bull Menninger Clin 62:195–214, 1998

Stevenson J, Meares R: An outcome study of psychotherapy for patients with borderline personality disorder. Am J Psychiatry 149:358–362, 1992

Tyrer P, Simmonds S: Treatment models for those with severe mental illness and comorbid personality disorder. Br J Psychiatry 44(suppl):15–18, 2003

Tyrer P, Gunderson JG, Lyons M, et al: Special feature: extent of comorbidity between mental state and personality disorders. J Personal Disord 11:242–259, 1997

Vaglum P, Friis S, Irion T, et al: Treatment response of severe and nonsevere personality disorders in a therapeutic community day unit. J Personal Disord 4:161–172, 1990

Van der Sande R, van Rooijen L, Buskens E, et al: Intensive in-patient and community intervention versus routine care after attempted suicide: a randomised controlled intervention study. Br J Psychiatry 171:35–41, 1997

Waldinger RJ, Gunderson JG: Effective Psychotherapy With Borderline Patients: Case Studies. Washington, DC, American Psychiatric Press, 1989

Widiger TA, Corbitt EM: Antisocial personality disorder, in DSM-IV Source Book, Vol 2. Edited by Widiger TA, Frances AJ, Pincus HA. Washington, DC, American Psychiatric Association, 1996, pp 703–716

Widiger TA, Weissman MM: Epidemiology of borderline personality disorder. Hosp Community Psychiatry 42:1015–1021, 1991

Wilberg T, Friis S, Karterud S, et al: Outpatient group psychotherapy: a valuable continuation treatment for patients with borderline personality disorder treated in a day hospital. A 3-year follow-up study. Nord J Psychiatry 52:213–221, 1998a

Wilberg T, Karterud S, Urnes O, et al: Outcomes of poorly functioning patients with personality disorders in a day treatment program. Psychiatr Serv 49:1562–1467, 1998b

Wilberg T, Urnes O, Friis S, et al: One-year follow-up of day treatment for poorly functioning patients with personality disorders. Psychiatr Serv 50:1326–1330, 1999

Winnicott DW: The Maturational Process and the Facilitating Environment. London, Hogarth Press, 1965

Winston A, Laikin M, Pollack J, et al: Short-term psychotherapy of personality disorders. Am J Psychiatry 151:190–194, 1994

10

Psychoanalysis and Psychodynamic Psychotherapy

Glen O. Gabbard, M.D.

The field of psychoanalysis emerged in the last decade of the nineteenth century as a means of treatment for hysterical symptoms. However, in a relatively short time the focus of psychoanalysis shifted toward long-standing character pathology. As early as 1908, Freud was inaugurating that shift when he wrote his classic paper "Character and Anal Eroticism" (Freud 1908/1959). Freud linked specific character traits, such as miserliness, obstinacy, and orderliness, with the anal psychosexual stage of development. Whereas he regarded neurotic symptoms as reflecting the return of repressed unconscious material, he viewed character traits as the end result of the successful use of repression as well as other defenses such as sublimation and reaction formation. As he moved in the direction of the structural model, he became aware that identification was of great importance in the formation of character. He recognized that some people can give

up a lost object only by identifying with the lost person, suggesting that one seminal aspect of the development of personality is identification with parents and others in the course of development.

Freud's work was expanded by Karl Abraham (1923/1948) when he developed a system of classifying character traits according to their linkage with oral, anal, and genital eroticism. However, it was Wilhelm Reich (1931) who was the true trailblazer in the psychoanalytic understanding of character. He developed the term *character armor* to describe the unconscious and ego-syntonic defensive style of patients who come to analytic treatment. He postulated that childhood conflicts were mastered with specific defense mechanisms. These defenses subsequently emerged in the psychoanalytic setting in the way patients entered the office, reclined on the couch, related to the analyst, and resisted the psychoanalytic process. Although neurotic symptoms were regarded as compromise formations that produced distress, Reich stressed that character traits were rarely sources of anxiety or emotional pain. This distinction continues into the present, when clinicians often remark how the character traits in patients with personality disorders often cause more distress in others than in the patient. However, this generalization understates the great extent to which many people with personality disorders suffer as a result of their character pathology.

CONCEPTUAL MODEL

Contemporary psychoanalysis is primarily geared to address character. The symptomatic neuroses of Freud's day are rare in today's clinical setting. Analysts focus on how distortions of self, compromises between wishes and defenses that oppose those wishes, and internal representations of self and others have forged the patient's personality (Gabbard 2000b). Psychodynamic psychotherapy, which is derived from psychoanalysis, may be used for Axis I conditions, such as panic disorder and major depression, but it is particularly useful to address the problems associated with Axis II disorders.

Psychoanalysts and dynamic therapists who treat personality disorders today must be biologically informed (Gabbard 2001). There is now abundant evidence that some personality traits are heritable (Cloninger et al. 1993; Livesley et al. 1993; Svrakic et al. 1993). The psychobiological model of Cloninger et al. (1993), for example, suggests that about 50% of personality is genetically based temperament, whereas another 50% is environmentally based character. These investigators stressed that the character variables, based on interactions with family members and peer groups, traumatic experiences, intrapsychic fantasy, and the cultural setting in which one develops, are highly influential in determining the subtype of personality disorder. Although not everyone

agrees with this particular model, psychoanalysts and psychotherapists alike must accept the limitations of the treatment they undertake. Genetically based temperament is unlikely to be altered by psychoanalysis or psychodynamic psychotherapy, but the areas of self-development, internal object relations, and the patient's effectiveness in coping with the environment may be profoundly affected by psychoanalytically oriented treatments. Temperament is highly stable over time, whereas the character dimensions tend to be malleable and undergo development throughout life (Svrakic et al. 1993).

From a psychoanalytic perspective, personality can be viewed as having five major components: 1) a biologically based temperament, 2) a set of internalized object relations, 3) an enduring sense of self, 4) a specific constellation of defense mechanisms, and 5) a characteristic cognitive style. Analysts and analytically oriented therapists would regard the achievement of a stable and positive sense of self and the establishment of mutually gratifying and enduring relationships as perhaps the two fundamental tasks of personality development (Blatt and Ford 1994). These two fundamental features of character evolve in a synergistic and dialectical relationship throughout the life cycle. Blatt (1992; Blatt and Ford 1994; Blatt et al. 2007) has stressed that character pathology often divides into two broad subgroups: anaclitic and introjective. The *anaclitic* type is mainly concerned with relationships with others, and these individuals have longings to be nurtured, protected, and loved. The *introjective* subtype, on the other hand, is primarily focused on self-development, and these individuals struggle with feelings of unworthiness, failure, and inferiority. They are highly self-critical, exceedingly perfectionistic, and competitive.

Because the work of psychoanalysis is heavily influenced by transference and countertransference developments in the treatment process, psychoanalytic clinicians tend to place a great deal of emphasis on how the patient's internal object relations are externalized in interpersonal relationships with others. The psychoanalytic setting is seen as a laboratory in which analysts can directly observe how their patients re-create their internal object world in the relationships they forge in the course of their daily lives. Hence, psychoanalytically oriented therapists tend to conceptualize the nature of the patient's psychopathology less in terms of DSM-IV-TR (American Psychiatric Association 2000) criteria and more in terms of what unfolds in the treatment relationship (Gabbard 1997a, 2001, 2007).

The character dimension of personality is usefully conceptualized as involving an ongoing attempt to actualize certain patterns of relatedness that largely reflect unconscious wishes. Through interpersonal behavior, patients try to impose on the clinician a particular way of responding and experiencing. Character traits, therefore, must be viewed as playing a fundamental role in actualizing an internal object relationship that is central to a wish-fulfilling fantasy in the patient (Sandler 1981). The key to understanding the patient's relationships outside the treatment, then, may be the observation of what develops in the transference-countertransference dimensions of the treatment process.

Developmental themes are at the heart of all psychoanalytic theories. Part of the conceptual model of personality disorders assumes that a child internalizes a self-representation in interaction with an object representation connected by an affect state. If, for example, a father repeatedly yells at his son, the child internalizes an object relations unit involving a critical, angry object, an inadequate and beleaguered self, and an affect of shame and smoldering resentment. At other times, when the father praises his son, the little boy may internalize a loving and admiring object, a good and praiseworthy self, and an affect state of glowing self-regard. These interactions are etched in neural networks and become repetitive patterns of relatedness (Westen and Gabbard 2002). Psy-

choanalysts and psychodynamic therapists understand the clinical setting as one in which patients attempt to re-create their internal object relationships through the externalization of these relatedness patterns formed in childhood.

The wish-fulfilling nature of actualizing internal object relationships is clear in the example of an internal self wishing to be loved and admired by an internal object. The wish is less apparent in those patients who establish one conflictual and self-defeating relationship after another. However, even a "bad" or tormenting object may provide safety and affirmation to a patient for a variety of reasons (Gabbard 2001; Sandler 1981). For abused children, for example, an abusive relationship may be safe in the sense that it is preferable to having no object at all or to being abandoned. A basic paradoxical situation arises in the lives of abused children, where the person to whom they look for safety and protection is also the abuser. They may have no alternative, then, but to seek safety in the shadow of one who has abused them. They may also assume that the only way of remaining connected to a significant figure of safety is to maintain an abuser–victim paradigm in the relationship. These relationships may be sought out by patients who were abused as children because they are reliable, predictable, and provide the patient with an ongoing sense of continuity and meaning. The devil one knows is generally perceived as better than the devil one does not know.

Some of the repetitive relationship patterns seen in patients with personality disorder are approximations of actual relationships these individuals had with real figures in the past. However, in some cases they involve wished-for relationships that never actually existed. Patients with severe childhood trauma, for example, often develop elaborate fantasies about a rescuer who will save them from abuse.

The mode of actualization within the clinical relationship is often referred to as *projective identification* (Gabbard 1995; Ogden

1979). Within this model, patients behave in a characterologically driven way that exerts interpersonal pressure on the therapist to conform to what is being projected onto him or her. In other words, a patient may "nudge" the analyst into assuming the role of an abuser in response to the patient's "victim" role. A patient who treats the therapist with contempt, for example, may engender countertransference anger or hate and lead the therapist to make sarcastic or devaluing comments to the patient.

Case Example

Mr. J was a 24-year-old graduate student who was struggling in his academic setting because he appeared to be threatened by success. He had all of the primary symptoms of obsessive-compulsive personality disorder (OCPD), and his highly perfectionistic expectations of himself led him to feel that he was always failing. In the course of analysis, he talked at great length about what a harsh taskmaster his father had been and how he was never able to live up to what his father expected of him. Eventually this pattern emerged in the transference, when the patient revealed that he feared that his analyst saw him as a failure as well. He felt the analyst was heavily invested in having him succeed in graduate school, and the patient was feeling that he could not possibly measure up to what his analyst expected. The analyst drew Mr. J's attention to how he had re-created with the analyst the same relationship he had with his father. The patient could readily see the connection, and he thanked the analyst for pointing it out. However, the analyst also recognized that the patient's deferential and ingratiating quality was a reaction formation to a good deal of resentment about feeling driven by others to succeed. The analyst thus interpreted that the patient had found a way to indirectly express his resentment at both his analyst and his father by thwarting their perceived hopes for his success in graduate school. By failing to pass his oral exam-

inations, he could have the fantasy of making his dad and his analyst suffer. Eventually the analyst was also able to point out to Mr. J that his graduate student advisor, another male about the age of his father, was also part of this same pattern of relatedness. Through interpretation, the analyst made the patient aware that he had placed this paternal figure in the same role as his father and his analyst.

In this model the patient's self-representation can elicit a corresponding object representation in the analyst. This model of character is closely related to the role relationship model of Horowitz (1988, 1991, 1998). In his theory, a person's schemas reflect unconscious self–other organizational units. These units are driven by powerful internal motives that lead away from feared outcomes and toward desired ends. Another way to view these schemas is as belief structures that have both form and content. They are often characterized, however, by conflicting desires and beliefs that become expressed in the transference relationship with the analyst.

In addition to the development of self in relation to objects in the formation of character, psychoanalytically oriented therapists study the unique set of defense mechanisms found in each patient as a key to diagnostic understanding and treatment. Defenses ward off awareness of unpleasant affect states and unacceptable aggressive or sexual wishes and preserve a sense of self-esteem in the face of narcissistic vulnerability. They may also serve to ensure safety when one is feeling threatened. A contemporary analytic perspective, however, would recognize that defense mechanisms do not merely change the relationship between an emotional state and an idea; they also influence the relationship between self and object (Vaillant and Vaillant 1999). Patients may be able to manage unresolved conflicts with important figures in their lives or with old objects from the past that haunt them in the present through the use of defenses. In patients with personality disorder for whom relationship difficulties are one of the major reasons for seeking treatment, dynamic clinicians conceptualize defenses as embedded in relatedness. Vaillant and Vaillant (1999) emphasized that the symptoms of patients with personality disorder often are designed to cope with unbearable relationships or unbearable people, whether in the present or in the past.

Psychoanalysts and psychodynamic therapists view the specific constellation of defenses that work in concert with characteristic patterns of object relations as having enormous importance for the diagnostic understanding of the patient. For example, someone with OCPD would use defensive operations such as reaction formation, intellectualization, undoing, and isolation of affect (Gabbard 2000c). These defenses tone down powerful affect states so that the patient is not in danger of losing control. These patients may be responsible, dutiful, and unfailingly courteous toward the analyst to be sure that no trace of aggression is revealed in their clinical interactions.

The fifth component of character—cognitive style—is intimately related to the patient's characteristic defenses. Persons with OCPD, for example, will come across as lacking flexibility and spontaneity in their thought processes because they are directed toward the control of all affect states. They will also address every detail of a situation in their pursuit of a perfect solution. Histrionic personality disorder patients, on the other hand, have a cognitive style that is directly linked to their excessive emotionality. Hence they avoid detail and will give impressionistic and global responses to questions that reflect the "feel" of a situation. These cognitive styles appear to be reasonably consistent across personality types (Shapiro 1965).

MAJOR PRINCIPLES OF TECHNIQUE

Psychoanalysis is traditionally conducted in 45- to 50-minute sessions four or five times a week and may last for several years. Most patients recline on the analyst's couch, although some prefer to sit for parts of the treatment when visual contact with the analyst is seen as necessary. The patient is asked to say whatever comes to mind in an effort to facilitate the process of free association. Patients generally have difficulty saying what comes to mind because of anxieties about what the analyst will think as well as shame about certain aspects of themselves that they find unacceptable.

The difficulties encountered in lying on a couch and saying whatever comes to mind four or five times a week inevitably lead to the development of transference and resistance, two of the major foci of psychoanalytic treatment. Resistance is not simply the reluctance to say what comes to mind. It is also a manifestation of the patients' unique defense mechanisms as they enter into the treatment process. In other words, defenses are intrapsychic mechanisms, but they become interpersonalized as resistances in the relationship with the analyst (Gabbard 2000c). Resistance also reveals significant internal object relationships. A contemporary view of resistances would include the fact that they are forces that oppose the optimal state of consciousness sought in analysis. In an ideal analytic process, patients develop a dual consciousness in which they relive certain experiences from their past in the transference to the analyst while also reflecting on those experiences and being curious about their meanings and origins (Friedman 1991).

Psychoanalysts view resistances not simply as obstacles to be avoided but as a major source of significant information about patients' characteristic defensive operations and their deeply ingrained personality traits. Analysts no longer spend most of their time in an archeological search for buried relics from the patient's past. Contemporary analysts focus more on the relationship between analyst and patient as a privileged view of how the patient's past has created certain patterns of conflict and problematic object relations in the present. In his 1914 paper, "Remembering, Repeating, and Working-Through," Freud (1914/1958) noted that what the patient cannot remember will be repeated in action in the patient's here-and-now behavior with the analyst, the original meaning of the term *acting-out*. Hence the patient's characterological pattern of internal object relations and the conflicts about those relationships unfold in front of the analyst without necessarily digging into childhood traumas to unlock hidden secrets.

While transference reflects the patient's past experiences with similar figures, it also incorporates the *real* aspects of the analyst. Hence transference is now considered to be a mixture of old relationships from the past and the new and real relationship with the analyst in the present. In other words, if an analyst chooses to be aloof, silent, and emotionally remote, the patient may well develop a transference to the analyst as a cold and unfeeling figure.

As the patient repeats long-standing patterns of relatedness during the sessions, the analyst is gradually drawn into a "dance." Through the process of projective identification described earlier, the analyst is transformed into a transference object. Not all analysts will react in the same way, and the specific features of the analyst's intrapsychic world will work in concert with what is being projected by the patient to shape the unique form of the analyst's countertransference. Some analysts may ignore the role being thrust on them or reject it. Others may defend against the role by assuming an opposite stance. Some analysts who are being pressured to take on the characteristics of a projected abusive object, for example, may become overly kind and empathic as a reaction formation to their growing feelings of sadism or anger.

In any case, a key aspect of the psychoanalytic treatment of patients with personality disorders is to maintain a free-floating responsiveness (Sandler 1981) to what is being evoked by the patient and to use this re-created "dance" as a way of understanding the patient's usual mode of object relatedness outside the treatment situation. When the role being evoked by the patient is unfamiliar and distressing to the analyst, such as the role of an abusive parent, some analysts may feel that an alien force has taken them over, and their subjective experience may be something along the lines of "I'm not behaving like myself" (Gabbard 2001). If the wished-for interaction being actualized by the patient is that of an idealized parent who is nurturing and understanding toward a needy child, the analyst may feel quite comfortable in the role and be unaware of its countertransference origins. One of the key components of technique, then, is for the analyst to clarify the nature of these unconscious relational patterns, acknowledging that they are jointly created, and then make them understandable to the patient. Transference-countertransference enactments may need to repeat themselves a number of times before they are apparent and can be interpreted to the patient.

Analysts listen to the development of themes in the associations of the patient. They carefully track patterns in the transference relationship that also emerge in narrative accounts of the patient's life in the present and in the past. As recurrent themes emerge, they begin to make these unconscious patterns more available to the patient's conscious awareness. A primary intervention is interpretation, which seeks to make connections or linkages for the patient that are largely outside the patient's awareness.

Psychodynamic psychotherapy is based on the same principles of technique but is less focused on interpretation of transference as the central intervention. Moreover, the frequency of sessions (usually from one to three per week) is less intense and the patient sits in a chair instead of reclining on a couch with the analyst out of view. Depending on the nature of the psychopathology, some patients require more support, more visual contact with the therapist, and less regression than what occurs typically in analysis. Patients with deficit-based pathology have often had extensive childhood deprivation or trauma. They may hear interpretations as attacks and feel shamed by them. In those situations, the therapist may need to use affirmative interventions (Killingmo 1989) that confirm exactly the way the patient is feeling and empathically validate the patient's right to feel that way. Many patients with this type of background may ultimately be able to use interpretations if the way is paved for them by validating and affirming interventions (Gabbard et al. 1994).

The goals of the treatment vary according to the patient's presenting complaints, the nature and severity of the psychopathology, and the clinician and analyst's theoretical model. Among those goals that are commonly established are resolution of conflict (Brenner 1976); a search for an authentic or *true self*, as Winnicott (1962) suggested; improved relationships as a result of a gain in understanding about one's internal object relationships (Gabbard 1996); an improved capacity to seek out appropriate selfobjects (Kohut 1984); the generation of new meanings within the therapeutic dialogue (Mitchell 1997); and an improved capacity for mentalization (Fonagy and Target 1996). (*Selfobjects* and *mentalization* are defined and discussed later in the chapter.) Regardless of the diverse goals, all psychoanalytically oriented treatment probably works through several modes of therapeutic action, of which one is the provision of insight through interpretation.

Another mode of therapeutic action is simply making observations from an outside perspective on what one sees in the patient (Gabbard 1997b). Patients cannot know how they come across to others because they are inside themselves. The therapist has the perspective of an object and therefore can help them see things that they do not see. Moreover, the "how to" of relatedness that is internalized in the earliest childhood relationships is embedded in implicit procedural memory (Gabbard and Westen 2003). Clinicians can see the automatic and unconscious

patterns of relatedness in action and help the patient become aware of these patterns. A therapist may observe, for example, that the patient looks ashamed whenever talking about his mother and will thus point that out to the patient. Fonagy (1999) stresses that a crucial avenue for therapeutic change may lie in a patient's increasing capacity to "find himself" in the therapist's mind. By consistently observing and commenting on the patient's feeling states and nonverbal communications, the patient may begin to assemble a portrait of himself or herself based on the analyst's observation and thereby develop increased capacity for mentalization. Consistent observations about the characterological patterns of the patient also make ego-syntonic character traits more ego-dystonic as the patient recognizes the problematic aspects of the traits as well as the interpersonal impact that the traits have on others.

In all forms of psychoanalysis and psychodynamic psychotherapy, another source of therapeutic action is internalization of the analyst or therapist and of the treatment relationship. Internalizing does not necessarily require the use of a conscious, declarative representation. The clinical relationship itself is accompanied by unconscious affective connections that have been referred to by Lyons-Ruth et al. (1998) as *implicit relational knowing*. This phenomenon refers to moments of meeting between clinician and patient that are not symbolically represented or dynamically unconscious in the ordinary sense. Some change occurs in the realm of procedural knowledge involving how to act, feel, and think in a particular relational context. As patients internalize the therapist's accepting and tolerant attitude, their superego is also modified so they are less self-critical and more accepting of their humanness.

From a cognitive neuroscience perspective, the internalization of the therapeutic relationship gradually builds a new neural network with a different type of object representation and a corresponding self-representation. The old networks are not completely obliterated by the treatment, but they are relatively weakened or deactivated while the new networks based on the treatment relationship are strengthened (Gabbard and Westen 2003).

All of these techniques and modes of therapeutic action are adapted to the individual patient and the type of personality disorder that most closely fits that patient. There is inevitably a trial-and-error component to this approach as one finds out which types of interventions are most suited to the patient's capacity to use psychoanalytically oriented treatment.

INDICATIONS AND CONTRAINDICATIONS

In determining for whom psychoanalysis and/or psychodynamic psychotherapy is indicated, two separate but related perspectives are necessary: 1) suitability according to the psychological characteristics of the patient, and 2) suitability according to diagnoses. Regardless of whether a patient meets diagnostic criteria for a specific personality disorder, the patient's psychological features may contraindicate the use of psychoanalysis or dynamic therapy.

The indications and contraindications for psychoanalysis and psychodynamic psychotherapy according to personality disorder are summarized in Table 10–1.

Foremost among the psychological characteristics necessary to recommend psychoanalytically oriented treatment is psychological mindedness. Although there are various components to this construct, the key components are the capacity to see meaningful connections between one's difficulties and one's inner world. The capacity to think in terms of analogy and metaphor is also crucial to psychological mindedness. In addition, there must be a curiosity about the origins of one's suffering and a strong motivation to endure anxiety and discomfort in the process of learning more about oneself.

Another feature that is necessary for analysis or dynamic therapy is the capacity to regress in the service of the ego. Patients must be able to let down their guard, relax their defenses, and get in touch with primitive and unpleasant emotional states to learn about what drives them to behave or think in the way they do. They must also have high tolerance for frustration, intact reality testing, reasonably good impulse control, and enough suffering to motivate them for the treatment.

Other signs of ego strength that make a person a reasonable candidate for psychoanalysis are the ability to sustain a job over a long period of time despite encountering difficulties and the capacity for enduring meaningful relationships with others. Finally, the presence of the capacity for mentalization based on secure attachment also is a positive sign for analyzability. *Mentalization* refers to one's ability to differentiate inner from outer states and to recognize that one's perceptions are only representations rather than accurate replicas of external reality. In other words, the patient is aware that his or her own and other people's ways of viewing the world are influenced by inner beliefs, feelings, and past experiences. This capacity may be present to a greater or lesser extent and exists on a continuum that is influenced by the nature of the relationship and the patient's early experience. Some patients with impaired mentalization may nevertheless be amenable to psychoanalysis and psychodynamic psychotherapy (Fonagy 2001).

Patients in a severe life crisis are rarely suited for psychoanalytically oriented treatment, although it may ultimately be appropriate after the crisis is over. Other contraindications are poor reality testing, poor impulse control, lack of psychological mindedness, little capacity for self-observation, cognitive impairment based on neurological dysfunction, extreme concreteness, and poor frustration tolerance (Gabbard 2004). These guidelines are helpful in assessing analyzability, but analysts recognize that they must retain a certain

Table 10–1.   Indications and contraindications for psychoanalysis and psychodynamic psychotherapy according to personality disorder diagnosis

Diagnosis	Suitability for psychoanalytically oriented treatment
Paranoid personality disorder	Rarely indicated
Schizoid personality disorder	May be indicated in exceptional circumstances
Schizotypal personality disorder	Contraindicated
Borderline personality disorder	Psychodynamic psychotherapy, particularly transference-focused psychotherapy and mentalization-based therapy, are efficacious
Narcissistic personality disorder	Strong indication for psychoanalysis or psychodynamic psychotherapy
Antisocial personality disorder	Contraindicated
Histrionic/hysterical personality disorders	Strongly indicated for hysterical personality disorders and for most patients with histrionic personality disorder
Obsessive-compulsive personality disorder	Strong indication for psychoanalysis or psychodynamic psychotherapy
Avoidant personality disorder	Indicated for cases that do not respond to brief cognitive-behavioral or behavior therapy treatments
Dependent personality disorder	Likely to do well in psychoanalysis if motivation is sufficient and usually responds well to psychodynamic therapy
Masochistic or self-defeating personality disorder	Strong indication for psychoanalysis or dynamic therapy

degree of humility because prediction of how a particular patient will do in the psychoanalytic process is less than perfect. Kantrowitz (1987), in a study of 22 patients in analysis, concluded that even with highly sophisticated psychological testing, clinicians cannot reliably predict who will do well in psychoanalysis. The following sections describe the indications and contraindications for psychoanalysis in patients with specific personality disorders.

Determining the appropriateness of psychoanalysis or psychodynamic therapy is also influenced by one's diagnostic understanding of the personality disorder, but this method, too, is imperfect in predicting outcomes. In the absence of randomized controlled trials of psychoanalytic treatment for the various per-

sonality disorders, clinicians must rely on clinical wisdom and the psychological characteristics favoring analyzability described above. Moreover, the presence of various comorbid conditions on Axis I, such as affective disorder, anxiety disorder, eating disorder, or substance abuse, may complicate psychoanalytic treatment even if the personality disorder itself is likely to be amenable to this approach. As a general principle, the Cluster C personality disorders appear to be amenable to dynamic therapy or psychoanalysis. Only a very small subgroup of patients with Cluster A personality disorders are likely to respond well to psychoanalytic efforts. Those patients with Cluster B personality disorders respond variably, depending on the diagnosis and the psychological characteristics.

Paranoid Personality Disorder

In a study of 100 patients who applied for psychoanalysis at the Columbia Psychoanalytic Center, Oldham and Skodol (1994) noted that 12 met research criteria for the diagnosis of paranoid personality disorder. Of those, only four were selected for analysis, and two of the four did not finish the analytic treatment. Their data suggested that most patients with paranoid personality disorder are not suited, but for a very small number with exceptional characteristics analysis may be worth a try. In general, paranoid patients do not have sufficient trust to allow for the development of an analytic process.

Schizoid and Schizotypal Personality Disorders

Schizotypal personality disorder is thought to be genetically linked with schizophrenia, and patients with schizotypal personality disorder are rarely, if ever, suitable for psychoanalysis or psychodynamic therapy. Patients with schizoid personality disorder, on the other hand, may in some cases be appropriate for analytically oriented treatment but rarely seek it. In the study by Oldham and Skodol (1994), only one person applying for psychoanalysis was diagnosed with schizoid personality disorder. The British psychoanalytic literature suggests that there may be a small number of patients who can be reached by psychoanalytic approaches, and a number of British analysts have reported on work with these patients (Balint 1979; Fairbairn 1954; Winnicott 1963/1965).

Borderline Personality Disorder

After surveying the entire literature on the treatment of borderline personality disorder, the American Psychiatric Association practice guideline concluded that psychotherapy, rather than psychoanalysis, in concert with medication, is probably the treatment of choice for the great majority of patients with borderline personality disorder. Problems of impulsivity and difficulties in maintaining a therapeutic alliance make psychoanalytic treatment extremely challenging for patients in this category. There are reports in the literature (Abend et al. 1983; Boyer 1977; Fonagy and Target 1996; Gabbard 1991) of patients with borderline pathology who were analyzed using the couch with somewhat modified forms of psychoanalytic technique. Borderline patients who can use an analytic process represent a very small subgroup and are probably closer to the Kernberg construct of borderline personality organization (Kernberg 1975) than a DSM-IV-TR borderline personality disorder. These patients are often conceptualized as part of the "widening scope" of psychoanalysis and generally require supportive interventions to make interpretation acceptable to the patient (Horwitz et al. 1996). Both mentalization-based therapy (MBT) (Bateman and Fonagy 1999, 2001, 2008) and transference-focused psychotherapy (TFP) (Clarkin et al. 2007) have been demonstrated efficacious in randomized controlled trials.

Narcissistic Personality Disorder

Most experts in the treatment of narcissistic personality disorder agree that psychoanalysis is the treatment of choice if the patient has the psychological and financial resources to undertake a commitment to psychoanalysis. Although the treatments are long and arduous, sometimes nothing short of this in-depth approach will touch a patient. In practice, many narcissistic patients are treated with psychodynamic psychotherapy, and clinical experience suggests that they may respond favorably if motivated. A frequent challenge in working with patients with narcissistic personality disorder is the common pattern of exaggerated self-importance, combined with devaluation of others, frequently leading to counter-transference reactions in the therapist.

Case Example

A patient with narcissistic personality disorder had been in psychodynamic psychotherapy for 5 weeks with a young therapist in training. The patient began one session by complaining about the therapist's relative youth. He asserted that the therapist seemed to be a beginner who probably did not know what he was doing. "Am I your first therapy case?" he taunted. The candidate replied, "What makes you ask that?" The patient laughed and said, "I'll bet your supervisor told you not to answer my questions, right?" The candidate, feeling he was being treated with contempt, became defensive and said, "No, I'm able to think for myself." The patient responded with further contempt, "I don't see much evidence of that." Without considering the potential consequences of his comment, the therapist blurted out, "Maybe you're too busy insulting me to notice." As soon as the words came out of his mouth, the therapist felt a deep sense of shame. He had allowed himself to be nudged into sarcasm by the patient's contempt.

Antisocial Personality Disorder

Because of lack of motivation, insufficient superego development, general dishonesty, and impulsivity, patients with antisocial personality disorder represent a contraindication to psychoanalysis or psychodynamic psychotherapy.

Histrionic and Hysterical Personality Disorders

The DSM-IV-TR construct of histrionic personality disorder represents a particular type of patient with personality disorder who is very close to the borderline diagnosis. In clinical practice, one frequently encounters a higher level of histrionic personality disorder that has traditionally been referred to as hysterical personality disorder (Gabbard 2000c). These patients represent a neurotically organized individual with reasonably good impulse control, mature triangular object relations, and an intact superego. Therefore, they are considered good candidates for psychoanalysis or psychodynamic psychotherapy. Those patients on the other end of the spectrum with histrionic personality disorder may require modified versions of psychoanalytic psychotherapy because they often cannot tolerate the intense affective states that are brought about in analytic treatment. Some histrionic patients, however, appear to be able to make use of psychoanalysis and dynamic therapy.

Obsessive-Compulsive Personality Disorder

Patients with OCPD, who must be differentiated from those with obsessive-compulsive disorder, are generally good candidates for psychoanalytically oriented treatments. While there are no data from rigorously controlled trials on the efficacy of psychoanalysis, psychodynamic therapy has been shown to be useful in Cluster C personality disorders, including OCPD (Svartberg et al. 2004).

Avoidant and Dependent Personality Disorder

Some patients with avoidant personality disorder appear to respond well to behavioral or cognitive-behavioral techniques (Alden 1989; Brown et al. 1995; Stravynski et al. 1982). However, when patients do not respond to brief behavioral or cognitive-behavioral treatments for avoidant personality disorder, they may do well in analysis or psychodynamic psychotherapy, particularly if they are motivated to understand the origins of their anxieties about intimate relationships with others.

Patients with dependent personality disorder may do well in either psychoanalysis or psychodynamic psychotherapy depending on their psychological mindedness, the extent of their suffering, and their motivation to change and understand themselves.

Masochistic or Self-Defeating Personality Disorder

Although not in the official DSM-IV-TR nomenclature, patients with predominantly self-defeating or masochistic symptom patterns are widely seen in clinical practice. For most of these patients, psychoanalysis or dynamic therapy is the treatment of choice, provided they have the psychological characteristics necessary for the treatment.

PSYCHOANALYTIC APPROACHES TO SPECIFIC PERSONALITY DISORDERS

As noted above, the psychoanalytically oriented therapist's technique needs to be tailored to the specific type of personality disorder. Although most personality disorders are mixed, in that they have traits of several different personality disorders, here we consider each of the personality disorders amenable to psychoanalysis and psychodynamic psychotherapy in its pure form for the sake of clarity. In actual practice, several technical approaches may need to be combined for patients who have different personality features in mixed personality disorder. The discussion here is confined to those personality disorders that are likely to benefit from psychoanalysis or psychodynamic psychotherapy approaches at least some of the time.

Schizoid Personality Disorder

Much of our understanding of the inner world of a patient with schizoid personality disorder derives from the work of the British object relations theorists. Balint (1979) viewed these patients as having a fundamental deficit in their ability to relate—a "basic fault" caused by significant inadequacies in the mothering they received as infants. He believed that the patient's difficulty in relating to others stems from this basic incapacity rather than from neurotic conflict. Fairbairn (1954), perhaps the foremost contributor to

our understanding of patients with schizoid personality disorder, viewed the schizoid retreat from object relations as a defense against a conflict between a wish to relate to others and a fear that one's neediness would harm others. The child who initially perceives its mother as rejecting may withdraw from the world; however, the infant's greed and neediness grow until they are experienced as insatiable. The child then fears that its greed will devour the mother, resulting in her disappearance. Relationships are experienced as dangerous and to be avoided.

The clinician who endeavors to treat patients with schizoid personality disorder must recognize that their fear of relationships will manifest itself in the transference and allow the patient the opportunity to retreat without making demands for more active participation. Winnicott (1963/1965) believed that the isolation of the patients with schizoid personality disorder preserves an important authenticity that is absolutely sacred to the evolving self of the patient: "There is an intermediate stage in healthy development in which the patient's most important experience in relation to the good or potentially satisfying object is the refusal of it" (p. 182). Hence the therapist must recognize that the schizoid withdrawal is a way to communicate with the "true self" within the patient instead of sacrificing that authenticity to artificial interactions with others, including the analyst, that would lead to a "false self" adaptation.

Although patients with schizoid personality disorder do not commonly seek help from a psychoanalytically oriented therapist, when they do, the therapist must provide the patient with a holding environment in which their frozen internal object relations will eventually "thaw" through the provision of a new experience of relatedness. The goal of the psychoanalytic approach, then, is more to provide a new relationship for internalization than to interpret unconscious conflict. Extraordinary patience is required for the treatment to take effect, and the patient must be allowed to go at his or her own pace. Therapists must recognize that their own agenda for change may get in the way of the patient's timetable for venturing out into a world of potentially dangerous relationships.

Borderline Personality Disorder

Borderline personality disorder has a greater research base than other personality disorders regarding the efficacy of psychodynamic psychotherapy. As noted earlier, both MBT and TFP have demonstrated efficacy in randomized controlled trials.

Mentalizing is defined as an understanding that other people's perceptions and behavior are related to their thoughts, wishes, feelings, and desires. In other words, they have a mind that interprets reality based on who they are—perceptions are not absolute truths, but impressions. This capacity varies considerably from person to person. Bateman and Fonagy (2004) base their MBT technique on the observation that patients with borderline personality disorder have a fragile mentalizing capacity that is vulnerable to interpersonal and social interactions. This difficulty relates to the patient's insecure capacity for attachment, which in turn can be linked to the insecure attachment to the caregiver during childhood. As a result, the attachment context of psychotherapy is essential to improve one's capacity for mentalizing. As one builds a solid therapeutic alliance with the therapist, one is also building a secure attachment base.

The MBT therapist spends a good deal of time during psychotherapy sessions on drawing the patient's attention to the patient's mental states. By systematically exploring what it is the patient feels from moment to moment, the therapist helps build a sense of self in the patient. The dyadic nature of psychotherapy provides the opportunity to generate multiple perspectives on situations that may seem absolute. The therapist repeatedly re-presents the patient's subjective experience in a way that frees the patient

from being locked into the reality of one exclusive view. In the MBT technique the focus is mainly on the patient's current state of mind. Transference interpretations that emphasize genetic reconstructions are generally not used. This approach stresses "mentalizing the transference." In other words, transference provides an opportunity to explore how the mind works with the therapist's assistance. The therapist encourages the patient to think about the present relationship with the therapist in the same way that other relationships are considered. Another mind is in the room with the patient, so that the patient's view can be contrasted with the therapist's view. The transference is used to demonstrate how the same behavior may be experienced differently and thought about differently by two different minds.

Bateman and Fonagy (1999, 2001, 2008) tested MBT in a randomized controlled trial in which 38 patients with borderline personality disorder were randomly assigned to a psychoanalytically oriented partial hospital program or to a control group. The partial hospitalization condition (treatment group) consisted of once-weekly individual psychoanalytic psychotherapy, thrice-weekly group psychotherapy, once-weekly expressive therapy informed by psychodrama techniques, a weekly community meeting, regular meetings with the case coordinator, and medication review by a resident psychiatrist. The control treatment consisted of regular psychiatric review an average of two times per month with a senior psychiatrist, inpatient admission as appropriate, outpatient and community follow-up, no psychotherapy, and medication similar to that received by the treatment group.

At 18-month follow-up, the investigators found a clear reduction in the proportion of the treatment groups patients who had attempted suicide in the previous 6 months. The average length of hospitalization increased dramatically in the control group during the last 6 months of the study, whereas it remained stable in the treatment group at around 4 days per 6 months. Self-reported state and trait anxiety both decreased substantially in the treatment group but remained unchanged in the control group. Depression scores also decreased significantly in the treatment group. Five years after discharge from MBT, the treatment group continued to show clinical and statistical superiority to the control group.

TFP was developed by Otto Kernberg, John Clarkin, and their colleagues at New York Presbyterian Hospital—Cornell Medical Center, Westchester Division (Clarkin et al. 2007). It is based on an object relations model of borderline psychopathology. Hence TFP emphasizes representations of self and others and how they are activated with the therapist and with others in significant relationships outside the therapy. Affect states connected with internal representations of self and others are also a major focus of the treatment. Controlling negative affect states by understanding their origins is central to the treatment. In addition, the therapist hopes to awaken positive affect, particularly through the protection of positive attachments to others. TFP establishes a contract regarding the expectations of the patient, the therapist, and the treatment. The therapist thus sets a frame designed to control destructive behavior and systematically examines patterns of relationships to others in the therapeutic relationship itself and in outside relationships. In contrast to MBT, TFP therapists interpret aggression in the transference relationship and link it to its genetic and intrapsychic origins.

TFP has been tested in a randomized controlled trial involving 90 patients with borderline personality disorder who were randomly assigned to one of three treatment groups: 1) TFP, 2) dialectical behavior therapy (DBT), or 3) supportive psychotherapy (SP). Six domains of outcome measures were assessed at 4-month intervals over a 12-month period by raters who were blind to treatment group. All three treatments appeared to have brought about positive change in multiple

domains to an approximately equivalent extent. In certain areas, though, TFP seemed to do better than the alternative treatments. It was associated with significant improvement in 10 of the 12 variables across the six symptom domains, compared with improvement in six variables with SP and five with DBT. Only TFP resulted in significant changes in impulsivity, irritability, verbal assault, and direct assault. Both TFP and DBT did better than SP in reducing suicidality. TFP also brought about a move from an insecure attachment classification to a secure one (Levy et al. 2006), a change not seen with the other two treatments. In addition, the TFP patients showed significantly greater changes in mentalizing capacity and in narrative coherence compared with those in other groups.

The research on borderline personality disorder suggests that more than one approach may be effective. Hence the clinician must tailor the therapeutic approach to the particular patient (Gunderson 2001; Gunderson and Links 2008). Some patients, for example, may find transference work disturbing and will prefer a focus on outside relationships or the acquisition of coping skills.

Narcissistic Personality Disorder

The technical approaches to narcissistic personality disorder tend to diverge along a dividing line marked by whether the clinician views the pathology as based on deficit, according to the self psychology of Kohut (1971), or as related to conflict, as described by Kernberg (1974a, 1974b, 1984). The differences between the two approaches are summarized in Table 10–2.

Kohut's approach to the psychoanalysis of narcissistic personality disorders used empathy as the cornerstone of the technique (Ornstein 1974, 1998). Kohut stressed the need to empathize with the patient's experiences of having numerous empathic failures at the hands of parents. In this regard, he advised analysts to accept the patient's comments in a "straight" manner, just as the pa-

Table 10–2. Techniques for treating narcissistic personality disorders: Kohut versus Kernberg

Kohut	Kernberg
Views mirror and idealizing transferences as two different poles of bipolar (Kohut 1977) or tripolar (Kohut 1984) self	Views mirror and idealizing as aspects of transference related to projection and reintrojection of patient's grandiose self
Accepts idealization of patient as normal developmental need	Interprets idealization as a defense
Empathizes with patient's feeling as an understandable reaction to failures of parents and others	Helps patient see his or her own contribution to problems in relationships
Accepts patient's comments at face value, viewing resistances as healthy psychic activities that safeguard the self	Confronts and interprets resistances as defensive maneuvers
Looks at the positive side of patient's experience	Examines both positive and negative aspects of patient's experience (if only positive experiences are emphasized, the patient may develop an increased fear of internal envy and rage)
Calls attention to patient's progress	Focuses on envy and how it prevents patient from acknowledging and receiving help
Has treatment goal of helping patient acquire ability to identify and seek out appropriate selfobjects	Has treatment goal of helping patient to develop guilt and concern and to integrate idealization and trust with rage and contempt

Source.   Based on Gabbard 2000c.

tient experiences them, rather than to interpret hidden meanings (Miller 1985). Kohut would accept this *idealizing transference* as a normal developmental need rather than interpreting what might lie beneath it. He viewed the mirror and idealizing transferences as the major developments in the analysis of narcissistic personality disorder. The *mirror transference* is an effort on the patient's part to capture the "gleam" in mother's eye by trying to impress the analyst. Sensitive to the patient's potential for self-fragmentation, Kohut would empathize with the patient's need to be affirmed and validated.

Kohut (1984) later postulated a third transference, the *twinship transference*. All three of these were regarded as the *selfobject*

transferences typical of narcissistic personality disorders. The analysis of those transferences is the major part of the technical approach. Kohut also strongly endorsed calling attention to the positive aspects of the patient's experience to avoid shaming or criticizing the patient and repeating the traumas of childhood. He would not hesitate to call attention to the patient's progress. The goal of the analysis was to help the patient acquire more appropriate and mature selfobjects with the full recognition that the patient could not possibly outgrow the need for selfobject responses, such as idealization, affirmation, and validation.

Kernberg's (1974a, 1974b) approach differs in that he sees the patient's grandiose self as a highly pathological and conflict-based solution that is not to be regarded as simply an arrested development of the normal self. He regards idealization as a defense against rage, contempt, and envy, and he advocates active interpretation of idealization. In general, Kernberg's approach is more confrontational than Kohut's, and he stresses the patient's greed and demandingness rather than his or her longings for affirmation. He also focuses to a greater extent on envy and how it prevents the patient from acknowledging and receiving help. Whereas Kohut views resistances as healthy psychic activities designed to safeguard the self, Kernberg confronts and interprets resistances as defensive maneuvers. He would see the goal of psychoanalysis as much broader than Kohut's. He would hope that the patient would develop a greater sense of guilt and concern while integrating idealization and trust with rage and contempt.

In actual practice, many psychoanalysts and dynamic therapists use elements of both Kernberg and Kohut in their approach to narcissistic patients. An empathic perspective, as described by Kohut, is often extremely helpful early in the treatment to form a therapeutic alliance with the patient so that the patient is willing to explore his or her inner world. Over time, patients often are more capable of responding to interpretation and confrontation when they feel a stable relationship has been established with the analyst. Both Kohut and Kernberg identify valid aspects of narcissistic pathology, but different types of narcissistic patients require different emphases.

Regardless of which technical strategy is chosen, clinicians treating narcissistic patients encounter formidable countertransference difficulties. They often have a sense that they are being used as a sounding board rather than a person with a separate internal world. They may need to tolerate long periods in which they feel they are peripheral to the narcissistic patient's associations. They may also note that with the hypervigilant va-

riety of narcissistic personality disorder (Gabbard 2000c), they feel coerced into focusing their attention completely on the patient during every moment of the session, and they may feel controlled into meeting the patient's unrealistic expectations of perfect attunement. If they fall short, they risk an explosion of narcissistic rage by a patient who sees a slight around every corner. Narcissistic patients may erupt with barrages of contempt and hatred when they feel they have not been given the attention they are due.

Hysterical/Histrionic Personality Disorders

Patients with hysterical personality disorder (i.e., the higher-functioning patients within the histrionic personality disorder rubric) generally are ideally suited for psychoanalysis and psychoanalytic therapy. They have internalized conflicts about relationships that can be examined in a solid therapeutic alliance with the analyst. They are generally committed to change and to improving their chronic difficulties in forming intimate relationships. The analyst may need to focus initially on the global and impressionistic cognitive style that prevents these patients from reflecting in detail on what is happening inside. Their displays of emotionality can be highly appealing and lead the analyst to feel a sense of obligation to rescue the patient. Nevertheless, for the analyst to be useful, the patient first needs to provide more details of the situations that create distress.

Superficial and shallow feelings may defend against more disturbing and more deeply experienced affects. Patients may need assistance in identifying their true feelings and the thoughts and events linked to them. They often feel buffeted by powerful feeling states and by external events. The analyst can help them to identify patterns in their lives that lead to particular types of emotional responses. Horowitz (1977) pointed out that these patients start to develop new patterns of perceiving relationships when they attend in more detail to themselves and others in their personal context. The analyst helps them see how they play an active role in perpetuating certain patterns of relating to others. They develop a capacity to compare the actual facts in an interpersonal situation with the internal patterns they superimpose on external situations.

Hysterical patients generally work well within the transference and use it as a primary vehicle for change. They may see the solution to their problem as simple identification with the analyst, and the analyst needs to confront the wish to bypass painful self-examination in the service of identification with the analyst. They also may fall in love with the analyst and feel that a loving relationship is in itself curative. However, the transference love needs to be carefully deconstructed in terms of its multiple meanings. It functions not only as a resistance to a deepening of the analytic process but also as an indirect expression of aggression, because it may create a frustrating situation for both analyst and patient. Hysterical patients often find themselves in triangular relationships in which they constantly repeat an oedipal romance that places them in the role of the excluded party. This pattern of longing for an unavailable romantic partner deserves a good deal of scrutiny in the course of the analysis, as it often reveals conflicts about truly separating from parents and establishing a life with a partner outside the family unit. Women with hysterical personality disorder are often "Daddy's girls," whereas men with the diagnosis are often called "Mama's boys." This attachment to the opposite-sex parent may keep them in a state of extended adolescence that prevents them from coming fully into their own. The analyst must systemically analyze their loyalty conflicts of this nature.

Those patients with histrionic personality disorder proper (i.e., the more disturbed variant within this category) may need a form of dynamic therapy that includes considerable support. Although many of the dynamics relate to the hysterical configuration, these patients tend to use primitive defenses; in addition, they have overwhelming separation anxiety and a lax superego. Some may be able to tolerate the frustration of the analytic setting if they have high intelligence, some degree of impulse control, and an ability to mentalize. However, many of these patients have much in common with patients who have borderline personality disorder and lack the requisite ego strengths to tolerate the process. If they are motivated to persevere in psychodynamic psychotherapy, much of what applies to the technique required with hysterical patients also applies to histrionic patients. However, they will require more ego support and greater postponement of interpretation to be effectively treated.

Obsessive-Compulsive Personality Disorder

Patients with OCPD are generally well suited for psychoanalysis or psychodynamic psychotherapy, but they must first overcome their anxieties about being out of control. Spontaneity and free association present them with a situation in which they must be open and drop their guard. Most obsessive-compulsive individuals have a host of rigid defenses to avoid spontaneity so they can avoid loss of control. Hence they will use resistances that reflect defensive operations such as isolation of affect, intellectualization, and reaction formation. The clinician may need to confront the tendency to use factual information as a way of avoiding emotional expression in the analysis.

OCPD patients may also attempt to be perfect, saying exactly the right thing and thereby pleasing the analyst or therapist. This wish to please may be a reaction formation against hostility about the power differential inherent in the analytic setting, the time constraints, and the fee. The analyst carefully analyzes elements of hostility and resentment and tries to bring them into the patient's awareness when possible.

Moreover, patients with OCPD are driven by harsh superego pressures, and they frequently externalize that superego onto the analyst. They assume the therapist will react with disapproval and criticism to any expressions of sexuality or aggression, and the therapist must interpret those fears as they emerge as resistances to being open with the therapist about what is happening in their lives and in their internal affective life. As the therapist conveys a sense of acceptance and tolerance, the patient gradually enters into a process of self-acceptance so that the superego is modified in the course of the analytic treatment.

Another major thrust in the treatment of these patients is helping them see that their compromise formations against aggression generally do not work. As they describe interactions with coworkers or intimate family members, the therapist needs to observe problematic patterns of relationships in which the patient tries to avoid any implications of anger. The analyst or therapist points out how their reaction formation against anger is imperfect, in that others sense the hostility and resentment below the surface, no matter how defended they are in their efforts to conceal anger. Part of the work also focuses on helping the patient realize the futility of pursuing perfection. As self-acceptance increases, expectations can be lowered and the patient can understand that the perfectionistic ideals come from long-standing feelings of being unloved as a child and no longer address the original situation that fostered them. Persons with OCPD are by nature competitive. They want to be the best at whatever they do, and they are constantly finding fault with the shortcomings of others. This pattern may well emerge in the transference, no matter how conscientiously the patient tries to conceal it from the therapist. Clinicians treating such patients may find themselves evoked into competitive power struggles with the patient about the amount of the bill, who is correct about a literary reference, and whose interpretation of a psychological situa-

tion is more accurate. Therapists need to be prepared to interpret this process (rather than enact it repeatedly) through the systematic interpretation of the rivalry. Obsessive-compulsive patients will then begin to recognize traces of sibling and oedipal rivalries of the past in contemporary relationships and will gain understanding of how these rivalries interfere with harmonious intimate relationships.

Avoidant Personality Disorder

Patients with avoidant personality disorder may be reluctant to seek help because the therapeutic relationship presents the same threats as other intimate relationships. They are prone to feeling shame, embarrassment, and humiliation associated with exposure. Shame is etymologically derived from the verb "to hide" (Nathanson 1987), and the avoidant patient often withdraws from interpersonal relationships and situations of exposure out of a wish to "hide out" from the highly unpleasant affect of shame. Hence, when they come to treatment, avoidant patients may "hide out" from the treater and try to avoid discussions of their fears.

This form of resistance, of course, is the crux of the treatment. The therapist needs to patiently explore what it is that the patient fears from engaging the therapist in sharing his or her anxieties and fantasies. What does the patient imagine the therapist will think about the patient's fears? Initially, this exploration may meet with clichés such as "rejection." As the analyst encourages the patient to elaborate more specific fantasies, core conflicts in the patient's internal object relationships begin to emerge. One may learn of experiences of humiliation from childhood that the patient is convinced will be repeated again and again. Another common theme in avoidant patients is that they are secretly thrilled with the possibility of "showing off," but they worry that their exhibitionistic display is self-centered and destructive to others. They may fear that they will become intoxicated with themselves if they are "center stage." They may also fear deep-seated resentment and anger at parents who shamed them. The inhibition of anger is frequently connected with the shame experience (Gabbard 2000c).

When psychoanalysts or therapists treat avoidant personality disorder, they may need to combine other measures as adjuncts. For example, patients who are reluctant to expose themselves to a feared situation may need to be encouraged to do so (Gabbard and Bartlett 1998; Sutherland and Frances 1995). In addition, a selective serotonin reuptake inhibitor may also help the patient overcome anxieties by addressing the biological temperament known as *harm avoidance.*

Dependent Personality Disorder

Insecure attachment is a hallmark of dependent personality disorder, and studies of these patients (West et al. 1994) have found a pattern of enmeshed attachment. Many of these patients grew up with parents who communicated in one way or another that independence was fraught with danger. They may have been rewarded for maintaining loyalty to their parents, who seemed to reject them in the face of any move toward independence. The central motivation of such patients is to obtain and maintain nurturing, supportive relationships.

Patients with dependent personality disorder who enter into psychoanalytically oriented treatment may present a formidable resistance that takes the form of transference longing. They may secretly or overtly hope that they can attach themselves forever to the therapist and solve their problem of having to face life as an independent individual. Hence the treatment setting poses a paradox: the patient must first develop dependency on the therapist to overcome problems with dependency (Gabbard 2000c).

Another variation on this dependence is that some of these patients will do whatever they can to get the therapist to tell them what to do. Their goal is often to continue a dependent attachment rather than to analyze. Clinicians must systematically help them examine the underlying anxieties associated with becoming independent.

These patients may also develop idealization of the therapist (Perry 1995). The transference serves as a resistance in this way because the portrayal of the therapist as omniscient is a way of turning over all responsibility for important decisions to the person treating them. Dependency may also be a way of managing anger and aggression—the so-called hostile dependency. Dependent clinging often masks aggression and can be regarded as a compromise formation in the sense that it defends against hostility while also expressing it. As many analysts know from firsthand experience, the person who is the object of the dependent patient's clinging may experience the patient's demands as hostile and tormenting (Gabbard 2000c).

The dependent patient's "dance" may evoke a number of countertransference reactions. Some clinicians may bask in the patient's idealizing transference and fail to confront the patient's lack of real change (Perry 1995). Others may try to take over for the patient and become authoritarian and directive as a response to frustration with the patient's failure to become independent. Some therapists may struggle with countertransference contempt or disdain. Termination may be a particularly problematic time in which transference-countertransference impasses and enactments occur. Therapists must steer a course between coercing the patient to terminate and avoiding the topic for fear of upsetting the patient.

Masochistic or Self-Defeating Personality Disorder

Even though masochistic or self-defeating personality disorder is not one of the DSM-IV-TR diagnostic entities on Axis II, it has a time-honored tradition in psychoanalysis. Masochistic character features are found in patients of both genders with striking frequency. Psychoanalytic practice is replete with examples of individuals who engage in self-defeating relationships, undermine their possibilities of vocational or financial success, and repeatedly evoke negative responses from others. The origins of this self-defeating pattern usually involve multiple determinants. Some patients are defending against dangerous competitive impulses, whereas others are presenting themselves as suffering and helpless in order to ensure care from others (Cooper 1993). Others may be actively mastering passively experienced childhood trauma by bringing on the adverse event through their own omnipotent control. They also may be reestablishing traumatic relationships as a way of maintaining familiarity and predictability instead of facing new anxieties.

Psychoanalytic work with masochistic patients attempts to lay bare the underlying psychodynamic themes and help patients see how their role as victim is one they repeatedly set up in their interactions with others. Many masochistic individuals are "grievance collectors" who wallow in self-pity but ultimately blame someone else for their predicament. They also have a secret omnipotence that shares a lot in common with narcissistic personality—namely, they feel that because they have suffered more extensively and more severely than others, they are therefore deserving of special treatment. This sense of entitlement to special martyred status may be tenaciously held on to despite the analyst's repeated interpretation of the wish.

A masochist requires a sadist to be complete, and a frequent development in the analysis of masochistic patients is that the analyst begins to enact "sadistic" attacks on the patient. These may take the form of accurately worded but aggression-fueled interpretations that make the patient worse, an example of negative therapeutic reaction (Gabbard 2004). Because the patient is deteriorating, the analyst may escalate the interpretive efforts, thus making the patient feel shamed and punished. The roles may be reversed as well—the patient may identify with the internal sadistic object and torment the analyst.

Analysts working with masochistic patients must be attuned to this development and help the patient see the gratification he or she derives from thwarting the analyst's efforts. This pleasure can often be traced back to a revenge fantasy in which the patient wishes to retaliate against parents who had excessive expectations (Gabbard 2000a). In some cases, patients may have felt that their parents wished to have them succeed so they would reflect well on the parents. Many masochistic patients seek to deprive their parents of that pleasure by repeatedly failing. In this way these patients may sacrifice their own lives because of the pleasure they take in vengeance against their parents. Analysts must help them see that they have re-created that situation in the analytic relationship and that it is ultimately self-defeating rather than "other-defeating."

Envy may also be a key component to the impasses that masochistic patients produce. To acknowledge receiving help from the analyst may make these patients riddled with envy that is tormenting to them. If they can simply collect one more grievance against the analyst as someone who is failing them, they can then avoid the envy of somebody who has the capacity to give and to be positive about life. Some masochistic patients do not want to reveal how much they have changed until after termination to ensure that the analyst derives no gratification from therapeutic success (Gabbard 2000a). Hence analysts must be wary of too much enthusiasm about changing the patient because that countertransference wish for success will activate the patient's self-defeating spiral. Often the optimal analytic posture is to help the patient understand what is happening while making it clear that how the patient chooses to apply the insight is ultimately up to the patient.

CONCLUSION

Psychoanalysis is a long and expensive treatment, but because of its intensity and duration, it may be capable of far-reaching changes that briefer therapies cannot approach. Defense mechanisms and representations of self and other may tenaciously resist change, and for some patients, only a systematic working through of these resistances will allow for structural, long-lasting change. The field of psychoanalysis must develop a greater research base to gain full credibility among the host of other treatments for personality disorders. A research design that will yield significant results has been outlined (Gabbard et al. 2002), but sources of funding in the current era remain scarce.

REFERENCES

Abend SM, Porder MS, Willick MS: Borderline Patients: Psychoanalytic Perspectives. New York, International Universities Press, 1983

Abraham K: Contributions to the theory of anal character (1923), in Selected Papers of Karl Abraham. London, Hogarth Press, 1948, pp 370–392

Alden L: Short-term structured treatment for avoidant personality disorder. J Consult Clin Psychol 56:756–764, 1989

American Psychiatric Association: Diagnostic and Statistical Manual of Mental Disorders, 4th Edition, Text Revision. Washington, DC, American Psychiatric Association, 2000

Balint M: The Basic Fault: Therapeutic Aspects of Regression. New York, Brunner/Mazel, 1979

Bateman A, Fonagy P: Effectiveness of partial hospitalization in the treatment of borderline personality disorder: a randomized controlled trial. Am J Psychiatry 156:1563–1569, 1999

Bateman A, Fonagy P: Treatment of borderline personality disorder with psychoanalytically oriented partial hospitalization: an 18-month follow-up. Am J Psychiatry 158:36–42, 2001

Bateman A, Fonagy P: Psychotherapy for Borderline Personality Disorder: Mentalization-Based Treatment. New York, Oxford University Press, 2004

Bateman A, Fonagy P: Eight-year follow-up of patients treated for borderline personality disorder: mentalization-based treatment versus treatment as usual. Am J Psychiatry 165:631–638, 2008

Blatt SJ: The differential effect of psychotherapy and psychoanalysis with anaclitic and introjective patients: the Menninger Psychotherapy Research Project revisited. J Am Psychoanal Assoc 40:691–724, 1992

Blatt SJ, Ford TQ: Therapeutic Change: An Object Relations Perspective. New York, Plenum, 1994

Blatt SJ, Besser A, Ford TQ: Two primary configurations of psychopathology and change in thought disorder in long-term intensive inpatient treatment of seriously disturbed young adults. Am J Psychiatry 164:1561–1567, 2007

Boyer LB: Working with a borderline patient. Psychoanal Q 46:386–424, 1977

Brenner C: Psychoanalytic Technique and Psychic Conflict. New York, International Universities Press, 1976

Brown EJ, Heimberg RG, Juster HR: Social phobias subtype and avoidant personality disorder: effect on severity of social phobia, impairment, and outcome of cognitive behavioral treatment. Behav Ther 26:467–486, 1995

Clarkin JF, Levy KN, Lenzenweger MF, et al: Evaluating three treatments for borderline personality disorder: a multi-wave study. Am J Psychiatry 164:922–928, 2007

Cloninger CR, Svrakic DM, Pryzbeck TR: A psychobiological model of temperament and character. Arch Gen Psychiatry 50:975–990, 1993

Cooper AM: Therapeutic approaches to masochism. J Psychother Pract Res 2:51–63, 1993

Fairbairn WRD: An Object-Relations Theory of the Personality. New York, Basic Books, 1954

Fonagy P: The process of change, and the change of processes: what can change in a "good" analysis? Keynote address to the spring meeting of Division 39 of the American Psychological Association, New York, April 16, 1999

Fonagy P: Attachment Theory and Psychoanalysis. New York, Other Press, 2001

Fonagy P, Target M: Playing with reality, I: theory of mind and the normal development of psychic reality. Int J Psychoanal 77:217–233, 1996

Freud S: Character and anal eroticism (1908), in The Standard Edition of the Complete Psychological Works of Sigmund Freud, Vol 9. Translated by Strachey J. London, Hogarth Press, 1959, pp 167–175

Freud S: Remembering, repeating and working-through (further recommendations on the technique of psycho-analysis II) (1914), in The Standard Edition of the Complete Psychological Works of Sigmund Freud, Vol 14. Translated by Strachey J. London, Hogarth Press, 1958, pp 145–156

Friedman L: A reading of Freud's papers on technique. Psychoanal Q 60:564–595, 1991

Gabbard GO: Technical approaches to transference hate in borderline patients. Int J Psychoanal 72:625–638, 1991

Gabbard GO: Countertransference: the emerging common ground. Int J Psychoanal 76:475–485, 1995

Gabbard GO: Love and Hate in the Analytic Setting. Northvale, NJ, Jason Aronson, 1996

Gabbard GO: Finding the "person" in personality disorders. Am J Psychiatry 154:891–893, 1997a

Gabbard GO: A reconsideration of objectivity in the analyst. Int J Psychoanal 78:15–26, 1997b

Gabbard GO: On gratitude and gratification. J Am Psychoanal Assoc 48:697–716, 2000a

Gabbard GO: Psychoanalysis, in Comprehensive Textbook of Psychiatry, 6th Edition, Vol 1. Edited by Kaplan HI, Sadock BJ. Baltimore, MD, Williams & Wilkins, 2000b, pp 431–478

Gabbard GO: Psychodynamic Psychiatry in Clinical Practice, 3rd Edition. Washington, DC, American Psychiatric Publishing, 2000c

Gabbard GO: Psychoanalysis and psychoanalytic psychotherapy, in Handbook of Personality Disorders. Edited by Livesley J. New York, Guilford, 2001, pp 359–376

Gabbard GO: Long-Term Psychodynamic Psychotherapy: A Basic Text. Washington, DC, American Psychiatric Publishing, 2004

Gabbard GO: Gabbard's Treatments of Psychiatric Disorders, 4th Edition. Washington, DC, American Psychiatric Publishing, 2007

Gabbard GO, Bartlett AB: Selective serotonin reuptake inhibitors in the context of an ongoing analysis. Psychoanalytic Inquiry 18:657–672, 1998

Gabbard GO, Westen D: Rethinking therapeutic action. Int J Psychoanal 84:823–841, 2003

Gabbard GO, Horwitz L, Allen JG, et al: Transference interpretation in the psychotherapy of borderline patients: a high-risk, high-gain phenomenon. Harv Rev Psychiatry 2:59–69, 1994

Gabbard GO, Gunderson JG, Fonagy P: The place of psychoanalytic treatments within psychiatry. Arch Gen Psychiatry 59:505–510, 2002

Gunderson JG: Borderline Personality Disorder: A Clinical Guide. Washington, DC, American Psychiatric Press, 2001

Gunderson JG, Links PS: Borderline Personality Disorder: A Clinical Guide, 2nd Edition. Washington, DC, American Psychiatric Publishing, 2008

Horowitz MJ: Structure and the processes of change, in Hysterical Personality. Edited by Horowitz MJ. New York, Jason Aronson, 1977, pp 329–399

Horowitz MJ: Introduction to Psychodynamics: A New Synthesis. New York, Basic Books, 1988

Horowitz MJ: Person Schemas and Maladaptive Interpersonal Patterns. Chicago, IL, University of Chicago Press, 1991

Horowitz MJ: Cognitive Psychodynamics: From Conflict to Character. New York, Wiley, 1998

Horwitz L, Gabbard GO, Allen JG, et al: Borderline Personality Disorder: Tailoring the Psychotherapy to the Patient. Washington, DC, American Psychiatric Press, 1996

Kantrowitz JL: Suitability for psychoanalysis. Yearbook of Psychoanalysis and Psychotherapy 2:403–415, 1987

Kernberg OF: Contrasting viewpoints regarding the nature and psychoanalytic treatment of narcissistic personalities: a preliminary communication. J Am Psychoanal Assoc 22:255–267, 1974a

Kernberg OF: Further contributions to the treatment of narcissistic personalities. Int J Psychoanal 55:215–240, 1974b

Kernberg OF: Borderline Conditions and Pathological Narcissism. New York, Jason Aronson, 1975

Kernberg OF: Severe Personality Disorders: Psychotherapeutic Strategies. New Haven, CT, Yale University Press, 1984

Killingmo B: Conflict and deficit: implications for technique. Int J Psychoanalysis 70:65–79, 1989

Kohut H: The Analysis of the Self. New York, International Universities Press, 1971

Kohut H: The Restoration of the Self. New York, International Universities Press, 1977

Kohut H: How Does Analysis Cure? Edited by Goldberg A. Chicago, IL, University of Chicago Press, 1984

Levy KN, Meehan KB, Clarkin JF, et al: Change in attachment patterns and reflective function in a randomized control trial of transference-focused psychotherapy for borderline personality disorder. J Consult Clin Psychol 74:1027–1074, 2006

Livesley WJ, Jang KL, Jackson DN, et al: Genetic and environmental contributions of dimensions of personality disorder. Am J Psychiatry 150:1826–1831, 1993

Lyons-Ruth K and Members of the Change Process Study Group: Implicit relational knowing: its role in development and psychoanalytic treatment. Infant Ment Health J 19:282–289, 1998

Miller JP: How Kohut actually worked. Progress in Self Psychology 1:13–30, 1985

Mitchell SA: Influence and Autonomy in Psychoanalysis. Hillsdale, NJ, Analytic Press, 1997

Nathanson DL: A timetable for shame, in The Many Faces of Shame. Edited by Nathanson DL. New York, Guilford, 1987, pp 1–63

Ogden TH: On projective identification. Int J Psychoanal 60:357–373, 1979

Oldham J, Skodol A: Do patients with paranoid personality disorder seek psychoanalysis? in New Psychoanalytic Perspectives. Edited by Oldham JM, Bohn S. Madison, CT, International Universities Press, 1994, pp 151–166

Ornstein PH: On narcissism: beyond the introduction, highlights of Heinz Kohut's contributions to the psychoanalytic treatment of narcissistic personality disorders. Annual of Psychoanalysis 2:127–149, 1974

Ornstein PH: Psychoanalysis of patients with primary self-disorder: a self psychological perspective, in Disorders of Narcissism: Diagnostic, Clinical, and Empirical Implications. Edited by Ronningstam EF. Washington, DC, American Psychiatric Press, 1998, pp 147–169

Perry JC: Dependent personality disorder, in Treatments of Psychiatric Disorders, Vol 2, 2nd Edition. Edited by Gabbard GO. Washington, DC, American Psychiatric Press, 1995, pp 2355–2366

Reich W: The characterological mastery of the oedipus complex. Int J Psychoanal 12:452–463, 1931

Sandler J: Character traits and object relationships. Psychoanal Q 50:694–708, 1981

Shapiro D: Neurotic Styles. New York, Basic Books, 1965

Stravynski A, Marks I, Yule W: Social skills, problems, and neurotic outpatients. Arch Gen Psychiatry 39:1378–1385, 1982

Sutherland SM, Frances A: Avoidant personality disorder, in Treatments of Psychiatric Disorders, Vol 2, 2nd Edition. Edited by Gabbard GO. Washington, DC, American Psychiatric Press, 1995, pp 2345–2353

Svartberg M, Stiles TC, Seltzer MH: Randomized, controlled trial of the effectiveness of short-term dynamic psychotherapy and cognitive therapy for Cluster C personality disorders. Am J Psychiatry 161:810–817, 2004

Svrakic DM, Whitehead C, Pryzbeck TR, et al: Differential diagnosis of personality disorders by the seven-factor model of temperament and character. Arch Gen Psychiatry 50:991–999, 1993

Vaillant GE, Vaillant LM : The role of ego mechanisms of defense in the diagnosis of personality disorders, in Making Diagnosis Meaningful: Enhancing Evaluation and Treatment of Psychological Disorders. Edited by Barron J. Washington, DC, American Psychological Association, 1999, pp 139–158

West M, Rose S, Sheldon-Keller A: Assessment of patterns of insecure attachment in adults and application to dependent and schizoid personality disorders. J Personal Disord 8:249–256, 1994

Westen D, Gabbard G: Developments in cognitive neuroscience, II: implications for theories of transference. J Am Psychoanal Assoc 50:99–134, 2002

Winnicott DW: The aims of psychoanalytic treatment, in The Maturational Processes and the Facilitating Environment. London, Hogarth Press, 1962, pp 166–170

Winnicott DW: Communicating and not communicating leading to a study of certain opposites, in The Maturational Processes and the Facilitating Environment: Studies in the Theory of Emotional Development. New York, International Universities Press, 1963/1965, pp 179–192

11

Mentalization-Based Treatment of Borderline Personality Disorder

Peter Fonagy, Ph.D., F.B.A.
Anthony W. Bateman, M.A., F.R.C.Psych.

Borderline personality disorder (BPD) is a complex psychiatric problem characterized by numerous deficits in cognitive, emotional, and behavioral functioning. These difficulties commonly include emotional instability, feelings of emptiness, impulsivity, suicidal ideation and gestures, enmeshed dysfunctional and volatile relationships, irrational anxieties about being abandoned by those one cares about, and paranoid thoughts (Lieb et al. 2004). These difficulties can be conceptualized as a dysfunction of self-regulation particularly in the context of social relationships. Both the difficulty with affect regulation and the catastrophic reaction to the loss of intensely emotionally invested social ties place BPD in the domain of attachment. A number of theorists have drawn on Bowlby's ideas in explanation of borderline pathology. Most specifically, Gunderson (1996) suggested that intolerance of aloneness was at the core of borderline pathology, and the inability of those with BPD to invoke a "soothing introject" was a consequence of early attachment failures. He carefully described typical patterns of borderline dysfunction in terms of exaggerated reactions of the insecurely attached infant; for example, clinging, fearfulness about dependency needs, terror of abandonment, and constant monitoring of the proximity of the caregiver. Lyons-Ruth and Jacobovitz (1999) focused on the disorganization of the attachment system in infancy as predisposing to later borderline pathology. Notably, they identified an insecure, as opposed to a secure, disorganized pattern as predisposing to conduct problems. Crittenden (1997) was particularly concerned with incorporating borderline individuals' deep ambivalence and fear of close relationships in her representation of adult attachment disorganization. Fonagy and colleagues (Fonagy and Bateman 2006a, 2006b; Fonagy et al. 2003) also used the framework of attachment theory but emphasized the crucial role played by attachment in the development of the capacity for mentalization and the way in which insecure disorganized attachment may generate vulnerability in the face of further turmoil and challenges.

We have discussed our developmental model of BPD in detail elsewhere (Bateman and Fonagy 2004; Fonagy et al. 2002, 2003). Essentially our account focuses around the development of the social affiliative system that we consider to drive many higher-order social-cognitive functions that in turn underpin interpersonal interaction, specifically in an attachment context. Four of these are of primary importance in understanding BPD: 1) affect representation and, related to this, affect regulation; 2) attentional control, also with strong links to the regulation of affect; 3) the dual arousal system involved in maintaining an appropriate balance between mental functions undertaken by the anterior and posterior portions of the brain; and 4) mentalization, a system for interpersonal understanding within the attachment context. Since these capacities evolve in the context of the primary caregiving relationships experienced by the child, in addition to the child's constitutional vulnerabilities, they are vulnerable to extremes of environmental deficiency as exemplified by severe neglect, psychological or physical abuse, childhood molestation, or other forms of maltreatment. If our understanding of others critically depends on whether as infants our own mental states were adequately understood by attentive adults, then there is ample opportunity for this developmental process to be disrupted. Our premise is that however this comes about, unstable or psychogenically/ defensively reduced mentalizing capacity is a core feature of BPD. Therefore, in order to be successful, any treatment must have mentalization as one of its foci or, at the very least, stimulate development of mentalizing as an epiphenomenon arising from other therapeutic initiatives.

In this chapter we briefly outline the theory of attachment and some empirical work linking BPD with dysfunctions of the attachment system. We consider BPD from an attachment theory perspective, and outline the modifications of classical attachment theory that have helped us to understand the disordered attachment of individuals with BPD. In particular, we emphasize the link between the development of the capacity of mentalization and the quality of attachment relationships, and link the failure of mentalization with symptoms of BPD. Finally, the treatment implications of our attachment theory–based model of BPD are discussed.

BRIEF OUTLINE OF ATTACHMENT THEORY

Bowlby's attachment theory has a biological focus (Bowlby 1969). Attachment readily reduces to a "molecular" level of infant behaviors, such as smiling and vocalizing, that alert the caregiver to the child's interest in socializing and bring the caregiver close to the child. Smiling and vocalizing are attachment behaviors, as is crying, which is experienced by most caregivers as aversive, and they engage the caregiver in caretaking behaviors. Bowlby emphasized the survival value of attachment in enhancing safety through proximity to the caregiver in addition to feeding, learning about the environment, and social interaction, as well as protection from predators. Bowlby (1969) considered the latter to be the biological function of attachment behavior. Attachment behaviors were seen as part of a "behavioral system" (a term Bowlby borrowed from ethology).

In the second volume of his *Attachment and Loss* trilogy, Bowlby established the set goal of the attachment system as maintaining the caregiver's accessibility and responsiveness, which he covered with a single term: *availability* (Bowlby 1973). *Availability* means confident expectation—gained from "tolerably accurately" (p. 202) represented experience over a significant time period—that the attachment figure will be available. The attachment behavioral system thus came to be underpinned by a set of cognitive mechanisms, discussed by Bowlby as representational models or by Craik (1943) as internal working models (Bretherton and Munholland 1999; Crittenden 1994; Main 1991; Sroufe 1996). Four representational systems are implied by the internal working models: 1) expectations of interactive attributes of early caregivers created in the first year of life and subsequently elaborated; 2) event representations by which general and specific memories of attachment-related experiences are encoded and retrieved; 3) autobiographical memories by which specific events are conceptually connected because of their relation to a continuing personal narrative and developing self-understanding; and 4) understanding of the psychological characteristics of other people and differentiating them from the characteristics of the self. It is in this last layer of the internal working models that we consider the dysfunctions of individuals with BPD to be most profound.

The second great pioneer of attachment theory, Mary Ainsworth (1969, 1985; Ainsworth et al. 1978), developed the well-known laboratory-based procedure of the Strange Situation for observing infants' internal working models in action. When infants are briefly separated from their caregivers in an unfamiliar situation, they show one of four patterns of behavior. Infants who display *secure* attachment explore readily in the presence of the caregiver, are anxious in the presence of the stranger and avoid her, are distressed by the caregiver's brief absence, rapidly seek contact with the caregiver afterward, and are reassured by this contact and return to their exploration. Some infants, designated as *anxious/avoidant*, appear to be made less anxious by separation, may not seek contact with the caregiver following separation, and may not prefer her over the stranger. *Anxious/resistant* infants show limited exploration and play, tend to be highly distressed by separation from the caregiver, and have great difficulty in settling afterward, showing struggling, stiffness, contin-

ued crying, or fuss in a passive way. The caregiver's presence or attempts at comforting fail to reassure, and the infant's anxiety and anger appear to prevent him or her from deriving comfort from proximity.

A fourth group of infants who show seemingly undirected behavior are referred to as *disorganized/disoriented* (Main and Solomon 1990). They show freezing, hand clapping, head banging, and a wish to escape the situation even in the presence of the caregiver (Lyons-Ruth and Jacobovitz 1999; van IJzendoorn et al. 1999). It is generally held that for such infants the caregiver has served as a source of both fear and reassurance, and thus arousal of the attachment behavioral system produces strong conflicting motivations.

Prospective longitudinal research has demonstrated that children with a history of secure attachment are independently rated as more resilient, self-reliant, socially oriented (Sroufe 1983; Waters et al. 1979), and empathic to distress (Kestenbaum et al. 1989), with deeper relationships and higher self-esteem (Sroufe 1983; Sroufe et al. 1990). Bowlby (1969) proposed that internal working models of the self and others provide prototypes for all later relationships. Such models are relatively stable across the life span (Collins and Read 1994).

Because internal working models function outside of awareness, they are change resistant (Crittenden 1990). The stability of attachment is demonstrated by longitudinal studies of infants assessed with the Strange Situation and followed up in adolescence or young adulthood with the Adult Attachment Interview (AAI; C. George, N. Kaplan, M. Main, "The Adult Attachment Interview," unpublished manuscript, Department of Psychology, University of California at Berkeley, 1985). This structured clinical instrument elicits narrative histories of childhood attachment relationships—the characteristics of early relationships, experiences of separation, illness, punishment, loss, maltreatment, or abuse. The AAI scoring system (M. Main, R. Goldwyn, "Adult Attachment

Rating and Classification System, Manual in Draft, Version 6.0," unpublished manuscript, University of California at Berkeley, 1994) classifies individuals into secure/autonomous, insecure/dismissing, insecure/preoccupied, or unresolved with respect to loss or trauma, which are categories based on the structural qualities of narratives of early experiences. Whereas *autonomous* individuals value attachment relationships, coherently integrate memories into a meaningful narrative, and regard these as formative, *insecure* individuals are poor at integrating memories of experience with the meaning of that experience. Those individuals who are *dismissing* of attachment show avoidance by denying memories and by idealizing or devaluing (or both idealizing and devaluing) early relationships. *Preoccupied* individuals tend to be confused, angry, or passive in relation to attachment figures, often still complaining of childhood slights, echoing the protests of the resistant infant. *Unresolved* individuals give indications of significant disorganization in their attachment relationship representation; this disorganization manifests in semantic or syntactic confusions in their narratives concerning childhood trauma or a recent loss.

Many studies have demonstrated that the AAI, administered to the mother or father, will predict not only the child's security of attachment to that parent but even more remarkably the precise attachment category that the child manifests in the Strange Situation (van IJzendoorn 1995). Thus, a dismissing AAI interview predicts avoidant Strange Situation behavior, whereas a preoccupied interview predicts anxious/resistant infant attachment. Lack of resolution of mourning (unresolved interviews) predicts disorganization in infant attachment (discussed later). Temperament (child-to-parent effects) seems an inadequate account of the phenomena, because the AAI of each parent, collected and coded before the birth of the child, predicts the attachment classification of the infant at 12 and 18 months (Fonagy et al. 1991b; Steele et al. 1996).

Evidence by Slade et al. (1999) provided an important clue about the puzzle of intergenerational transmission of attachment security. They demonstrated that autonomous (secure) mothers on the AAI represented their relationship with their toddlers in a more coherent way than dismissing and preoccupied mothers. Mothers interviewed with the AAI who demonstrated a strong capacity to reflect on their own and their own caregiver's mental states in the context of recollecting their own attachment experiences were far more likely to have children securely attached to them—a finding that we have linked to the parent's capacity to foster the child's self-development (Fonagy et al. 1993). We have also found that mothers in a relatively high-stress (deprived) group characterized by single-parent families, parental criminality, unemployment, overcrowding, and psychiatric illness would be far more likely to have securely attached infants if their capacity to be reflective (psychologically minded) in relation to their attachment histories was high (Fonagy et al. 1994).

The disorganized/disoriented infant category appears to have the strongest predictive significance for later psychological disturbance (Carlson 1998; Lyons-Ruth 1996; Lyons-Ruth et al. 1993; Ogawa et al. 1997). A number of studies (Lyons-Ruth 1995; Lyons-Ruth et al. 1989; Shaw and Vondra 1995; Shaw et al. 1997) have suggested that disorganized attachment is a vulnerability factor for later psychological disturbance in combination with other risk factors. A study with a large sample ($N=223$) confirmed that those whose attachment classification was disorganized in infancy or atypical at age 24 months were most likely to be rated high on externalizing behavior at 3.5 years (Vondra et al. 2001). A meta-analysis of studies of disorganized attachment based on 2,000 mother–infant pairs (van IJzendoorn et al. 1999) estimated its prevalence at 14% in middle-income samples and 24% in low-income groups. Similarly, adolescent mothers tended to have an overrepresentation of disorganized infants (23%) as well as fewer secure infants (40% versus 62%) and more avoidant infants (33% versus 15%). The stability of the classification of disorganized attachment is fair ($r = 0.36$) (van IJzendoorn et al. 1999), with some indication that lack of stability may be accounted for by increases in the number of disorganized infants between 12 and 18 months (Barnett et al. 1999; Vondra et al. 1999).

Quite a lot is known about the causes of disorganized attachment. The prevalence of attachment disorganization is strongly associated with family risk factors such as maltreatment (Carlson et al. 1989) and major depressive disorder (Lyons-Ruth et al. 1990; Teti et al. 1995). In addition, there is an extensively proven association between disorganization of attachment in the baby and unresolved mourning or abuse in the mother's own personal experience, revealed in the AAI (van IJzendoorn 1995). Three studies have helped to clarify this superficially mysterious association between slips in the mother's narrative about past trauma and bizarre behavior by the infant in the Strange Situation with her. Jacobovitz et al. (1997) reported a strong association between such slips in the AAI before the child was born and observations of frightened or frightening behavior toward the baby at 8 months. These behaviors included extreme intrusiveness, baring teeth, and entering apparently trancelike states. If the mother's unresolved trauma happened before she was 17 years old, her frightened or frightening behavior was more evident. Interestingly, these unresolved mothers did not differ from the rest of the sample in terms of other measures of parenting such as sensitivity and warmth. Maternal frightened or frightening behavior predicted infant attachment disorganization, but the strongest predictor was maternal dissociated behavior (Schuengel et al. 1999). In an independent investigation, Lyons-Ruth et al. (1999b) also found that frightened and frightening behavior predicted infant disorganization, particularly when the mother strongly misinterpreted the baby's attach-ment cues and when the mother gave conflicting messages that both elicited and rejected attachment.

Both cross-sectional and longitudinal investigations indicate that disorganized infant attachment shifts into controlling attachment behavior in middle childhood (van IJzendoorn et al. 1999). Observational studies suggest that disorganized children are less competent in playing with other children, in conflict resolution (Wartner et al. 1994), and in consistency of interaction with different peers (Jacobovitz and Hazen 1999).

In terms of the long-term consequences of attachment classification from childhood, studies only partially confirm initial hopes of theorists and researchers. There can be little doubt that something is carried forward. Prediction from insecure-disorganized attachment is particularly powerful for various adverse outcomes, including psychiatric disorder. The pathways of association are by no means straightforward (Sroufe et al. 1999). For individuals with extremely harsh or chaotic early caregiving, the process of attentional, emotional, and symbolic regulation might be derailed, and the integration of self-states across behavioral states may never be fully achieved. Because early attachment disturbance makes itself felt as a dysfunction of self-organization (stress regulation, attention regulation, and mentalization)—and because these capacities are needed to deal with social stress— relationship disturbance in the early years, together with additional social pressures, does predict psychological disturbance.

PROBLEMS WITH A SIMPLE ATTACHMENT MODEL

There is no doubt that borderline individuals are insecure in their attachment, but descriptions of insecure attachment from infancy or adulthood provide an inadequate clinical account for several reasons: 1) Anxious attachment is very common; in working-class nonclinical population samples, the majority of children are classified as anxiously attached, with a high proportion classified as disorganized (Broussard 1995). 2) Anxious patterns of attachment in infancy correspond to relatively stable adult strategies (Main et al. 1985), yet the hallmark of the disordered attachments of borderline individuals is the absence of stability (Higgitt and Fonagy 1992). 3) In both delinquent and borderline individuals there are variations across situations or types of relationships; the delinquent adolescent is, for example, aware of the mental states of others in his gang, and the borderline individual is at times hypersensitive to the emotional states of mental health professionals and family members. 4) The clinical presentation of borderline patients frequently includes a violent attack on the patient's own body or that of another human being. It is likely that the propensity for such violence must include an additional component that predisposes such individuals to act upon bodies rather than upon minds.

To the extent that we assume that abnormal patterns of attachment arise as a consequence of abnormalities in child rearing, it is somewhat of an embarrassment that prospective studies of maltreatment often fail to yield powerful personality effects beyond the contextual (e.g., life events; Widom 1999). A more important problem is that all adult attachment measures are hopelessly confounded with symptoms and traits. Thus, for example, in Meyer et al.'s (2001) study of Pilkonis's (1988) borderline attachment prototype, the correlation between the attachment prototype and symptomatology was so high that only one of these variables could be used in the regression because of colinearity problems. Similarly, the AAI coding for fearful preoccupied categories calls for statements about fear of loss that are also symptomatic of a diagnosis of BPD.

The model of attachment in use by attachment theorists places greatest importance on early experience, yet the social experiences of individuals with BPD are likely to be distorted by later rather than earlier social encounters. It is unclear in most theories proposing attachment as an explanatory variable how early attachment and later maltreatment might interact. As we have seen, controlling for attachment styles does not account for temperamental and characterological differences between BPD and non-BPD patients. Impulsivity and negative affectivity/emotional dysregulation characterize BPD best (Gurvits et al. 2000; Paris 2000; Silk 2000; Trull 2001a). Many attachment measures such as the AAI rely on autobiographical memory. In fact, in the AAI specific memories are coded as indicators of insecurity. Studies of autobiographical memory of borderline patients suggest that they have a tendency to produce overly general memories (Startup et al. 2001), which again underscores the difficulty of establishing independent measures of BPD status and attachment.

AN ATTACHMENT THEORY OF BORDERLINE PERSONALITY DISORDER

Disorganization of Attachment

The caregiver's sensitivity to the child's mental state is strongly associated with secure attachment and the development in the child of the capacity to mentalize—that is, to represent the behavior of self and others in terms of underlying mental states (Fonagy and Target 1997; Fonagy et al. 1991a; Meins and Fernyhough 1999; Meins and Russell 1997; Meins et al. 1998, 2001; Raikes and Thompson 2006; Symons, 2004). Mentalizing is a relatively new term for a concept as ancient as philosophy of mind. *Mentalizing* is akin to what Olson (1994) construes as subjectivity—that is, "the *recognition* that what is in the mind is in the mind...the recognition of one's own and others' mental states as mental states" (p. 234). The term *mentalizing* was introduced into the psychoanalytic literature some decades ago (Brown 1977; Compton 1983; De M'Uzan 1973; Lecours and Bouchard 1997) and came to be applied to the understanding of autism as a neurobiologically based failure of psychosocial development (Frith et al. 1991; Morton 1989). Fonagy and colleagues opened the door to wider clinical applications of this developmental research in showing how mentalizing plays a significant role in diverse forms of developmental psychopathology (Fonagy 1991, 1995; Fonagy and Target 1997; Fonagy et al. 2002; Target and Fonagy 1996), and we continue expanding these clinical applications here.

True to its origins in psychoanalysis, mentalizing intertwines with the related concepts of psychological mindedness (Appelbaum 1973; Namnum 1968), observing ego, and potential space (Bram and Gabbard 2001; Ogden 1985; Winnicott 1971). Mentalizing also overlaps with the venerable concepts of empathy and insight. We do not propose replacing these traditional concepts with mentalizing but rather argue that theory and research on mentalizing anchor this network of clinical concepts in evolutionary biology, neurobiology, contemporary developmental research, and attachment theory.

High levels of parental reflective function (capacity for mentalization) are associated with good outcomes in terms of secure attachment in the child. The converse, then, is that low levels of reflective function generate insecure and perhaps disorganized attachment. The latter category of attachment in infancy is most likely to be associated with self-harming or aggressive and potentially violent behavior later in development. A study by Grienenberger et al. (2001) showed that mothers with low levels of mentalization (or reflective function) on the Parent Development Interview (an interview assessing the parent's mental representation of the child) are more likely to show intrusiveness, fearfulness, withdrawing, and other behaviors shown to generate disorganized attachment in the infant (Lyons-Ruth et al. 1999b). The suggestion here is that poor mentalization of the infant in the mother permits

behaviors that undermine the healthy development of the infant's representational capacities (particularly the organization of affect and the organization of focused attention or effortful control) (Fonagy and Target 2002), which in turn can undermine attachment processes, leading to the development of a disorganized self, parts of which are experienced as "alien" or not really belonging to the self. In the absence of the capacity for mentalization, the coherence of this self can only be ensured by primitive psychological strategies such as projective identification. It is the impact of attachment disorganization on the self that might be most important for us in understanding BPD.

Establishment of the Alien Self

An important complication arises if the processes that normally generate an agentive self fail. In early childhood the failure to find another being behaving contingently with one's internal states can create a desperation for meaning as the self seeks to find itself in the other. This desperation leads the individual to take in noncontingent reflections from the object. Unfortunately, as these reflections do not map onto anything within the child's own experience, they cannot function as totally effective experiences of the self. As Winnicott (1967) noted, inaccurate mirroring leads the child to internalize representations of the parent's state rather than a usable version of his or her own experience. This creates what we have termed an *alien experience* within the self: ideas or feelings are experienced as part of the self that do not seem to belong to the self (Fonagy et al. 1995, 2000). These representations of the other internalized as part of the self probably originate in early infancy, when the mother's reflective function at least partially but regularly failed the infant.

This alien other, the residue of maternal nonresponsiveness, probably exists in seed form in all our self-representations, because we have all experienced neglect to a greater or lesser extent (Tronick and Gianino 1986). Normally, however, parts of the self-representation that are not rooted in the internalized mirroring of self-states are nevertheless integrated into a singular, coherent self-structure by the capacity for mentalization. The representational agentive self creates an illusion of coherence within our representations of ourselves by attributing agency, accurately or inaccurately assuming that mental states invariably exist to explain experience. Dramatic examples of this capacity for mentalization were noted long ago in studies of individuals with neural lesions, such as individuals with surgical bisections of the corpus callosum, so-called split-brain patients (Gazzaniga 1985). When presented with emotionally arousing pictures in the hemifield without access to language, they would find improbable mentalized accounts for their heightened emotional state.

Controlling Internal Working Model

The normal process of attributing agency through putative mental states preconsciously works in the background of our minds to lend coherence and psychological meaning to our lives, our actions, and our sense of self. Individuals whose capacity for mentalization is not well developed may need to use controlling and manipulative strategies to restore coherence to their sense of self. The alien aspects of the self may be externalized into an attachment figure. Using processes often described in the clinical literature as "projective identification," the attachment figure is manipulated into feeling the internalized emotions as part of the self but not entirely "of the self." These are not self-protective maneuvers in the sense of needing to shed feelings that the individual cannot acknowledge; rather, they protect the self from the experience of incongruence or incoherence that has the potential to generate far deeper anxieties (see Kernberg 1982, 1983; Kohut 1977). Apparently coercive, manipu-

lative behavior reflects the individual's inability to contain the incoherence of his or her self-structure. Unfortunately, in performing this function—in becoming, for example, angry and punitive in response to unconscious provocation—the attachment figure is in the worst possible state to help restore the afflicted individual's mentalizing function because he or she has lost touch with the individual's mental world. Thus the controlling internal working model further undermines the child's capacity to establish an agentive self-structure.

To state it simply, disorganized attachment is rooted in a disorganized self. Attachment research has demonstrated the sequelae of disorganized attachment in infancy to be extreme controlling and dominating behavior in middle childhood (see Solomon and George 1999; Green and Goldwyn 2002). The individual, when alone, feels unsafe and vulnerable because of the proximity of a torturing and destructive representation from which he or she cannot escape because it is experienced from within rather than from without the self. Unless the individual's relationship permits externalization, he or she feels almost literally at risk of disappearance, psychological merging, and the dissolution of all relationship boundaries. The need to externalize the alien part of the self may serve inadvertently to re-create relationships in which the persecutor is "generated" outside, in the shape of relationships of emotional turmoil and significant negativity.

Failure of Mentalization

Disturbed interpersonal relatedness is a key aspect of BPD related to temperamental attributes of negative affectivity and impulsivity (Gurvits et al. 2000; Paris 2000; Silk 2000; Trull et al. 2000; Domes et al. 2006) and psychosocial experiences of maltreatment (e.g., Trull 2001b; Zanarini et al. 1997; Zlotnick et al. 2001). Studies that have attempted to find the underlying dimensions of borderline phenomenology tended to identify either two

(Rosenberg and Miller 1989) or three factors (Clarkin et al. 1993; Sanislow et al. 2000). These factors normally include a dimension of disturbed relatedness, emotional dysregulation and impulsivity, or behavioral dyscontrol. At least the first of these may be related to a deficit in the capacity for accurate perception of the respective mental states of self and other and self–other differentiation (Fonagy et al. 2000; Gunderson 2001). Deficits of this aspect of interpersonal perception have been demonstrated in analogue studies using film clips (e.g., Arntz and Veen 2001), affect recognition and alexithymic symptoms (e.g., Sayar et al. 2001), and narratives of childhood experiences (Fonagy et al. 1996; Vermote et al. 2004). Individuals with BPD exhibit emotional hyperresponsiveness (see summary in Herpertz 2003; Leichsenring and Sachsse 2002) and deficits in emotion recognition and the capacity for empathy (Bland et al. 2004; Guttman and Laporte 2002; Soloff et al. 2003; Wagner and Ambrosini 2001). But the deficit in social cognition is evidently not straightforward; it is situation and context dependent. For example, impaired recognition of integrated emotional stimuli has been shown to be associated with interpersonal antagonism, particularly suspiciousness and assaultiveness (Minzenberg et al. 2006). It seems that when an individual with BPD is emotionally aroused and as their relationship with another moves into the sphere of attachment, thereby intensifying the relationship, their ability to think about the mental state of another can rapidly disappear (see Fonagy and Bateman 2006a, 2006b for further discussion of this point).

A deficit of interpersonal awareness implies an underlying failure of effective and stable self–other differentiation at the level of distinguishing respective mental states. Some of the brain abnormalities identified in BPD patients correspond to a failure of representation of self-states being a key dysfunction. Some evidence suggests that the anterior cingulate cortex plays a key role in mentalizing the self, at least in the domain of emotional

states (Damasio 1999; Frith and Frith 1999; Lane et al. 1997, 1998). Lane (2000) proposed more specifically that implicit self-representations (i.e., phenomenal self-awareness) can be localized to the dorsal anterior cingulate, whereas explicit self-representations (i.e., reflection) can be localized to the rostral anterior cingulate. Moreover, intriguing findings regarding mirror neurons suggest that representations of self and others bearing on interpretation of intentional action promote mentalization by virtue of shared anatomical circuitry (Brothers 1997; Gallese 2000, 2001; Jeannerod 1997). Activation of the medial prefrontal cortex (including the ventromedial prefrontal cortex overlapping the orbitofrontal cortex) has been demonstrated in a series of neuroimaging studies in conjunction with a wide range of theory of mind inferences in both visual and verbal domains (Fletcher et al. 1995; Gallagher et al. 2000; Goel et al. 1995; Happe et al. 1996; Klin et al. 2000). It appears likely that extensive prefrontal cortex (i.e., orbitofrontal extending into more dorsal medial cortex) is involved in mentalizing interactively in a way that requires implicitly representing the mental states of others.

Impact of Trauma

Key to understanding severe personality disorder is the inhibition of mentalization, perhaps prototypically in response to trauma. Patients with BPD defensively avoid thinking about the mental states of self and others, because these experiences have led them to experiences of unbearable pain in the course of maltreatment (Fonagy 1991). Especially in individuals in whom the capacity for mentalization is already weak, trauma may bring about a complete collapse.

Both clinical and experimental evidence supports the view that trauma commonly brings about a partial and temporary collapse of mentalization. The disorganizing effects of trauma on attention and stress regulation are well known (Allen 2001). The capacity for mentalization is undermined in a significant proportion of individuals who have experienced trauma. Maltreated toddlers have difficulty in learning to use internal state words (Beeghly and Cicchetti 1994; Cicchetti and Beeghly 1987). Neglected children have greater difficulty in discriminating facial emotional expression, and physically abused children show a response bias toward angry expression and greater variance in their interpretation of facial affect (Pollak et al. 2000). A study of sexually abused Canadian girls demonstrated that children with sexual abuse histories had lower reflective functioning (RF) scores on the childhood attachment interviews in relation to self than demographically matched control subjects (Normandin et al. 2002). In the same study, dissociation was shown to be closely related to the low RF of abused children. Whereas 75% of those with low RF on the child attachment interview scored high in dissociation, only 20% of those with high RF could be said to be dissociating. Young adults who have been maltreated experience greater difficulty with the Reading the Mind in the Eyes Test (a relatively simple measure of implicit mentalization that involves identifying photographs with one of four mental states) (Fonagy et al. 2001).

Considerable evidence supports the claim that individuals with a history of abuse who are also limited in their capacity to think about mental states in themselves and others in the AAI are highly likely to have a diagnosis of BPD (Fonagy et al. 1996). Other researchers have replicated this finding with other samples showing trauma. For example, in the Kortenberg-Leuven Process-Outcome Study of inpatient treatment of personality disorder (Vermote et al. 2004), a significant negative correlation was reported between RF measured on the Object Relations Inventory (Blatt et al. 1996) and Structured Clinical Interview for DSM-IV Axis II Personality Disorders diagnosis of BPD, and an even stronger correlation was found with clinical observation of self-harm.

Although psychological trauma is a functional route to impaired mentalizing, neuro-

biological approaches underscore how trauma may compromise the development of cerebral structures that support mentalizing. Schore (2001) reviewed extensive evidence that secure attachment relationships are essential to the normal development of the prefrontal cortex and thus to affect regulation. Hence, early maltreatment, which is associated with extremely compromised (disorganized) attachment (Barnett et al. 1999; Lyons-Ruth and Jacobovitz 1999; Lyons-Ruth et al. 1999a, 1999b), is most likely to undermine the development of cortical structures key to mentalization.

Arnsten (1998; Arnsten et al. 1999) and Mayes (2000, 2002) have linked extreme stress to altered dynamics in arousal regulation in a way that is highly pertinent to trauma. They described how increasing levels of norepinephrine and dopamine interact with each other and differentially activate receptor subtypes so as to shift the balance between prefrontal executive control and posterior-subcortical automatic control over attention and behavior. Mild to moderate levels of arousal are associated with optimal prefrontal functioning and thus with employment of flexible mental representations and response strategies conducive to complex problem solving. On the other hand, extreme levels of arousal trigger a neurochemical switch that shifts the individual into posterior cortical-subcortical dominance such that vigilance, the fight-or-flight response, and amygdala-mediated memory encoding predominate. In effect, high levels of excitatory stimulation (at α_1 adrenergic and D_1 dopaminergic receptors) take the prefrontal cortex offline. This switch in attentional and behavioral control is adaptive in the context of danger that requires rapid automatic responding. Yet Mayes (2000) pointed out that early stressful and traumatic experiences may permanently impair the dynamic balance of arousal regulation, altering the threshold for this switch process. Thus, sensitized individuals may be prone to impaired prefrontal functioning in the face of stress, with automatic posterior-subcortical responding taking control of attention and behavior and undermining flexible mental representations and coping. In line with this suggestion is the observation that *N*-acetyl-aspartate, a marker of neural integrity, is lowered in the anterior cingulate region of the medial prefrontal cortex of maltreated children and adolescents (De Bellis et al. 2000).

These proposals regarding impaired arousal regulation and shifting the balance of prefrontal-posterior cortical functioning are consistent with neuroimaging studies employing symptom provocation in persons with posttraumatic stress disorder (PTSD). Such induced posttraumatic states are associated with diminished medial prefrontal and anterior cingulate activity (Bremner et al. 1999a, 1999b; Lanius et al. 2001; Rauch et al. 1996; Shin et al. 2001). A similar observation was reported in a positron emission tomography study comparing sexually abused women who had PTSD with women with a similar history who did not. The women with PTSD were found to have lower levels of anterior cingulate blood flow during traumatic imagery (Shin et al. 1999). This finding suggests that some BPD symptoms may be connected to an impairment of medial prefrontal cortical functioning (Zubieta et al. 1999). Van der Kolk et al. (1996) viewed findings showing deactivation in Broca's area in posttraumatic states as indicative of "speechless terror" and concluded that in such states, "the brain is 'having' its experience. The person may feel, see, or hear the sensory elements of the traumatic experience, but he or she may be physiologically prevented from translating this experience into communicable language" (p. 131). Thus, dysfunctional arousal may play a part in the reemergence of the subjective state we have described as psychic equivalence. *Psychic equivalence* is a developmentally primitive mode of experiencing the subjective world before mentalization has fully developed. The 2-year-old child is convinced that all that is in his mind is equivalent to that which exists outside and all that is out-

side must by definition exist in his mind, because his mind is functionally equivalent to the material world (Fonagy and Target 1996; Target and Fonagy 1996). The complement to this state is the pretend mode of experiencing subjectivity, in which the child feels that nothing that he experiences as subjective has any possible connection with reality.

We propose a synergy among psychological defenses, neurobiological development, and shifts in brain activity during posttraumatic states such that mentalizing activity is compromised. The shift in the balance of cortical control locks the traumatized person into either 1) the psychic equivalence mode, associated with an inability to employ alternate representations of the situation (i.e., functioning at the level of primary rather than secondary representations), much less the ability to explicate the state of mind (meta-representation); or 2) the pretend mode, associated with states of dissociative detachment.

Exposure of the Alien Self

When mirroring fails in infancy, the child internalizes a noncontingent mental state as part of a representation within the psychological self. These internalizations sit within the self without being connected to it by a set of meanings. It is this incoherence within the self-structure that we referred to as an "alien self" (Fonagy and Target 2000). As we have said, such incoherencies in self-structure may not only characterize profoundly neglected children. The coherence of self that we all experience is somewhat illusory. This illusion is normally maintained by the continuous narrative commentary on behavior that mentalization provides, which fills in the gaps and makes us feel that our experiences are meaningful. In the absence of a robust mentalizing capacity, with disorganized patterns of attachment, the disorganization of the self-structure is clearly revealed.

When trauma inhibits mentalization, the self is suddenly experienced as incoherent.

Parts within the trauma survivor feel like the self yet also feel substantively different, sometimes even persecutory. The persecutory nature of the alien part of the self arises as a sequel to maltreatment in childhood, adolescence, or even adulthood. Anna Freud (1936) described the process by which the child aims to gain control over powerful, hostile external forces through identification with the aggressor. If the cohesion of the self-structure has been weakened by limited interpersonal interpretive function and the discontinuity within the self represented by the alien part of the self is well established, identification with the maltreater is most likely to occur with the help of this alien part of the self-structure. In slight disagreement with Anna Freud, we do not look at this process as an identification, because that would imply (following Sandler's [1987] clarification of the concept) a change in the shape of the self in the direction of achieving more significant similarities with the abusive figure. It is more like a kind of "colonization" of the alien part of the self by the child's or adolescent's image of the mental state of the abuser.

The aim of the strategy is to gain a sense of control over the uncontrollable. This attempt at control is ultimately a highly maladaptive solution, because the persecution from the maltreating person is now experienced from within. A part of the self-structure is thought to wish to destroy the rest of the self. This experience of persecution from within may be one aspect of the massive impact that maltreatment can have on the self-esteem of those subject to abuse (e.g., Mullen et al. 1996). They feel that they are evil because they have internalized evil into the part of the self that is most readily decoupled from the self but nevertheless is felt as part of the self. A way of coping with the intolerable pain that this self-persecutory self within the self represents is through externalization into the physically proximal other. The part of the self that is so painful is forced outside and another physical being is manipulated and cajoled until they behave in a way that en-

ables the individual to feel that they no longer own the persecutory alien part of the self. At the simplest level, the world then becomes terrifying because the persecutory parts are experienced as outside. At a more complex level, it is felt essential that the alien experiences are owned by another mind, so that another mind is in control of these parts of the self. This defensive externalization might help to explain why, strikingly, persons with BPD frequently find themselves in interpersonal situations in which they are maltreated or abused by their partners.

Given that the relationship between childhood maltreatment and BPD is complex, the statistics on the sequelae of childhood sexual abuse seem quite relevant to this point. Victims of childhood abuse who are revictimized are most likely to have severe mental health problems, including (as we have seen frequently) BPD. According to one study, 49% of abused women compared with 18% of women without the experience of sexual abuse had been battered by their partners (Briere and Runtz 1987). In a large study with a sample representative of San Francisco (Russell 1986), between 38% and 48% of abused women (depending on the severity of abuse) had physically abusive husbands compared with 10%–17% of nonabused women. This finding should in no sense be taken to mean that the men involved in the battering are any less culpable. Individuals with experiences of maltreatment appear to be drawn to individuals who are likely to maltreat them, we would argue, in order to increase the opportunity of externalizing intolerable mental states concerning themselves. As thus might be expected, many sexual assaults experienced by college-age survivors of sexual abuse occur at the hands of a known individual (Gidycz et al. 1995). Indeed, one survey demonstrated that 81% of the adult sexual assaults experienced by revictimized women were perpetrated by male acquaintances of the survivors (Cloitre et al. 1997).

Another person is essential to create the illusion of coherence. BPD patients require rather than enjoy relationships. Relationships are necessary to stabilize the self-structure but are also the source of greatest vulnerability because in the absence of the other, when the relationships break down or if the other shows independence, the alien self returns to wreak havoc (persecute from within) and to destabilize the self-structure. Vulnerability is greatest in the context of attachment relationships. Past trauma leaves an impoverished internal working model from the point of view of clear and coherent representations of mental states in self and other. This representational system is activated by the attachment relationship with the consequence that the mental states of the other are no longer clearly seen. The physical other is desperately needed to free the self from its inwardly directed violence, but only as long as it acts as the vehicle for the patient's self-state. When this process occurs, dependence on the other is total. Substitution is inconceivable, no matter how destructive or hopeless the relationship might seem from the outside.

Self-Harm

We can now begin to understand the violence committed by certain individuals with BPD against others or themselves. For such individuals, self-harm may entail a fantasy of eradicating the alien part of the self unconsciously imagined to be part of their body. Self-mutilators report a range of conscious motivations, including self-punishment, tension reduction, improvement in mood, and distraction from intolerable affects (Favazza 1992; Herpertz 1995). Following the act of self-harm, the individual mostly reports feeling better and relieved (Favazza 1992; Herpertz 1995; Kemperman et al. 1997). We suggest that in the absence of a person who may act as a vehicle for the alien part of the self, a person with BPD achieves self-coherence through the externalization of this part of the self into a part of their body. Attempts at self-harm are acts carried out in a mode of psychic

equivalence when a part of the body is considered isomorphic with the alien part of the self at the same time as creating a respite from intolerable affects. Attempts at self-mutilation are more common when the patient is in isolation or after the loss of an other who, up to that point, could fulfill the task of being a vehicle for the persecuting alien part of the self.

Suicide

Clinical and epidemiological studies have demonstrated that between 55% and 85% of those who self-mutilate also attempt suicide (Dulit et al. 1994; Stanley et al. 1992), and BPD carries a suicide risk of around 5%–10% (Fyer et al. 1988; Stone et al. 1987). Most consider attempted suicide to be on a continuum of lethality with other types of deliberate self-harm (e.g., Linehan 1986). We understand suicide attempts as at the extreme of attempts at self-mutilation often consequent on experience of loss of the other. In such states, feelings of despair, hopelessness, and depression predominate. The loss of the other as a vehicle for the alien parts of the self—the disruption of the process of externalization—signals the destruction of the constitutional, or real, part of the self. Hence, the sense of despair is not from the loss of the object who normally would not have been a genuine attachment figure in the first place but from the anticipated loss of self-cohesion. The act of suicide is at least in part an act in the psychic equivalence mode aimed at destroying the alien part of the self (hence the continuum with self-harm). When BPD patients attempt suicide, their subjective experience is decoupled from reality (in the pretend mode of subjectivity), and in a sense they believe they (or their true selves) will survive the attempt but their alien selves will be destroyed forever. Consistent with our view is evidence that suicide attempters with BPD features perceive their suicidal attempts as less lethal, with a greater likelihood of rescue and with less certainty of death (Stanley et al. 2001). In fact, in some patients suicide is felt as "a secure base," a reunion with a state that can reduce existential fear.

Impulsive Acts of Violence

The same models of pathology that account for self-harming behavior are generally held to be applicable to certain categories of acts of interpersonal violence (Dutton 1995; Fonagy 1999; Fonagy et al. 1997; Gilligan 1997; Meloy 1992). In BPD we see interpersonal violence of an explosive or affective type (Vitiello and Stoff 1997) that is often associated with antisocial personality disorder. Identification with the aggressor leads to the colonization of the alien part of the self by the maltreating figure, and vulnerability to a malevolent mind brings with it the defensive inhibition of mentalizing capacity. Acts of violence themselves are usually the consequence of a failure of the externalization of the alien self. When the other refuses to be a vehicle for intolerable self-states—he or she refuses to be cowed or humiliated—the vulnerable mind of such an individual turns to interpersonal destruction. An important trigger for violence is the experience of "ego-destructive shame." The lack of a coherent sense of agentive self creates a massive vulnerability to humiliation in such individuals. This humiliation is felt when the other refuses to accept a role of complete passivity and through manifesting agency presents unbearable humiliation to the violent mind. The challenge is unbearable in the mode of psychic equivalence, in which shame is experienced not just as an idea or feeling but as having the actual power to destroy the self. The destruction of the other through violence is an expression of the hoped-for destruction of the alien self; it is an act of hope or liberation and is often associated with elation and only later with regret. The absence of mentalization at these moments is of course of further assistance.

TREATMENT IMPLICATIONS OF THE ATTACHMENT MODEL

It should be apparent from this discussion about attachment and BPD that the focus in treatment needs to be on stabilizing the sense of self and helping the patient maintain an optimal level of arousal. To this end, we have defined some core underpinning techniques to be used in the context of group and individual therapy and labeled them mentalization-based treatment (MBT; Bateman and Fonagy 2004, 2006). The initial task in MBT is to stabilize emotional expression because without improved control of affect there can be no serious consideration of internal representations. Although the converse is true to the extent that without stable internal representations there can be no robust control of affects, identification and expression of affect are targeted first simply because they represent an immediate threat to continuity of therapy as well as potentially to the patient's life. Uncontrolled affect leads to impulsivity, and only once this affect is under control is it possible to focus on internal representations and to strengthen the patient's sense of self.

To implement MBT effectively, greater activity on the part of the therapist is required, with more collaboration and openness than is implied in the classical analytic stance. In psychodynamic treatment of BPD patients, the therapist has to become what the patient needs him or her to be—the vehicle for the alien self, the carrier of alternative but not destabilizing perspectives. Yet to become the alien self is to be lost to the patient as a provider of different perspectives and therefore to be of no help to the patient. The therapist must aim to achieve a state of equipoise between the two—allowing him- or herself to do as required yet trying to retain as clearly and coherently as possible an image of his or her own state of mind alongside that of the patient. This mental attitude is what we have called the mentalizing stance of the therapist.

Enhancing Mentalization, Retaining Mental Closeness, and Working With Current Mental States

A therapist needs to maintain a mentalizing stance in order to help a patient develop a capacity to mentalize. Self-directed mentalistic questions are a useful way of ensuring that a focus on mentalizing is maintained. Why is the patient saying this now? Why is the patient behaving like this? What might I have done that explains the patient's state? Why am I feeling as I do now? What has happened recently in the therapy or in our relationship that may justify the current state? The therapist will be asking him- or herself these typical questions within the mentalizing therapeutic stance and is perfectly at liberty to ask these out loud in a spirit of inquiry. This approach pervades the entire treatment setting. Thus in group therapy, techniques focus on encouraging patients to consider the mental states and motives of other members as well as their own: "Why do you think that she is feeling as she does?" The therapist is not looking for complex "unconscious" reasons but rather the answers that common sense or folk psychology would suggest to most reasonable people.

Focusing the therapist's understanding of his or her interactions with the patient on the patient's current mental state will allow the therapist to link external events, however small, to powerful internal states that are otherwise experienced by the patient as inexplicable, uncontrollable, and meaningless. A focus on psychological process and the "here and now" rather than on mental content in the present and past is implicit in this approach. Little therapeutic gain results from continually focusing on the past. Recovering memories is now recognized as a somewhat risky aim with BPD patients (Brenneis 1997; Sandler and Fonagy 1997). We would wish to add that another risk involves the possibility of encouraging BPD patients to enter a pretend-psychic equivalent mode of relating, in which they (unbeknownst to the therapist)

no longer use the same circumspect subjective criteria of historical accuracy that most of us use but rather assume that because they experience something in relation to a childhood (usually adult) figure, it is bound to be true. To avoid these risks, the focus of MBT needs to be on the present state and how it remains influenced by events of the past rather than on the past itself. If the patient persistently returns to the past, the therapist needs to link back to the present, move the therapy into the here and now, and consider the present experience.

An important indicator of underlying process and the here and now is the manifest affect that is specifically targeted, identified, and explored within an interpersonal context in MBT. The challenge for the professional working with the patient is to maintain a mentalizing therapeutic stance in the context of countertransference responses that may provoke the therapist to react rather than to think. Understanding within an interpersonal context why the situation arose in the first place, why such an externalization became necessary, is the likely immediate solution to this challenge. Retaining mental closeness is done simply by representing accurately the current or immediately past feeling state of the patient and its accompanying internal representations and by strictly and systematically avoiding the temptation to enter into conversation about matters not directly linked to the patient's beliefs, wishes, and feelings.

It could be argued that the focus on mentalization in MBT is akin to the emphasis on cognitions in cognitive-behavioral treatments and that the exploration of affects is similar to the stress on affect control in dialectical behavior therapy (Linehan et al. 1991, 1999, 2002). There is some truth in this observation, but we would argue that the techniques used in those therapies are often effective because they enhance mentalizing; the success that they have is through the stimulation of exploration of the mind and the joint attention given to mental processes. Our interventions are more firmly rooted within the interpersonal context and understood within that framework, and they are perhaps more inherently integrative in taking not only the specific mental processes and behavior of the patient into account but also the relational context. Furthermore, we explicitly use transference to explore the meaning of the patient's experience, and we now turn to discuss this approach.

Transference, Interpretation, and Bearing in Mind the Deficits

Bearing in mind the limited processing capacities of BPD patients in relation to attachment issues, patients cannot be assumed to have a capacity to work with conflict, to express feelings through verbalization, to use metaphor, to resist actions, and to reflect on content, all of which form part of standard psychoanalytic process. These attributes depend on a stable self-structure and ability to form secondary (symbolic) and perhaps tertiary representations (e.g., your feelings about my thoughts about your wishes) that buffer feelings, explain ideas, and give context and meaning to interpersonal and intrapsychic processes. Borderline patients' enfeebled mentalizing capacity and emergence of psychic equivalence means that feelings, fantasies, thoughts, and desires are experienced with considerable force because they cannot be symbolized, held in a state of uncertainty, or given secondary representation with meaning. Under these circumstances the use of metaphor and the interpretation of conflict are more likely to induce bewilderment and incomprehension than to heighten the underlying meaning of the discourse, so the use of these techniques is minimized in MBT. This technical stance has important implications for the use of transference.

Our overall approach owes much to that of Otto Kernberg, John Clarkin, Frank Yeomans, and their groups (Clarkin et al. 1996, 1998, 1999; Kernberg 1992; Kernberg et al. 2002). In many respects, the model of the mind that underpins our approach is the one brilliantly advanced by Kernberg over the past few decades (Kernberg 1975, 1976, 1980, 1984). However, there are also important differences, and nowhere are these differences more apparent than in our approach to the transference. In the transference focused psychotherapy (TFP) model, patients are seen as reestablishing dyadic relations with their therapists that reflect rudimentary representations of self–other relationships of the past (so-called part–object relationships). Thus, TFP considers the externalization of these self-object-affect triads to be at the heart of therapeutic interventions. We do not differ from the TFP therapist in emphasizing the externalization process, but we are far less concerned with the apparent relationship that is thus established between patient and therapist. In our model, the role relationships established by the patient through the transference relationship are considered preliminary to the externalization of the parts of the self the patient wishes to disown. In order to achieve a state of affairs where the alien part of the self is experienced as outside rather than within, the patient needs to create a "relationship" with the therapist through which this externalization may be achieved. The patient subtly and unconsciously manipulates the therapist to experience particular intense feelings, sometimes quite specific thoughts. These originally belong to the patient, but after a period of coercive interactions they are reassuringly seen by him to be outside, in the therapist's mind. Once the externalization is achieved, the patient has no interest in the relationship with the therapist and may in fact wish to repudiate it totally. At these moments the therapist may feel abandoned. Some instances of boundary violations may be related to the therapist's difficulty in coping with the implicit rejection entailed by the patient's wish to distance himself from the disowned part of his mind. Focusing the patients' attention on the dyad that is established through the externalization can be seen as undermining their attempts to separate from the disowned part of themselves. This focus can be counterproductive, leading the patient to prematurely terminate the treatment.

Effectiveness of Mentalization-Based Treatment

Our initial study (Bateman and Fonagy 1999) of MBT compared its effectiveness in the context of a partial hospital program with routine general psychiatric care for patients with BPD. Treatment took place within a routine clinical service and was implemented by mental health professionals without full psychotherapy training who were offered expert supervision. Results showed that patients in the partial hospital program showed a statistically significant decrease on all measures in contrast with the control group, which showed limited change or deterioration over the same period. Improvement in depressive symptoms, decrease in suicidal and self-mutilatory acts, reduced inpatient days, and better social and interpersonal function began after 6 months and continued to the end of treatment at 18 months.

The 44 patients who participated in the original study were assessed at 3-month intervals after completion of the trial using the same battery of outcome measures (Bateman and Fonagy 2001). Results demonstrated that patients who had received partial hospital treatment not only maintained their substantial gains but also showed a statistically significant continued improvement on most measures in contrast with the control group of patients, who showed only limited change during the same period. Because of continued improvement in social and interpersonal function, these findings suggest that longer-term rehabilitative changes were stimulated.

Finally, an attempt was made to assess health care costs associated with partial hospital treatment compared with treatment within general psychiatric services (Bateman and Fonagy 2003). Health care utilization of all patients who participated in the trial was assessed using information from case notes

and service providers. Costs were compared 6 months prior to treatment, during 18 months of treatment, and at 18-month follow-up. No cost differences were found between the groups during pretreatment or treatment. During the treatment period, the costs of partial hospital treatment were offset by less psychiatric inpatient care and reduced emergency department treatment. The trend for costs to decrease in the experimental group during follow-up was not duplicated in the control group, suggesting that specialist partial hospital treatment for BPD is no more expensive than general psychiatric care and leads to considerable cost savings after the completion of 18 months' treatment.

All patients who participated in the partial hospital treatment trial have now been followed up with 8 years after initial randomization (Bateman and Fonagy 2008). The primary outcome for this long-term follow-up study was in learning of the number of suicide attempts. But in light of the limited improvement related to social adjustment in follow-along studies, we were concerned with establishing whether the social and interpersonal improvements found at the end of 36 months had been maintained and whether additional gains in the area of vocational achievement had been made in either group. Patients treated in the MBT program remained better than those receiving treatment as usual (TAU). Although, while they maintained their initial gains at the end of treatment, their general social function remained somewhat impaired. Nevertheless, many more were employed or in full-time education than the comparison group, and only 14% still met diagnostic criteria for BPD compared with 87% of the patients in the comparison group who were available for interview.

A number of important questions have arisen from this research. First, although we operationalized treatment for research purposes, a more detailed manual was required if we were to demonstrate that treatment was generalizable across settings and practitioners and could be applied with fidelity by generically trained mental health staff. Second, in common with other treatments of BPD, it remains unclear what exactly are the effective ingredients of treatment. The partial hospital program is a complex, multifaceted intervention including analytic and expressive therapies, and there is inevitably a "milieu" effect. We were unable to show that the target of our interventions, mentalization, had been enhanced in patients treated within the partial hospital program compared with control patients because of the complexity of measuring reflective function. For research purposes Fonagy et al. (1998) have now operationalized the ability to apply a mentalizing interpretational strategy as reflective function. Individuals are not expected to articulate this theoretically but to demonstrate it in the way they interpret events within attachment relationships. Individuals differ in the extent to which they are able to go beyond observable phenomena to give an account of their own or others' actions in terms of beliefs, desires, plans, and so on, and in BPD patients this capacity is reduced.

We have operationalized MBT as an outpatient adaptation to answer some of these questions. Outpatient treatment removes the milieu aspect of therapy and focuses solely on mentalization within individual and group analytic therapy. Treatment consists of an individual and group psychoanalytic session once a week, a total of 2.5 hours of psychotherapy, and is part of a randomized controlled trial that is under way at present. Again, treatment is implemented by generic mental health practitioners trained in MBT who are offered expert supervision. Even if this program turns out to be reasonably effective, the research into MBT and other treatments for BPD is only just beginning.

CONCLUSION

MBT may not be radically different from other forms of intervention widely practiced by psychotherapists and other mental health professionals in the various contexts in which individuals with BPD are being treated. We claim no originality for the intervention. How could we? MBT represents the relatively unadulterated implementation of a combination of developmental processes readily identified in all our histories: a) the establishment of an intense (attachment) relationship based on contingent mirroring of the mental states of patients, and b) the coherent re-presentation of their feelings and thoughts so that patients are able to identify themselves as thinking and feeling in the context of powerful bonds and high levels of emotional arousal. In turn, the recovery of mentalization helps patients regulate their thoughts and feelings, which then makes relationship and self-regulation a realistic possibility. Although we would claim to have identified a particular method that makes the delivery of this therapeutic process possible, we make no claims of uniqueness. Many situations can likely bring about symptomatic and personality change by this mechanism. The goal of further research is to identify increasingly effective and cost-effective methods for generating change in this excessively difficult group. In pursuing this goal there may indeed be nothing quite so practical as a good theory, such as the theory of human bonding.

REFERENCES

Ainsworth MDS: Object relations, dependency and attachment: a theoretical review of the infant-mother relationship. Child Dev 40:969–1025, 1969

Ainsworth MDS: Attachments across the lifespan. Bull N Y Acad Med 61:792–812, 1985

Ainsworth MDS, Blehar MC, Waters E, et al: Patterns of Attachment: A Psychological Study of the Strange Situation. Hillsdale, NJ, Erlbaum, 1978

Allen JG: Interpersonal Trauma and Serious Mental Disorder. Chichester, England, Wiley, 2001

Appelbaum SA: Psychological-mindedness: word, concept and essence. Int J Psychoanal 54:35–46, 1973

Arnsten AFT: The biology of being frazzled. Science 280:1711–1712, 1998

Arnsten AFT, Mathew R, Ubriani R, et al: Alpha-1 noradrenergic receptor stimulation impairs prefrontal cortical cognitive function. Biol Psychiatry 45:26–31, 1999

Arntz A, Veen G: Evaluations of others by borderline patients. J Nerv Ment Dis 189:513–521, 2001

Barnett D, Ganiban J, Cicchetti D: Maltreatment, emotional reactivity and the development of type D attachments from 12 to 24 months of age. Monogr Soc Res Child Dev 64:172–192, 1999

Bateman A, Fonagy P: Effectiveness of partial hospitalization in the treatment of borderline personality disorder: a randomized controlled trial. Am J Psychiatry 156:1563–1569, 1999

Bateman A, Fonagy P: Treatment of borderline personality disorder with psychoanalytically oriented partial hospitalization: an 18-month follow-up. Am J Psychiatry 158:36–42, 2001

Bateman A, Fonagy P: Health service utilization costs for borderline personality disorder patients treated with psychoanalytically oriented partial hospitalization versus general psychiatric care. Am J Psychiatry 160:169–171, 2003

Bateman A, Fonagy P: Psychotherapy for Borderline Personality Disorder: Mentalization Based Treatment. New York, Oxford University Press, 2004

Bateman AW, Fonagy P: Mentalization-Based Treatment for Borderline Personality Disorder: A Practical Guide. New York, Oxford University Press, 2006

Bateman A, Fonagy P : Eight-year follow-up of patients treated for borderline personality disorder: mentalization-based treatment versus treatment as usual. Am J Psychiatry 165:631–638, 2008

Beeghly M, Cicchetti D: Child maltreatment, attachment, and the self system: emergence of an internal state lexicon in toddlers at high social risk. Dev Psychopathol 6:5–30, 1994

Bland AR, Williams CA, Scharer K, et al: Emotion processing in borderline personality disorders. Issues Ment Health Nurs 25:655–672, 2004

Blatt SJ, Stayner D, Auerbach JS, et al: Change in object and self representations in long-term, intensive, inpatient treatment of seriously disturbed adolescents and young adults. Psychiatry: Interpersonal and Biological Processes 59:82–107, 1996

Bowlby J: Attachment and Loss, Vol 1: Attachment. London, Hogarth Press and the Institute of Psycho-Analysis, 1969

Bowlby J: Attachment and Loss, Vol 2: Separation: Anxiety and Anger. London, Hogarth Press and the Institute of Psycho-Analysis, 1973

Bram AD, Gabbard GO: Potential space and reflective functioning: towards conceptual clarification and preliminary clinical implications. Int J Psychoanal 82:685–699, 2001

Bremner JD, Narayan M, Staib LH, et al: Neural correlates of memories of childhood sexual abuse in women with and without posttraumatic stress disorder. Am J Psychiatry 156:1787–1795, 1999a

Bremner JD, Staib LH, Kaloupek D, et al: Neural correlates of exposure to traumatic pictures and sound in Vietnam combat veterans with and without posttraumatic stress disorder: a positron emission tomography study. Biol Psychiatry 45:806–816, 1999b

Brenneis CB: Recovered Memories of Trauma: Transferring the Present to the Past. Madison, CT, International Universities Press, 1997

Bretherton K, Munholland KA: Internal working models in attachment relationships: a construct revisited, in Handbook of Attachment: Theory, Research and Clinical Applications. Edited by Cassidy J, Shaver PR. New York, Guilford, 1999, pp 89–114

Briere J, Runtz M: Post-sexual abuse trauma: data and implications for clinical practice. J Interpers Violence 2:367–397, 1987

Brothers L: Friday's Footprint: How Society Shapes the Human Mind. New York, Oxford University Press, 1997

Broussard ER: Infant attachment in a sample of adolescent mothers. Child Psychiatry Hum Dev 25:211–219, 1995

Brown DG: Drowsiness in the countertransference. Int Rev Psychoanal 4:481–492, 1977

Carlson EA: A prospective longitudinal study of attachment disorganization/disorientation. Child Dev 69:1107–1128, 1998

Carlson V, Cicchetti D, Barnett D, et al: Disorganised/disoriented attachment relationships in maltreated infants. Dev Psychol 25:525–531, 1989

Cicchetti D, Beeghly M: Symbolic development in maltreated youngsters: an organizational perspective, in Atypical Symbolic Development: New Directions for Child Development, Vol 36. Edited by Cicchetti D, Beeghly M. San Francisco, CA, Jossey-Bass, 1987, pp 5–29

Clarkin JF, Hull JW, Hurt SW: Factor structure of borderline personality disorder criteria. J Personal Disord 7:137–143, 1993

Clarkin J, Foelsch PA, Kernberg OF: Manual for the Inventory of Personality Organization. Ithaca, NY, Cornell University Medical College, 1996

Clarkin JF, Yeomans F, Kernberg OF: Psychodynamic Psychotherapy of Borderline Personality Organization: A Treatment Manual. New York, Wiley, 1998

Clarkin JF, Kernberg OF, Yeomans F: Transference-Focused Psychotherapy for Borderline Personality Disorder Patients. New York, Guilford, 1999

Cloitre M, Scarvalone P, Difede J: Posttraumatic stress disorder self and interpersonal dysfunction among sexually retraumatized women. J Trauma Stress 10:437–452, 1997

Collins NR, Read SJ: Representations of attachment: the structure and function of working models, in Advances in Personal Relationships, Vol 5: Attachment Process in Adulthood. Edited by Bartholomew K, Perlman D. London, Jessica Kingsley, 1994, pp 53–90

Compton A: The current status of the psychoanalytic theory of instinctual drives, I: drive concept, classification, and development. Psychoanal Q 52:364–401, 1983

Craik K: The Nature of Explanation. Cambridge, England, Cambridge University Press, 1943

Crittenden PM: Internal representational models of attachment relationships. Infant Ment Health J 11:259–277, 1990

Crittenden PM: Peering into the black box: an exploratory treatise on the development of self in young children, in Rochester Symposium on Developmental Psychopathology, Vol 5: Disorders and Dysfunctions of the Self. Edited by Cicchetti D, Toth SL. Rochester, NY, University of Rochester Press, 1994, pp 79–148

Crittenden PM: Toward an integrative theory of trauma: a dynamic-maturation approach, in Rochester Symposium on Developmental Psychopathology, Vol 8: Developmental Perspectives on Trauma. Edited by Cicchetti D, Toth SL. Rochester, NY, University of Rochester Press, 1997, pp 33–84

Damasio A: The Feeling of What Happens: Body and Emotion in the Making of Consciousness. New York, Harcourt Brace, 1999

De Bellis MD, Keshavan MS, Spencer S, et al: N-acetyl-aspartate concentration in the anterior cingulate of maltreated children and adolescents with PTSD. Am J Psychiatry 157:1175–1177, 2000

De M'Uzan M: A case of masochistic perversion and an outline of a theory. Int J Psychoanal 54:455–467, 1973

Domes G, Winter B, Schnell K, et al: The influence of emotions on inhibitory functioning in borderline personality disorder. Psychol Med 36:1163–1172, 2006

Dulit RA, Fyer MR, Leon AC, et al: Clinical correlates of self-mutilation in borderline personality disorder. Am J Psychiatry 151:1305–1311, 1994

Dutton DG: Male abusiveness in intimate relationships. Clin Psychol Rev 15:567–581, 1995

Favazza AR: Repetitive self-mutilation. Psychiatr Ann 22:60–63, 1992

Feeney JA, Noller P: Attachment style as a predictor of adult romantic relationships. J Pers Soc Psychol 58:281–291, 1990

Fletcher PC, Happe F, Frith U, et al: Other minds in the brain: a functional imaging study of "theory of mind" in story comprehension. Cognition 57:109–128, 1995

Fonagy P: Thinking about thinking: some clinical and theoretical considerations in the treatment of a borderline patient. Int J Psychoanal 72:1–18, 1991

Fonagy P: Playing with reality: the development of psychic reality and its malfunction in borderline patients. Int J Psychoanal 76:39–44, 1995

Fonagy P: Male perpetrators of violence against women: an attachment theory perspective. Journal of Applied Psychoanalytic Studies 1:7–27, 1999

Fonagy P, Bateman A: Mechanisms of change in mentalization-based treatment of BPD. J Clin Psychol 62:411–430, 2006a

Fonagy P, Bateman A: Progress in the treatment of borderline personality disorder. Br J Psychiatry 188:1–3, 2006b

Fonagy P, Target M: Playing with reality, I: theory of mind and the normal development of psychic reality. Int J Psychoanal 77:217–233, 1996

Fonagy P, Target M: Attachment and reflective function: their role in self-organization. Dev Psychopathol 9:679–700, 1997

Fonagy P, Target M: Playing with reality, III: the persistence of dual psychic reality in borderline patients. Int J Psychoanal 81:853–874, 2000

Fonagy P, Target M: Early intervention and the development of self-regulation. Psychoanalytic Inquiry 22:307–335, 2002

Fonagy P, Steele H, Moran G, et al: The capacity for understanding mental states: the reflective self in parent and child and its significance for security of attachment. Infant Ment Health J 13:200–217, 1991a

Fonagy P, Steele H, Steele M: Maternal representations of attachment during pregnancy predict the organization of infant-mother attachment at one year of age. Child Dev 62:891–905, 1991b

Fonagy P, Steele M, Moran GS, et al: Measuring the ghost in the nursery: an empirical study of the relation between parents' mental represenlations of childhood experiences and their infants' security of attachment. J Am Psychoanal Assoc 41:957–989, 1993

Fonagy P, Steele M, Steele H, et al: Theory and practice of resilience. J Child Psychol Psychiatry 35:231–257, 1994

Fonagy P, Leigh T, Kennedy R, et al: Attachment, borderline states and the representation of emotions and cognitions in self and other, in Rochester Symposium on Developmental Psychopathology, Vol 6: Cognition and Emotion. Edited by Cicchetti D, Toth SL. Rochester, NY, University of Rochester Press, 1995, pp 371–414

Fonagy P, Leigh T, Steele M, et al: The relation of attachment status, psychiatric classification, and response to psychotherapy. J Consult Clin Psychol 64:22–31, 1996

Fonagy P, Target M, Steele M, et al: The development of violence and crime as it relates to security of attachment, in Children in a Violent Society. Edited by Osofsky JD. New York, Guilford, 1997, pp 150–177

Fonagy P, Target M, Steele H, et al: Reflective-Functioning Manual, Version 5.0, for Application to Adult Attachment Interviews. London, University College London, 1998

Fonagy P, Target M, Gergely G: Attachment and borderline personality disorder: a theory and some evidence. Psychiatr Clin North Am 23:103–122, 2000

Fonagy P, Stein H, White R: Dopamine receptor polymorphism and susceptibility to sexual, physical and psychological abuse: preliminary results of a longitudinal study of maltreatment. Paper presented at the 10th Biannual Meeting of the Society for Research in Child Development, Minneapolis, MN, April 2001

Fonagy P, Gergely G, Jurist E, et al: Affect Regulation, Mentalization and the Development of the Self. New York, Other Press, 2002

Fonagy P, Target M, Gergely G, et al: The developmental roots of borderline personality disorder in early attachment relationships: a theory and some evidence. Psychoanalytic Inquiry 23:412–459, 2003

Freud A: The Ego and the Mechanisms of Defence. New York, International Universities Press, 1936

Frith CD, Frith U: Interacting minds: a biological basis. Science 286:1692–1695, 1999

Frith U, Morton J, Leslie AM: The cognitive basis of a biological disorder: autism. Trends Neurosci 14:433–438, 1991

Fyer MR, Frances AJ, Sullivan T, et al: Suicide attempts in patients with borderline personality disorder. Am J Psychiatry 145:737–739, 1988

Gallagher IIL, IIappe F, Brunswick N, et al: Reading the mind in cartoons and stories: an fMRI study of "theory of mind" in verbal and non-verbal tasks. Neuropsychologia 38:11–21, 2000

Gallese V: The acting subject: toward the neural basis of social cognition, in Neural Correlates of Consciousness. Edited by Metzinger T. Cambridge, MA, MIT Press, 2000, pp 325–333

Gallese V: The "shared manifold" hypothesis: from mirror neurons to empathy. Journal of Consciousness Studies 8:33–50, 2001

Gazzaniga MS: The Social Brain: Discovering the Networks of the Mind. New York, Basic Books, 1985

Gidycz CA, Hanson K, Layman MJ: A prospective analysis of the relationships among sexual assault experiences: an extension of previous findings. Psychol Women Q 19:5–29, 1995

Gilligan J: Violence: Our Deadliest Epidemic and Its Causes. New York, Grosset/Putnam, 1997

Goel V, Grafman N, Sadato M, et al: Modeling other minds. Neuroreport 6:1741–1746, 1995

Green J, Goldwyn R: Annotation: attachment disorganisation and psychopathology: new findings in attachment research and their potential implications for developmental psychopathology in childhood. J Child Psychol Psychiatry 43:835–846, 2002

Grienenberger J, Kelly K, Slade A: Maternal reflective functioning and the caregiving relationship: the link between mental states and mother–infant affective communication. Paper presented at the Biennial Meetings of the Society for Research in Child Development, Minneapolis, MN, April 2001

Gunderson JG: The borderline patient's intolerance of aloneness: insecure attachments and therapist availability. Am J Psychiatry 153:752–758, 1996

Gunderson JG: Borderline Personality Disorder: A Clinical Guide. Washington, DC, American Psychiatric Press, 2001

Gurvits IG, Koenigsberg HW, Siever LJ: Neurotransmitter dysfunction in patients with borderline personality disorder. Psychiatr Clin North Am 23:27–40, 2000

Guttman H, Laporte L: Alexithymia, empathy, and psychological symptoms in a family context. Compr Psychiatry 43:448–455, 2002

Happe F, Ehlers S, Fletcher P, et al: "Theory of mind" in the brain: evidence from a PET scan study of Asperger syndrome. Neuroreport 8:197–201, 1996

Herpertz SC: Self-injurious behavior: psychopathological and nosological characteristics in subtypes of self-injurers. Acta Psychiatr Scand 91:57–68, 1995

Herpertz SC: Emotional processing in personality disorder. Curr Psychiatry Rep 5:23–27, 2003

Higgitt A, Fonagy P: The psychotherapeutic treatment of borderline and narcissistic personality disorder. Br J Psychiatry 161:23–43, 1992

Jacobovitz D, Hazen N: Developmental pathways from infant disorganization to childhood peer relationships, in Attachment Disorganization. Edited by Solomon J, George C. New York, Guilford, 1999, pp 127–159

Jacobovitz D, Hazen N, Riggs S: Disorganized mental processes in mothers, frightening/frightened caregiving and disoriented/disorganized behavior in infancy. Paper presented at the Biennial Meetings of the Society for Research in Child Development, Washington, DC, April 1997

Jeannerod M: The Cognitive Neuroscience of Action. Oxford, England, Blackwell, 1997

Kemperman I, Russ MJ, Shearin E: Self-injurious behavior and mood regulation in borderline patients. J Personal Disord 11:146–157, 1997

Kernberg OF: Borderline Conditions and Pathological Narcissism. New York, Jason Aronson, 1975

Kernberg OF: Object Relations Theory and Clinical Psychoanalysis. New York, Jason Aronson, 1976

Kernberg OF: Internal World and External Reality: Object Relations Theory Applied. New York, Jason Aronson, 1980

Kernberg OF: Self, ego, affects and drives. J Am Psychoanal Assoc 30:893–917, 1982

Kernberg OF: Object relations theory and character analysis. J Am Psychoanal Assoc 31:247–271, 1983

Kernberg OF: Severe Personality Disorders: Psychotherapeutic Strategies. New Haven, CT, Yale University Press, 1984

Kernberg OF: Aggression in Personality Disorders and Perversions. New Haven, CT, Yale University Press, 1992

Kernberg OF, Clarkin JF, Yeomans FE: A Primer of Transference Focused Psychotherapy for the Borderline Patient. New York, Jason Aronson, 2002

Kestenbaum R, Farber E, Sroufe LA: Individual differences in empathy among preschoolers' concurrent and predictive validity, in Empathy and Related Emotional Responses: New Directions for Child Development. Edited by Eisenberg N. San Francisco, CA, Jossey-Bass, 1989, pp 51–56

Klin A, Schultz R, Cohen DJ: Theory of mind in action: developmental perspectives on social neuroscience, in Understanding Other Minds: Perspectives From Developmental Cognitive Neuroscience, 2nd Edition. Edited by Baron-Cohen S, Tager-Flusberg H, Cohen DJ. New York, Oxford University Press, 2000, pp 357–388

Kohut H: The Restoration of the Self. New York, International Universities Press, 1977

Lane RD: Neural correlates of conscious emotional experience, in Cognitive Neuroscience of Emotion. Edited by Lane RD, Nadel L. New York, Oxford University Press, 2000, pp 345–370

Lane RD, Ahern GL, Schwartz GE, et al: Is alexithymia the emotional equivalent of blindsight? Biol Psychiatry 42:834–844, 1997

Lane RD, Reiman EM, Axelrod B, et al: Neural correlates of levels of emotional awareness: evidence of an interaction between emotion and attention in the anterior cingulate cortex. J Cogn Neurosci 10:525–535, 1998

Lanius RA, Williamson PC, Densmore M, et al: Neural correlates of traumatic memories in posttraumatic stress disorder: a functional MRI investigation. Am J Psychiatry 158:1920–1922, 2001

Lecours S, Bouchard M-A: Dimensions of mentalisation: outlining levels of psychic transformation. Int J Psychoanal 78:855–875, 1997

Leichsenring F, Sachsse U: Emotions as wishes and beliefs. J Pers Assess 79:257–273, 2002

Lieb K, Zanarini MC, Schmahl C, et al: Borderline personality disorder. Lancet 364:453–461, 2004

Linehan M: Suicidal people: one population or two? Ann N Y Acad Sci 487:16–33, 1986

Linehan MM, Armstrong HE, Suarez A, et al: Cognitive-behavioral treatment of chronically parasuicidal borderline patients. Arch Gen Psychiatry 48:1060–1064, 1991

Linehan MM, Schmidt H, Dimeff LA, et al: Dialectical behavior therapy for patients with borderline personality disorder and drug-dependence. Am J Addict 8:279–292, 1999

Linehan MM, Dimeff LA, Reynolds SK, et al: Dialectical behavior therapy versus comprehensive validation therapy plus 12-step for the treatment of opioid dependent women meeting criteria for borderline personality disorder. Drug Alcohol Depend 67:13–26, 2002

Lyons-Ruth K: Broadening our conceptual frameworks: can we reintroduce relational strategies and implicit representational systems to the study of psychopathology? Dev Psychol 31:432–436, 1995

Lyons-Ruth K: Attachment relationships among children with aggressive behavior problems: the role of disorganized early attachment patterns. J Consult Clin Psychol 64:32–40, 1996

Lyons-Ruth K, Jacobovitz D: Attachment disorganization: unresolved loss, relational violence and lapses in behavioral and attentional strategies, in Handbook of Attachment Theory and Research. Edited by Cassidy J, Shaver PR. New York, Guilford, 1999, pp 520–554

Lyons-Ruth K, Zoll D, Connell DB, et al: Family deviance and family disruption in childhood: associations with maternal behavior and infant maltreatment during the first two years of life. Dev Psychopathol 1:219–236, 1989

Lyons-Ruth K, Connell DB, Grunebaum HU: Infants at social risk: maternal depression and family support services as mediators of infant development and security of attachment. Child Dev 61:85–98, 1990

Lyons-Ruth K, Alpern L, Repacholi B: Disorganized infant attachment classification and maternal psychosocial problems as predictors of hostile-aggressive behavior in the preschool classroom. Child Dev 64:572–585, 1993

Lyons-Ruth K, Bronfman E, Atwood G: A relational diathesis model of hostile-helpless states of mind: expressions in mother–infant interaction, in Attachment Disorganization. Edited by Solomon J, George C. New York, Guilford, 1999a, pp 33–70

Lyons-Ruth K, Bronfman E, Parsons E: Atypical attachment in infancy and early childhood among children at developmental risk, IV: maternal frightened, frightening, or atypical behavior and disorganized infant attachment patterns. Monogr Soc Res Child Dev 64:67–96, 1999b

Main M: Metacognitive knowledge, metacognitive monitoring, and singular (coherent) vs. multiple (incoherent) model of attachment: findings and directions for future research, in Attachment Across the Life Cycle. Edited by Parkes CM, Stevenson-Hinde J, Marris P. London, Tavistock/Routledge, 1991, pp 127–159

Main M, Solomon J: Procedures for identifying infants as disorganized/disoriented during the Ainsworth Strange Situation, in Attachment During the Preschool Years: Theory, Research and Intervention. Edited by Greenberg M, Cicchetti D, Cummings EM. Chicago, IL, University of Chicago Press, 1990, pp 121–160

Main M, Kaplan N, Cassidy J: Security in infancy, childhood and adulthood: a move to the level of representation. Monogr Soc Res Child Dev 50:66–104, 1985

Mayes LC: A developmental perspective on the regulation of arousal states. Semin Perinatol 24:267–279, 2000

Mayes LC: A behavioral teratogenic model of the impact of prenatal cocaine exposure on arousal regulatory systems. Neurotoxicol Teratol 24:385–395, 2002

Meins E, Fernyhough C: Linguistic acquisitional style and mentalising development: the role of

maternal mind-mindedness. Cogn Develop 14:363–380, 1999

Meins E, Russell J: Security and symbolic play: the relation between security of attachment and executive capacity. Br J Dev Psychol 15:63–76, 1997

Meins E, Fernyhough C, Russell J, et al: Security of attachment as a predictor of symbolic and mentalising abilities: a longitudinal study. Soc Dev 7:1–24, 1998

Meins E, Fernyhough C, Fradley E, et al: Rethinking maternal sensitivity: mothers' comments on infants' mental processes predict security of attachment at 12 months. J Child Psychol Psychiatry 42:637–648, 2001

Meloy RJ: Violent Attachments. Northvale, NJ, Jason Aronson, 1992

Meyer B, Pilkonis PA, Proietti JM, et al: Attachment styles and personality disorders as predictors of symptom course. J Personal Disord 15:371–389, 2001

Minzenberg MJ, Poole JH, Vinogradov S: Social-emotion recognition in borderline personality disorder. Compr Psychiatry 47:468–474, 2006

Morton J: The origins of autism. New Scientist 1694:44–47, 1989

Mullen PE, Martin JL, Anderson JC, et al: The long-term impact of the physical, emotional, and sexual abuse of children: a community study. Child Abuse Negl 20:7–21, 1996

Namnum A: The problem of analyzability and the autonomous ego. Int J Psychoanal 49:271–275, 1968

Normandin L, Ensink K, Kernberg P: The role of trauma in the development of borderline personality disturbance in children. Paper presented at the Transference Focused Psychotherapy for Borderline Personality Disorder Symposium, New York, November 2002

Ogawa JR, Sroufe LA, Weinfield NS, et al: Development and the fragmented self: longitudinal study of dissociative symptomatology in a nonclinical sample. Dev Psychopathol 9:855–879, 1997

Ogden T: On potential space. Int J Psychoanal 66:129–141, 1985

Olson DR: The World on Paper. Cambridge, England, Cambridge University Press, 1994

Paris J: Childhood precursors of borderline personality disorder. Psychiatr Clin North Am 23:77–88, 2000

Pilkonis P: Personality prototypes among depressives. J Personal Disord 2:144–152, 1988

Pollak SD, Cicchetti D, Hornung K, et al: Recognizing emotion in faces: developmental effects of child abuse and neglect. Dev Psychol 36:679–688, 2000

Raikes HA, Thompson RA: Family emotional climate, attachment security, and young children's emotional knowledge in a high risk sample. Br J Dev Psychol 24:89–104, 2006

Rauch SL, van der Kolk BA, Fisler RE, et al: A symptom provocation study of posttraumatic stress disorder using positron emission tomography and script-driven imagery. Arch Gen Psychiatry 53:380–387, 1996

Rosenberg PH, Miller GA: Comparing borderline definitions: DSM-III borderline and schizotypal personality disorders. J Abnorm Psychol 98:161–169, 1989

Russell DEH: The Secret Trauma: Incest in the Lives of Girls and Women. New York, Basic Books, 1986

Sandler J: From Safety to the Superego: Selected Papers of Joseph Sandler. New York, Guilford, 1987

Sandler J, Fonagy P (eds): Recovered Memories of Abuse: True or False? London, Karnac Books, 1997

Sanislow CA, Grilow CM, McGlashan TH: Factor analysis of DSM-III-R borderline personality criteria in psychiatric inpatients. Am J Psychiatry 157:1629–1633, 2000

Sayar K, Ebrinc S, Ak I: Alexithymia in patients with antisocial personality disorder in a military hospital setting. Isr J Psychiatry Relat Sci 38:81–87, 2001

Schore AN: Effects of a secure attachment relationship on right brain development, affect regulation, and infant mental health. Infant Ment Health J 22:7–66, 2001

Schuengel C, Bakermans-Kranenburg M, van IJzendoorn M: Frightening maternal behaviour linking unresolved loss and disorganised infant attachment. J Consult Clin Psychol 67:54–63, 1999

Shaw DS, Vondra JI: Infant attachment security and maternal predictors of early behavior problems: a longitudinal study of low-income families. J Abnorm Child Psychol 23:335–357, 1995

Shaw DS, Owens EB, Vondra JI, et al: Early risk factors and pathways in the development of early disruptive behavior problems. Dev Psychopathol 8:679–700, 1997

Shin LM, McNally RJ, Kosslyn SM, et al: Regional cerebral blood flow during script-driven imagery in childhood sexual abuse-related PTSD: a PET investigation. Am J Psychiatry 156:575–584, 1999

Shin LM, Whalen PJ, Pitman RK, et al: An fMRI study of anterior cingulate function in posttraumatic stress disorder. Biol Psychiatry 50:932–942, 2001

Silk KR: Borderline personality disorder: overview of biologic factors. Psychiatr Clin North Am 23:61–75, 2000

Slade A, Belsky J, Aber JL, et al: Mother's representation of their relationships with their toddlers: links to adult attachment and observed mothering. Dev Psychol 35:611–619, 1999

Soloff PH, Kelly TM, Strotmeyer SJ, et al: Impulsivity, gender, and response to fenfluramine challenge in borderline personality disorder. Psychiatry Res 119:11–24, 2003

Solomon J, George C: Attachment Disorganization. New York, Guilford, 1999

Sroufe LA: Infant–Caregiver Attachment and Patterns of Adaptation in Preschool: The Roots of Maladaption and Competence, Vol 16. Hillsdale, NJ, Erlbaum, 1983

Sroufe LA: Emotional Development: The Organization of Emotional Life in the Early Years. New York, Cambridge University Press, 1996

Sroufe LA, Egeland B, Kreutzer T: The fate of early experience following developmental change: longitudinal approaches to individual adaptation in childhood. Child Dev 61:1363–1373, 1990

Sroufe LA, Carlson E, Levy AK, et al: Implications of attachment theory for developmental psychopathology. Dev Psychopathol 11:1–13, 1999

Stanley B, Winchel R, Molcho A, et al: Suicide and the self-harm continuum: phenomenological and biochemical evidence. Int Rev Psychiatry 4:149–155, 1992

Stanley B, Gameroff MJ, Michalsen V, et al: Are suicide attempters who self-mutilate a unique population? Am J Psychiatry 158:427–432, 2001

Startup M, Heard H, Swales M, et al: Autobiographical memory and parasuicide in borderline personality disorder. Br J Clin Psychol 40:113–120, 2001

Steele H, Steele M, Fonagy P: Associations among attachment classifications of mothers, fathers, and their infants. Child Dev 67:541–555, 1996

Stone MH, Hurt SW, Stone DK: The PI 500: long-term follow-up of borderline inpatients meeting DSM-III criteria, I: global outcome. J Personal Disord 1:291–298, 1987

Symons DK: Mental state discourse, theory of mind, and the internalization of self-other understanding. Dev Rev 24:159–188, 2004

Target M, Fonagy P: Playing with reality, II: the development of psychic reality from a theoretical perspective. Int J Psychoanal 77:459–479, 1996

Teti D, Gelfand D, Isabella R: Maternal depression and the quality of early attachment: an examination of infants, preschoolers and their mothers. Dev Psychol 31:364–376, 1995

Tronick EZ, Gianino AF: The transmission of maternal disturbance to the infant, in Maternal Depression and Infant Disturbance. Edited by

Tronick EZ, Field T. San Francisco, CA, Jossey-Bass, 1986, pp 5–11

Trull TJ: Relationships of borderline features to parental mental illness, childhood abuse, Axis I disorder, and current functioning. J Personal Disord 15:19–32, 2001a

Trull TJ: Structural relations between borderline personality disorder features and putative etiological correlates. J Abnorm Psychol 110:471–481, 2001b

Trull TJ, Sher KJ, Minks-Brown C, et al: Borderline personality disorder and substance use disorders: a review and integration. Clin Psychol Rev 20:235–253, 2000

van der Kolk PA, McFarlane AC, Weisaeth L (eds): Traumatic Stress: The Effects of Overwhelming Experience on Mind, Body, and Society. New York, Guilford, 1996

van IJzendoorn MH: Adult attachment representations, parental responsiveness, and infant attachment: a meta-analysis on the predictive validity of the Adult Attachment Interview. Psychol Bull 117:387–403, 1995

van IJzendoorn MH, Scheungel C, Bakermans-Kranenburg MJ: Disorganized attachment in early childhood: meta-analysis of precursors, concomitants and sequelae. Dev Psychopathol 22:225–249, 1999

Vermote R, Vertommen H, Corveleyn J, et al: The Kortenberg-Louvain Process-Outcome Study. Paper presented at the IPA Congress, New Orleans, LA, March 2004

Vitiello B, Stoff DM: Subtypes of aggression and their relevance to child psychiatry. J Am Acad Child Adolesc Psychiatry 36:307–315, 1997

Vondra JI, Hommerding KD, Shaw DS: Atypical attachment in infancy and early childhood among children at developmental risk, VI: stability and change in infant attachment in a low-income sample. Monogr Soc Res Child Dev 64:119–144, 1999

Vondra JI, Shaw DS, Swearingen L, et al: Attachment stability and emotional and behavioral regulation from infancy to preschool age. Dev Psychopathol 13:13–33, 2001

Wagner KD, Ambrosini PJ: Childhood depression: pharmacological therapy/treatment (pharmacotherapy of childhood depression). J Clin Child Psychol 30:88–97, 2001

Wartner UG, Grossman K, Fremmer-Bombrik E, et al: Attachment patterns at age six in South Germany: predictability from infancy and implications for pre-school behaviour. Child Dev 65:1014–1027, 1994

Waters E, Wippman J, Sroufe LA: Attachment, positive affect, and competence in the peer group: two studies in construct validation. Child Dev 50:821–829, 1979

Widom CS: Posttraumatic stress disorder in abused and neglected children grown up. Am J Psychiatry 156:1223–1229, 1999

Winnicott DW: Mirror-role of the mother and family in child development, in The Predicament of the Family: A Psycho-Analytical Symposium. Edited by Lomas P. London, Hogarth Press, 1967, pp 26–33

Winnicott DW: Playing and Reality. London, Tavistock, 1971

Zanarini MC, Williams AA, Lewis RE, et al: Reported pathological childhood experiences associated with the development of borderline personality disorder. Am J Psychiatry 154:1101–1106, 1997

Zlotnick C, Mattia J, Zimmerman M: Clinical features of survivors of sexual abuse with major depression. Child Abuse Negl 25:357–367, 2001

Zubieta JK, Chinitz JA, Lombardi U, et al: Medial frontal cortex involvement in PTSD symptoms: a SPECT study. J Psychiatr Res 33:259–264, 1999

12

Dialectical Behavior Therapy

Barbara Stanley, Ph.D.
Beth S. Brodsky, Ph.D.

Dialectical behavior therapy (DBT) was developed in the early 1990s by Marsha Linehan as a treatment specifically for suicidal and self-injuring individuals with borderline personality disorder (BPD) (Linehan 1993a), a population with a broad range of serious problems in addition to suicidality (Kehrer and Linehan 1996). A form of cognitive-behavioral psychotherapy, DBT can be adapted for use in other personality disorders, particularly those in which there is significant behavioral and emotional dyscontrol (Stanley et al. 2001). However, other than its use in BPD to date, most adaptations of DBT have been directed toward Axis I diagnoses, such as eating disorders (Telch et al. 2001), or

special segments of the psychiatric population, such as adolescents (Rathus and Miller 2002) or geriatric patients (Lynch et al. 2003).

DBT has been evaluated in several efficacy studies, and it is currently undergoing a large-scale evaluation under our direction, funded by the National Institute of Mental Health (NIMH), at the New York State Psychiatric Institute/Columbia University Department of Psychiatry. In this chapter, we summarize DBT as described in the two published treatment manuals (Linehan 1993a, 1993b) and as we apply it in our efficacy study (Stanley et al. 2007).

DBT was developed in response to the need for empirically supported psychothera-

This work was supported in part by National Institute of Mental Health grants R01 MH61079, MH062665, and P20AA015630 to Dr. Stanley.

The authors would like to thank Alex Chapman, Ph.D., postdoctoral fellow in Behavior Research and Therapy Clinics, under the direction of Marsha Linehan, Ph.D., of the University of Washington, for his thoughtful comments on an earlier draft of this chapter.

pies for chronically suicidal individuals with BPD. Although originally developed for the self-injuring, it is also used in the segment of the BPD population that does not exhibit self-harm behaviors (Robins et al. 2001). Treatment retention of individuals with BPD is a well-known and significant problem, as is their lack of progress and dissatisfaction with their therapies. At the time when DBT was developed, empirical support for existing therapies, including supportive and psychodynamically oriented treatment, was lacking. Cognitive-behavioral therapy (CBT) showed efficacy in patients with depression and anxiety disorders, but individuals with BPD had trouble tolerating standard CBT (Dimeff and Linehan 2001). CBT places a strong emphasis on change strategies that, by themselves, are very difficult for individuals with BPD to accept and utilize. BPD patients tend to experience an almost exclusive focus on change as criticism and invalidation of their suffering rather than its intent as helpful. This approach, in turn, exacerbates their already harsh self-criticism and contributes to their poor retention rate in therapy.

In attempting to tackle this problem, DBT explicitly emphasizes the need to balance change strategies with acceptance and validation techniques. This balance is important for two primary reasons. First, acceptance and change, in and of themselves, are important ingredients in any successful psychotherapy. Many problems and issues confronted in psychotherapy cannot be changed. An obvious example is past history and childhood experiences. Patients are sometimes entrenched in a place of nonacceptance about their past and consequently are unable to move beyond a stance that it "should not have happened." Second, acceptance and change have a dynamic interplay that creates a *dialectic*. Increased acceptance enables greater change, and more change allows for increased tolerance and acceptance of what cannot be changed.

This chapter describes the theoretical underpinnings of DBT, provides an overview of the components of standard DBT treatment as developed for individuals with BPD who experience self-injurious and suicidal behavior, discusses basic DBT techniques and strategies, reviews the empirical findings of its efficacy, and provides case material demonstrating crucial aspects of the treatment. The intent of this chapter is to provide an overview of DBT and illustrate how it uniquely addresses the difficulties specific to the treatment and retention of individuals with BPD. For a comprehensive description of DBT, the treatment manuals (Linehan 1993a, 1993b) should be consulted.

THEORETICAL PERSPECTIVES

Biosocial Theory of Borderline Personality Disorder

DBT was developed from a particular theoretical perspective on the nature of BPD (Linehan 1987, 1993a). BPD is viewed as a disorder of *dysregulation*—dysregulation of behavior, affect, cognition, and interpersonal relationships. The chronic suicidal behavior characteristic of many individuals with BPD is seen as a consequence of these dysregulations. The biosocial theory (Linehan 1993a) on which DBT rests attributes the dysregulation to a transaction between an inborn emotional vulnerability and an emotionally invalidating childhood environment. The biologically based emotional vulnerability is characterized by an intense, quick reaction to emotionally evocative stimuli in the environment, along with a slow return to baseline after emotional arousal. The invalidating environment consists of caretakers who may punish, ignore, reject, and/or disregard the child's emotional experience and therefore do not provide conditions in which the individual can learn to regulate emotional experiences. A transaction between these two elements—in which 1) the emotional sensitivity leads to increased perception of threat in interpersonal situations and 2) the invalidating response from the environment exacerbates the emotional vulnerability—results in a propensity to dysregulation. Linehan (1993a) also applies learning theory to explain how the emotionally vulnerable individual develops self-destructive behaviors to obtain a nurturing response from the invalidating environment. As the behaviors escalate, they are intermittently reinforced, making them very difficult to unlearn.

The most egregious example of an invalidating environment would be one involving sexual abuse, physical abuse, or neglect. Besides being a clear example of invalidation of the child's needs, the experience of childhood abuse and neglect is often characterized by much inconsistency and conflict as the child experiences both nurturing and abuse/neglect from the same caretaker. Given the high prevalence of reported childhood abuse among individuals with BPD (Brodsky et al. 1995; Herman et al. 1989; Ogata et al. 1990), the biosocial theory maintains that abuse cannot be ignored as contributory to the etiology of BPD. Nor is abuse thought to have been present in all individuals who develop BPD. Less explicit forms of invalidation such as repeated dismissal or denial of a child's emotional experience and reinforcement of maladaptive coping mechanisms can also lead to severe impairment in self-regulation (Stanley and Brodsky 2005). For example, if children who cry in response to disappointments are repeatedly told "You have nothing to cry about," the result is often not what is intended—that is, to make them feel better. Instead, if it is a frequent occurrence, children begin to mistrust their inner states and become unable to read their own emotional cues. Children begin to question whether in fact there is something to cry about and become confused about their internal sense of upset and uncertain about what they are feeling. If carried forward into adulthood, their emotional experiences remain somewhat mysterious to them. Emotions are misperceived, misread, mistrusted, and experienced as an unidentifiable jumble of upset.

It is important to note that this theoretical stance does not ascribe "weights" to how much biological vulnerability and environmental invalidation is necessary to yield BPD. If an individual has a biological predisposition to emotional sensitivity, vulnerability, and reactivity, he or she is likely to be more easily hurt. Patients with preexisting vulnerability experience hurt more deeply, react more strongly, and have a greater propensity to feel invalidated. Thus, it can be challenging to provide a validating and supportive environment for the emotionally sensitive child. Finally, it is also important to underscore the fact that this theoretical perspective awaits empirical validation. Although some research has begun to examine this theory of BPD, at this point it remains a theoretical perspective, and it may be shown ultimately that either biological predispositions or environmental factors are the overriding determinants of BPD. Nevertheless, like other forms of psychotherapy, DBT was developed from a theoretical orientation, but its techniques and applicability are not dependent on it.

Treatment Theoretical Underpinnings

DBT is a theoretically and philosophically coherent treatment, with dialectical philosophy at its core, embedded within which is behavioral science (learning principles) and Zen mindfulness practice (Linehan 1993a). These perspectives have direct applicability in the treatment techniques and the understanding of patients and their problems.

LEARNING PRINCIPLES

The predominant theoretical approach of DBT is learning principles. An exhaustive review of learning principles is beyond the scope of this review, but in brief, behaviors are understood as maintained through either operant or classical conditioning. This distinction serves to shape the way in which behavior change should be approached. If a maladaptive behavior is understood as maintained through operant conditioning, removal of reinforcers is called for. Alternatively, positive reinforcement of adaptive behaviors can be implemented. If a maladaptive behavior is maintained through respondent (classical) conditioning, loosening the connection between the conditioned and unconditioned stimuli is important.

Although learning principles are prominent in all forms of CBT, some forms of CBT emphasize the importance of, and therefore focus on, the role of cognitions. Other forms of CBT place an emphasis on behavior. For example, the CBT developed by Beck emphasizes the importance of distorted cognitions (Beck et al. 2003). Exposing and examining these faulty cognitions then becomes an important focus of the treatment. Correcting them is believed to be the pathway to change. Alternatively, DBT places a greater emphasis on emotion. Given the behavioral perspective, DBT defines cognition as behavior. DBT focuses on understanding that reinforcers maintain a maladaptive behavior and attempts to loosen the links that lead to the behavior through a variety of means. This focus does not imply that DBT never examines distorted cognitions or that Beck's CBT never examines behavioral reinforcers. Instead, CBT varies in its approach to problems, as do the variety of psychodynamically oriented psychotherapies.

DBT aims to provide increased support for patients to remain safe on an outpatient basis as well as support for the therapist working with the chronically suicidal outpatient. This goal is achieved through applying learning principles toward capability and motivation enhancement of both patient and therapist. Patient capability is enhanced through the teaching of adaptive skillful behaviors, and motivation is enhanced through the reinforcement of progress and nonreinforcement of maladaptive behaviors. For the therapist, a DBT outpatient consultation team is a source of support and guidance as well as an aid to keep the therapist focused on the treatment goals and format.

MINDFULNESS ORIENTATION

Certain aspects of Eastern philosophy are integral to DBT (Robins 2002), particularly a focus on acceptance and the importance of mindfulness practice. Linehan (1997) observed that an exclusive focus on change in behavior therapy is experienced as invalidating by traumatized or rejection-sensitive individuals, and it can result in early dropout or resistance to change within the treatment. Therefore, the DBT strategy involves acceptance of whatever is valid about the individual's current behaviors, viewing these behaviors as the patient's best efforts to cope with unbearable pain. However, Linehan (1997) also noted that ignoring the need for change is just as invalidating because it does not take the problems and negative consequences of the patient's behavior seriously. This can lead to hopelessness and suicidality. Thus, acceptance and validation are combined with change strategies. The balance of change with acceptance is one of the most unique aspects of the dialectical approach (described in the next section) and is solidly based in the Zen mindfulness perspective. Change is achieved through the tension and resolution of this essential conflict between acceptance of individuals as they are right now and the demand that they change. Thus, the dialectical strategy encourages cognitive restructuring from an "either/or" to a "yes/and" perspective—directly addressing the dichotomous thinking that is characteristic of individuals with BPD and that often leads to maladaptive behaviors (Linehan 1997).

Mindfulness practice teaches controlling the mind to stay in the present moment without judgment. This practice is extremely useful in helping patients remain in the present rather than focusing on past worries or future fears. As patients fight urges to hurt themselves, mindfulness practice is useful in helping them distract themselves from urges, and it ultimately helps them to reduce the intensity of their urges.

DIALECTICAL APPROACH

DBT is based on a dialectical perspective representing a reconciliation of opposites by arriving at a synthesis of these opposites. A dialectical worldview is the overarching perspective in DBT and is manifest in the strategies and assumptions of the treatment. Therapists create a balance between accepting the patients' dysfunctions and helping patients modify their thinking and behavior. The dialectical philosophy leads to the following assumptions that underlie DBT. The first explicit assumption is that patients are doing the best they can. At the same time, patients want to improve, but they need to do better, try harder, and be more motivated to change. A second assumption is that patients may not have caused all of their own problems, but they have to solve them anyway. An additional assumption is that patients cannot fail in therapy; rather, if failure occurs, it is the treatment that fails (Linehan 1993a, 1997).

These philosophical assumptions serve to enhance motivation and inform the therapeutic stance at all times (Cialdini et al. 1975; Freedman and Fraser 1966). For example, the first assumption encourages a nonjudgmental approach and discourages negative thinking on the therapist's part in the face of ongoing difficult patient behavior. The second assumption validates the need for change, without blame or judgment, and promotes effective problem solving. Furthermore, it also underscores the belief that the therapist cannot save the patient—the patient must do most of the work with the help of the therapist. The therapist's role is to encourage self-care rather than to take care of the patient. If the patient does not make progress, gets worse, or drops out of treatment, the burden of the failure is assumed by the therapy— that is, that the therapy was not successful in

enhancing motivation, and it removes blame from the patient regarding lack of motivation. This approach is particularly helpful to patients who experience tremendous, crippling self-blame that can inhibit taking chances and extending themselves in both therapy and life generally.

TREATMENT COMPONENTS: A TWO-PRONGED APPROACH

DBT consists of two components in which patients participate: individual psychotherapy and group skills training. This approach derives from a point of view not only that individuals need to understand their maladaptive patterns of behavior as they occur in individual psychotherapy but that they also have certain deficits that can best be overcome by developing a means of compensation and skills. These patients often report that they know *why* they "do what they do" but they "do not know what to do instead" or how to get themselves to do what they know they should do. Although the first half of this statement may be only partially correct, the second half is almost always true. A two-pronged approach to treatment acknowledges this problem by adopting a stance that patients may need to be taught coping strategies and skills in a more explicit manner than is typically done with patients who have personality disorders. Thus, this approach suggests that both an understanding of maladaptive patterns of thinking and behavior and skill development are useful in treating patients with personality disorders. Personality disorders are seen, in part, as deficits in certain skill areas that prevent the person from behaving in an effective manner. In addition to these two forms of patient contact, a consultation team for DBT therapists is considered an integral aspect of the treatment.

Individual Therapy

Patients attend at least one, sometimes two, individual therapy sessions of 50–60 minutes each week. Double sessions of 90–110 minutes can be utilized (Linehan 1993a). Although not always possible, it is desirable to have the flexibility to alter session lengths depending on the patient's needs and the task at hand. For example, patients who have difficulty opening up or who have trouble closing up at the end of sessions may benefit from longer sessions for a period of time until they develop the capacity to transition in and out of sessions. Also, there are times when the type of treatment work benefits from longer sessions. When conducting trauma exposure sessions, longer session lengths are required. Alternatively, some patients have difficulty tolerating the intense closeness that can be experienced in individual treatment for more than brief periods of time. While this capacity to tolerate closeness is being worked on with the patient, allowing briefer sessions avoids premature termination.

The individual therapy session is structured by the treatment hierarchy and a number of behavioral techniques. Any life-threatening behaviors (target 1) are the top priority and must be addressed within an individual session if they have occurred. Therapy-interfering behaviors (target 2) are the second in priority and are the first priority in the absence of life-threatening behaviors. As long as target 1 and 2 behaviors are either absent or addressed within a session, quality-of-life issues may also be targeted within any given session. The patient is required to keep a daily record of behaviors, level of misery, and suicidal ideation on what is called a *diary card* (Linehan 1993b) (described in more detail later). Therapist and patient review the diary card together and use it to create an agenda for the session. If the patient engaged in self-injury, a behavioral analysis (described later) is required.

Skills Training

Skills training is generally based on learning theory and utilizes behavioral principles such as shaping, modeling, repeated prac-

tice, behavior rehearsal, homework, and reinforcement of socially appropriate behaviors. Behavior change is facilitated by the combination of the direct instruction of information, modeling of behaviors by role models, prompting of specific behaviors, and positive reinforcement of successive approximations toward the desired goal. The specific goal or behavior to be changed will differ depending on the patient's presenting problem. The teaching of skillful behaviors with which to replace the maladaptive ones is a major component of capacity enhancement in DBT. Attending a weekly skills training group in which skills are taught within a didactic framework, preferably by a therapist other than the individual therapist, is an essential component of the treatment. The group serves to introduce and teach the concepts of skills, and it provides an opportunity to interact with other patients who are also learning skills. A skills training manual (Linehan 1993b) describes the skills and how to teach them and contains worksheets and homework assignments to facilitate learning. In vivo skills coaching is conducted in such a way as to enhance patient capability and motivation.

The first step in the process of skills training is the assessment of the skill deficit, which in DBT takes place in the individual therapy session. Once the specific deficit has been identified, skills training may be implemented. Direct instruction on the skill to be learned begins the training. This instruction gives the patient the required knowledge to perform the skill. Next is modeling, by the therapist or skills trainer, of the skill behavior to be learned. Modeling has many functions for the patient (Spieglar and Guevremont 1998). First, it teaches the patient a new behavior through observation of a model. Second, the patient is prompted to perform a behavior after observing a model engage in the behavior. Third, the patient is motivated to engage in similar behavior after observing the favorable consequences it receives, which is the concept of *vicarious reinforce-*

Table 12–1. Dialectical behavior therapy skills training modules

I.   Mindfulness
     A. Focus on the moment
     B. Awareness without judgment

II. Distress tolerance
     A. Crisis survival strategies
     B. Radical acceptance of reality

III. Emotion regulation
     A. Observe and identify emotional states
     B. Validate and accept one's emotions
     C. Decrease vulnerability to negative emotions
     D. Increase experience of positive emotions

IV. Interpersonal effectiveness
     A. Assertiveness training
     B. Cognitive restructuring
     C. Balance objectives with maintaining relationships and self-esteem

ment. Lastly, after observing a person who is serving as a model safely engaging in the anxiety-provoking behavior, the patient's anxiety is decreased.

After the skill has been modeled for the patient, it is the patient's turn to perform the behavior, often referred to as *behavior rehearsal.* The first step is prompting or reminding the patient to perform a behavior. Next is the process of shaping, which is the reinforcing of components of the target behavior that are successively closer approximations of the actual target behavior. Feedback is given to the patient regarding success, and there is reinforcement of the behavior results. After the skill has been rehearsed or practiced, the patient is then asked to participate in a roleplay situation that requires use of the skill. Outside of skills training sessions, patients may be asked to complete homework assignments that will require more use of the skill. Eventually, this repeated practice will lead to mastery of the targeted skill or behavior.

Linehan (1993b) outlined four specific skills training modules that target the four areas of dysregulation of BPD: mindfulness skills address cognitive dysregulation, distress tolerance skills address behavioral dysregulation, emotion regulation skills address affect dysregulation, and interpersonal effectiveness skills address dysregulation of interpersonal relationships (Table 12–1).

Although the modules were developed for BPD, they have broad applicability to other problems and disorders, such as avoidant, dependent, and paranoid personality disorders (Stanley et al. 2001). The individual modules have been designed to remedy a specific dysfunction; however, they reinforce each other, thus creating a comprehensive treatment of the "whole patient."

The first module is core *mindfulness* skills training, which focuses on dysregulations of self and cognition. Mindfulness skills are based on Eastern Zen Buddhist principles. Patients are taught techniques for focusing their thoughts and attention on the present, establishing attentional control, and coupling awareness with nonjudgmental thinking. The goal is to help the patient establish a lifestyle of mental awareness and inner connectivity.

The second module is *distress tolerance* skills training, which focuses on teaching skills to help the patient tolerate and deal with problems such as impulsivity and suicidal ideation. The fundamental goal of this module is learning the skills of both distracting from a distressing situation and accepting situations when they cannot be changed. Distress tolerance skills focus on how to live through a crisis situation without engaging in destructive behaviors. Crisis survival strategies include self-soothing and distracting techniques, pro-and-con analyses, and strategies for accepting reality rather than fighting it.

The third skill module is *emotion regulation,* which teaches the necessary skills to control dysregulated experiences and expressions of anger, anxiety, fear, and depression as well as dysregulated positive emotions such as love and joy. Emotion regulation skills include observing and identifying emotional states and validating and accepting one's emotional reactions. There are also techniques for decreasing vulnerability to negative emotions and increasing the experience of positive emotions.

Finally, the fourth module is *interpersonal effectiveness* training, which exposes borderline patients to effective strategies for mending interpersonal conflict. Interpersonal effectiveness skills incorporate assertiveness training techniques with cognitive restructuring. Patients are encouraged and taught to challenge distorted cognitions related to interpersonal interactions and to identify and stay mindful of their goals within these interactions. They learn techniques for effectively making requests or saying no to unwanted demands and balancing their objectives with maintaining relationships and self-esteem.

Case Example

Ms. K is a highly intelligent 28-year-old woman working as a secretary and studying for her bachelor's degree. She lives with her boyfriend of 6 years; the two were in couples therapy seeking help in deciding whether to get married. Ms. K was referred by the couples therapist to individual therapy for the treatment of binge-eating disorder: the patient's obesity and out-of-control binge eating were interfering with the couple's sex life. During the course of individual psychotherapy, it became apparent that the patient was exhibiting symptoms of BPD that were contributing to the primary difficulties in her relationship with her boyfriend. Her binge eating was an impulsive behavior that was often triggered by fears of abandonment, feelings of emptiness, and identity diffusion, and the binge eating was a self-soothing mechanism for feelings of uncontrollable rage. The patient was also having difficulties in her relationships with supervisors at work due to a tendency to idealize, and then devalue, those in authority and to feel used and victimized and view the supervisors with suspicion when under

stress. The individual therapist identified the need for the patient to develop more skillful coping mechanisms to replace the binge eating and impaired interpersonal functioning and referred her for adjunct DBT skills training. Although Ms. K was not initially interested in changing her interpersonal behaviors, because she viewed her difficulties with her supervisors as external to herself, she was highly motivated to gain control over her eating and agreed to undergo skills training.

Ms. K immediately took to the skills training. She found the mindfulness skills extremely helpful in allowing her to observe and describe urges to binge, which gave her increasing control over her eating behaviors. She learned distress tolerance skills that helped her distract from and also tolerate the feelings of anger and emptiness without resorting to binge eating. She was able to use the support of the other group members to observe her interpersonal patterns, and she became more willing to try new ways of interpreting the behaviors of others. She described it thus: "Mindfulness skills helped me more clearly distinguish between my thoughts and behaviors in an interpersonal interaction and what the contribution of the other person was."

STAGES OF TREATMENT AND TREATMENT HIERARCHY

DBT has four stages of treatment. Stage 1 specifically targets the reduction of life-threatening behavior and is therefore the most researched and of particular interest to clinicians who treat the chronic suicidality of BPD patients on an outpatient basis. Within the context of treating self-injury, other behavioral, interpersonal, cognitive, and emotional difficulties are also addressed. These include behaviors that interfere with the therapy and interpersonal difficulties. Once a patient has control over self-injurious behaviors, the patient enters into stage 2. Stage 2 in DBT helps patients increase emotional experiencing. Because many individuals with BPD have a history of childhood abuse (Brodsky et al. 1995; Herman et al. 1989), exposure-based procedures are used to treat the residue of childhood trauma (Foa 1997). Other quality-of-life issues, such as self-actualization in social and vocational arenas, become the target of treatment during stage 3. Finally, stage 4 treatment focuses on increasing joy and a sense of completeness and connectedness.

HIERARCHY OF TREATMENT GOALS

A standard hierarchy of goals is built into stage 1 DBT (Table 12–2). The primary goal is the reduction of life-threatening behaviors. The first task of the clinician is to establish a commitment from the patient to accept this hierarchy of goals, particularly the primary one of reducing self-injury. The sessions in which this commitment is negotiated are considered the pretreatment phase.

A second goal in stage 1 is the reduction of therapy-interfering behaviors. Such behaviors include lateness, missed sessions (of individual and/or skills groups), failure to keep a diary card (described later), and any other behavior on the part of the patient or therapist that interferes with the therapy. The third goal is the reduction of quality-of-life-interfering behaviors, such as interpersonal difficulties and personal and vocational functioning.

Table 12–2. Hierarchy of dialectical behavior therapy goals in stage 1

1. Reduction of life-threatening behaviors

2. Reduction of therapy-interfering behaviors

3. Reduction of quality-of-life-interfering behaviors

Case Example

Ms. L is a 28-year-old, single white woman living with two roommates in a major metropolitan area. She was referred to DBT from a day program she had been attending for 3 months following hospitalization for a suicide attempt. The suicide attempt consisted of a serious overdose of her roommate's benzodiazepines, which Ms. L took impulsively after an argument with her boyfriend. She had lost consciousness, was found by her roommate, and was taken to the emergency department where she received gastric lavage. She regained consciousness after a few hours, and other vital signs were not affected.

At the time of the attempt, Ms. L was taking art courses and looking for a position as an office worker. In the past, after graduating from college, she had worked as an administrative assistant at a bank for about 2 years until she became depressed, somewhat paranoid, and angry. She would miss work frequently and get into altercations with coworkers when she was there. As she described it, "I stopped coming to work because I felt as if my boss was deliberately trying to give me a hard time." She was referred to DBT because she had been diagnosed with BPD and was intermittently suicidal. She experienced suicidal ideation, she occasionally engaged in self-injury consisting of cutting her inner arm without intent to die, her mood fluctuated from depression to anger to feelings of emptiness, and she had interpersonal difficulties due to increased guardedness and suspiciousness when she was under stress. She reported a severe history of repeated sexual abuse at the hands of her stepfather between the ages of 8 and 12. When drunk he would enter her room at night and would frighten her into having intercourse and remaining quiet about it. This abuse ended when her mother and stepfather divorced. Ms. L suspected that her mother knew about the abuse but was uncertain that this was the case. She developed an inability to trust her own perceptions and had a very conflicted relationship with her mother, whom she perceived as weak and in need of protection. Ms. L had a treatment history of not regularly attending therapy and not remaining with one particular therapy treatment for more than a few months. She reported on intake that she had never found therapy very helpful and never felt that she could allow herself to trust a therapist to understand or help her.

Following the DBT hierarchy, the therapist identified treatment goals with Ms. L. Target 1 was the reduction of life-threatening behaviors. For Ms. L, these were suicide attempts in the form of overdoses, nonsuicidal self-cutting behaviors, and suicidal ideation. Target 2 was the correction of treatment-interfering behavior; Ms. L needed to attend therapy and skills training group sessions consistently and on time and with diary card and skills homework prepared. Target 3 would attend to quality-of-life issues—in this case, finding and maintaining employment.

The main challenge was to obtain Ms. L's commitment to the goal of reducing self-injury. From the patient's perspective, the self-injury was not problematic. She would vacillate between feeling that "having to live with the horrible feelings and memories is just too much to bear and suicide feels like the only way out" and feeling that "I don't think I will do something stupid like that [overdosing on pills] again; I'm not suicidal anymore." Her stated goal for treatment was to work through her childhood trauma, which was the main cause of her unhappiness and hopelessness.

Every time the therapist asked Ms. L to commit to the goal of reducing her self-injury, she would respond, "You just don't get it," start crying, and withdraw from interaction. Ms. L was experiencing the focus on change of her behavior as invalidation of her trauma history. Thus, the therapist implemented the "foot in the door" rather than the "door in the face" techniques. This intervention required a major focus on validation—of the pain, the

hopelessness, and the horror of her childhood abuse.

The use of validation strategies over a number of sessions allowed Ms. L to feel that the therapist understood the disruption that her trauma history caused her in all areas of her life, despite the insistence on reducing her self-injury. The therapist explained that she was very interested in working with Ms. L on healing from the trauma. However, Ms. L needed first to be able to control the life-threatening behaviors and increase her adaptive coping strategies for dealing with the painful feelings surrounding the trauma. Ms. L and the therapist eventually made a commitment to work together to reduce her self-injury.

Consistent attendance to therapy was identified as a second goal of treatment. Finding employment would be a third, a quality-of-life goal that they would work toward in the absence of self-injury or therapy-interfering behavior. Although Ms. L agreed to focus on reduction of self-injury as the primary goal, the therapist agreed to balance this focus with understanding that the suicidal feelings and self-injury were validations of Ms. L's pain. Several times during the course of Ms. L's treatment she would miss a session only to return and insist that she needed to focus on the trauma and not on the reduction of her self-injury. Later analysis revealed that she had felt invalidated by too strong an emphasis on change in the previous session. At these times, the commitment needed to be revisited on both sides: Ms. L's commitment to reducing her behaviors, and the therapist's commitment to balancing change with validation.

This case demonstrates the DBT treatment hierarchy and how it is implemented when working with patients. In Ms. L's case, the patient was experiencing an overwhelming number of problems simultaneously. Having a treatment hierarchy provided both the patient and the therapist with a "road map" for the treatment and helped to prevent the continual "putting out of fires" that can characterize many treatments with BPD individuals. This latter approach often comes at the expense of working on longer-term goals and issues that will equip the individual for leading a more functional and independent life.

MAJOR TREATMENT TECHNIQUES AND STRATEGIES

A broad range of techniques is employed in DBT. An exhaustive review is beyond the scope of this chapter. Instead, in this section we give some examples of the major tools and techniques to give the reader a sense of how the treatment is conducted.

Behavioral Analysis

A major change technique used in the individual session is the step-by-step behavioral analysis of self-injurious or therapy-interfering behaviors. The dialectical approach to behavioral analysis is unique to DBT. This approach involves identifying the vulnerability the patient brings to the situation, the precipitating event, and the reinforcing consequences of the self-injurious behavior. The positive consequences for the patient, such as immediate relief from unbearable emotional pain, are highlighted and validated. The patient and therapist then collaborate in reconstructing the series of events (thoughts, feelings, actions, and environmental events) that led to the self-injury. The therapist asks for as much detail as possible and weaves solutions or alternative skillful behaviors the patient might have used into the thread of the analysis. Behavioral analysis is a useful tool for gaining understanding into the emotional and behavioral events that lead to an unwanted behavior and for generating specific solutions. It is also built into DBT as an aversive consequence of the maladaptive behavior. The expectation of spending a good portion of the next therapy session involved in a painstaking analysis of a self-injurious act often serves as a deterrent.

Crisis Management, Coaching, and Intersession Contact

Therapist availability between sessions is critical when treating suicidal patients. In DBT, in vivo skills coaching is conducted by the individual therapist to provide the necessary support for learning new behaviors "in the moment." Patients are encouraged to call or page individual therapists between sessions when they are fighting urges to self-injure and require help in implementing a substitute skillful behavior. During these phone contacts, the therapist and patient decide on a number of skillful ways of handling the current stressful situation. Skills coaching through phone consultation is also a strategy for encouraging the generalization of skillful behavior to other life situations.

Rather than resulting in constant calling by the patient, phone contacts are focused and limited to skills coaching and relationship repair. If the patient calls but is not really interested in problem solving, the therapist indicates availability when the patient is interested in skills coaching and quickly ends the contact. If skills coaching is agreed on, therapist and patient quickly review which skills the patient has already tried, and the therapist "cheerleads" and helps the patient generate a plan to try new skills. The therapist praises the patient for calling and validates the difficulty of tolerating the pain and trying a new behavior. These contacts are generally brief and goal directed, often result in the prevention of self-injury, and therefore are positively reinforcing for the therapist (if not the patient).

The 24-hour rule of DBT states that patients cannot call the therapist for 24 hours after they have engaged in self-injury. This rule does not apply to scheduled appointments. If a patient calls the therapist after the fact, the therapist, once ascertaining that the patient is safe from further self-harm, expresses regret that they cannot speak for the next 24 hours. The therapist wishes out loud that the patient had called sooner so he or she could have received skills coaching and support. The therapist then expresses the desire to hear from the patient as soon as the 24-hour period is past. Thus, patients are encouraged to call before they engage in self-injurious behavior, giving the therapist a chance to intervene. The rationale for this rule is to avoid reinforcement of life-threatening behavior and to provide the opportunity for reinforcement of appropriate help-seeking behavior.

If a patient uses between-session contact inappropriately and begins to burn out the therapist, it is addressed as a therapy-interfering behavior—addressed by conducting behavioral analyses, generating solutions, and applying skills to the reduction of the behavior.

Case Example

Ms. M is a 24-year-old female with a history of more than 20 brief psychiatric hospitalizations for suicidality. In response to her distress, Ms. M often takes overdoses of available medications and then goes or is taken to the emergency department. These visits usually result in hospitalization, which Ms. M finds both helpful (because it gives her a rest from the troubles of her life) and disruptive (because of the negative reactions of family and friends and because she misses work and other responsibilities). Ms. M expressed a desire not to be hospitalized anymore. The therapist suggested that developing a safety plan would help in the short term while skills and strategies were being developed to handle distress.

About 6 months into Ms. M's treatment, she paged her therapist on a Sunday morning because she had taken a "handful" (10–12) of pills to help her calm down after being very upset by an interaction with her boyfriend. The patient said she could not remember exactly which pills she took. It is important to note that although the "24-hour rule" emphasizes the importance of asking for help prior to engaging in a self-injurious behavior, the safety of the patient is evaluated and a safety plan is developed at any point that the patient

contacts the therapist. Ms. M's boyfriend had called her at the last minute the previous evening to cancel their plans because he wanted to see a friend first and then meet later. She became very angry with him and told him not to bother coming at all. She then felt very lonely and guilty that she had yelled at him. She became agitated, lying awake all night thinking that he would leave her. She then took the pills to help her get to sleep.

The therapist reminded the patient that it might have been helpful to page the therapist before taking the pills, evaluated the patient's current safety, and determined with the patient that she should go to the emergency department to get a medical evaluation. Ms. M expressed a desire to be admitted to the hospital because she was tired and needed a rest. She stated that she did not really want to kill herself but was not sure she could prevent herself from taking pills again and that she wanted to go to the hospital to "get away from things" and have a rest. The therapist validated her feelings of wanting a rest but also reminded her of all that they had been working on and expressed the wish that Ms. M would stay out of the hospital so that they could have their outpatient appointment the next day. The therapist offered to do whatever she could to help the patient tolerate staying out of the hospital and not resort to taking another overdose. The therapist reminded Ms. M that it was her choice whether to present herself to the emergency department as in need of hospitalization. The therapist encouraged Ms. M to call from the emergency department so that the therapist could either coach her to stay out of the hospital or engage the hospital staff to make them aware of the treatment goals.

Ms. M called as requested—she had been medically cleared but still wanted to be hospitalized for a rest. The therapist spoke with emergency staff and asked them to evaluate her suicidality. The therapist also encouraged them to make their decision to hospitalize based on the current level of suicidality rather than the patient's desire to be hospitalized. The therapist indicated that she would be willing to see Ms. M the next day as an outpatient and work with her to keep her safe outside the hospital. Ms. M called later that day, complaining that the emergency staff had made her wait 10 hours and she just wanted to go home. The therapist let Ms. M know that she was looking forward to seeing her the next day for their appointment.

This case illustrates how a DBT approach works both to ensure the safety of a potentially suicidal patient in crisis and to encourage the patient to stay out of the hospital and continue building a life worth living. This vignette also describes the way in which DBT encourages managing the contingencies in the environment (working with the emergency department staff) in order not to reinforce less skillful behavior and to promote more skillful behavior (i.e., encouraging Ms. M to figure out a way to control her suicidal urges and to stay out of the hospital and resume outpatient therapy).

Diary Cards

Patients use diary cards to keep track of all target 1 problems (life-threatening and self-injurious behaviors as well as behaviors that have an impact on target 1 problems) on a daily basis. Some examples of these problems might be overall mood, use of nonprescribed substances, urges to self-injure, and adherence to medication regimens. In addition, the therapist and patient decide together about any other important behaviors, urges, and feelings to track. These may include eating disorders, urges to physically hurt other people, and impulsive behaviors such as shoplifting.

The diary card serves as the means for setting the session agenda and is reviewed with the patient at the outset of each session. These cards are particularly useful for patients who experience frequent episodes of dissociation or who tend to remember only what happened in their current mood states. The cards are also helpful for patients who

feel a great deal of shame about their behaviors. If the shameful behaviors are not recorded on the card, patients often feel too embarrassed to bring them up. Surprisingly, although some patients do not record all relevant behaviors and urges on the cards, it seems easier for patients to be truthful and record these items on the cards than to take the initiative of bringing up these behaviors and urges in a session. Diary cards jog the memory of patients and often result in having available information that would never have been brought up or recollected.

VALIDATION

Validation is a strategy that is used in many forms of psychotherapy including supportive, psychodynamic, and client-centered therapies. Linehan (1993a) presented the essence of validation in the context of DBT psychotherapy: "The therapist communicates to the client that her responses make sense and are understandable within her current life context or situation. Validation strategies require the therapist to search for, recognize, and reflect to the client the validity inherent in her response to events" (p. 223). Validation is at the core of the acceptance/change dialectic and is a crucial aspect of the therapeutic approach in DBT. Linehan therefore delineated five levels of validation: 1) listening and observing; 2) accurate reflection; 3) articulating the unverbalized; 4) validating in terms of sufficient, but not necessarily valid, causes; 5) validating as reasonable "in the moment."

Validation is much less frequently utilized in CBT. In DBT, discussions of the patient's emotional experiences, suffering, and difficulty with changing are some of the occasions for using validation. The basic function of validation is to communicate to patients that their responses are understandable and make sense within their current life situation or context (Linehan 1993a). Validation should never be patronizing, and it should never validate that which is invalid. Validation is composed of three steps: 1) active observing of what the patient is reporting; 2) reflection of the patient's feelings, thoughts, and behaviors in a nonjudgmental and nonauthoritarian manner, whereby the therapist phrases the reflection not as a pronouncement but more as a question; and 3) direct validation of the validity and "understandability" of the patient's response.

Balancing Change and Acceptance

There is an ongoing focus on maintaining a balance between change and acceptance strategies within each intervention and over the course of the treatment. Validation and acceptance without a change focus can lead to demoralization that things will never be any different. An approach that focuses too intensely on change can make a patient feel poorly understood and criticized. This effect, in turn, can increase a patient's self-blame and lead to early treatment dropouts.

Consultation Team

An assumption of DBT is that therapists treating suicidal individuals with BPD also need support. An integral aspect of DBT is the role of the consultation team to which therapists can bring any problems they are experiencing with their patients. The consultation team assumes a dialectic stance and provides both suggestions and support. In addition, the team provides a valuable function of helping therapists stay on track and follow the treatment hierarchy as prescribed. It is important to note that this consultation team is more similar to a supervision team than a patient's "treatment team." In the DBT model, team members in a day hospital or an inpatient setting tend not to have meetings jointly with the patient in order to avoid "splitting" or to avoid presenting a unified front to patients—

which can be experienced as overwhelming and intimidating to patients. Instead, each staff member's experience with the patient is treated as valid and a synthesis of their experiences is sought. Furthermore, staff members are treated in the therapy as any other person in the patient's life. Therefore, instead of intervening and talking to the other staff member about a patient's complaint or upset, the therapist coaches a patient in how to handle the complaint directly with the staff member. For example, if a patient in DBT complains bitterly to the therapist that the psychiatrist is often late to appointments and the patient finds it enraging, the therapist's first approach is to help the patient express the feelings about the lateness directly to the psychiatrist rather than the therapist discussing it with the psychiatrist.

Efficacy Data

DBT was originally tested in a randomized, controlled clinical trial (Linehan et al. 1991, 1993, 1994; Shearin and Linehan 1992). The 1-year DBT treatment compared with treatment as usual showed significant effects in three areas: 1) suicidal behavior and self-mutilation, 2) maintenance in treatment, and 3) amount of inpatient treatment. DBT subjects engaged in significantly fewer self-injurious acts than treatment-as-usual subjects. This effect was most marked in the first 4 months of treatment. DBT patients also had significantly fewer severe self-injurious acts, in terms of medical consequences, than treatment-as-usual patients. Also, DBT patients had greater retention in individual therapy compared with treatment-as-usual patients (84% remaining in DBT treatment) and had significantly fewer days of hospitalization per person. In addition, DBT showed greater reduction in anger and improved functioning (Linehan et al. 1994). There were no group differences on measures of depression, hopelessness, suicidal ideation, or reasons for living. On 1-year follow-up, Linehan et al. (1993) found that DBT subjects had significantly fewer suicidal and self-mutilating behaviors, less anger, fewer psychiatric inpatient days, and better social adjustment than treatment-as-usual subjects.

DBT has also been tested as a 6-month treatment in two small sample studies (Koons et al. 2001; Stanley et al. 1998). Stanley et al. (1998), in a pilot study, found that individuals in DBT demonstrated decreased rates of self-injurious behavior and urges to self-injure and decreased hopelessness and subjective depression over the course of a 6-month treatment. Treatment retention was very high, with a 95% completion rate. Koons et al. (2001), in an outpatient study of female veterans with BPD, found that those in DBT had lower rates of self-injury, suicidal ideation, hopelessness, anger, and depression when compared with a treatment-as-usual group. In addition, Verheul et al. (2003) conducted a 12-month trial comparing DBT with treatment as usual in the Netherlands. This trial of 58 females with BPD found that DBT had a better retention rate and greater reductions in self-injury and other forms of self-damaging impulsive behavior. Suicide attempt rates were low in both groups and approached but did not reach significance, with 7% of the DBT group making suicide attempts compared with 26% of the treatment-as-usual group.

DBT has also been adapted for inpatient settings (Simpson et al. 1998; Swenson et al. 2001; Turner 2000). Barley et al. (1993) conducted a partial replication of DBT's efficacy in a pre/post design by showing a reduction in rates of suicidal behavior and self-mutilation incidents with DBT. Monthly rates of self-destructive behavior on an inpatient unit were compared before and after the introduction of DBT with rates on a similar general adult inpatient unit using a non-DBT treatment. Mean monthly rates of self-injurious behavior on the DBT unit were significantly lower after the introduction of DBT, whereas rates on the non-DBT unit were not significantly altered during the same time period. Therefore, DBT appears to be effective in treating the more serious behavioral aspects of BPD, namely suicidal behavior and self-mutilation. In addition, Bohus et al. (2000), in an uncontrolled inpatient trial of DBT, found that parasuicidal females with BPD showed decreased self-injury, depression, dissociation, and anxiety postdischarge. Although there are no trials of patients with other personality disorders, efficacy data have been shown for DBT with domestic violence partners (Fruzzetti and Levensky 2000) and in bulimia (Safer et al. 2001), binge eating (Telch et al. 2001), hyperactivity (Hesslinger et al. 2002), and substance use disorders (Linehan et al. 1999, 2002; van den Bosch et al. 2002). Also, adaptations and efficacy in special populations have been explored, including forensic patients (McCann et al. 2000; Trupin et al. 2002), the elderly depressed (Lynch et al. 2003), and adolescents (Miller et al. 1997; Rathus and Miller 2002). Further treatment outcome studies comparing DBT with other forms of psychotherapy and/or psychopharmacological treatment are currently under way (Linehan et al. 2006). See Scheel (2000) and Robins and Chapman (2004) for a comprehensive critical review of empirical findings regarding DBT for all disorders.

CONCLUSION

DBT is a cognitive-behavioral treatment that has demonstrated efficacy in BPD. It has also been adapted to other disorders and specialized populations. Although it has not yet been adapted to other personality disorders, it is likely to be useful in those disorders in which impulsivity and behavioral dyscontrol are prominent.

REFERENCES

Barley WD, Buie SE, Peterson EW, et al: Development of an inpatient cognitive-behavioral treatment program for borderline personality disorder. J Personal Disord 7:232–240, 1993

Beck AT, Freeman A, Davis DD: Cognitive Therapy of Personality Disorders, 2nd Edition. New York, Guilford, 2003

Bohus M, Haaf B, Stiglmayr C, et al: Evaluation of inpatient dialectical behavior therapy for borderline personality disorder: a prospective study. Behav Res Ther 38:875–888, 2000

Brodsky BS, Cloitre M, Dulit RA: Relationship of dissociation to self-mutilation and childhood abuse in borderline personality disorder. Am J Psychiatry 152:1788–1792, 1995

Cialdini RB, Vincent JE, Lewis SK, et al: Reciprocal concessions procedure for inducing compliance: the door-in-the-face technique. J Pers Soc Psychol 31:206–215, 1975

Dimeff L, Linehan M: Dialectical behavior therapy in a nutshell. The California Psychologist 34:10–13, 2001

Foa EB: Psychological processes related to recovery from a trauma and an effective treatment for PTSD. Ann N Y Acad Sci 821:410–424, 1997

Freedman JL, Fraser SC: Compliance without pressure: the foot-in-the-door technique. J Pers Soc Psychol 4:195–202, 1966

Fruzzetti AE, Levensky ER: Dialectical behavior therapy for domestic violence: rationale and procedures. Cogn Behav Pract 7:435–447, 2000

Herman JL, Perry JC, van der Kolk BA: Childhood trauma in borderline personality disorder. Am J Psychiatry 146:490–495, 1989

Hesslinger B, Tebartz van Elst L, Nyberg E, et al: Psychotherapy of attention deficit hyperactivity disorder in adults: a pilot study using a structured skills training program. Eur Arch Psychiatry Clin Neurosci 252:117–184, 2002

Kehrer CA, Linehan MM: Interpersonal and emotional problem-solving skills and parasuicide among women with borderline personality disorder. J Personal Disord 10:153–163, 1996

Koons C, Robins CJ, Tweed JL, et al: Efficacy of dialectical behavior therapy in women veterans with borderline personality disorder. Behav Ther 32:371–390, 2001

Linehan MM: Dialectical behavior therapy: a cognitive-behavioral approach to parasuicide. J Personal Disord 1:328–333, 1987

Linehan MM: Cognitive-Behavioral Treatment of Borderline Personality Disorder. New York, Guilford, 1993a

Linehan MM: Skills Training Manual for Treating Borderline Personality Disorder. New York, Guilford, 1993b

Linehan MM: Dialectical behavior therapy for borderline personality disorder. J Calif Alliance Ment Ill 8:44–46, 1997

Linehan MM, Armstrong HE, Suarez A, et al: Cognitive-behavioral treatment of chronically parasuicidal borderline patients. Arch Gen Psychiatry 48:1060–1064, 1991

Linehan MM, Heard HL, Armstrong HE: Naturalistic follow-up of a behavioral treatment for chronically parasuicidal borderline patients. Arch Gen Psychiatry 50:971–975, 1993

Linehan MM, Tutek D, Heard HL, et al: Interpersonal outcome of cognitive-behavioral treatment for chronically suicidal borderline patients. Am J Psychiatry 5:1771–1776, 1994

Linehan MM, Schmidt H, Dimeff LA, et al: Dialectical behavior therapy for patients with borderline personality disorder and drug-dependence. Am J Addict 8:279–292, 1999

Linehan MM, Dimeff LA, Reynolds SK, et al: Dialectical behavior therapy versus comprehensive validation therapy plus 12-step for the treatment of opioid dependent women meeting criteria for borderline personality disorder. Drug Alcohol Depend 67:13–26, 2002

Linehan MM, Comtois KA, Murray AM, et al: Two-year randomized controlled trial and follow-up of dialectical behavior therapy vs. therapy by experts for suicidal behaviors and borderline personality disorder. Arch Gen Psychiatry 63:757–766, 2006

Lynch TR, Morse JQ, Mendelson T, et al: Dialectical behavior therapy for depressed older adults: a randomized pilot study. Am J Geriatr Psychiatry 11:33–45, 2003

McCann RA, Ball EM, Ivanoff A: DBT with an inpatient forensic population: the CMHIP forensic model. Cogn Behav Pract 7:447–456, 2000

Miller AL, Rathus JH, Linehan MM, et al: Dialectical behavior therapy adapted for suicidal adolescents. Journal of Practical Psychiatry and Behavioral Health 3:78–86, 1997

Ogata SN, Silk KR, Goodrich S, et al: Childhood sexual and physical abuse in adult patients with borderline personality disorder. Am J Psychiatry 147:1008–1013, 1990

Rathus JH, Miller AL: Dialectical behavior therapy adapted for suicidal adolescents. Suicide Life Threat Behav 32: 146–157, 2002

Robins CJ: Zen principles and mindfulness practice in dialectical behavior therapy. Cogn Behav Pract 9:50–57, 2002

Robins CJ, Chapman AL: Dialectical behavior therapy: current status, recent developments, and future directions. J Personal Disord 18:73–89, 2004

Robins CJ, Ivanoff AM, Linehan MM: Dialectical behavior therapy, in Handbook of Personality Disorders: Theory, Research, and Treatment. Edited by Livesley WJ. New York, Guilford, 2001, pp 117–139

Safer DL, Telch CF, Agras WS: Dialectical behavior therapy for bulimia nervosa. Am J Psychiatry 158:632–634, 2001

Scheel KR: The empirical basis of dialectical behavior therapy: summary, critique, and implications. Clin Psychol Sci Pract 7:68–86, 2000

Shearin EN, Linehan MM: Patient-therapist ratings and relationship to progress in dialectical behavior therapy for borderline personality disorder. Behav Ther 23:730–741, 1992

Simpson EB, Pistorello J, Begin A, et al: Use of dialectical behavior therapy in a partial hospital program for women with borderline personality disorder. Psychiatr Serv 49:669–673, 1998

Spieglar MD, Guevremont DC: Contemporary Behavior Therapy, 3rd Edition. Pacific Grove, CA, Brooks/Cole Publishing, 1998

Stanley B, Brodsky B: Suicidal and self-injurious behavior in borderline personality disorder: the self-regulation action model, in Understanding and Treating Borderline Personality Disorder: A Guide for Professionals and Families. Edited by Gunderson JG, Hoffman PD. Washington, DC, American Psychiatric Publishing, 2005, pp 43–63

Stanley B, Ivanoff A, Brodsky B, et al: Comparison of DBT and treatment as usual in suicidal and self-mutilating behavior. Paper presented at the Annual Meeting of the Association for the Advancement of Behavior Therapy, Washington, DC, November 1998

Stanley B, Bundy E, Beberman R: Skills training as an adjunctive treatment for personality disorders. J Psychiatr Pract 7:324–335, 2001

Stanley B, Brodsky B, Nelson JD, et al: Brief dialectical behavior therapy (DBT-B) for suicidal behavior and non-suicidal self-injury. Arch Suicide Res 11:337–341, 2007

Stanley B, Brodsky BS, Wilson S, et al: Efficacy of dialectical behavior therapy and fluoxetine for suicidal behavior and self-injury in borderline personality disorder: a randomized controlled trial. In press

Swenson CR, Sanderson C, Dulit RA, et al: The application of dialectical behavior therapy for patients with borderline personality disorder on inpatient units. Psychiatr Q 72:307–324, 2001

Telch CF, Agras WS, Linehan MM: Dialectical behavior therapy for binge eating disorder. J Consult Clin Psychol 69:1061–1065, 2001

Trupin EW, Stewart DG, Beach B, et al: Effectiveness of dialectical behaviour therapy program for incarcerated female juvenile offenders. Child and Adolescent Mental Health 7:121–127, 2002

Turner RM: Naturalistic evaluation of dialectical behavior therapy-oriented treatment for borderline personality disorder. Cogn Behav Pract 7:413–419, 2000

van den Bosch LMC, Verheul R, Schippers GM, et al: Dialectical behavior therapy of borderline patients with and without substance abuse problems: implementation and long-term effects. Addict Behav 27:911–923, 2002

Verheul R, van den Bosch LMC, Koeter MWJ, et al: Dialectical behavior therapy for women with borderline personality disorder. Br J Psychiatry 182:135–140, 2003

13

Group Treatment

William E. Piper, Ph.D.
John S. Ogrodniczuk, Ph.D.

This chapter focuses on group treatment for personality disorders. Group treatment is a general type of therapy, similar to individual therapy or family therapy. Group therapies may take many different forms based on their theoretical and technical orientations. Because of the presence of multiple patients, group therapies have certain unique features that distinguish them from other general types of therapy. These unique features may facilitate or complicate the treatment of personality disorders. Similarly, personality disorders have certain features that may facilitate or complicate their treatment with group therapies.

Initially, this chapter considers these facilitating and complicating features of group therapies and personality disorders. Next, forms of group treatment that differ in format, intensity, and objectives are considered, followed by a discussion of research support for group treatments. The perceived usefulness of group treatment for each of the 10 DSM-IV-TR (American Psychiatric Associa-

tion 2000) personality disorders is reviewed, and two case examples of patients treated with one of the most powerful forms of group treatment—day treatment—are presented. Finally, a number of conclusions are offered.

GROUP FEATURES THAT FACILITATE TREATMENT OF PERSONALITY DISORDERS

Because personality disorders are serious long-term conditions that are resistant to change, powerful treatments are needed. Group treatments are capable of mobilizing strong forces for change, such as peer pressure. The group, which is sometimes referred to as a *cohesive social microcosm*, can exert considerable pressure on patients to participate. It is capable of eliciting the typical maladaptive behaviors of each patient. The other patients can observe, provide feedback, and offer suggestions for change. The patient can subsequently practice adaptive behavior. This process is commonly referred to as *interpersonal learning*. Other patients may learn through observation and imitation. Simply recognizing that other patients share one's difficulties (*universality*) and helping other patients with their problems (*altruism*) can be therapeutic. These various processes (cohesion, interpersonal learning, imitation, universality, and altruism) are regarded as powerful unique therapeutic factors of group treatment (Yalom and Leszcz 2005).

There are other facilitative features of group treatment as well. Paralyzing negative transference toward the therapist is less likely to occur in group therapy compared with individual therapy because the situation is less intimate, and strong affects such as rage are diluted and expressed toward other patients. Similarly, feedback from the therapist in the individual therapy situation may be dismissed as biased, but this is much less likely to occur in response to feedback from several peers in a therapy group. In addition, because of the variety of affects expressed by different patients, integration of positive and negative affects is facilitated.

GROUP FEATURES THAT COMPLICATE TREATMENT OF PERSONALITY DISORDERS

Group features may also produce complications. Some patients with personality disorders resent sharing the therapist and feel neglected and deprived. In the group situation, regressive behavior such as emotional outbursts, aggressive actions, or suicidal threats are more difficult to manage and contain than in individual therapy. Groups are prone to scapegoating; patients with personality disorders provide many provocations. There are a number of concerns in the group situation, relative to individual therapy, that many patients with personality disorders find troublesome, including loss of control, individuality, understanding, privacy, and

safety (Piper and Ogrodniczuk 2004). The therapist is subject to such concerns as well.

PERSONALITY DISORDER FEATURES THAT FACILITATE GROUP TREATMENT

The predominant feature of patients with personality disorders that facilitates group treatment is their strong tendency to openly demonstrate interpersonal psychopathology through behavior in the group. Compared with patients with many Axis I disorders, patients with personality disorders are more likely to demonstrate rather than describe their interpersonal problems. Although this also occurs in individual therapy, the stimuli from multiple patients precipitate pathological interpersonal behavior more intensely and quickly in group therapy. This behavior can be clearly recognized and dealt with immediately in the group. A second facilitative feature of patients with some personality disorders (e.g., dependent, histrionic, borderline) is that they are "other seeking." They tend to value the connections in the group.

PERSONALITY DISORDER FEATURES THAT COMPLICATE GROUP TREATMENT

Many of the behaviors characteristic of those with personality disorders complicate group treatment. Because these behaviors are often offensive to members of the group, they tend to weaken cohesion and distract members from working. Usually, such patients challenge the guidelines and norms that have been established in the group. Examples of antitherapeutic behaviors include minimal disclosure, excessive disclosure, scapegoating, extra-group socializing, absenteeism, lateness, and premature termination.

When a patient's antitherapeutic behaviors persist in the group over time, the behaviors may be conceptualized as roles. The persons occupying the roles are commonly labeled as "difficult" patients in the group therapy literature (Bernard 1994; Rutan and Stone 2001). These difficult patients are often those with personality disorders. Examples of difficult roles and the DSM-IV-TR personality disorders often associated with them are the silent or withdrawn role (schizoid, schizotypal, paranoid, avoidant); the monopolizing role (histrionic, borderline, narcissistic); the boring role (narcissistic, obsessive-compulsive); the therapist helper role (histrionic, dependent); the challenger role (antisocial, borderline, obsessive-compulsive); and the help-rejecting complainer role (borderline, narcissistic, histrionic). Although these roles are occupied by individual persons, they frequently express something that other patients wish to have expressed and therefore are supported by others in the group. Among the personality disorders regularly seen in outpatient groups, patients with borderline and narcissistic personality disorders are usually viewed as the most difficult to treat and manage (Leszcz 1989; Tuttman 1990). For that reason, a combination of group therapy and individual therapy is often recommended.

DIFFERENT FORMS OF GROUP TREATMENT

Forms of group treatment differ in structure (format), intensity, and objectives. Four forms can be distinguished: short-term outpatient group therapy, long-term outpatient group therapy, day treatment, and inpatient/residential treatment.

Short-Term Outpatient Group Therapy

Short-term outpatient group therapy often involves a single session per week for 20 or fewer weeks. Certain focal symptoms (e.g., depression) or behaviors (e.g., affect expression, social skills) are targeted for change.

These groups are usually not intensive in nature. They do not attempt to change the basic personality traits or personality structure that characterize personality disorders. Many examples are described in the literature, including supportive groups for patients who experience complicated grief (Piper et al. 2001) or for patients who are undergoing organ transplantation (Abbey and Farrow 1998).

Long-Term Outpatient Group Therapy

Long-term outpatient group therapy consists of one or two sessions per week for at least 1–2 years. It focuses on the interpersonal world of the patient. It is intensive in nature and over time involves confrontation and interpretation of the patient's core conflicts, defensive style, and long-term maladaptive behaviors. It attempts to change the basic personality traits and personality structure that characterize personality disorders. Long-term outpatient group therapy is regarded as an appropriate and effective group treatment for personality disorders, especially when used in combination with long-term individual psychotherapy. The latter allows stabilization of the patient and an opportunity to disclose private and sensitive information that would be difficult to reveal in the group setting initially, although over time such revelation becomes possible. This group approach assumes that over time the group comes to represent a social microcosm in which the interpersonal difficulties of the patients become vividly illustrated by the interpersonal behavior of the patients in the group. Two well-known texts that focus on long-term group psychotherapy are those of Rutan and Stone (2001) and Yalom (1995).

Day Treatment

Day treatment is a form of partial hospitalization. It is designed for patients who do not require full-time hospitalization and who are unlikely to benefit a great deal from outpatient group therapy. Day treatment patients have often had an unsuccessful course of outpatient group therapy. Patients typically participate in a variety of therapy groups for several hours each day for 3–5 days per week. The therapy groups are often from different technical orientations. For example, behavioral and cognitive interventions can be used in structured, skills-oriented groups; whereas dynamic interventions are used in unstructured, insight-oriented groups. Family and couples interventions may also be employed. Day treatment is an intensive form of therapy. Its goals include relief of symptoms, reduction of problematic behaviors, modification of maladaptive character traits, and facilitation of psychological maturation.

Several other features contribute to making day treatment a powerful treatment. First is the intensity of the group experience. Patients participate in a number of different groups each day. Second, the groups vary in size, structure, objectives, and processes. This variety provides a comprehensive approach. Third, the different groups are integrated and synergistic. Patients are encouraged to think about the entire system. Fourth, patients benefit from working with multiple staff members and a large number of other patients. Fifth, day treatment capitalizes on the traditional characteristics of a therapeutic community (democratization, permissiveness, communalism, reality confrontation). These features strengthen cohesion, which helps patients endure difficult periods of treatment. The structure of day treatment programs encourages patients to be responsible, engenders mutual respect between patients and staff, and facilitates patients' participation in the treatment of their peers. Well-known approaches to day treatment programs are described by Bateman and Fonagy (1999) and Piper et al. (1996).

Inpatient/Residential Treatment

As in day treatment, hospital inpatient wards and residential treatment centers commonly provide a variety of group treatment patient activities. Inpatient/residential treatments include admission groups, community groups, patient governance groups, insight groups, occupational therapy groups, support groups, and discharge groups. Although groups are a highly visible set of activities in acute treatment settings, they tend to be regarded as a minor part of the treatment regimen. Instead, psychotropic medications that are used to calm the patient and facilitate problem solving regarding the acute crisis are viewed as the dominant treatment. Two different approaches to inpatient treatment are described by Rosen et al. (2001).

In North America, the lengths of stay in acute hospital settings have been decreasing significantly in response to escalating costs. Today, length of stay in such settings has come to mean short-term crisis management often of a week or less. Similarly, the cost of long-term care, (e.g., several months to a year) in retreat settings that in the past provided powerful milieu therapies has become prohibitive, with many centers having closed down or greatly scaled down in size. Others have accommodated to the changing health care environment but have preserved intensive hospital interdisciplinary treatment, carried out for an average length of stay of about 6 weeks (e.g., The Menninger Clinic). Another example of residential treatment is that which occurs in some prisons. Some institutions have treatment programs for inmates with antisocial personality disorder (ASPD) who have been convicted of crimes. Some experts have objected to residential care for personality disorders on the grounds that it promotes dependency. An approach to working with patients in residential treatment groups is described by Kibel (2003).

RESEARCH SUPPORT FOR THE GROUP TREATMENT OF PERSONALITY DISORDERS

There is a striking absence of evaluative research on treatments for personality disorders. In the case of group treatments, the number of studies are few indeed. There are very few randomized clinical trials of psychosocial treatments. However, the trials that have been published provide encouraging findings. In this section, we summarize findings from several of the recent clinical trials. Outpatient group therapy studies are followed by partial hospitalization studies.

Randomized Clinical Trials

Cappe and Alden (1986) compared brief (8 weekly 2-hour sessions) behavioral group therapy with a waiting list control condition for a sample of 52 patients with avoidant personality disorder. The patients who were treated with a combination of graduated exposure training and interpersonal process training improved significantly more than patients who received only graduated exposure and patients on the waiting list. In a similar trial, Alden (1989) compared three variations of brief behavioral group therapy (10 weekly 2.5-hour sessions) with a waiting list control condition for a sample of 76 patients with avoidant personality disorder. All three treatment conditions demonstrated greater improvement than the waiting list control condition. However, the author noted that despite significant improvements, the patients did not achieve normal functioning.

Linehan et al. (1991) compared dialectical behavior therapy (DBT), which involved 2.5 hours of group skills training and 1 hour of individual therapy per week for 1 year, with regular community treatment (usually individual therapy) for a sample of 44 patients with borderline personality disorder. DBT resulted in greater reductions in symptoms and parasuicidal and dysfunctional behaviors, decreased dropouts, fewer and shorter inpatient admissions, and improved work status compared with regular treatment. However, no differences were evident on self-reported levels of depression, hopelessness, or suicidal ideation. Although useful, the authors argued that treatment of 1 year's duration was not sufficient.

Marziali and Munroe-Blum (1994) compared time-limited interpersonal group therapy, which consisted of weekly 90-minute sessions for 25 weeks and biweekly sessions for the next 10 weeks (30 sessions in total), with open-ended, weekly individual therapy for a sample of 79 patients with borderline personality disorder. All patients demonstrated significant improvement on outcome measures, with no difference between the two treatment conditions. However, both conditions suffered high dropout rates.

Piper et al. (1993) compared time-limited day treatment, which consisted of group treatment in the form of a diverse set of daily group therapies for 7 hours per day, 5 days per week, for 18 weeks, with a waiting list control condition for a sample of 120 patients with affective and personality disorders. The most prevalent personality disorders were dependent and borderline. Day treatment patients demonstrated greater improvement on a comprehensive set of seven outcome variables that included symptoms, interpersonal behavior, self-esteem, and life satisfaction. The control condition patients evidenced little improvement—that is, minimal spontaneous remission. Improvements for the day treatment patients were maintained at 8-month follow-up.

Bateman and Fonagy (1999) compared psychoanalytically oriented day treatment, which consisted of a combination of group and individual therapies for 5 days a week for a maximum of 18 months, with a standard care control condition, which consisted of infrequent meetings with a psychiatrist but no formal therapy, for a sample of 44 patients with borderline personality disorder. Day treatment patients showed significant improvements that exceeded minimal change for standard care on a variety of outcome variables, including suicide attempts and acts of self-mutilation and self-reports of depression, anxiety, general symptoms, interpersonal functioning, and social adjustment. Subsequent to discharge from day treatment, patients were provided with 18 months of psychoanalytically oriented outpatient group therapy. Following completion of this treatment regimen, these patients were compared to the treatment-as-usual patients. Day treatment patients maintained their earlier gains and in some cases improved on them (Bateman and Fonagy 2001). Five years following the completion of the outpatient group therapy, the two patient groups were compared again. The patients who received day treatment and outpatient group therapy continued to have superior performance on a number of outcome indicators, yet their general social performance remained impaired (Bateman and Fonagy 2008).

Herbert et al. (2005) compared standard cognitive-behavioral group therapy (CBGT) and CBGT with social skills training (SST) for patients with social anxiety disorder. Although the study was focused on social anxiety disorder, 75% of the sample also met criteria for avoidant personality disorder. Improvements on a variety of outcome indexes occurred for both treatments; however, significantly greater gains were made with the combination of CBGT and SST.

Blum et al. (2008) compared Systems Training for Emotional Predictability and Problem Solving (STEPPS), a 20-week CBGT for outpatients with borderline personality disorder, with treatment as usual. STEPPS differs from typical CBGT in that it teaches and trains key members of patients' support networks to use a consistent approach and language with the patient. Patients treated with STEPPS made greater improvements in impulsivity, affectivity, mood, and global functioning. However, there were no differences in suicide attempts, self-harm acts, or hospitalization.

Naturalistic Studies

Findings from a number of carefully conducted naturalistic outcome studies that focused on the group treatment of personality disorders also have been published. These tend to be pre/post, single-condition studies or studies with nonrandomly assigned conditions. These studies involved outpatient group therapy (Budman et al. 1996), day treatment (Hafner and Holme 1996; Tasca et al. 1999; Wilberg et al. 1998, 1999), and residential treatment (Chiesa et al. 2003). In general, the findings from these naturalistic studies were consistent with those of randomized clinical trials in providing evidence of favorable outcomes for patients with personality disorders, in particular those with borderline personality disorder. Most of the randomized clinical trials and naturalistic studies focused on group treatments from a psychodynamic or cognitive-behavioral orientation. A recent meta-analytic review that focused on both group and individual treatments of personality disorders from psychodynamic and cognitive-behavioral orientations concluded that both orientations were effective treatments (Leichsenring and Leibing 2003).

Clinical Reports

Clinical reports of successful group treatments of patients with personality disorders are the most prevalent type of evidence in the literature. They provide the basis for most recommendations about the suitability of specific personality disorders for group treatment. The following section reflects conclusions from a number of reviews that are based primarily on clinical reports (Azima 1993; Gunderson and Gabbard 2001; Robinson 1999; Sperry 1999). There is considerable consensus among these reviews.

FORMS OF GROUP TREATMENT FOR SPECIFIC PERSONALITY DISORDERS

Cluster A

Schizoid Personality Disorder

There is agreement that some patients with schizoid personality disorder can definitely benefit from group treatment, which involves social learning stemming from consistent exposure to other patients. Difficulties can involve passivity and silence, which may irritate other patients.

Schizotypal Personality Disorder

Group therapy may play an invaluable role in patients with schizotypal personality disorder, particularly in increasing socialization skills. Difficulties can arise if the patient's peculiarities are bizarre and difficult for other patients to tolerate. Prolonged silence can also be problematic. Preparation in individual therapy can be very helpful.

Paranoid Personality Disorder

Patients with paranoid personality disorder usually do not do well in a group because of their hypersensitivity, suspiciousness, and misinterpretation of others' comments. Feedback from other group members can be very powerful if the patient remains in the group and is receptive to feedback.

Cluster B

Borderline Personality Disorder

Group therapy can be extremely effective for borderline personality disorder patients and is often combined with individual therapy. This appears to be the case for (DBT, which includes a weekly group therapy session (Linehan et al. 1991). The group treatment is psychoeducational with an emphasis on strengthening interpersonal skills, distress tolerance/reality acceptance skills, and emotion regulation skills. (More detail about DBT can be found in Chapter 12 of this volume, "Dialectical Behavior Therapy.") In group therapy, both transference and countertransference are diffused, and thus it is more tolerable for both parties. As a result, interpretations may be better tolerated in group therapy. Nevertheless, the patient's tendency to express anger and other strong affects in an unpredictable manner can lead

to rejection and scapegoating. Such patients are very challenging to treat.

Narcissistic Personality Disorder

Group therapy for patients with narcissistic personality disorder is usually regarded as problematic. Lack of empathy, a sense of entitlement, and hunger for admiration are not engaging characteristics of this disorder. Scapegoating is common. Dropout rates are high. If the patient can be convinced to stay, much useful learning can occur. Group therapy is often combined with individual therapy.

Histrionic Personality Disorder

For those with histrionic personality disorder, group therapy can definitely be helpful. Such patients can help energize the group. However, there is a better prognosis for those with less dramatic behavior. Difficulties follow if the patient slips into the role of monopolizer or help-rejecting complainer.

Antisocial Personality Disorder

Outpatient group therapy is not suitable for patients with ASPD, although some intensive residential programs and therapeutic community programs in prisons have reported successes (Dolan 1998; Warren and Dolan 1996).

Cluster C

Avoidant Personality Disorder

Group therapy can be extremely useful for those with avoidant personality disorder because such patients are usually well motivated. Often the therapy group follows a course of individual therapy.

Dependent Personality Disorder

For patients with dependent personality disorder, group therapy is regarded as an effective treatment, and some believe that it is the treatment of choice because the patients' dependent cravings can be gratified and their overclinging can be confronted (Azima 1993). Group therapy provides many opportunities for these patients to learn to be more independent and expressive.

Obsessive-Compulsive Personality Disorder

Group therapy can be helpful for some obsessive-compulsive patients. Difficulties involve the patient's tendencies to act as an additional therapist and to be stubborn and too work oriented. This behavior usually results in resentment from the other patients.

Summary

Thus, according to the clinical literature, schizoid, schizotypal, borderline, histrionic, avoidant, and dependent personality disorders are regarded as particularly suitable for group treatment. In contrast, paranoid, narcissistic, and obsessive-compulsive personality disorders are regarded as difficult to treat. Most group treatments are contraindicated for ASPD. Although single personality disorders, such as borderline, are often addressed in the clinical literature, it is quite common for patients to meet criteria for several personality disorders (Dolan et al. 1995), and this comorbidity complicates treatment. Research evidence from the individual therapy literature has shown that the number of personality disorders a patient is diagnosed with is inversely related to favorable outcome (Ogrodniczuk et al. 2001).

The following illustration summarizes the treatment of a patient with dependent personality disorder and narcissistic traits in an intensive (7 hours per day, 5 days per week), time-limited (18 weeks), group-oriented day treatment program with a daily census of approximately 35 patients. This powerful program is fully described in Piper et al. (1996).

Case Example

Mr. N was a 50-year-old, unemployed divorcé who lived with his 75-year-old widowed mother. His father had died 7 years previously. Mr. N presented with feelings of discontent about his life. He had a pervasive feeling of having failed in his relationships and in the workplace. He was diagnosed as having a dependent personality disorder with significant narcissistic traits. He was experiencing a difficult phase of his life. At Mr. N's admission, the therapist's etiological formulation read as follows:

Patient's hereditary factors may be indicated by his father's depression at age 50. In terms of psychosocial factors, his current distress seemed to have been triggered by recent negative criticism at work and a growing perception of failure. His feelings likely intensified through unsuccessful attempts at farming, entrepreneurship, and sales. He experienced both feelings of inadequacy and rage because others were unable to recognize his special and unique qualities. The belief that he should be a strong role model seemed to start in his family of origin, where he was the eldest. His efforts to succeed were not acknowledged by either parent. There seemed to be a lack of support for expressing his opinions or making decisions. He felt controlled by his mother. Neither parent seemed receptive of his viewpoints. His unconscious life seemed dominated by negative self-images and experiences of rejection, devaluation, and control.

In relationships with women, Mr. N tried to see himself as the strongest and most deserving of attention. He perceived himself as giving to women and being there for them but avoided thinking about how much he needed from them. He was drawn to women like his mother, whom he saw as emotional, controlling, and unable to meet his needs. He dealt with these relationships in the same way his father had dealt with his mother—by being submissive and by walking away from conflicts. In so doing, however, Mr. N became resentful and furious toward women. He also acknowledged avoiding closeness with women. In his last serious relationship, 10 years earlier, he had hoped that he had found his idealized mother-figure. The woman was seen as caring, easygoing, and submissive. Mr. N felt deeply betrayed when she suddenly left after 2 years. Following this breakup, he may have had a major depression. He avoided dealing with his emotions by becoming preoccupied with pastimes such as woodwork and music. He eventually returned to another woman, his mother, where he has continued to feel controlled and neglected but was unable to recognize his conflicting needs for closeness and independence. This conflict contributed to his feelings of frustration and inadequacy.

In summary, Mr. N was described as a dependent man whose lack of self-assertion in relation to women had contributed to failure in intimate relationships. His craving for perfectly attuned attention and responsiveness to his physical and emotional needs also interfered with his relationships. The result was a growing sense of dissatisfaction with his life.

On admission to the day treatment program, Mr. N received the following DSM-IV-TR diagnostic profile:

Axis I: Phase-of-life problem
Axis II: Dependent personality disorder with significant narcissistic traits
Axis III: None
Axis IV: Negative criticism at work
Axis V: Global assessment of functioning
      Current: 60
      Highest during past year: 70

Mr. N formulated in his own words the following problem areas that he most wanted to work on in treatment: 1) Work problems: "I have failed in the past and am afraid to try again, to get back into it"; 2) Relationships: "I am afraid to get involved"; "I need a wife and a family, but I have built up walls."

Summary of Mr. N's Experience in the Day Treatment Program

Mr. N's paternalism and grandiosity emerged early in his treatment. He quickly assumed the role of giving advice to fellow patients and lending an ear to those in distress. At the same time, his difficulty identifying his own feelings and needs was evident. He frequently treated the female members of the group with a mixture of devaluation and condescension for their inability to respond to his needs in the group. He often sat next to the male psychiatrist in the large psychotherapy group but had difficulty elaborating on the possible reasons for his need to be near the male leader of the program.

The staff members and fellow patients consistently confronted him about his tendency to create distance by giving advice and by not elaborating on personal issues. He gradually became able to talk about the failures in his life and began to express feelings of hurt, anger, shame, and guilt. During the middle phase of the 18-week program, in an interview with his mother, he expressed his feelings of anger toward her for her controlling and neglectful ways. He explained his needs to separate emotionally and physically from her and for her to recognize his needs. In therapy groups, he was able to understand how his conflictual relationship with his mother had resembled his relationships with other women in his life. He began to see that his advice giving was part of a ploy to create dependency on him so that his needs and demands could be catered to. He was deeply conflicted about dependency in relation to women. Difficulty acknowledging his own dependency drove him to make women dependent on him while at the same time he resented his role in supporting them. His fear of independence interfered with his ability to assert himself with his mother and with other significant women.

During the final phase of treatment, loss issues became predominant. His youngest daughter confronted him about his emotional distance as a father. This confrontation enabled Mr. N to begin exploration of unresolved grief in relation to his own father. Not only was he faced with the loss of his father through death but also through emotional distance during his early developmental years. In the therapy groups, Mr. N began to see that his giving advice to fellow patients had been done partly in the hope that he would receive similar support and caring from the staff members and from the male psychiatrist in particular, who represented his father. He also began to recognize that his escalating and sometimes frantic demands, enacted especially with the female group members, reflected his needs for confirmation of his self-worth and the availability of someone to complete his fragmented self-image.

Outcome

At the time of his discharge, Mr. N still was living with his mother but had definite plans to move out. He did not elaborate on his intentions regarding his current girlfriend. He found a temporary job and intended to return to a career in sales. Mr. N showed considerable improvement on measures of general symptomatic distress, mood level, self-esteem, and defensive functioning. He demonstrated moderate improvements in areas reflecting sexual, family, and social functioning as well as life satisfaction. He also made significant improvements in the two problem areas identified at the beginning of treatment.

We believe that the success of Mr. N's treatment can, in part, be attributed to the basic therapeutic features of day treatment, which include exposure to multiple patients and multiple staff members in a variety of therapy groups for several hours each day over several months. The diversity of groups allows patients to begin to participate in one group in which they feel comfortable before actively participating in others. It also provides a comprehensive approach to treatment. The experience provides many opportunities for the unique features of group treatment (cohesion, interpersonal learning, imitation, universality, altruism) to have their effects. The time-limited program in which Mr. N participated created pressure to work hard in a relatively short period of time in his life.

Case Example

Ms. O was a 26-year-old, single nursing assistant who lived on her own. She sought help because of repeated destructive relationships with men and an inability to tolerate male authority figures, especially at work. A recent confrontation with a male supervisor, in which she had become extremely angry, weepy, and confused, precipitated the crisis that prompted her to seek help. At admission, the therapist's etiological formulation read as follows:

Ms. O's family of origin was divided as a result of the emotional distance between her father and mother. Mother was seen as overinvolved, dependent, and verbally abusive toward Ms. O. Her father was seen as distant and emotionally unavailable to her. She tried hard to win his approval and acceptance through the pursuit of academics and sports, but her efforts went unnoticed. Ms. O's father abandoned the family for another woman when Ms. O was age 13 years. She felt deserted and responsible for his leaving. She developed a persistent feeling of being a bad person. Unable to vent her anger and rage at her father for leaving and at her mother for letting him go, she instead became her mother's protector. At school, she was a protector of the underdog. This role continued into her adult life and into her work environment. As a result, she frequently came into considerable conflict with authority figures. There was evidence of triangulation in Ms. O's relationships in which she symbolically ended up fighting for her mother against her father. There was also a strong preoedipal pattern to her history. This pattern was manifested in the theme of destruction throughout her adult life: the self-abuse through bulimic behavior, alcohol abuse, and physical abuse by her boyfriends. Her desperation for a relationship with her father may have hidden a deep sense of emotional neglect at the hands of her inadequate mother.

In summary, Ms. O was described as an emotionally labile woman whose pervasive sense of inadequacy culminated in frequent acts of self-destruction. Her oppositional disposition toward authority figures and fear of intimacy with men often interfered with her relationships. This disposition resulted in a growing sense of instability in her mood and her relationships.

On admission to the day treatment program, Ms. R received the following DSM-IV-TR diagnostic profile:

Axis I: Bulimia nervosa, cyclothymia, alcohol dependence (in remission)
Axis II: Borderline personality disorder with significant dependent traits
Axis III: None
Axis IV: Discord with boss, discord with parents and sibling
Axis V: Global assessment of functioning
             Current: 52
             Highest during past year: 65

Ms. O formulated the following problem areas in her own words that she most wanted to work on in treatment: 1) "to be able to deal with my depression and mood swings"; 2) "to improve my relationships with others"; and 3) "to understand and stop my eating disorder."

Summary of Ms. O's Experience in the Day Treatment Program

Representative of Ms. O's functioning outside of the treatment setting, her passage through the day treatment program was stormy. Early in treatment, she demonstrated difficulty adhering to the limits defined by the therapists. She missed groups and spent considerable time counseling other patients during breaks. Within the groups, she would focus on other patients' problems rather than her own. She was openly scathing of the therapists' perceived failure to do the right thing for the patients. However, she would move in quickly to defend them when they were confronted by other patients.

Through consistent confrontation and limit setting on the part of the therapists, Ms. O began to explore her feelings of rejection and of being uncared for by her family. Ms. O found herself becoming attached to two male patients. This attachment enabled her to explore her mixed feelings toward her father and brother. She also began to consider how she had assumed the role of the bad child in her family and had been scapegoated by her brother. However, she showed considerable reluctance to be open with her feelings toward her mother.

Ms. O experienced considerable stress as she entered the termination phase of treatment. Her symptoms returned with full force as she was confronted with losing the group, a deep reminder of the loss of her family when her father left. She once again began to test the limits of the therapists' tolerance through absenteeism and counseling fellow patients outside designated group hours. The other group members confronted Ms. O about her defiant behavior and helped her recognize it as a repetition of old maladaptive patterns: she loses important people in her life because she is a "bad" person. Contained by the group, she was able to talk about her painful feelings in relation to losing the two male patients to whom she had become attached. She was also able to confront her father to let him know for the first time of her feelings of rejection. Ms. O also began to recognize that her intolerance of authority and oppositional behavior were manifestations of the conflict between her wish to be accepted and cared for and her fear of being rejected.

Outcome

Upon her discharge from the day treatment program, Ms. O returned to work but continued to experience an uneasy relationship with her supervisor. She showed moderate improvements on measures of interpersonal functioning and general symptomatic distress. She also made modest improvements in two of the three problem areas that she identified at the beginning of treatment. Regarding her bulimia, there was little improvement. It was concluded that although the groups were helpful for Ms. O, the 18-week time limit was insufficient to deal effectively with her multiple, long-standing problems. Long-term group treatment was suggested.

CONCLUSION: EVIDENCE OF EFFICACY AND EFFECTIVENESS

The number of randomized clinical trials that have been conducted to evaluate the efficacy, effectiveness, and utilization of group treatments for those with personality disorders is small, but growing and they have definitely demonstrated the benefits of the various forms of group therapy. It appears that many of the successful treatments are combinations of interventions, some of which are group treatments; for example DBT and the STEPPS treatment package. In a number of ways, the components complement each other.

It is likely that the successes that group treatments have achieved are related to unique features arising from the presence of peers in groups. Group influence is a powerful agent. It becomes even more powerful in programs such as day treatment in which patients participate in a large number of groups that focus on different aspects of the patient's difficulties and capitalize on synergistic effects (Ogrodniczuk and Piper 2001).

The primary implication of the findings from the studies reviewed in this chapter is that group therapy should be considered an effective treatment for patients with personality disorders, including those that are typically regarded as difficult to treat (e.g., those with borderline personality disorder). Selection of appropriate group therapy is not a straightforward task, becasuse many clinical research issues related to the group treatment of personality disorders are still unanswered. Important considerations include:

- The locus of the group (i.e., inpatient or outpatient; in a hospital, a residential setting, or in private practice)
- The time frame for the group (i.e., long-term or short-term)
- The theoretical paradigm of the group, which will affect the goals of the group

- The composition of the group (i.e., whether it will be a group for patients with mixed diagnoses or a homogeneous group for those with a specific disorder)
- The role of group therapy in the patient's treatment regimen (i.e., whether group therapy will be the only treatment the patient receives or part of a more comprehensive regimen that includes other interventions provided either concurrently or sequentially)

There are a number of guiding principles for the successful implementation of group therapy services for patients with personality disorder. We believe that clinicians should:

- Attend carefully to referral sources, because inappropriate referrals can be a significant burden on resources.
- Select patients with attention to optimal patient–treatment matching. The use of different groups will depend on the patient's degree of interpersonal deficit, motivations for treatment, ability to form relationships with the therapist and other group members, and aptitude for particular types of work (e.g., insight-oriented work vs. SST).
- Provide pre-therapy preparation. Group work can be difficult and is often foreign to many patients. Preparing patients for the work of the group can contribute significantly to the benefit that patients derive from the group.
- Encourage personal responsibility in the patients, given that the group is only as good as the contributions from its members.
- Facilitate patient participation in the group because passivity can lead to other problems within the group, such as scapegoating.

Successful provision of group therapy services also involves avoiding certain pitfalls that historically have plagued many programs. These include attempting to treat inappropriate patients–for example, those who are too acutely disturbed or those who are too chronically disabled to engage in therapeutic tasks. Also, attempting to treat a mixture of patients with conflicting needs in the same group can limit the benefit that patients receive from participating in the group. Predicting who will do well in group therapy, however, is never a perfect science. Some patients who are regarded as high risk inevitably surprise us and do well. Excluding all patients who do not fully meet one's selection criteria means that such patients would be prevented from receiving a beneficial treatment. We do not want to deprive all high-risk patients of an opportunity to benefit, even though we know a number of such patients will not. With further research, we can begin to develop more clear ideas about how much risk or how many high-risk patients to accept in a group. Having one or two high-risk patients in a group is far different from having many.

Personality disorders are serious long-term conditions that are resistant to change and difficult to treat. Group therapy may have unique advantages for the treatment of patients with personality disorders. It offers a level of intensiveness and containment that is unmatched in individual therapy and capitalizes on the therapeutic features of group participation (e.g., universality, thus facilitating treatment of the chronic emotional and behavioral difficulties experienced by these patients). Research increasingly demonstrates that a variety of group therapies are effective for patients with personality disorders. Yet, the research literature is insufficient for making specific recommendations regarding which types of groups (e.g., duration, orientation, setting) to offer to which types of patients. Nevertheless, clinicians should feel confident in recommending and/or providing group therapy to patients with personality disorders. Group therapy is a cost-efficient and cost-effective mental health intervention and fits well within the current service paradigm that demands more for less.

REFERENCES

Abbey S, Farrow S: Group therapy and organ transplantation. Int J Group Psychother 48:163–185, 1998

Alden L: Short-term structured treatment for avoidant personality disorder. J Consult Clin Psychol 57:756–764, 1989

American Psychiatric Association: Diagnostic and Statistical Manual of Mental Disorders, 4th Edition, Text Revision. Washington, DC, American Psychiatric Association, 2000

Azima FJ: Group psychotherapy with personality disorders, in Comprehensive Group Psychotherapy. Edited by Kaplan HI, Sadock BJ. Baltimore, MD, Williams & Wilkins, 1993, pp 393–406

Bateman A, Fonagy P: Effectiveness of partial hospitalization in the treatment of borderline personality disorder: a randomized controlled trial. Am J Psychiatry 156:1563–1569, 1999

Bateman A, Fonagy P: Treatment of borderline personality disorder with psychoanalytically oriented partial hospitalization: an 18-month follow-up. Am J Psychiatry 158:36–42, 2001

Bateman A, Fonagy P: Eight-year follow-up of patients treated for borderline personality disorder: mentalization-based treatment versus treatment as usual. Am J Psychiatry 165:631–638, 2008

Bernard HS: Difficult patients and challenging situations, in Basics of Group Psychotherapy. Edited by Bernard HS, MacKenzie KR. New York, Guilford, 1994, pp 123–156

Blum N, St. John D, Pfohl B, et al: Systems Training for Emotional Predictability and Problem Solving (STEPPS) for outpatients with borderline personality disorder: a randomized controlled trial and 1-year follow-up. Am J Psychiatry 165:468–478, 2008

Budman SH, Demby A, Soldz S: Time-limited group psychotherapy for patients with personality disorders. Int J Group Psychother 46:357–377, 1996

Cappe RF, Alden LE: A comparison of treatment strategies for clients functionally impaired by extreme shyness and social avoidance. J Consult Clin Psychol 54:796–801, 1986

Chiesa M, Fonagy P, Holmes J: When less is more: an exploration of psychoanalytically oriented hospital-based treatment for severe personality disorder. Int J Psychoanal 84:637–650, 2003

Dolan B: Therapeutic community treatment for severe personality disorders, in Psychopathy: Antisocial, Criminal, and Violent Behavior.

Edited by Millon T, Simonsen E. New York, Guilford, 1998, pp 407–430

Dolan B, Evans C, Norton K: Multiple Axis II diagnoses of personality disorder. Br J Psychiatry 166:107–112, 1995

Gunderson JG, Gabbard GO: Personality Disorders in Treatments of Psychiatric Disorders, 3rd Edition. Edited by Gabbard GO. Washington, DC, American Psychiatric Publishing, 2001, pp 2222–2368

Hafner RJ, Holme G: The influence of a therapeutic community on psychiatric disorder. J Clin Psychol 52:461–468, 1996

Herbert JD, Gaudiano BA, Rheingold AA, et al: Social skills training augments the effectiveness of cognitive behavioral group therapy for social anxiety disorder. Behav Ther 36:125–138, 2005

Kibel HD: Interpretive work in milieu groups. Int J Group Psychother 53:303–329, 2003

Leichsenring F, Leibing E: The effectiveness of psychodynamic therapy and cognitive behavior therapy in the treatment of personality disorders: a meta-analysis. Am J Psychiatry 160:1223–1232, 2003

Leszcz M: Group psychotherapy of the characterologically difficult patient. Int J Group Psychother 39:311–335, 1989

Linehan MM, Armstrong HE, Suarez A, et al: Cognitive-behavioral treatment of chronically parasuicidal borderline patients. Arch Gen Psychiatry 48:1060–1064, 1991

Marziali E, Munroe-Blum H: Interpersonal Group Psychotherapy for Borderline Personality Disorder. New York, Basic Books, 1994

Ogrodniczuk JS, Piper WE: Day treatment for personality disorders: a review of research findings. Harv Rev Psychiatry 9:105–117, 2001

Ogrodniczuk JS, Piper WE, Joyce AS, et al: Using DSM Axis II information to predict outcome in short-term individual psychotherapy. J Personal Disord 15:126–138, 2001

Piper WE, Ogrodniczuk JS: Brief group therapy, in Handbook of Group Counseling and Psychotherapy. Edited by DeLucia-Waack J, Gerrity DA, Kalodner C, et al. Beverly Hills, CA, Sage, 2004, pp 641–650

Piper WE, Rosie JS, Azim HFA, et al: A randomized trial of psychiatric day treatment for patients with affective and personality disorders. Hosp Community Psychiatry 44:757–763, 1993

Piper WE, Rosie JS, Joyce AS, et al: Time Limited Day Treatment for Personality Disorders: Integration of Research and Practice in a Group Program. Washington, DC, American Psychological Association, 1996

Piper WE, McCallum M, Joyce AS: Patient personality and time-limited group psychotherapy for complicated grief. Int J Group Psychother 51:525–552, 2001

Robinson DJ: Field Guide to Personality Disorders. Port Huron, MI, Rapid Psychler, 1999

Rosen D, Stukenberg KW, Sacks S: The group-as-a-whole relations model of group psychotherapy. Bull Menn Clin 65:471–488, 2001

Rutan JS, Stone WN: Psychodynamic Group Psychotherapy, 3rd Edition. New York, Guilford, 2001

Sperry L: Cognitive Behavior Therapy of DSM-IV Personality Disorders: Highly Effective Interventions for the Most Common Personality Disorder. Philadelphia, PA, Brunner/Mazel, 1999

Tasca GA, Balfour L, Bissada H, et al: Treatment completion and outcome in a partial hospitalization program: interactions among patient variables. Psychother Res 9:232–247, 1999

Tuttman S: Principles of psychoanalytic group therapy applied to the treatment of borderline and narcissistic disorders, in The Difficult Patient in Group: Group Psychotherapy With Borderline and Narcissistic Disorders. Edited by Roth BE, Stone WN, Kibel HD. Madison, CT, International Universities Press, 1990, pp 7–29

Warren F, Dolan B: Treating the "untreatable": therapeutic communities for personality disorders. Therapeutic Communities: International Journal for Therapeutic and Supportive Organizations 17:205–216, 1996

Wilberg T, Karterud S, Urnes O, et al: Outcomes of poorly functioning patients with personality disorders in a day treatment program. Psychiatr Serv 49:1462–1467, 1998

Wilberg T, Urnes O, Friis S, et al: One-year follow-up of day treatment for poorly functioning patients with personality disorders. Psychiatr Serv 50:1326–1330, 1999

Yalom ID: The Theory and Practice of Group Psychotherapy, 4th Edition. New York, Basic Books, 1995

Yalom ID, Leszcz M: The Theory and Practice of Group Psychotherapy, 5th Edition. New York, Basic Books, 2005

14

Somatic Treatments

Paul H. Soloff, M.D.

BASIC ASSUMPTIONS UNDERLYING PHARMACOTHERAPY IN THE PATIENT WITH PERSONALITY DISORDER

A pharmacological approach to the treatment of personality disorders is based on the effects of medications on neurotransmitter functions that mediate expression of state symptoms and trait vulnerabilities related to basic personality dimensions. In terms of neurotransmitter function, the distinction between Axis I and Axis II disorders is arbitrary. Symptoms characteristic of patients with personality disorder may be mediated, in part, by the same neurotransmitter systems as similar symptoms in Axis I disorders. For example, ideas of reference, paranoid ideation, and mild thought disorder in patients with schizotypal personality disorder may be mediated in part by the same dopaminergic neurotransmitter systems as more severe forms of thought disorder. Both respond to dopaminergic blockade with neuroleptic agents. Symptom severity may be related to other disease-specific genetic or biological differences in these disorders. For

example, schizotypal personality disorder is not the same as schizophrenia.

Pharmacotherapy in personality disorders is narrowly focused on those few dimensions that command the most clinical attention, such as affective dysregulation (e.g., labile, depressed, angry, or anxious moods), cognitive-perceptual symptoms ("psychoticism"), and impulsive aggression. These symptoms prompt urgent care because they mediate suicidal behavior, self-injury, or assault, and result in emergency department visits or hospitalization. As a result, most drug trials have been conducted in patients with borderline, schizotypal, and antisocial personality disorders.

Pharmacological interventions directed toward dimensions of personality disorders is a relatively new concept. The empirical literature, although growing, is still woefully inadequate. The work group that developed the practice guideline for treating borderline personality disorder (BPD) (American Psychiatric Association 2001) identified approximately 60 published reports on pharmacotherapy of BPD; half were randomized controlled trials (RCTs) and the rest were open-label or small sample studies. Since then, additional RCTs have been published, including new trials with second-generation antipsychotic drugs and anticonvulsants. Interpreting this literature requires an appreciation of the unique difficulties in conducting pharmacotherapy trials with personality disorder patients. Examples of these difficulties include the following:

1. Before the introduction of structured diagnostic interviews, clinician diagnoses of personality disorders were notoriously unreliable, raising questions about validity of diagnoses and generalizability of results. Some early reports used definitions of personality disorders no longer accepted in the modern nomenclature (e.g., emotionally unstable character disorder [Rifkin et al. 1972]). Structured interviews for personality disorder diagnoses, corresponding to DSM definitions, are now the accepted gold standard for randomized controlled studies.
2. By definition, personality disorders are Axis II diagnoses. Comorbidity with Axis I disorders is common and must be controlled in any research design.
3. Overlapping symptoms in definitions of Axis I and II disorders often make differential diagnosis and determination of etiology of symptoms difficult (e.g., mood instability in BPD and bipolar II disorder). The relationship between depression and BPD has generated controversy, because it is often unclear whether the depressed patient with BPD has one disorder or two (Gunderson and Philips 1991; Koenigsberg et al. 1999; Soloff et al. 1991).
4. Comorbidity with Axis II "near neighbors" is often unavoidable.
5. Because personality disorder diagnoses are defined as syndromes, there is marked heterogeneity in the symptom presentations within any given personality disorder. Target symptoms for pharmacotherapy must be quantified by standardized assessment measures tailored to specific personality disorder symptoms. For example, the Affective Lability Scale may be more appropriate than the Hamilton Rating Scale for Depression (Ham-D) when antidepressants are being used to stabilize mood fluctuations rather than to treat a comorbid major depression.

6. Symptoms in the patient with personality disorder may be stress-related and transient, resolving with time alone or with crisis intervention therapy. A placebo condition is required to control for spontaneous remission of symptoms in drug trials. The need for placebo control raises additional problems, such as patient compliance and cooperation with an extended drug trial. Impulsive-aggressive patients assigned to placebo, for example, may not complete the study (Hollander et al. 2001).
7. Measurement of efficacy against trait vulnerabilities, such as impulsive aggression, must be done in appropriately long time frames, because the base rates of targeted behaviors (e.g., assaults, suicide gestures) may be low in a short time frame.
8. Dropout rates are typically high and must be carefully considered in evaluating study results (Kelly et al. 1992). Inability to retain the patient in a therapeutic trial may be attributable to the patient's instability or the unacceptability of the treatment.

A pharmacological approach to treatment of personality disorders is symptom-specific and based on modifying neurotransmitter function in cognitive, affective, and impulsive-behavioral symptom domains. Both acute state symptoms (such as anger and anxiety) and trait vulnerabilities (such as impulsivity and dysregulated affect) are targets for treatment. Pharmacotherapy is not a primary treatment for problems of character or maladaptive interpersonal relationships, which are the focus of psychotherapy. Patients engaged in effective psychotherapy (e.g., dialectical behavior therapy [DBT]), may not require adjunctive medication; however, for the very unstable symptomatic patient, appropriate use of medication may facilitate adherence to psychotherapy. To underscore the empirical nature of this treatment, it is important to note that the U.S. Food and Drug Administration has not approved any medication for treatment of any personality disorder. All recommendations made in this chapter are based on review of empirical studies and are, by definition, off-label uses.

PHARMACOTHERAPIES

Neuroleptics

Neuroleptics have been studied more extensively than any other medication class used in the treatment of personality disorder. Randomized controlled studies have included inpatients, outpatients, and adult and adolescent patients treated with a wide variety of first-generation and second-generation (atypical) antipsychotic agents. Most of these studies have been conducted in patients with BPD and/or schizotypal personality disorder. Neuroleptic medications, used in low dosages, are the treatment of first choice for cognitive-perceptual symptoms, especially stress-related ideas of reference, transient paranoid ideas, and illusions. Neuroleptic medications are also recommended for control of anger and hostility and have some efficacy in managing impulsive aggression. Neuroleptics have a broad spectrum of effects and reduce symptom severity across all symptom domains, including affective and impulsive-behavioral symptoms.

Cognitive disturbance was the rationale for treatment in the earliest case reports and open-label trials. Patients often had both borderline and schizotypal symptom presentations. Many first-generation antipsychotic drugs were studied, including haloperidol, perphenazine, thiothixene (Brinkley et al. 1979, Hymowitz et al. 1986), thioridazine (Teicher et al. 1989), and flupenthixol (Kutcher

et al. 1995). Dosages were typically in the lower range of clinical usage. While these drugs appeared helpful in treating schizotypal symptoms, such as ideas of reference, paranoid ideation, and illusions, they also demonstrated a much broader spectrum of efficacy against depression, anxiety and anger, impulsive-behavioral symptoms, and global symptom severity.

Random-assignment, parallel comparison studies comparing two neuroleptics without placebo controls also demonstrated a broad spectrum of efficacy in patients with BPD. Leone (1982) found that loxapine succinate (mean dosage, 14.5 mg/day) or chlorpromazine (mean dosage, 110 mg/day) produced improvement in depressed mood, anxiety, anger-hostility, and suspiciousness. Serban and Siegel (1984) reported that thiothixene (mean dose [±standard deviation (SD)], 9.4 mg [±7.6 mg]) or haloperidol (mean dose [±SD], 3.0 mg [±0.8 mg]) produced improvements in anxiety, depression, derealization, paranoia (ideas of reference), and general symptoms in patients with BPD and schizotypal personality disorder. A global measure of borderline psychopathology also improved with thiothixene.

Studies involving RCTs confirmed the broad spectrum of efficacy for low-dose neuroleptics, although efficacy against schizotypal symptoms and psychoticism, anger, and hostility were most consistently noted. Goldberg et al. (1986) studied outpatients with either BPD or schizotypal personality disorder. They required each patient to have at least one mild psychotic symptom, introducing a bias toward cognitive-perceptual symptoms. Patients received thiothixene (mean dosage, 8.67 mg/day) for up to 12 weeks and reported significant improvement over placebo in psychotic cluster symptoms—specifically, illusions and ideas of reference—but also in self-rated obsessive-compulsive and phobic anxiety symptoms. The more severely symptomatic the patient was at baseline, the better the patient responded to thiothixene.

Cowdry and Gardner (1988) conducted a complex, placebo-controlled, four-drug crossover study among outpatients with BPD using trifluoperazine (mean dosage, 7.8 mg/day) as the neuroleptic condition, with each trial lasting 6 weeks. Patients were also required to meet criteria for hysteroid dysphoria, an affective syndrome defined by histrionic traits, mood reactivity, rejection sensitivity, and atypical depressive symptoms, and to have a history of extensive behavioral dyscontrol, introducing a bias toward affective and impulsive-behavioral symptoms. Those patients who were able to stay on trifluoperazine for 3 weeks or longer (7 of 12 patients) were among the best mood responders in the study, with significant improvement over placebo on physician ratings of depression, anxiety, rejection sensitivity, and suicidality.

Soloff et al. (1986, 1989) studied acutely ill inpatients with BPD defined by the Diagnostic Interview for Borderline Patients and compared haloperidol with amitriptyline and placebo in a 5-week trial. Symptom severity was an inclusion criterion, defined by a Global Assessment Scale (GAS) score of less than 50 and either a Ham-D score of 17 or greater (measuring depression) or a score of 66 or greater on the Inpatient Multidimensional Psychiatric Scale (assessing psychoticism). Patients receiving haloperidol (mean dosage, 4.8 mg/day) showed significantly more improved symptom severity across all symptom domains than those receiving placebo. Severity of schizotypal symptoms was a predictor of favorable response. In the final analysis of this study (Soloff et al. 1989), haloperidol was significantly superior to placebo on global measures, self- and observer-rated depression, anger and hostility, schizotypal symptoms, psychoticism, and actual impulsive behaviors on the ward—in effect, a broad spectrum of symptom presentations. Haloperidol was equal to amitriptyline against depressive symptoms.

A second study by the same group, using the same design but comparing haloperidol with phenelzine and placebo, failed to replicate the broad spectrum efficacy of haloperidol (mean dosage, 3.93 mg/day). BPD patients in the nonreplicating study spent less time in the hospital and were significantly less impaired (Soloff et al. 1993). At baseline, they had less schizotypal symptoms, psychoticism, and impulsive ward behavior than did patients in the first study (Soloff et al. 1989). By chance, patients randomized to haloperidol in the nonreplicating study also were more depressed than those assigned to phenelzine and had more comorbid major depressive disorder (MDD) (Soloff et al. 1993). Efficacy for haloperidol was limited to hostile belligerence and impulsive-aggressive behaviors.

Cornelius et al. (1993) followed the sample used in the Soloff et al. (1989) study in a continuation study of responders maintained on their original medication assignments for 16 weeks following an initial 5 weeks of acute treatment. Intolerance of medication over time resulted in significant noncompliance and dropout. The 22-week attrition rates were 87.5% for haloperidol, 65.7% for phenelzine, and 58.1% for placebo. Analysis of endpoint data (all subjects carried forward) revealed significant continuing improvement on haloperidol compared with placebo only in the treatment of irritability, with a trend in total hostility. Patients on haloperidol reported significant worsening in depressive symptoms over time, which was attributed in part to the side effect of akinesia. Clinical improvement was modest and of limited clinical importance. This study illustrates the difficulties of continuation treatment with high-potency neuroleptics in the patient with personality disorder.

In a 6-month study, Montgomery and Montgomery (1982) controlled for noncompliance by using depot flupenthixol decanoate 20-mg injections once a month in a study of recurrently parasuicidal patients with borderline and histrionic personality disorders. Patients receiving flupenthixol demonstrated significant decreases in suicidal behaviors by 4 months compared with the placebo group.

The introduction of second-generation neuroleptics greatly increases clinicians' options for treating the patient with personality disorder. In an open-label trial, Frankenburg and Zanarini (1993) reported that clozapine (mean dosage [±SD], 253.3 mg/day [±163.7 mg/day]) improved positive and negative psychotic symptoms and global functioning in 15 patients with BPD and comorbid Axis I psychotic disorder not otherwise specified (NOS) who had been intolerant of, or whose illness had been refractory to, other neuroleptic trials. Patients were recruited from a larger study of patients with treatment-resistant psychotic symptoms, raising the question of whether their symptoms were truly part of the Axis II disorder. Improvement was modest but statistically significant. These concerns were addressed by Benedetti et al. (1998), who excluded all Axis I psychotic disorders from a cohort of patients with treatment-refractory BPD. Target symptoms included "psychotic-like" paranoid ideation and referential thinking (which were transient and stress-related), visual illusions, hypnagogic phenomena, and odd beliefs (which "never reached a clear-cut delusional or hallucinatory quality"). Patients' symptoms had been refractory to 4 months of prior treatment with medication and psychotherapy. In a 4-month trial of 12 patients treated with clozapine (mean dosage [±SD], 43.8 mg/day [±18.8 mg/day]) and concurrent psychotherapy, Benedetti et al. (1998) reported that low-dose clozapine improved symptoms in all domains—cognitive-perceptual, affective, and impulsive-behavioral. Clozapine may also have utility in treatment of self-mutilation and aggression in Axis I psychotic patients with comorbid Axis II BPD (Chengappa et al. 1995, 1999).

Clozapine, arguably the most effective of the atypical agents, is associated with lowered white blood cell counts, jeopardizing the body's immune response—a rare but dangerous side effect. Because of this risk,

weekly white blood cell counts must be obtained for the first 6 months of treatment and biweekly thereafter for the duration of clozapine therapy. Fortunately, newer second-generation neuroleptics (e.g., olanzapine, risperidone, quetiapine, aripiprazole) are less difficult to use than clozapine and are better tolerated than first-generation agents. Open-label and RCTs are now published describing the efficacy of each of these agents in BPD or schizotypal personality disorder.

Rocca et al. (2000) reported that risperidone (mean dosage, 3.27 mg/day) produced improvement in aggression, hostility and suspicion, depressive symptoms, and overall global functioning in an open-label trial of 8 weeks' duration in patients with BPD. In an RCT, Koenigsberg et al. (2003) found that low dosages of risperidone (to 2 mg/day), compared with placebo, produced significant improvement by 3 weeks of treatment in negative and positive symptoms of psychoticism in patients with schizotypal personality disorder, sustained through a 9-week trial.

Open-label trials of olanzapine (mean dose, 9.32 mg) in patients with schizotypal personality disorder have produced improvement in measures of psychoticism (Brief Psychiatric Rating Scale [BPRS]); depressed mood (Beck Depression Inventory [BDI], Ham-D); impulsive aggression (Overt Aggression Scale [OAS]); and overall global functioning (GAS) in much longer trials of 26 weeks' duration (although only 8 of 11 patients completed the full trial) (Keshavan et al. 2004). Schulz et al. (1999) conducted an 8-week open-label, dose-finding study of olanzapine in patients with BPD and comorbid dysthymia. Patients received an average dosage (±SD) of 7.5 mg/day (± 2.61 mg/day), with a range of 2.5–10 mg. Significant improvement was reported in all global scales including general symptom severity (Hopkins Symptom Checklist–90 [SCL-90]); hostility (Buss-Durkee Hostility Inventory); impulsivity (Barratt Impulsiveness Scale); depression (BPRS, the Depression Scale of the SCL-90 [SCL-90-DEP]); and in interpersonal sensitivity, psychoticism, anxiety, and anger/hostility (SCL-90). Zanarini and Frankenburg (2001) improved on this design in a 6-month placebo-controlled, RCT study of olanzapine in patients with BPD (mean dosage [±SD], 5.33 mg/day [±3.43 mg/day]). They reported significant improvement over placebo in the areas of interpersonal sensitivity, anxiety, anger and hostility, paranoia (all SCL-90), dissociation, positive symptoms of psychoticism (Positive and Negative Syndrome Scale [for schizophrenia] [PANSS]), and global function (Global Assessment of Functioning [GAF] Scale).

In a 12-week RCT, Bogenschutz and Nurnberg (2004) found that olanzapine (2.5–20 mg/day) was superior to placebo in improving global functioning on a Clinical Global Impression (CGI) Scale modified for patients with BPD. Zanarini et al. (2004) compared three medication treatments in patients with BPD: olanzapine (mean dosage [SD], 3.3 mg/day [±1.8 mg/day]), fluoxetine (mean dosage [±SD], 15.0 mg/day [±6.5 mg/day]) and olanzapine-fluoxetine combination (mean dosage [±SD] fluoxetine, 12.7 mg/day [±5.9 mg/day] plus olanzapine 3.2 mg/day [±1.5 mg/day]). They assessed symptomatic changes in depressed mood (on the Montgomery-Åsberg Depression Rating Scale) and impulsive aggression (on the Overt Aggression Scale—Modified [OAS-M]) over an 8-week trial. While all three interventions produced some improvement, olanzapine monotherapy and the olanzapine-fluoxetine combination were superior to fluoxetine over time on both measures. Treatment with a neuroleptic alone, olanzapine monotherapy, was superior to combined antidepressant and neuroleptic medication (combination condition) in treating depressive symptoms. Fluoxetine monotherapy was associated with reductions in both impulsive aggression and severity of depression.

Soler et al. (2005) combined DBT with an RCT study of olanzapine and placebo in a 12-week trial of BPD patients with moderate to high degrees of clinical severity. Patients re-

ceiving concurrent olanzapine (mean dosage [±SD], 8.83 mg/day [±3.8 mg/day]) did significantly better than patients receiving placebo on measures of depression (Ham-D), anxiety (Hamilton Anxiety Rating Scale [Ham-A]), and impulsivity/aggressive behavior. This study allowed patients to continue psychoactive medications established prior to the study. While preexisting medication use was similar in the two groups and held constant for the 12-week trial, the presence of additional medications potentially confounds results.

Efficacy and safety data have been widely reported for the use of olanzapine in routine treatment of BPD, using oral formulations. A recent prospective observational study described the urgent use of intramuscular olanzapine (10 mg) for treatment of acute agitation in patients with BPD seen in an emergency room setting (Damsa et al. 2007). All patients had refused oral medications and 20 patients (80%) required physical restraint. Diagnostic assessments were conducted (by a separate research staff) after treatment had resolved the agitation. Symptomatic improvement, assessed on the PANSS–Excited Component (PANSS-EC) , the Agitated Behavior Scale, and the Clinical Global Impression–Severity of Illness (CGI-S) were assessed at baseline, 2 hours postinjection and 12–24 hours later. Although several patients required a second dose (5 mg), and one patient required a third dose (5 mg), statistically significant improvement occurred after 2 hours in all three assessment measures (though no further significant change occurred 12–24 hours later). Aside from asymptomatic decreases in blood pressure, there were no significant medical complications.

As newer atypical neuroleptics are introduced, offering more favorable side-effect profiles (e.g., in terms of weight gain and metabolic syndrome), they have also been assessed for efficacy in BPD. In an RCT study of aripiprazole (15 mg/day) in patients with BPD, Nickel et al. (2006) found significant improvement for drug over placebo across all scales of the SCL-90, most notably on obsessive-compulsion, insecurity in social contacts, depression, anxiety, aggressiveness/hostility, phobic anxiety, paranoid thinking, and psychoticism. Additionally, subjects on aripiprazole showed significantly greater improvement on the Ham-D and Ham-A scales and on four State-Trait Anger Expression Inventory (STAXI) scales (i.e., the same broad spectrum of effects described for earlier neuroleptic trials). Open-label trials also suggest that quetiapine may have broad spectrum efficacy in treating patients with BPD. In dosages ranging from 251 to 540 mg/day, and durations of 12 weeks, three recent open-label studies demonstrated efficacy for quetiapine on a broad spectrum of symptom measures assessing affective, cognitive, and impulsive-behavioral symptoms (Bellino et al. 2006, Perrella et al. 2007, Villeneuve and Lemelin 2005).

In these acute treatment studies, low-dose neuroleptics produced improvement in treatment trials extending from 5 weeks to 6 months. A role for low-dose neuroleptics in continuation and maintenance therapies of the patient with personality disorder has yet to be established through multiple controlled-treatment trials.

Antidepressants

Selective Serotonin Reuptake Inhibitors and Related Medications

Selective serotonin reuptake inhibitor (SSRI) antidepressants are the drugs of first choice in the treatment of both affective dysregulation and impulsive-aggressive behavior in patients with personality disorder. Symptoms of affective dysregulation include marked lability of mood (intense, reactive, angry, depressive, or anxious feelings). (Anger may be a reflection of affective dysregulation or accompany impulsive aggression. In extreme expression, anger can be expressed behaviorally as temper tantrums,

physical assaults, property destruction, or self-injury.) Rejection sensitivity and depressive "mood crashes" result from a similar disinhibition of mood. (Impulsive aggression is discussed later in greater detail.)

BPD has been studied most intensively with antidepressants because of the prominence of affective dysregulation as a major component of temperament. Mood instability, "mood crashes," and "rejection-sensitive dysphoria" are familiar clinical terms describing this trait vulnerability. Some investigators view the affective dysregulation of the BPD patient as a subclinical manifestation of an affective disorder, evidence that some variants of BPD may be part of the broader affective disorders spectrum (Akiskal et al. 1985). Reviewing the antidepressant literature, one should keep in mind that studies in which there is a lack of control for comorbid Axis I depression would be expected to demonstrate a favorable response for antidepressant treatments but may not reflect the pharmacological responsiveness of the Axis II syndrome.

Early case experience and small open-label trials with fluoxetine, sertraline, and venlafaxine (a mixed SSRI/norepinephrine uptake blocker) indicated efficacy against affective, impulsive-behavioral, and even cognitive-perceptual symptoms in patients with BPD. Aggression and irritability, depressed mood, and self-mutilation responded to fluoxetine (up to 80 mg), venlafaxine (up to 400 mg), or sertraline (up to 200 mg) in treatment trials of 8–12 weeks' duration (Cornelius et al. 1990; Kavoussi et al. 1994; Markovitz and Wagner 1995; Markovitz et al. 1991; Norden 1989). An unexpected finding in these early open-label reports was that improvement in impulsive behavior appeared rapidly, often within the first week of treatment, and disappeared as quickly with discontinuation or noncompliance (Coccaro and Kavoussi 1997). Improvement in impulsive aggression appeared to be independent of effects on depression and anxiety and occurred regardless of whether the patient had comorbid MDD. Failure to respond to one SSRI did not predict poor response to all SSRIs. For example, some patients with illness that was refractory to fluoxetine (80 mg) have proved responsive to a subsequent trial of sertraline. Similarly, some patients whose illness failed to respond to sertraline, paroxetine, or fluoxetine in a first trial have proved responsive to venlafaxine (Markovitz 1995). In one study, higher doses (e.g., to the point of inducing tremor) and a longer trial (24 weeks) of sertraline converted half of sertraline nonresponders to responders (Markovitz 1995).

Following these open-label reports, two placebo-controlled, randomized studies were reported in patients with BPD (Markovitz 1995; Salzman et al. 1995). Neither study is easily generalizable. Salzman et al. (1995) conducted a 12-week trial of fluoxetine (20–60 mg/day) in 27 highly functional subjects (not identified as patients) with BPD or borderline-trait disturbances. The subjects had a mean baseline GAS score of 74. One advantage of this mildly symptomatic sample was the absence of other Axis I or II comorbid diagnoses. Exclusion criteria also included recent suicidal behavior, self-mutilation, substance abuse, or current severe aggressive behavior—that is, behaviors typical of BPD patients seeking treatment. This strategy limits generalizability to more seriously ill patients, but it allows for a test of efficacy against symptoms unencumbered by comorbidity. For subjects who completed the study ($n=22$), significant improvements were reported for subjects receiving fluoxetine compared with those receiving placebo in self- and observer-rated anger, depression, and global function. A large placebo response was noted. Improvement in anger was found to be independent of changes in depressed mood. Improvement in this highly functional sample was modest, with no subject improving more than 20% on any measure.

Markovitz (1995) studied 17 patients (9 receiving fluoxetine, 8 receiving placebo) for 14 weeks; those receiving fluoxetine were given dosages ranging from 20 mg/day to 80 mg/day. This sample was noteworthy for the high rate of comorbid Axis I affective disorders (10 with MDD, 6 with bipolar disorder), anxiety disorders, and somatic complaints (e.g., headaches, premenstrual syndrome, irritable bowel syndrome). Although this sample is more typical of an impaired BPD patient population, comorbidity with affective and anxiety disorders confounds interpretation of results, because SSRIs are effective for these disorders independent of BPD. Patients receiving fluoxetine improved significantly more than those receiving placebo on measures of depression and anxiety and on global measures. Measures of impulsive aggression were not included in this study. Anecdotally, some patients with premenstrual syndrome and headaches noted improvement in these somatic presentations with fluoxetine, whereas none improved with placebo.

A double-blind, placebo-controlled study by Coccaro and Kavoussi (1997) focused attention on impulsive aggression as a dimensional construct (i.e., a symptom domain found across personality disorder categories but especially characteristic of BPD and other Cluster B personality disorders). They recruited 40 male subjects, not identified as patients, with prominent impulsive aggression as a behavioral disturbance in the context of a DSM-III-R (American Psychiatric Association 1987) personality disorder. Personality disorder diagnoses included 11 (28%) eccentric cluster disorders, 19 (48%) dramatic cluster disorders, and 16 (40%) anxious cluster disorders. There was a high rate of comorbidity with dysthymic disorder or depression NOS, although MDD and bipolar disorder were excluded. Anxiety disorders and alcohol and drug abuse were also prominent. Following a 12-week double-blind, placebo-controlled trial of fluoxetine (20–60 mg), subjects receiving fluoxetine had significantly greater improvement than those receiving placebo on specific measures of verbal aggression and aggression against property. Improvement was significant by week 10, with first trends ($P=0.06$) appearing by week 4. Improvement in irritability appeared by week 6, again with an early trend apparent by week 4. Global improvement, favoring fluoxetine, was significant by week 4. As in the open-label trials and the Salzman et al. (1995) study, these investigators found that the effects on aggression and irritability did not appear due to improvement in mood or anxiety symptoms. More recently introduced SSRIs appear to have similar properties. An open-label, 8-week study using citalopram (mean dosage, 45.5 mg/day) in patients with Cluster B personality disorder or intermittent explosive disorder (but no MDD) also demonstrated significant decreases in irritable (impulsive) aggression (Reist et al. 2003).

Rinne et al. (2002) reported a double-blind, placebo-controlled trial of fluvoxamine in female patients with BPD treated for 6 weeks at 150 mg and then followed in a "half-crossover" design (all patients on active drug) for 6 weeks with a 12-week open-label continuation. Significant improvement with fluvoxamine was found only in a scale measuring rapid mood shifts, with the most improvement in the first 6 weeks. There were no significant changes in anger or impulsivity. The authors suggested that effects on anger and impulsivity may be related to gender—that is, more easily demonstrated in male patients (as in the Coccaro and Kavoussi [1997] study mentioned previously), who may respond preferentially to an SSRI. However, in the Zanarini et al. (2004) study (in the earlier section "Neuroleptics"), fluoxetine monotherapy was associated with reductions in both impulsive aggression and severity of depression among female subjects with BPD.

An important negative study was reported by Simpson et al. (2004), who added a placebo-controlled RCT study of fluoxetine (to 40 mg/day) to a 12-week course of DBT in women with BPD recruited from a 5-day DBT-based partial hospital program. The addition of fluoxetine to DBT produced no significant advantage over DBT with placebo on standardized measures of depression, anxiety, aggression, dissociation, anger, and global functioning. Within the fluoxetine group, there were no significant pre-/posttreatment improvements (while the placebo group improved significantly in clinician-rated global functioning and depression, with meaningful reductions in anxiety and dissociation). By chance, the fluoxetine group had significantly higher pretreatment GAF scores compared with placebo (mean dosage [±SD], 49.39 mg/day [±9.10 mg/day]) Admission to a 5-day partial program suggests acuteness of symptomatic decompensation and moderate to severe functional impairment. In the absence of a "no treatment" control group, the effect of DBT cannot be distinguished from the effects of time alone. Nonetheless, this study suggests that addition of fluoxetine to an effective form of psychotherapy was not helpful in this symptomatic BPD sample.

In summary, these studies show efficacy for SSRI antidepressants against affective symptoms in the patient with personality disorder, specifically depressed mood (Markovitz 1995; Salzman et al. 1995; Zanarini et al. 2004), anger (Salzman et al. 1995), and anxiety (Coccaro and Kavoussi 1997; Markovitz 1995), and against impulsive-behavioral symptoms, specifically, verbal and indirect aggression (Coccaro and Kavoussi 1997). Global symptom severity also improves (Coccaro and Kavoussi 1997; Markovitz 1995; Salzman et al. 1995). Effects on impulsive aggression (Coccaro and Kavoussi 1997) and anger (Salzman et al. 1995) are independent of effects on affective symptoms, including depressed mood (Coccaro and Kavoussi 1997; Salzman et al. 1995) and anxiety (Coccaro and Kavoussi 1997). The study by Simpson et al. (2004) cautions that pharmacotherapy may not improve outcomes in the context of an effective form of psychotherapy.

Monoamine Oxidase Inhibitors

Monoamine oxidase inhibitor (MAOI) antidepressants (phenelzine, tranylcypromine) are second-line treatments for depressed mood in the patient with personality disorder, especially "atypical" depression so common in the patient with BPD. They may also be helpful in reducing social anxiety and hypersensitivity in patients with avoidant personality disorder in the context of social phobia (Liebowitz et al. 1986).

Although empirical support for MAOI antidepressants (phenelzine, tranylcypromine) in the BPD patient is similar to that of the SSRI antidepressants, this class of medications is considered a second choice because of dietary restrictions, drug interactions, and safety concerns (e.g., risk of hypertensive crises). (We are not aware of any studies using the new transdermal formulation of the MAOI selegiline [Emsam] in patients with BPD.) Patients must be willing to comply with the tyramine-free diet and abstain from certain classes of medication (e.g., many decongestants, meperidine, some older antihypertensives) and drugs of abuse (especially cocaine and amphetamines) or risk acute hypertensive crisis. Only cooperative and compliant patients should be considered for MAOI therapy. Many BPD patients do test the dietary limits through minor indiscretions as a manipulative gesture in the context of psychotherapy; however, few are willing to risk a heart attack or stroke in order to test the psychiatrist. (One sophisticated BPD patient of mine intentionally ate a large portion of quiche Lorraine, made with excellent aged cheeses, resulting in a hypertensive headache, a visit to the emergency department, and a late-night call to her psychiatrist saying, "It looked like a piece of pie!") With proper patient selection and instruction, hypertensive crisis is rare, most frequently precipitated by the accidental use of over-the-counter decongestant medication (e.g., pseudoephedrine) or drugs of abuse (e.g., cocaine). Fear of MAOIs among inexperienced clinicians, especially psychiatrists trained after the advent of SSRIs, has greatly reduced their use, even in disorders for which they have clear advantages (e.g., atypical pattern depression, refractory depression).

Tricyclics or Heterocyclics

The utility of tricyclic antidepressants (TCAs) for the treatment of affective dysregulation or mood symptoms in BPD or other personality disorders is highly questionable. When a clear diagnosis of major depression can be made, therapy should be directed at the Axis I disorder. Where atypical depression is present, the MAOI antidepressants may be preferred. At best, the response to TCA (e.g., amitriptyline) appears modest in magnitude. Paradoxical behavioral toxicity to amitriptyline has been reported in some inpatients with BPD, consisting of increased suicide threats, paranoid ideation, demanding and assaultive behaviors, and an apparent disinhibition of impulsive behavior (Soloff et al. 1986, 1987). A choice of antidepressant for Axis I major depression comorbid with BPD should take this literature into consideration. The possibility of behavioral toxicity, and the known lethality of TCAs in overdose, supports the preferential use of an SSRI or related antidepressant as treatment of first choice for the affective dysregulation of the patient with personality disorder.

Anxiolytics

Anxiety is a common and chronic complaint among many patients with personality disorders and is a defining characteristic of the "anxious/fearful" Cluster C disorders (avoidant, dependent, and obsessive-compulsive personality disorders). Although anxiety is widely treated as a symptom independent of any Axis I diagnosis, there is a paucity of studies of anxiolytic use in patients ascertained specifically for personality disorder diagnoses. For example, studies of alprazolam efficacy for avoidant personality traits (mean dosage, 2.9 mg/day × 8 weeks) are reported in the context of treating social phobia (Reich et al. 1989).

Cowdry and Gardner (1988) included alprazolam, a short-acting, high-potency benzodiazepine, in their double-blind, placebo-controlled crossover study of female BPD outpatients with comorbid hysteroid dysphoria and extensive histories of dyscontrol (self-mutilation, overdoses, rage episodes). Patients received an dosage of 4.7 mg/day on average of alprazolam for a 6-week trial. Use of alprazolam was associated with serious episodes of behavioral dyscontrol involving drug overdoses, self-mutilation, and throwing a chair at a child. Seven of 12 (58%) patients receiving alprazolam had episodes of serious behavioral dyscontrol compared with 1 of 13 patients receiving placebo (8%). Four alprazolam trials were stopped by the blind investigator, whereas none of the placebo trials required early termination (Gardner and Cowdry 1985). Alprazolam has been associated with emergence of extreme anger and hostile behavior, including physical assaultiveness, in patients with panic disorder, agoraphobia, obsessive-compulsive disorder, and major depression. These patients had histories of "chronic anger and resentment whose overt expression was well suppressed" (Rosenbaum et al. 1984). However, open-label case experience suggests that alprazolam may be helpful against anxiety in carefully selected patients with BPD (Faltus 1984).

Open-label case experience has also been reported in patients with BPD using clonazepam, a long-half-life (18–50 hours) benzodiazepine with anticonvulsant properties similar to carbamazepine and serotonin-enhancing properties similar to lithium carbonate (Freinhar and Alvarez 1985). Clonazepam is helpful as an adjunctive agent in the treatment of impulsivity, violent outbursts, and anxiety in a variety of disorders, including bipolar mania, schizoaffective disorder, schizophrenia, and BPD. Its efficacy may be related to an increase in serotonin levels and increased serotonin synthesis and function (Chouinard 1987).

Benzodiazepines in general warrant careful supervision because of the potential for abuse and the development of pharmacological tolerance with prolonged use. The use of benzodiazepine anxiolytics in patients with BPD should be limited to patients who fail to respond to other antianxiety treatments (e.g., SSRI antidepressants) and who are at low risk for abuse. Short-half-life benzodiazepine anxiolytics (e.g., alprazolam) should be used with great caution because of the risk of behavioral disinhibition or impulsive aggression. Patients with histories of behavioral disinhibition who are in need of anxiolytic treatment may be treated with clonazepam, a long-half-life benzodiazepine. There are no currently available studies of nonbenzodiazepine anxiolytics in patients with personality disorder diagnoses in the absence of Axis I anxiety disorders.

Lithium Carbonate and Anticonvulsant Mood Stabilizers

Lithium carbonate and the anticonvulsant mood stabilizers phenytoin, carbamazepine, divalproex sodium, and lamotrigine have all been studied in patients with personality disorders for the treatment of impulse dyscontrol. These studies have been conducted in patients with borderline and antisocial personality disorders in whom behavioral impulsivity and impulsive aggression were prominent characteristics. A separate literature, although relevant, describes the successful use of anticonvulsants (e.g., carbamazepine) in the treatment of intermittent explosive disorder and "rage outbursts" independent of personality diagnosis (Mattes 1990). Efficacy of anticonvulsants against aggression in patients with personality disorder (e.g., borderline or antisocial) may be independent of electroencephalographical abnormalities (Reeves et al. 2003).

An early hypothesis concerning the origin of impulse dyscontrol suggested that explosive anger and impulsive aggression were mediated by the same neural mechanisms involved in seizure disorders (Barratt 1972). This hypothesis led to trials of the anticonvulsant phenytoin as a treatment for impulsive aggression and nonepileptic rage in a variety of settings and populations. The results of many early studies were inconclusive, due in part to methodological problems involving diagnosis and assessment of aggression. Nonetheless, in some studies phenytoin has proved effective as an antiaggressive agent. Barratt et al. (1997) conducted a double-blind, placebo-controlled crossover study in a correctional facility using inmates with antisocial personality disorder but no Axis I comorbidity. Using structured interviews for diagnoses and standardized measures for aggression, these investigators demonstrated that phenytoin (in dosages up to 300 mg/day) significantly reduced impulsive-aggressive behavior but not premeditated aggression.

Lithium was also shown to have antiaggressive efficacy in chronically assaultive male prisoners in a placebo-controlled crossover study in which subjects received at least 1 month of lithium therapy (Sheard et al. 1976) and in longer-term open-label trials with incarcerated aggressive prisoners (Tupin et al. 1973) and aggressive delinquents followed both in institutional settings and as outpatients (Sheard 1975). Decreases in aggressive behaviors were documented through objective behavioral measures. Diagnoses of patients in these studies were not controlled and included patients with schizophrenia in the Tupin et al. (1973) study and diverse personality disorders among the adult and adolescent delinquent subjects in the Sheard study (Sheard 1971, 1975). Subsequently, case reports reported both mood-stabilizing and antiaggressive effects of lithium in individual patients defined as having BPD (LaWall and Wesselius 1982; Shader et al. 1974).

Links et al. (1990) compared lithium with desipramine in 17 outpatients with BPD in a double-blind, placebo-controlled crossover study. All patients received lithium for 6 weeks (with 4 weeks at constant dose) at an average dosage of 985.7 mg/day and received concurrent psychotherapy. Among 10 patients completing both lithium and placebo treatments, therapists' blind ratings indicated greater improvement during the lithium trial, although patients' self-ratings did not reflect significant differences between lithium and placebo treatment. The authors noted that therapists were favorably impressed by decreases in impulsivity during the lithium trial. There was a trend for patients receiving lithium to report less anger and suicidal symptoms than patients receiving desipramine.

Carbamazepine has been studied in two double-blind, placebo-controlled studies using very different patient samples and resulting in inconsistent findings.

In the first study, Gardner and Cowdry (1986b; Cowdry and Gardner 1988) studied female BPD outpatients who also had comorbid hysteroid dysphoria and extensive histories of behavioral dyscontrol. Patients received 6-week trials of medication, with 4 weeks at steady dosage (mean, 820 mg/day). Among the 11 patients who completed both a placebo and a carbamazepine trial, patients showed less behavioral dyscontrol and less severe types of behavioral dyscontrol during the carbamazepine trials. Comparing all patients, there were fewer suicide attempts or other major dyscontrol episodes during the carbamazepine trials (1 in 14 patients) compared with the placebo trials (7 of 11 patients, $P=0.005$). Patients receiving carbamazepine also showed improvement in anxiety, anger, and euphoria by physician's assessments, although patients did not report improved mood. There was a significant decrease in impulsivity and suicidality during the carbamazepine trials compared with the placebo trials.

In an earlier report from the same study, Gardner and Cowdry (1986a) reported development of melancholia during carbamazepine treatment as an untoward effect in 3 of 17 (18%) patients.

In the second study, de la Fuente and Lotstra (1994) failed to replicate the findings of efficacy for carbamazepine in BPD that were noted in the Cowdry and Gardner studies (1988). De la Fuente and Lotstra (1994) conducted a double-blind, placebo-controlled trial of carbamazepine among inpatients in whom BPD was the main diagnosis. They rigorously excluded patients with any comorbid Axis I disorder, a history of epilepsy, or electroencephalographical abnormalities. Unlike the studies of Cowdry and Gardner (1988), patients were not selected for histories of behavioral dyscontrol. In the study by de la Fuente and Lotstra (1994), 20 patients (10 receiving carbamazepine and 10 receiving placebo) were studied in the hospital with medication trials of up to 32 days in duration. Carbamazepine dosages were adjusted to yield plasma levels in the low therapeutic range. There were no significant differences between carbamazepine and placebo on measures of affective or cognitive-perceptual symptoms, impulsive-behavioral "acting-out," or global assessments. The two patients who failed to complete the study dropped out because of "acting-out" behaviors. Both were receiving carbamazepine.

Divalproex sodium has been used in open-label trials targeting the agitation and aggression of BPD patients in a state hospital setting (Wilcox 1995) and the mood instability and impulsivity of BPD patients in an outpatient clinic (Stein et al. 1995). Wilcox (1995) reported a 68% decrease in time in seclusion and improvement in anxiety, tension, and global symptom scores (BPRS) among 30 BPD patients receiving divalproex sodium for 6 weeks in a state hospital setting. Patients did not have "psychiatric comorbid conditions" (by clinical assessment), although five had abnormalities on the electroencephalogram (EEG) (with no seizure disorders). Patients received dosages titrated to plasma levels of 100 µg/mL. Concurrent psychotropic medications were allowed. Both divalproex sodium and the abnormal EEG were predictive of improvement, although only the medication effect was significant. The author noted that anxiety played a role in the agitation of these patients and that both the antiaggressive and antianxiety effects of divalproex sodium were instrumental in decreasing agitation and time in seclusion.

Stein et al. (1995) treated 11 cooperative outpatients with BPD with divalproex so-

dium, which was titrated to plasma levels of 50–100 µg/mL. Among eight patients completing the study, half were responders on a measure of global improvement. Improvement was noted in physicians' ratings of mood, anxiety, anger, impulsivity, and rejection sensitivity; in patients' ratings of global improvement (SCL-90); and in observed irritability (OAS-M).

Kavoussi and Coccaro (1998) also reported significant improvement in impulsive aggression and irritability after 4 weeks of divalproex sodium in 10 patients with impulsive aggression in the context of a DSM-IV (American Psychiatric Association 1994) personality disorder. Eight patients completed the 8-week study; six had a 50% or greater reduction in aggression and irritability (OAS-M). All patients had previously failed a trial of fluoxetine (up to 60 mg for 8 weeks) prior to taking divalproex sodium.

Frankenburg and Zanarini (2002) conducted a 6-month, double-blind, placebo-controlled trial of divalproex sodium (average dose [±SD], 850 mg [±249 mg]) in female patients meeting criteria for both BPD and bipolar II disorder. Analyses at 8 weeks and endpoint (using analysis of last observation carried forward) demonstrated divalproex to be superior to placebo on measures of interpersonal sensitivity, anger/hostility (SCL-90), and impulsive aggression (OAS-M). Comorbidity with bipolar II disorder makes this study difficult to generalize to personality disorder patients without bipolar spectrum illness. However, the similarity in symptoms between bipolar II disorder and BPD suggests clinical usefulness of divalproex sodium trials with either disorder.

Using an RCT design, Hollander et al. (2001) enrolled 16 outpatients with BPD (and no Axis I depression or bipolar diagnoses) and compared divalproex sodium with placebo in a 10-week randomized, controlled study. Dropout rates were high, involving 50% of those receiving divalproex sodium and 100% of those receiving placebo, due to lack of efficacy or impulsive decisions. No placebo patient was a responder. Patients receiving divalproex sodium improved significantly on global functioning (GAS, Clinical Global Impressions—Improvement of Illness), with nonsignificant trends for improvement in aggression and depressed mood. Hollander et al. (2003) followed this study with an expanded RCT study that included a broader spectrum of Cluster B patients. This expanded study also demonstrated significant treatment effects for divalproex sodium against irritability and aggression compared with placebo in Cluster B patients in a multisite trial of 12 weeks' duration. (The study also included other comparison groups with impulse-control disorders, intermittent explosive disorder, and post-traumatic stress disorder.) Differences between Cluster B patients receiving divalproex and those receiving placebo were significant in the last 4 weeks of the trial. Improvements in impulsive aggression were greater for the Cluster B patients than for groups of patients with other impulsive disorders. Treatment effects were enhanced by excluding patients with premeditated aggression rather than impulsive aggression.

In a follow-up analysis of this study, focusing exclusively on patients with BPD, Hollander et al. (2005) reported that divalproex-treated patients responded significantly better than placebo-treated patients on measures of state aggression (OAS), trait impulsiveness (Barratt Impulsiveness Scale), affective instability (depression and hypomania on the Young Mania Rating Scale and on the Ham-D). Importantly, they noted that high pretreatment levels of trait impulsivity (Barratt Impulsiveness Scale) and state aggression (OAS) were related to better responsiveness to divalproex. The effects of impulsivity and aggression on treatment response appeared to be independent of each other.

As newer anticonvulsant medications have been released, they have been tested against affective instability and impulsive aggression in patients with BPD; these symptoms bear a close resemblance to symptoms in the bipolar spectrum.

Oxcarbazepine, an anticonvulsant related to carbamazepine, was studied in an open-label trial with patients with BPD (Bellino et al. 2005). Patients received 1,200–1,500 mg/day for 12 weeks. Significant improvement was noted in global functioning (CGI-S) and BPRS mean scores, Ham-A, and four subscales of the Borderline Personality Disorder Severity Index, including impulsivity, affective instability, interpersonal relationships, and outbursts of anger. As with previous trials of mood stabilizers in BPD (e.g., lithium, carbamazepine, divalproex), oxcarbazepine may be helpful in managing symptoms of affective instability and impulsivity.

Nickel and colleagues reported two RCTs of topiramate, specifically targeting aggression in medication-free female subjects (Nickel et al. 2004) and male subjects (Nickel et al. 2005) with BPD. After 8 weeks on topiramate (up to 250 mg/day by week 6), patients in both studies receiving active drug had significantly greater improvement on state anger, trait anger, anger-out, and anger control subscales of the STAXI compared with patients receiving placebo. Weight loss was a common side effect of topiramate. Women receiving topiramate lost an average of 5.7 lb (vs. 0.7 lb, placebo), while men lost 11.4 lb (vs. 0.7 lb, placebo). A third study by the same group compared topiramate (up to 200 mg/day by week 6) to placebo in female BPD subjects assessed for general psychopathology (on the SCL-90), for health-related quality of life (Short-Form 36-Item Health Survey [SF-36]), and on the Inventory of Interpersonal Problems (IIP; Loew et al. 2006). Compared with patients receiving placebo, patients taking topiramate showed significant improvement after 10 weeks on SCL-90 subscales of Somatization, Interpersonal Sensitivity, Anxiety, Hostility, Phobic Anxiety, and Global Symptom Severity. Additionally, patients receiving topiramate had significantly better outcomes on all eight quality-of-life indicators on the SF-36, and four of the subscales of the IIP. Women receiving topiramate lost an average of 12.5 lb in this study (vs. 3.1 lb, placebo.)

Working within the same group, Tritt et al. (2005) studied the efficacy of lamotrigine (200 mg/day by week 6) on aggression in women with BPD, applying the same methods as described by Nickel et al. (2004, 2005) for topiramate. At the end of the 8-week drug trial, subjects receiving lamotrigine had significantly more improvement than subjects receiving placebo on all five anger subscales of the STAXI. Weight loss did not differ significantly between groups, nor did any subjects develop a serious skin rash.

Meta-Analyses and Evidence-Based Practice

Meta-analyses are rapidly becoming a major source for recommendations on "evidence-based practice." Meta-analyses identify significant effects of a given treatment within multiple treatment trials and ask at what rate the treatment can be expected to produce the effect. Typically, a large number of databases are first surveyed for studies meeting predetermined inclusion criteria (e.g., RCT studies with placebo controls, standardized assessments, low attrition rates). Effect sizes for the results of treatment on specific symptoms (e.g., depression, hostility) are calculated from predetermined outcome measures and statistically compared between studies. In the pooling of data, important clinical distinctions may be lost, including differing methods of diagnosis, different settings, confounding variables (such as concurrent treatments), and assessment by multiple diverse outcome measures. The results of the meta-analyses are dependent on how one defines the treatment targets and selects the outcome measures. In symptom-specific analyses, the grouping of target symptoms for analysis is critical (e.g., does anger belong with affective instability or impulsive aggression?). In an ideal model, all studies would use the same outcome measure for each target symptom, allowing meaningful comparison of effect sizes between studies. As this is not realistic practice, diverse outcome measures that purport to assess similar traits are often compared. (Conversely, studies may be excluded from the analysis for not using comparable measures.) Pharmacotherapy literature in BPD does not presently lend itself well to such an approach. Compared with literature in depression or schizophrenia, there are relatively few RCT studies in BPD, meaning insufficient power for analyses of critical core features (such as suicidality). Few studies of a given drug (or drug class) use comparable methods in terms of dose, duration, and, most importantly, outcome measures. Dropout rates tend to be high in studies of BPD, often reflecting poor acceptability of treatment (an exclusion criterion for some meta-analyses). Despite these limitations, meta-analyses are becoming a more frequently cited tool for making recommendations concerning evidence-based practice and are appearing in the pharmacotherapy literature on treating BPD.

Nose et al. (2006) conducted a meta-analysis of published RCT studies in patients with BPD. Among 84 potentially relevant RCT studies, only 22 placebo-controlled comparisons met inclusion criteria for the meta-analysis. Outcome categories included core traits of BPD: affective instability and anger, impulsivity and aggression, unstable interpersonal relationships, suicidality, and global function. Data extracted from four antidepressant studies and six mood stabilizer studies found efficacy against affective instability and anger. Antipsychotics (represented by three studies) had a positive effect on impulsivity and aggression. (In contrast, six antidepressant trials and three mood stabilizer studies showed no significant effects.) Antipsychotics also had positive effects on unstable interpersonal relationships (three studies) and global functioning (seven studies). The study did not target cognitive-perceptual symptoms for analysis. Among specific drugs, evidence was strong for the efficacy of fluoxetine against affective instability and impulsivity, for topiramate and lamotrigine against anger, and olanzapine for its effect on global functioning.

In marked contrast, the Cochrane Collaboration group, which conducts meta-analyses across many medical treatments, surveyed 28 databases and identified only 10 RCT studies in BPD meeting their rigorous inclusion criteria for meta-analysis (Binks et al. 2006). Though the review was also published in 2006 , no RCT study published after 1995 met their inclusion criteria. The Cochrane review was largely negative. However, they found evidence that antidepressants may improve scores on anger and perhaps depression (though not conclusively) and that MAOIs may help those with hostility, but not reduce borderline symptoms or improve global functioning. They found no advantages over placebo for antipsychotics (three studies), but some favorable change in global outcomes for one mood stabilizer, divalproex. The Cochrane report concluded: "If offered medication, people with BPD should know that this is not based on good evidence from trials. That does not mean it may not do considerable good and there is not indication of significant harm" (Binks et al. 2006, p. 19). It is important for clinicians to understand the methodology, strengths, and weaknesses of this kind of analysis, which will certainly claim influence in defining practice guidelines in the future.

ELECTROCONVULSIVE THERAPY

Electroconvulsive therapy (ECT) is indicated for the treatment of Axis I psychiatric disorders that have proved refractory to pharmacotherapy and are known to respond to ECT. The vast majority of patients referred for ECT have an affective spectrum disorder, although patients with schizoaffective disorder and schizophrenia may also benefit. On rare occasions, ECT may be a treatment of first choice for responsive Axis I disorders when clinical presentation requires urgency (e.g., catatonia), when pharmacotherapy poses unacceptable risk (e.g., neuroleptic malignant syndrome), or by patient preference (rein-

forced by past success). Depressed patients with prominent personality disorders are often not referred for ECT because of a widespread belief among practitioners that their illness is refractory to this somatic treatment. The literature on the efficacy of ECT for the depressed patient with personality disorder is remarkably inconclusive. Methodological differences between studies make generalization difficult.

The prejudice against the use of ECT treatment for depressed personality disorder patients may be traced back to early case reports and clinical series that described diminished responsiveness to ECT in patients with "neurotic" depression, a broadly defined construct of low diagnostic reliability incorporating many traits now attributed to comorbid personality disorder. Patients with "hysterical personality features" and BPD had poor outcomes with ECT (Kramer 1982; Lazare and Klerman 1968). Following the introduction of structured interviews for Axis I and II disorders and standardized outcome measures, empirical studies began to temper this view.

Pfohl et al. (1984) studied 41 inpatients with DSM-III (American Psychiatric Association 1980) MDD and comorbid Axis II personality disorder and compared them with 37 patients with MDD alone. Patients received somatic treatment by antidepressant medication or ECT, with all treatment decisions made by their attending physicians. Standard ratings of mood (Ham-D, BDI) and global functioning (GAS) were done before treatment and at discharge from the hospital. Depressed patients with comorbid personality disorder receiving antidepressant medications were less improved at discharge than patients with MDD alone; however, there was no difference between groups for patients receiving ECT.

This result was extended in a naturalistic study of outcomes in the treatment of 228 depressed inpatients. Black et al. (1988) reported that depressed patients with personality disorder receiving adequate antidepressant medication were less likely to recover than patients with MDD alone. However, there were no differences between groups in recovery after ECT. Depressed patients with personality disorder were less likely to be referred for ECT and generally received less aggressive treatment. In an expanded study involving 1,471 depressed inpatients, Black et al. (1991) found that the presence of a personality disorder diagnosis was a significant statistical predictor of poor outcome for hospital treatment in general (with antidepressant medication or ECT). Depressed patients with a personality disorder diagnosis were 50% less likely to be recovered at hospital discharge than patients with MDD without a personality disorder. (There was no analysis by separate treatment groups.)

Zimmerman et al. (1986) found no significant differences in immediate response to ECT treatment (on Ham-D, BDI, or GAS) between DSM-III MDD patients with and without a comorbid personality disorder. Patients had similar pretreatment symptom severity on Ham-D, BDI, and GAS and received similar (although uncontrolled) ECT treatments and pharmacotherapy. Follow-up (by phone) at 6 months indicated more episodes of rehospitalization and higher symptom scores in the personality disorder group. Although starting with similar improvement at hospital discharge, patients with personality disorder were less likely to maintain recovery compared with the depressed patients with no personality disorder.

Casey and Butler (1995) and Casey et al. (1996) studied ECT treatment in 40 inpatients with DSM-III-R MDD who were examined for personality disorder using Tyrer's Personality Assessment Schedule posttreatment. Patients were rated pretreatment, posttreatment, and every 6 weeks for 6 months and at 1 year after discharge using an outcome measure of mood (Ham-D-21) and social functioning (Social Functioning Schedule). A 12-month follow-up rated patients globally according to medication usage and patient status. ECT practice and con-

current antidepressant medication usage were uncontrolled, although patients in both groups had similar numbers of treatments (5 with personality disorder and 5.2 with no personality disorder) and days in the hospital. Depressed patients with personality disorder had acutely poorer outcomes on both the depression and social functioning scale following ECT treatment compared with depressed patients with no personality disorder. The presence or absence of a personality disorder was the strongest predictor of the Social Functioning Schedule outcome, explaining 31% of variance at discharge. Significant differences between groups on Ham-D disappeared by the first 6-week follow-up and for the Social Functioning Schedule by 12 weeks. There were no differences between groups in rehospitalizations after 6 or 12 months. The authors concluded that the presence of a personality disorder adversely affects early symptomatic recovery after ECT but not longer-term outcome.

Blais et al. (1998) obtained personality testing pre- and post-ECT in a small study sample ($N = 16$) of depressed patients to determine changes in significant personality traits with ECT. Using the self-rated Millon Clinical Multiaxial Inventory—II, the investigators found significant changes (improvement) in four personality scales with ECT treatment: avoidant, histrionic, aggressive/sadistic, and schizotypal. Changes in passive-aggressive and borderline personality scale scores tended toward improvement but fell short of significance. Other personality scales appeared stable and did not change with ECT. Controlling for pretreatment depression scores, only a pretreatment diagnosis of BPD predicted posttreatment depression scores (on the BDI), with higher pretreatment BPD scores predicting poorer outcome.

Feske et al. (2004) reported that outcome differences following ECT for depressed patients with a comorbid personality disorder depended on the type of personality disorder. They divided 139 patients with a primary diagnosis of unipolar MDD into groups with comorbid BPD (*n*=20), other personality disorders (*n*=42), or no comorbid personality disorder (*n*=77). ECT methods and concurrent medication were controlled by a standard protocol. Patients with comorbid BPD showed a poorer acute response to ECT than the other two groups, who did not differ significantly.

In a review of this literature, DeBattista and Mueller (2001) concluded that 40%–75% of patients with MDD and comorbid personality disorder have a 50% decrease in depression scale scores with ECT, an efficacy equal to response rates among other patients with treatment-resistant depression without personality disorder comorbidity. However, increased relapse rates, rehospitalization, and psychosocial dysfunction (6 months to 1 year posttreatment) suggest that underlying personality disorder affects long-term outcome.

A major confounding factor in these studies is difficulty separating affective symptoms of the depressive disorder from those intrinsic to the personality disorder. For example, the affective dysregulation ("mood crashes"), low self-esteem, pessimism, chronic suicidality, and self-injurious behaviors of the patient with BPD are often misconstrued as Axis I affective pathology and assessed by outcome measures (e.g., BDI, Ham-D) that may correlate highly with diagnostic criteria. Not infrequently, a clinician will target these personality traits for ECT treatment, resulting in a predictably poor outcome. A recommendation for ECT in the personality disorder patient with comorbid MDD, especially the BPD patient, must be guided by the presence and severity of verifiable neurovegetative symptoms such as sleep disturbance, appetite disturbance, weight change, low energy, anhedonia, and loss of libido. These symptoms should be confirmed by outside observers because they provide an objective gauge of treatment response. Periodic use of an objective rating scale, such as the Ham-D, facilitates documentation of change over the

course of treatment. The greatest challenge for the clinician is not when to institute a course of ECT in the depressed personality disorder patient but when to stop ECT. As the neurovegetative symptoms of MDD resolve, the patient may continue to report personality characteristics that reflect the Axis II pathology and are not responsive to ECT. For example, low self-esteem can be an acute symptom of MDD or a chronic personality trait. Knowledge of the patient's personality functioning prior to the onset of MDD is critical to knowing when the "baseline" has been achieved. Many personality disorder patients with illness termed "refractory" to ECT for persistence of depressive complaint are, in fact, already in remission of their Axis I disorder and exhibiting their chronic characterological complaints and behaviors.

CONCLUSION

Pharmacotherapy is an important adjunctive treatment in the overall management of the patient with severe personality disorder. Symptoms of cognitive-perceptual disturbance, affective dysregulation, and impulsive-behavioral dyscontrol are appropriate targets for medication trials. Problems of character and of interpersonal dynamics are the domain of the psychotherapies and will not respond to medication. Because personality disorders are dimensional syndromes, a symptom-specific approach is warranted, potentially involving multiple medications. It is important to study the effects of each medication before adding a second or third agent. Ineffective medications should be discontinued. Expectations of efficacy should be modest and residual symptoms are the rule.

Pharmacotherapy of the personality disorders is still a relatively new and evolving practice. Current recommendations are based on a woefully small database of drug trials. The patient with personality disorder is best served by a comprehensive treatment approach involving psychotherapy, symptom-specific medication management, and psychoeducation for the patient and family.

REFERENCES

Akiskal HS, Chen SE, Davis GC, et al: Borderline: an adjective in search of a noun. J Clin Psychiatry 46:41–48, 1985

American Psychiatric Association: Diagnostic and Statistical Manual of Mental Disorders, 3rd Edition. Washington, DC, American Psychiatric Association, 1980

American Psychiatric Association: Diagnostic and Statistical Manual of Mental Disorders, 3rd Edition, Revised. Washington, DC, American Psychiatric Association, 1987

American Psychiatric Association: Diagnostic and Statistical Manual of Mental Disorders, 4th Edition. Washington, DC, American Psychiatric Association, 1994

American Psychiatric Association: Practice Guideline for the Treatment of Patients with Borderline Personality Disorder. Washington, DC, American Psychiatric Association, 2001

Barratt ES: Impulsiveness and anxiety: toward a neuropsychological model, in Anxiety: Current Trends in Theory and Research. Edited by Spielberger C. New York, Academic Press, 1972, pp 195–222,

Barratt ES, Stanford M, Felthous AR, et al: The effects of phenytoin on impulsive and premeditated aggression: a controlled study. J Clin Psychopharmacol 17:341–349, 1997

Bellinio S, Paradiso E, Bogetto F: Oxcarbazepine in the treatment of borderline personality disorder: a pilot study. J Clin Psychiatry 66:1111–1115, 2005

Bellino S, Paradiso E, Bogetto F: Efficacy and tolerability of quetiapine in the treatment of borderline personality disorder: a pilot study. J Clin Psychiatry 67:1042–1046, 2006

Benedetti F, Sforzini L, Colombo C, et al: Low dose clozapine in acute and continuation treatment of severe borderline personality disorder. J Clin Psychiatry 59:103–107, 1998

Binks CA, Fenton M, McCarthy L, et al: Pharmacologic interventions for people with borderline personality disorder. Cochrane Database of Systematic Reviews 2006, Issue 1. Art. No. CD005653. DOI: 10.1002/14651858. CD005653

Black DW, Bell S, Hulbert J, et al: The importance of Axis II in patients with major depression: a controlled study. J Affect Disord 14:115–122, 1988

Black DW, Goldstein RB, Nasrallah A, et al: The prediction of recovery using a multivariate model in 1,471 depressed inpatients. Eur Arch Psychiatry Clin Neurosci 241:41–45, 1991

Blais MA, Matthews J, Schouten R, et al: Stability and predictive value of self-report personality traits pre- and post-electroconvulsive therapy: a preliminary study. Comp Psychiatry 39:231–235, 1998

Bogenschutz MP, Nurnberg GH: Olanzapine versus placebo in the treatment of borderline personality disorder. J Clin Psychiatry 65:104–109, 2004

Brinkley JR, Beitman BD, Friedel RO: Low dose neuroleptic regimes in the treatment of borderline patients. Arch Gen Psychiatry 36:319–326, 1979

Casey P, Butler E: The effects of personality on the response to ECT in major depression. J Personal Disord 9:134–142, 1995

Casey P, Meagher D, Butler E: Personality, functioning, and recovery from major depression. J Nerv Ment Dis 184:240–245, 1996

Chengappa KNR, Baker RW, Sirri C: The successful use of clozapine in ameliorating severe self mutilation in a patient with borderline personality disorder. J Personal Disorder 9:76–82, 1995

Chengappa KNR, Ebeling T, Kang JS, et al: Clozapine reduces severe self-mutilation and aggression in psychotic patients with borderline personality disorder. J Clin Psychiatry 60:477–484, 1999

Chouinard G: Clonazepam in acute and maintenance treatment of bipolar affective disorder. J Clin Psychiatry 48:29–36, 1987

Coccaro EF, Kavoussi RJ: Fluoxetine and impulsive-aggressive behavior in personality disordered subjects. Arch Gen Psychiatry 54:1081–1088, 1997

Cornelius JR, Soloff PH, Perel JM, et al: Fluoxetine trial in borderline personality disorder. Psychopharmacol Bull 26:151–154, 1990

Cornelius JR, Soloff PH, Perel JM, et al: Continuation pharmacotherapy of borderline personality disorder with haloperidol and phenelzine. Am J Psychiatry 150:1843–1848, 1993

Cowdry RW, Gardner DL: Pharmacotherapy of borderline personality disorder: alprazolam, carbamazepine, trifluoperazine and tranylcypromine. Arch Gen Psychiatry 45:111–119, 1988

Damsa C, Adam E, De Gregorio F, et al: Intramuscular olanzapine in patients with borderline personality disorder: an observational study in an emergency room. Gen Hosp Psychiatry 29:51–53, 2007

DeBattista C, Mueller K: Is electroconvulsive therapy effective for the depressed patient with comorbid borderline personality disorder. J ECT 17:91–98, 2001

de la Fuente JM, Lotstra F: A trial of carbamazepine in borderline personality disorder. Eur Neuropsychopharmacol 4:479–486, 1994

Faltus FJ: The positive effect of alprazolam in the treatment of three patients with borderline personality disorder. Am J Psychiatry 141:802–803, 1984

Feske U, Mulsant BH, Pilkonis PA, et al: Clinical outcome of ECT in patients with major depression and comorbid borderline personality disorder. Am J Psychiatry 161: 2073–2080, 2004

Frankenburg FR, Zanarini MC: Clozapine treatment of borderline patients: a preliminary study. Compr Psychiatry 34:402–405, 1993

Frankenburg FR, Zanarini MC: Divalproex sodium treatment of women with borderline personality disorder and bipolar II disorder: a double blind placebo controlled pilot study. J Clin Psychiatry 63:442–446, 2002

Freinhar JP, Alvarez WA: Clonazepam: a novel therapeutic adjunct. Int J Psychiatry Med 15:321–328, 1985

Gardner DL, Cowdry RW: Alprazolam-induced dyscontrol in borderline personality disorder. Am J Psychiatry 142:98–100, 1985

Gardner DL, Cowdry RW: Development of melancholia during carbamazepine treatment in borderline personality disorder. J Clin Psychopharmacol 6:236–239, 1986a

Gardner DL, Cowdry RW: Positive effects of carbamazepine on behavioral dyscontrol in borderline personality disorder. Am J Psychiatry 143:519–522, 1986b

Goldberg SC, Schulz SC, Schulz PM, et al: Borderline and schizotypal personality disorders treated with low dose thiothixene vs. placebo. Arch Gen Psychiatry 43:680–686, 1986

Gunderson JG, Philips KA: A current view of the interface between borderline personality disorder and depression. Am J Psychiatry 148:967–975, 1991

Hollander E, Allen A, Lopez RP, et al: A preliminary double blind, placebo-controlled trial of divalproex sodium in borderline personality disorder. J Clin Psychiatry 62: 199–203, 2001

Hollander E, Tracy KA, Swann AC, et al: Divalproex in the treatment of impulsive aggression: efficacy in Cluster B personality disorders. Neuropsychopharmacology 28:1186–1197, 2003

Hollander E, Swann AC, Coccaro EF, et al: Impact of trait impulsivity and state aggression on divalproex versus placebo response in borderline personality disorder. Am J Psychiatry 162:621–624, 2005

Hymowitz P, Frances A, Jacobsberg LB, et al: Neuroleptic treatment of schizotypal personality disorders. Compr Psychiatry 27:267–271, 1986

Kavoussi RJ, Coccaro EF: Divalproex sodium for impulsive aggressive behavior in patients with personality disorder. J Clin Psychiatry 59:676–680, 1998

Kavoussi RJ, Liu J, Coccaro EF: An open trial of sertraline in personality disordered patients with impulsive aggression. J Clin Psychiatry 55:137–141, 1994

Kelly T, Soloff PH, Cornelius JR, et al: Can we study (treat) borderline patients: attrition from research and open treatment. J Personal Disord 6:417–433, 1992

Keshavan M, Shad M, Soloff PH, et al: Efficacy and tolerability of olanzapine in the treatment of schizotypal personality disorder. Schizophr Res 71:97–101, 2004

Koenigsberg HW, Anwunah I, New AS, et al: Relationship between depression and borderline personality disorder. Depress Anxiety 10:158–167, 1999

Koenigsberg HW, Reynolds D, Goodman M, et al: Risperidone in the treatment of schizotypal personality disorder. J Clin Psychiatry 64:628–634, 2003

Kramer BA: Poor response to electroconvulsive therapy in patients with a combined diagnosis of major depression and borderline personality disorder (letter). Lancet 2:1048, 1982

Kutcher S, Papatheodorou G, Reiter S, et al: The successful pharmacologic treatment of adolescents and young adults with borderline personality disorder: a preliminary open trial of fluopenthixol. J Psychiatry Neurosci 20:113–118, 1995

LaWall JS, Wesselius CL: The use of lithium carbonate in borderline patients. J Psychiatr Treat Eval 4:265–267, 1982

Lazare A, Klerman GL: Hysteria and depression: the frequency and significance of hysterical personality features in hospitalized depressed women. Am J Psychiatry 124 (suppl):48–56, 1968

Leone N: Response of borderline patients to loxapine and chlorpromazine. J Clin Psychiatry 43:148–150, 1982

Liebowitz MR, Fyer AJ, Gorman JM, et al: Phenelzine in social phobia. J Clin Psychopharmacol 6:93–98, 1986

Links P, Steuiner M, Boiago I, et al: Lithium therapy for borderline patients: preliminary findings. J Personal Disord 4:173–181, 1990

Loew TH, Nickel MK, Muehlbacher M, et al: Topiramate treatment for women with borderline personality disorder. A double-blind, placebo controlled study. J Clin Psychopharmacology 26:61–66, 2006

Markovitz PJ: Pharmacotherapy of impulsivity, aggression and related disorders, in Impulsivity and Aggression. Edited by Hollander E, Stein D. New York, Wiley, 1995, pp 263–287

Markovitz PJ, Wagner SL: Venlafaxine in the treatment of borderline personality disorder. Psychopharmacol Bull 31:773–777, 1995

Markovitz PJ, Calabrese JR, Schulz SC, et al: Fluoxetine in the treatment of borderline and schizotypal personality disorders. Am J Psychiatry 148:1064–1067, 1991

Mattes JA: Comparative effectiveness of carbamazepine and propranolol for rage outbursts. J Neuropsychiatry Clin Sci 2:159–164, 1990

Montgomery SA, Montgomery D: Pharmacologic prevention of suicidal behavior. J Affect Disord 4:291–298, 1982

Nickel MK, Nickel C, Mitterlehner FO, et al: Topiramate treatment of aggression in female borderline personality disorder patients: a double-blind, placebo controlled study. J Clin Psychiatry 65:1515–1519, 2004

Nickel, MK, Nickel C, Kaplan P, et al: Treatment of aggression with topiramate in male borderline patients: a double-blind, placebo-controlled study. Biol Psychiatry 57:495–499, 2005

Nickel MK, Muehlbacher M, Nickel C, et al: Aripiprazole in the treatment of patients with borderline personality disorder: a double blind placebo-controlled study. Am J Psychiatry 163:833–838, 2006

Norden MJ: Fluoxetine in borderline personality disorder. Prog Neuropsychopharmacol Biol Psychiatry 13:885–893, 1989

Nose M, Cipriani A, Biancosino B, et al: Efficacy of pharmacotherapy against core traits of borderline personality disorder: meta-analysis of randomized controlled trials. Int Clin Psychopharmacol 21:345–353, 2006

Perrella C, Carrus D, Costa E, et al: Quetiapine for the treatment of biorderline personality disorder: an open-label study. Prog Neuropsychopharmacol Biol Psychiatry 31:158–163, 2007

Pfohl B, Stangl D, Zimmerman M: The implications of DSM-III personality disorders for patients with major depression. J Affect Disord 7:309–318, 1984

Reeves RR, Struve FA, Patrick G: EEG does not predict response to valproate treatment of aggression in patients with borderline and antisocial personality disorders. Clin Electroencephalogr 34:84–86, 2003

Reich J, Noyes R, Yates W: Alprazolam treatment of avoidant personality traits in social phobic patients. J Clin Psychiatry 50:91–95, 1989

Reist C, Nakamura K, Sagart E, et al: Impulsive-aggressive behavior: open-label treatment with citalopram. J Clin Psychiatry 64:81–85, 2003

Rifkin A, Quitkin F, Carillo C, et al: Lithium carbonate in emotionally unstable character disorder. Arch Gen Psychiatry 27:519–523, 1972

Rinne T, van den Brink W, Wouters L, et al: SSRI treatment of borderline personality disorder: a randomized, placebo controlled clinical trial for female patients with borderline personality disorder. Am J Psychiatry 159:2048–2054, 2002

Rocca P, Marchiaro L, Cocuzza E, et al: Treatment of borderline personality disorder with risperidone. J Clin Psychiatry 63:241–244, 2000

Rosenbaum JF, Woods SW, Groves JE, et al: Emergence of hostility during alprazolam treatment. Am J Psychiatry 141:792–793, 1984

Salzman C, Wolfson AN, Schatzberg A, et al: Effect of fluoxetine on anger in symptomatic volunteers with borderline personality disorder. J Clin Psychopharmacol 15:23–29, 1995

Schulz SC, Camlin KL, Berry SA, et al: Olanzapine safety and efficacy in patients with borderline personality disorder and comorbid dysthymia. Biol Psychiatry 46:1429–1435, 1999

Serban G, Siegel S: Response of borderline and schizotypal patients to small doses of thiothixene and haloperidol. Am J Psychiatry 141:1455–1458, 1984

Shader RI, Jackson AH, Dodes LM: The anti-aggressive effects of lithium in man. Psychopharmacologia (Berl) 40:17–24, 1974

Sheard MH: Effects of lithium on human aggression. Nature, March 12, 1971, pp 113–114

Sheard MH: Lithium in the treatment of aggression. J Nerv Ment Dis 160:108–118, 1975

Sheard MH, Marini JL, Bridges CI, et al: The effect of lithium on impulsive aggressive behavior in man. Am J Psychiatry 133:1409–1413, 1976

Simpson EB, Yen S, Costello E, et al: Combined dialectal behavior therapy and fluoxetine in the treatment of borderline personality disorder. J Clin Psychiatry 65:379–385, 2004

Soler J, Pascual JC, Campins J, et al: Double blind, placebo controlled study of dialectal behavior therapy plus olanzapine for borderline personality disorder. Am J Psychiatry 162:1221–1224, 2005

Soloff PH, George A, Nathan S, et al: Progress in pharmacotherapy of borderline disorders. Arch Gen Psychiatry 43:691–697, 1986

Soloff PH, George A, Nathan RS, et al: Behavioral dyscontrol in borderline patients treated with amitriptyline. Psychopharmacol Bull 23:177–181, 1987

Soloff PH, George A, Nathan RS, et al: Amitriptyline vs haloperidol in borderlines: final outcomes and predictors of response. J Clin Psychopharmacol 9:238–246, 1989

Soloff PH, Cornelius J, George A: The depressed borderline: one disorder or two? Psychopharmacol Bull 27:23–30, 1991

Soloff PH, Cornelius J, George A, et al: Efficacy of phenelzine and haloperidol in borderline personality disorder. Arch Gen Psychiatry 50:377–385, 1993

Stein DJ, Simeon D, Frenkel M, et al: An open trial of valproate in borderline personality disorder. J Clin Psychiatry 56:506–510, 1995

Teicher MH, Glod CA, Aronson SJ, et al: Open assessment of the safety and efficacy of thioridazine in the treatment of patients with borderline personality disorder. Psychopharmacol Bull 25:535–549, 1989

Tritt K, Nickel C, Lahmann C, et al: Lamotrigine treatment of aggression in female borderline patients: a randomized, double-blind, placebo-controlled study. J Psychopharmacol 19:287–291, 2005

Tupin JP, Smith DB, Clanion TL, et al: The long term use of lithium in aggressive prisoners. Compr Psychiatry 14:311–317, 1973

Villeneuve E, Lemelin S: Open-label study of atypical neuroleptic quetiapine for treatment of borderline personality disorder: impulsivity as main target. J Clin Psychiatry 66:1298–1303, 2005

Wilcox JA: Divalproex sodium as a treatment for borderline personality disorder. Ann Clin Psychiatry 7:33–37, 1995

Zanarini MC, Frankenburg F: Olanzapine treatment of female borderline patients: a double-blind placebo controlled pilot study. J Clin Psychiatry 62:849–854, 2001

Zanarini MC, Frankenburg FR, Parachini EA: A preliminary, randomized trial of fluoxetine, olanzapine, and the olanzapine-fluoxetine combination in women with borderline personality disorder. J Clin Psychiatry 65:903–907, 2004

Zimmerman M, Coryell W, Pfohl B, et al: ECT response in depressed patients with and without a DSM-III personality disorder. Am J Psychiatry 143:1030–1032, 1986

15

Therapeutic Alliance

Donna S. Bender, Ph.D.

Any patient beginning treatment enters a relationship, whether it is for a short time during a hospital stay or over many years in long-term psychotherapy. This relationship with the clinician has the potential for improving the patient's quality of life, perhaps through the alleviation of symptoms or more profoundly through shifts in character structure. It is sometimes difficult to determine a priori who will benefit from what treatment with whom, but one factor has stood out in the research lexicon as the most robust predictor of outcome: therapeutic alliance (Horvath and Greenberg 1994; Horvath and Symonds 1991; Orlinsky et al. 1994).

Because establishing a productive alliance arises within the matrix of a relationship between patient and therapist, when considering personality disorders one must note that most such disorders are associated in some way with significant impairment in interpersonal relations. Speaking about the nature of relationships of individuals characterized by certain types of personality pa-

thology, Masterson (1988) has stated the following:

> Each type of pathology produces its own confusion and its own distorted version of loving and giving. The borderline patient defines love as a relationship with a partner who will offer approval and support for regressive behavior.... The narcissist defines love as the ability of someone else to admire and adore him, and to provide perfect mirroring.... Psychopaths seek partners who respond to their manipulations and provide them with gratification. The schizoid...finds love in an internal, autistic fantasy. (pp. 110–111)

In fact, several studies have shown that rather than categorical diagnosis, it is the preexisting quality of the patient's relationships that most significantly affects the quality of the therapeutic alliance (Gibbons et al. 2003; Hersoug et al. 2002; Piper et al. 1991). Consequently, the clinician must consider an individual's characteristic way of relating so

289

that appropriate interventions can be employed to effectively retain and involve the patient in the treatment, regardless of modality. Forming an alliance is often difficult, however, particularly in work with patients with severely narcissistic, borderline, or paranoid proclivities, because troubled interpersonal attitudes and behaviors will also infuse the patient's engagement with the therapist. For example, narcissistic patients may not be able to allow the therapist to act as a separate, thinking person for quite a long time, whereas someone with borderline issues may exhibit wildly fluctuating emotions, attitudes, and behaviors, thwarting the potential helpfulness of the clinician.

DEFINITION OF THERAPEUTIC ALLIANCE

The concept of the therapeutic alliance is often traced back to Freud, who observed very early in his work the need to convey interest and sympathy to the patient to engage her or him in a collaborative treatment endeavor (Meissner 1996; Safran and Muran 2000). Freud (1912/1946) also delineated an aspect of the transference—the unobjectionable positive transference—which is an attachment that should not be analyzed because it serves as the motivation for the patient to collaborate: "The conscious and unobjectionable component of [positive transference] remains, and brings about the successful result in psychoanalysis as in all other remedial methods" (p. 319). This statement is an early precursor to the modern empirical evidence showing that alliance is related to treatment outcome across modalities.

There are several contemporary definitions of alliance that we might consider to further our discussion of treating patients with personality disorders. One conceptualization, using psychoanalytic language, was posited by Gutheil and Havens (1979): The patient's ability to form a rational alliance arises from "the therapeutic split in the ego

which allows the analyst to work with the healthier elements in the patient against resistance and pathology" (p. 479). This definition is useful vis-à-vis personality disorders in two regards: 1) the recognition that there will be pathological parts of the patient's personality functioning that may serve to thwart the attempted helpfulness of the clinician, and 2) the need for the clinician to be creative in enlisting whatever adaptive aspects of the patient's character may avail themselves for the work of the treatment.

Another definition that was developed in an attempt to transcend theoretical traditions is Bordin's (1979) identification of three interdependent components of the alliance: bond, tasks, and goals. The *bond* is the quality of the relationship formed in the treatment dyad that then mediates whether the patient will take up the *tasks* inherent in working toward the *goals* of a particular treatment approach. At the same time, the clinician's ability to negotiate the tasks and goals with the patient will also affect the nature of the therapeutic bond. This multifaceted view of the alliance underscores the complexity of the factors involved (Safran and Muran 2000).

Arguably, if the goal of treatment is fundamental character change, the Bordin definition of alliance specifies necessary, but not sufficient, elements. Adler (1980) observed that patients with borderline and narcissistic difficulties may not be able to establish a mature working alliance until much later in a successful treatment. Others who typically work with more disturbed patients have noted that establishing a therapeutic alliance may be one of the primary goals of the treatment and that there may be different phases in alliance development as treatment progresses. Gunderson (2000) observed the following alliance stages in the course of conducting long-term psychotherapy with patients with borderline personality disorder:

1) Contractual (behavioral): initial agreement between the patient and therapist on treatment goals and their roles in achieving them (Phase I); 2) Relational

(affective/empathic): emphasized by Rogerian client-centered relationships; patient experiences the therapist as caring, understanding, genuine, and likable (Phase II); 3) Working (cognitive/motivational): psychoanalytic prototype; patient joins the therapist as a reliable collaborator to help the patient understand herself or himself; its development represents a significant improvement for borderline patients (Phases III–IV). (p. 41)

Progression through these stages, if successful, typically takes a number of years. The implication is that to reach a point at which work leading to substantive and enduring personality change can occur may require a lengthy initial alliance-building period. As Bach (1998) noted, "Perhaps the primary problem in engaging the difficult patient is to build and retain what Ellman (1991) has called analytic trust. These difficult patients have generally lost their faith not only in their caregivers, spouses, and other objects but also in the world itself as a place of expectable and manageable contingencies" (p. 185).

ALLIANCE STRAINS AND RUPTURES

Although a strong positive alliance can predict a successful treatment outcome, the converse is also true: problems in the treatment alliance may lead to premature termination if not handled in a sensitive and timely manner. Evidence has shown that strains and ruptures in the alliance are often related to unilateral termination (Samstag et al. 1998). Thus, negotiating ruptures in the alliance is another issue that has garnered increasing attention in the psychotherapy literature. For example, Strauss et al. (2006) demonstrated that skillfully addressing ruptures strengthens the alliance, leading to better treatment outcome for a group of patients with avoidant or obsessive-compulsive personality disorder.

Disruptions in the alliance are inevitable and occur more frequently than may be readily apparent to the clinician (Safran and Muran 2000). One study (Hill et al. 1993) asked patients to report about thoughts and feelings that they were not expressing to their therapists. Most things that were not discussed were negative, and even the most experienced therapists were aware of uncommunicated negative material only 45% of the time. It has also been suggested, however, that therapist awareness of patients' negative feelings may actually create problems; therapists, rather than being open and flexible in response, may at times become defensive and negative or may become more rigid in applying treatment techniques (Safran et al. 2001).

Safran and Muran (2000) outlined a model specifying two subtypes of ruptures: withdrawal and confrontation. Withdrawals are sometimes fairly subtle. One example is a therapist who assumes the treatment is progressing but may be unaware that a patient is withholding important information because of lack of trust or fear of feeling humiliated. Other types of withdrawal behaviors include such things as intellectualizing, talking excessively about other people, or changing the subject. Withdrawal behaviors may be more common in patients who are overly compliant at times, such as those with dependent or obsessive-compulsive personality disorder or those who are uncomfortable about interpersonal relations, such as patients with avoidant personality disorder.

Confrontations, on the other hand, are usually more overt, such as complaining about various aspects of therapy or criticizing the therapist. Some may be rather dramatic, such as a patient who storms out of session in a rage or leaves an angry message on the therapist's answering machine. Confrontation ruptures are likely to be more frequently experienced with more brittle patients such as those with borderline, narcissistic, or paranoid personality disorder. In any event, clinicians are best served by being alert to ruptures and adopting the attitude that these are often excellent opportunities to engage the patient in a collaborative effort to observe and learn about that patient's own style (Horvath and Greenberg 1994).

ALLIANCE CONSIDERATIONS BY DSM CLUSTER

For ease of discussion, this section is organized by DSM-IV-TR (American Psychiatric Association 2000) personality disorder diagnostic clusters to address particular alliance-relevant issues associated with each. However, there is increasing evidence that the DSM categories and clusters do not adequately capture the complexity of character pathology traits and symptoms. For instance, patients often meet criteria for at least two personality disorders, perhaps spanning different clusters, such as the co-occurrence of schizotypal personality disorder with borderline personality disorder or borderline personality disorder with avoidant personality disorder (McGlashan et al. 2000). In other cases, a patient may not meet full criteria for any one disorder but has prominent features associated with one or several personality disorders.

Thus, in practical terms, a clinician considering salient elements of the therapeutic alliance should determine which aspects of a patient's personality pathology are dominant or in ascendance at intake and at various points over the course of treatment. That being said, it has been suggested that the nature of the alliance established early in the treatment is more powerfully predictive of outcome (Horvath and Luborsky 1993). One example of the relationship of early alliance and outcome regarding personality disorders was demonstrated in a study of long-term psychotherapy with a group of patients with borderline personality disorder: therapist ratings of the alliance at 6 weeks predicted subsequent dropouts (Gunderson et al. 1997). As Horvath and Greenberg (1994) noted: "It seems reasonable to think of alliance development in the first phase of therapy as a series of windows of opportunity,

decreasing in size with each session" (p. 3). Thus, Table 15–1 summarizes by personality disorder the tendencies that may serve to challenge early collaboration building as well as aspects that a clinician might use to engage the patient.

Cluster A

Cluster A—the so-called odd/eccentric cluster—comprises schizotypal, schizoid, and paranoid personality disorders. What is most relevant for alliance building is the profound impairment in interpersonal relationships associated with these disorders. Because there are often pronounced paranoid or alienated features, people with these characteristics often do not seek treatment unless dealing with acute Axis I problems such as substance abuse. For those who are treatment seeking, there is evidence that these patients have great difficulty establishing a working alliance (e. g., Lingiardi et al. 2005).

Schizotypal

Schizotypal phenomena are thought by some to exist on the schizophrenia spectrum, given the associated disordered cognitions and bizarre beliefs. Because it is almost always the case that such individuals have one or no significant others outside family members, it is often assumed that schizotypal individuals have no desire to become involved in relationships. However, in many cases, it is more a matter of being excruciatingly uncomfortable around people rather than a lack of interest in connection. This discomfort may not be readily apparent, so establishing an alliance with such patients may require being attentive to clues about what is not being said. The therapist may be a player in some elaborated fantasy that is making it difficult for the patient to find some minimum level of comfort. A study by Bender et al. (2003) assessed various attributes of how patients with personality disorder think about their therapists. Interestingly, results showed that patients with schizotypal personality disorder had the highest level of mental involvement with therapy outside the session, missing their therapists and wishing for friendship while also feeling aggressive or negative. One man with schizotypal personality disorder (who had also become attached to the female research assistant) revealed the following view of his therapist:

> Very beautiful and attractive in a sense that I yearn to have a sexual relationship with her. She's very smart and educated. She knows what she wants out of life and I wish I were working for I could take her out to the movies and dinner. She turns me on and I desperately want to make love to her eternally. She's my life and knowing she doesn't feel the same, I live in dreams. (Bender et al. 2003, p. 231)

Schizoid

Benjamin (1993) noted that schizoid personality is more consistently associated with a lack of desire for intimate human connection. She described that some people with schizoid character can be found living very conventional lives on the surface, having families, jobs, and so on. However, usually things are arranged such that people are kept at an emotional distance. There may also be a pronounced lack of conflict, with associated affective coldness or dullness such that a truly schizoid person is unlikely to become anxious or depressed and thus is usually totally lacking any motivation to seek treatment. However, Akhtar (1992) suggested that underlying all of this apparent detachment is an intense neediness for others and the capability of interpersonal responsiveness with a few carefully selected people. Patients who may have more access to these latter attributes have a greater likelihood of forming an alliance in therapy if they choose to seek treatment.

Paranoid

The "paranoid" label largely speaks for itself. Paranoid individuals are incessantly loaded for bear and see bears where others do not—that is, they are vigilantly on the lookout for perceived slights, finding offense in even the most benign of circumstances. Alliance-building challenges are obvious. However, it has also been noted that paranoid individuals are often acting in defense of an extremely fragile self-concept and may possibly be reached over time in treatment with an approach that includes unwavering affirmation and careful handling of the many possible ruptures (Benjamin 1993).

Cluster B

The "dramatic" cluster includes borderline, narcissistic, histrionic, and antisocial personality disorders. Each of these character styles is associated in some way with pushing the limits, and great care is needed by clinicians to avoid crossing inappropriate lines in a quest to build an alliance. Thus, many Cluster B patients present some of the most daunting treatment challenges.

Borderline

Kernberg (1967) described the borderline personality as being riddled with aggressive impulses that constantly threaten to destroy positive internal images of the self and others. According to this model, the person with borderline personality disorder does not undergo the normal developmental process of psychological integration but rather, as a defensive attempt to deal with aggression, creates "splits" in his or her mind to protect the good images from the bad. This splitting leads to a fractured self-concept and the identity problems associated with this disorder. Thus, one can expect the alliance-building work to be rather rocky because these patients frequently exhibit pronounced emotional upheaval, self-destructive acting-out, and views of the therapist that alternate between idealization and denigration. Within relationships, such individuals are very needy and demanding, often straining the boundaries of the treatment relationship and exerting pressure on clinicians to behave in ways they normally would not. Re-

Table 15–1. Alliance-relevant aspects of each personality disorder style

Personality disorder trait cluster	Alliance challenges	Points of possible engagement in treatment
Schizotypal	Suspiciousness/paranoia Profound interpersonal discomfort Bizarre thinking	Possible motivation for human connection
Schizoid	Social detachment Emotional aloofness	Underlying neediness and sensitivity
Paranoid	Expectations of harm or exploitation Hypersensitivity to perceived criticism Inclination to withdraw or attack	Underlying need for affirmation
Borderline	Unstable emotional and cognitive states Extremely demanding Proneness to acting-out	Relationship seeking Responds to warmth and support
Narcissistic	Need for constant positive regard Contempt for others Grandiose sense of entitlement	Responds over time to empathy and affirmation
Histrionic	Attempts to charm and entertain Emotionally labile Unfocused cognitive style	Relationship seeking Responds to warmth and support
Antisocial	Controlling Tendency to lie and manipulate No empathy or regard for others Use of pseudoalliance to gain some advantage	May engage in treatment if in self-interest or if Axis I symptoms cause sufficient distress
Avoidant	Expectations of criticism or rejection Proneness to shame and humiliation Reluctance to disclose information	Responds to warmth/empathy Desire for relationships in spite of vulnerabilities

Table 15–1. Alliance-relevant aspects of each personality disorder style (*continued*)

Personality disorder trait cluster	Alliance challenges	Points of possible engagement in treatment
Dependent	No value placed on independence/taking initiative Submission leading to pseudoalliance	Friendly and compliant Likely to stay in treatment
Obsessive-compulsive	Need for control Perfectionistic toward self and others Fear of criticism from therapist Restricted affect Stubbornness	Conscientious Use of intellectualization may be helpful at times Will try to be a "good patient"

search has demonstrated that such pressures can impair the clinician's ability to reflect on his or her mental states and those of the patient (Diamond et al. 2003). Furthermore, clinicians who work with such patients must be able to tolerate and productively discuss anger and aggression. However, because patients with borderline personality disorder are, in most cases, relationship seeking, this is a positive indicator for engagement in treatment.

One treatment study of borderline patients (Waldinger and Gunderson 1984) examined alliance development over time. Psychodynamic psychotherapy was employed using largely noninterpretive interventions in the initial alliance-building period (the issue of intervention choice is discussed further later in the chapter). The authors observed that a strong alliance and good treatment outcome were linked to two factors: 1) a solid commitment by the participating therapist to remain engaged in the treatment until significant gains had been made by the patients; and 2) special emphasis on facilitating the patients' expression of aggression and rage without fear of retaliation. Other studies (e.g., Bennett et al. 2006; Horwitz et al. 1996) that have undertaken detailed analysis of alliance ruptures in the treatment of patients with borderline personality disorder have demonstrated the importance of the therapist vigilantly attending to the alliance. Horwitz et al. (1996) noted that "clinical observation of our cases revealed that the repair of moment-to-moment disruptions in the alliance often was the key factor in maintaining the viability of the psychotherapy" (p. 173).

Narcissistic

Narcissistic character traits have received considerable attention in the clinical literature. Kohut (1977) described individuals in whom there is a fundamental deficit in the ability to regulate self-esteem without resorting to omnipotent strategies of overcompen-

sation or overreliance on admiration by others. Some people who are narcissistically vulnerable have difficulty maintaining a cohesive sense of self because of ubiquitous shame, resulting from a sense that they fundamentally fall short of some internal ideal. They look for constant reinforcement from others to bolster their fragile self-images. This combination of traits has been referred to alternatively as *vulnerable, deflated,* or *covert narcissism.*

On the other side of the narcissistic "coin"—what the DSM narcissistic personality disorder diagnosis captures—are people who are intensely grandiose, seeking to maintain self-esteem through omnipotent fantasies and defeating others. They defend against needing others by maintaining fusions of ideal self, ideal other, and actual self-images. Thus, there is an illusion maintained whereby this type of narcissistic person has a sense that because he or she is perfect, love and admiration will be received from other "ideal people," and thus there is no need to associate with inferiors. In its most extreme form, this manifestation of character pathology has been referred to as *malignant narcissism* (Kernberg 1984).

It is obvious that such personality traits pose significant challenges in alliance building. It is often the case that the patient will need to keep the therapist out of the room, so to speak, for quite a long time by not allowing him or her to voice anything that represents an alternative view to that of the patient's. For such patients, other people, including the therapist, do not exist as separate individuals but merely as objects for gratifying needs. The clinician must tolerate this state of affairs, sometimes for a lengthy period of time. Meissner (1996) observed, "Establishing any degree of trust with such patients may be extremely difficult, but not impossible, for a consistent respect for their vulnerability and a recognition of their need not to trust may in time undercut their defensive need" (p. 228).

Histrionic

A patient with histrionic personality needs to be the center of attention and may behave in seductive ways in an attempt to keep the clinician entertained and engaged. At the same time, emotional expressions are often shallow and greatly exaggerated, and the histrionic patient assumes a deep connection and dependence very quickly. Details are presented in vague and overgeneralized ways. There is very little tolerance for frustration, resulting in demands for immediate gratification. As opposed to the more well-integrated, higher-functioning, neurotic "hysterical personality" often written about in the psychoanalytic literature, the histrionic personality disorder organization more closely resembles the borderline personality disorder organization. Particular borderline aspects include a tendency to utilize splitting defenses, rather than repression, and a marked degree of identity diffusion (Akhtar 1992). The attention-seeking attribute can be helpful in establishing a preliminary alliance. However, as with patients with borderline pathology, the clinician must be prepared to manage escalating demands and dramatic acting-out.

Antisocial

Antisocial personality is associated with ongoing violation of society's norms, manifested in such behaviors as theft, intimidation, violence, or making a living in an illegal fashion such as by fraud or selling drugs. Also narcissistic by definition, people with antisocial personality disorder (ASPD) have little or no regard for the welfare of others. Clearly, this personality disorder is found extensively among inmates within the prison system. Stone (1993) suggested that there are gradations of the antisocial style, with the milder forms being more amenable to treatment. However, within the broader label of *antisocial* is a subset of individuals who are considered to be psychopathic. Psychopaths are sadistic and manipulative pathological liars; show no empathy, compassion, or remorse for hurting others; and take no responsibility for their actions. The most dramatic form is manifested by individuals who torture or murder their victims. Those who perpetrate such violence reside on the extreme end of the spectrum of antisocial behavior and would be the most difficult to treat.

In keeping with the notion that there is a spectrum of antisocial psychopathology, empirical evidence shows that some ASPD patients are capable of forming a treatment alliance resulting in positive outcome (Gerstley et al. 1989). Consequently, it has been recommended by some that a trial treatment of several sessions be applied with ASPD patients who may typically be assumed to be untreatable. However, there is always the risk that such patients, particularly within an institutional context (e.g., a hospital or prison), may exhibit a pseudoalliance to gain certain advantages (Gabbard 2005). For example, there could be a disingenuous profession of enhanced self-understanding and movement toward reform as an attempt to manipulate the therapist into recommending inappropriate privileges.

There is some indication that depression serves as a moderator in the treatment of ASPD patients. One study demonstrated that depressed ASPD patients are more likely to benefit from treatment compared with nondepressed ASPD patients (Shea et al. 1992). Thus, the presence of depression may serve as motivation for these patients to seek and comply with treatment.

Sadomasochistic Character

Cases in which difficult patients take a prominent role in orchestrating situations to sabotage a potentially helpful treatment are ubiquitous in the clinical literature. This type of dynamic points to an additional element commonly overlooked in treatments in general but of particular relevance when trying to establish and maintain an alliance with patients with character pathology: sadomasochism. Most dramatically overt in patients with borderline, narcissistic, and/or antisocial issues, relational tendencies that are anywhere from tinged to saturated by sadomasochistic trends span the spectrum of personality disorder pathology. The presence of sadomasochistic patterns does not mean that overt sexual perversions will be present, although they may be, but that the patient has characteristic ways of engaging others in a struggle in which one party is suffering at the hands of the other. Patients with a sadomasochistic approach to relationships make it very difficult for the clinician working in any modality to be a helpful agent of change (see Chapter 10 of this volume, "Psychoanalysis and Psychodynamic Psychotherapy"). Furthermore, it is sometimes the case with such patients that at the foundation of the alliance is a very subtle, or not so subtle, sadomasochistic enactment.

For example, a patient may, on the surface, be agreeing with the therapist's observations but is actually experiencing them as verbal assaults while masochistically suffering in silence and showing no improvement in treatment. There is the patient who is highly provocative, attempting to bait the therapist into saying and doing things that may prove to be counterattacks. There are also patients who act out in apparently punishing ways, such as attempting suicide using a newly prescribed medication when it seemed as though the treatment was progressing.

Bach (1994) described a sadomasochistic way of relating as arising as "a defense against and an attempt to repair some traumatic loss that has not been adequately mourned" (p. 4). This trauma could have come in the form of an actual loss of a parent, loss of love as a result of abuse or neglect, or some experience of loss of the self due to such things as childhood illness or circumstances leading to overwhelming anxiety. From this perspective, the cruel behavior of the sadist may, for instance, be an attempt to punish the object for threatened abandonment. The masochistic stance involves a way of loving someone who gives

ill treatment—the only way of maintaining a connection is through suffering (Berliner 1947). Early in development, this way of loving is self-preservative—the sadism of the love object is turned upon the self as a way of maintaining a needed relationship (Menaker 1953). However, in an adult, this masochistic solution, with its always-attendant aggressive-sadistic elements, serves to cause significant interpersonal dysfunction.

Case Example

A single woman in her forties, Ms. P, was referred for psychotherapy after she had gone to see four or five other therapists, staying for only several sessions maximum because she found them all to be incompetent in some way. An avid reader of self-help literature, she considered herself an expert on the helping professions. Highly intelligent and extremely articulate, Ms. P was aspiring to be a filmmaker. She had gone through a series of "day jobs" with corporations, reporting that her women supervisors were always untalented, unreasonable, and critical of her. Her interpersonal relations were always tumultuous, her moods very unstable, and it was apparent that she had been grappling with narcissistic and borderline personality disorder issues for decades.

Sadomasochistic trends became apparent very quickly. In the first meeting, Ms. P launched the first of many critiques, reporting that she had found the therapist's greeting to be too upbeat but then also criticizing the therapist for not reassuring her that she would have a successful treatment. She ultimately announced that the therapist was "gifted," so she would continue with this treatment, but there were many sessions in which she would find fault or deliver lectures on technique and theory. At the same time, she was extremely brittle and incapable of reflecting on this type of behavior, feeling as a victim if there was any vague hint that she might be doing something questionable. Thus, while attacking the therapist, she was doing it in the service of collecting grievances and, as Berliner

(1947) observed about such patients, she "would rather be right than happy" (p. 46). Hence, both the sadistic and masochistic sides of the same coin were in evidence.

With patients such as this one, it is very important to be able to tolerate the expression of aggression. Consequently, to maintain an alliance with this very difficult woman, the therapist had to constantly assess whether the attacks represented a rupture in the alliance that had to be addressed or whether Ms. P simply needed to give voice to some of her tremendous anger at the world. In the instances it was judged that the alliance was in jeopardy, the therapist would discuss Ms. P's reaction to the therapist's interventions, acknowledging Ms. P's distress and telling Ms. P that the therapist would reflect on what had led her to make such comments. Ms. P usually found great relief in this approach, appreciating the therapist's willingness to reflect on the situation.

What is central is that the therapist withstood being portrayed as bad or incompetent in the patient's mind without retaliating as though it were true. If the therapist had had a different psychology, it would have been rather easy to take up the role of sadist in all of this, perhaps wrapped in the flag of "interpreting her aggression"; however, Ms. P and this therapist were a good match, because such retributive behavior would have been a sadomasochistic enactment and would have caused Ms. P to take a hasty departure.

Cluster C

The "anxious/fearful" cluster comprises avoidant, dependent, and obsessive-compulsive personality disorders. Patients who are most closely characterized by Cluster C disorders are emotionally inhibited and averse to interpersonal conflict and are often considered to be the treatable "neurotics" on the spectrum of personality disorders. These patients frequently feel very guilty and internalize blame for situations even when it is clear there is none. This latter tendency often facilitates alli-

ance building, because the patient is willing to take some responsibility for his or her dilemma and will somewhat more readily engage in a dialogue with the therapist to sort it all out, compared with patients with more severe Cluster A or B diagnoses (Stone 1993).

Dependent

Fearing abandonment, dependent patients tend to be very passive, submissive, and needy of constant reassurance. They go to great lengths not to offend others, even at great emotional expense, agreeing with others' opinions when they really do not or volunteering to do unsavory chores to stay in someone's good graces. In the context of treatment, dependent patients are easily engaged, at least superficially, but often withhold a great deal of material for fear of alienating the therapist in some way. The following is an example of how this might play out (Benjamin 1993).

> A patient [with dependent personality disorder] was chronically depressed, and the doctor tried her on a new antidepressant. She did not improve and had a number of side effects, but did not mention them to the doctor. Fortunately, the doctor remembered to ask for the specific side effects. The patient acknowledged the signs, and the doctor wrote a prescription for a different antidepressant. The patient was willing to acknowledge the signs of problems…, but she did not offer the information spontaneously. The doctor asked her why she did not say anything. She explained, "I thought that maybe they were just part of the way the drug worked…. I figured you would know what was best." (p. 405)

Benjamin also observed that one difficulty in working in psychotherapy with such patients is the reinforcement gained by the patient's behavior. That is, because the passivity and submissiveness usually result in being taken care of, despite the associated cost, dependent patients are loath to see the value in asserting some independence. Furthermore, there is a deeply ingrained assumption by these patients that they are actually incapable of functioning more independently and that being more assertive will be experienced by others as alienating aggressiveness. Thus, a therapist must be very alert to the withdrawal types of strains and ruptures, such as withholding information, as well as to the challenge to the alliance that may occur when the therapist attempts to encourage more independence.

Avoidant

The avoidant individual is extremely interpersonally sensitive, afraid of being criticized, and constantly concerned about saying or doing something foolish or humiliating. In spite of an intense desire to connect with others, an avoidant person does not let anyone get close unless absolutely sure the person likes him or her. Because of this acute sensitivity, there is some evidence that some avoidant patients are somewhat difficult to retain in treatment. One study showed that a group of avoidant patients was significantly more likely to drop out of a short-term supportive-expressive treatment compared with obsessive-compulsive personality disorder patients (Barber et al. 1997). Clinicians who work with avoidant patients need to be constantly mindful of the potentially shaming effects of certain comments but can also work with the patient's underlying hunger for attachment to enlist them in building an alliance.

Furthermore, there is preliminary evidence supporting the notion that at least some patients diagnosed with avoidant personality disorder are actually better characterized as vulnerable narcissists. These patients covertly crave admiration to bolster their fragile self-esteem and secretly or unconsciously feel entitled to it rather than simply being afraid of not being liked or accepted (Dickenson and Pincus 2003). Gabbard (2005) also referred to this style as *hypervigilant narcissism*, emphasizing extreme interpersonal sensitivity, other-directedness, and shame proneness aspects. An underlying unrecognized narcissism in avoidant personality disorder has significant treatment implications, changing the nature of the forces affecting the alliance as well as shaping the types of treatment interventions that are indicated.

Obsessive-Compulsive

The obsessive-compulsive character is associated with more stable interpersonal relationships than some other styles, but typical defenses are centered on repression, with patterns of highly regulated gratification and ongoing denial of interpersonal and intrapsychic conflicts (Shapiro 1965). Self-willed and obstinate, with a constant eye toward rules and regulations, people with obsessive-compulsive attributes guard against any meaningful consideration of their impulses toward others. Maintaining control over internal experience and the external world is a top priority, so rigidity is often a hallmark of this character type. Except in its most severe manifestations, obsessive-compulsive character pathology is less impairing than some of the others and more readily ameliorated by treatment. Although stubborn and controlling and averse to considering emotional content, obsessive-compulsive individuals also generally try to be "good patients" and so can be engaged in a constructive alliance that is less rocky compared with other types of personality disorder patients.

Case Example

Mr. Q, a 25-year-old graduate student in philosophy, began a twice-weekly psychotherapy. His presenting complaint was difficulty with completing work effectively, particularly writing tasks, due to excessive anxiety and obsessionality (he met criteria for obsessive-compulsive personality disorder and generalized anxiety disorder). When he came for treatment, he was struggling to make progress on his master's thesis. Although Mr. Q socialized quite a bit, he reported that intimate relationships often felt "wooden." He was usually overcommitted, with an endless list of "shoulds" that he would constantly mentally review and remind himself how much he was failing to satisfy his obligations. A central theme throughout treatment was his tendency to be self-denigrating, loathing himself as a person deserving of punishment in some way yet being extremely provocative (sadomasochistic trends). He also held very strong political beliefs, sure that his way of viewing things was superior to others'.

Establishing a productive alliance with Mr. Q was not easily accomplished at first. In the early phase of treatment, he was extremely controlling and challenging in sessions, talking constantly and tangentially, often losing the core point of his statements because of a need to present excessive details. Any statement the therapist made was experienced as an intrusion or interruption. For example, if the therapist attempted to be empathic using a word Mr. Q had not used, such as saying, "That sounds difficult," he would respond, "Difficult? I don't know if I'd choose the word difficult. Challenging, maybe, or daunting, but not difficult." Thus, for a number of months in the initial phase of the treatment, the therapist chose her words carefully, which eventually paved the way for increased dialogue about his problems. Mr. Q also began to tolerate a discussion of his emotional life, a topic that previously had been very threatening to him.

Passive-Aggressive

Some of the aspects of this latter case example may be described as passive-aggressive, particularly the patient's tendency to excessively procrastinate in doing his work. Passive-aggressive traits include argumentativeness, scorning authority, resistance to carrying out social and occupational responsibilities, angry pessimism, alternating between defiance and contrition, envy, and exaggerated complaints about personal misfortune. These attributes pose challenges to the formation of an effective therapeutic alliance because

these patients are likely to expect that the treatment holds no promise of helping, and they behave in ways that contribute to that outcome. The passive-aggressive (negativistic) personality disorder diagnosis was included in Cluster C in DSM-III-R (American Psychiatric Association 1987) but was subsequently shifted to the appendix of disorders needing further study in DSM-IV (American Psychiatric Association 1994). Some experts on phenomenology argue that this diagnosis is clinically very useful and should be restored to the DSM list of personality disorders (e.g., Wetzler and Morey 1999).

ALLIANCE CONSIDERATIONS WITHIN DIFFERENT TREATMENT PARADIGMS

Clearly, no matter what treatment paradigm one adopts for working with personality disorder patients, attention to the alliance is of utmost importance. Thoughts and feelings on the part of the therapist must be monitored closely, because interactions with difficult patients may often be provocative, inducing reactions that must be carefully managed. (Refer to Chapter 16, "Boundary Issues," for a discussion of some of the most serious consequences of treatments gone awry.) Although this topic is usually discussed as countertransference in the psychoanalytic/psychodynamic tradition, it is also quite applicable across all treatments (Gabbard 1999).

Treatment approach and technique must be flexible so that interventions can be made appropriate to the individual patient's style. Otherwise, the alliance may be jeopardized and the patient will not benefit or may leave treatment altogether. For example, Spinhoven et al. (2007) found an interaction between alliance and therapeutic techniques, influencing course and outcome of a group of patients with borderline personality disorder. Furthermore, it is likely that noticeable improvements in symptoms and functioning in patients with personality disorders will require a significantly longer period of treatment than is required for patients with no character pathology. Although the application of specific treatment approaches is discussed at length in other chapters of this book, it is worth mentioning here a few alliance-relevant considerations pertaining to each broad treatment context.

Psychodynamic Psychotherapy/ Psychoanalysis

One long-standing issue within the psychodynamic psychotherapy tradition is the application of particular techniques. Interpretation of the transference was long considered the heart of the psychoanalytic approach. However, as the application of this treatment evolved and clinicians gained more experience with more disturbed patients—most notably those with borderline and narcissistic trends—it became apparent that, in many cases, transference interpretations with such patients were often counterproductive. Refraining from making deep, interpretive interventions early on is consistent with notions of writers such as Winnicott (1965) and Kohut (1984) who asserted that certain, more disturbed, patients cannot tolerate such interpretations in the initial phase of treatment.

Gabbard (2005) stressed the importance of understanding that there is usually a mixture of supportive and expressive (interpretive) elements in every analysis or psychodynamic psychotherapy. That is, the expressive, insight-oriented mode of assisting patients in uncovering unconscious conflicts, thoughts, or affects through interpretation or confrontation may be appropriate at times, whereas a more supportive approach of bolstering the patient's defenses and coping abilities is preferable in other circumstances.

For instance, it may be difficult to focus on more insight-oriented interventions with a patient with borderline impairments until that patient is assisted in achieving a safe, more stable alliance. Similarly, the severely narcissistically impaired patient may not be able to accept the analyst's interpretations of his or her unconscious motivations for quite a long time, so that supportive, empathic communications may be more effective interventions in building an alliance by helping the patient feel heard and understood. Conversely, some obsessional patients may benefit earlier in treatment by interpretations of the repressed conflicts that may underlie the symptoms.

The results of the Psychotherapy Research Project of The Menninger Foundation, which included patients with personality disorders, led Wallerstein (1986) to conclude that both expressive and supportive interventions can lead to character change. At the same time, there is empirical evidence supporting the notion that a fairly solid alliance must be present to effectively utilize transference interpretations per se. Bond et al. (1998) demonstrated with a group of personality disorder patients in long-term treatment that for those patients whose alliance was weak, transference interpretations caused further impairment to the alliance. Conversely, the alliance was strengthened by transference interpretations when already solidly established. At the same time, supportive interventions and discussions of defensive operations resulted in moving the therapeutic work forward with both the weak and strong alliance groups of patients.

These findings are consistent with a study conducted by Horwitz et al. (1996) exploring the effect of supportive and interpretive interventions on the therapeutic alliance with a group of patients with borderline personality disorder. The authors concluded that although many times therapists are eager to pursue transference interpretations, such interventions are "high-risk, high-gain" and need to be employed carefully. They may damage the alliance with patients who are vulnerable and prone to feelings of shame and humiliation. Therefore, there must be flexibility in adjusting technique according to the dynamics of a particular patient at a particular time given the patient's capacities and vulnerabilities, appropriately balancing both supportive and expressive interventions.

Case Example

Ms. R sought treatment when she was in her early 30s. She was referred for psychotherapy from her graduate school's counseling center. Ms. R presented in a major depressive episode and met eight out of a possible nine criteria for borderline personality disorder. The initial phase of the twice-weekly psychodynamic treatment focused on her depression and helping her to stabilize sometimes-devastating affective instability. She also reported intermittent, but not life-threatening, instances of cutting herself, particularly after some unsatisfactory encounter with a friend or colleague.

The patient's lack of object constancy, her affective instability, and a fragmented sense of self contributed to great variations in the nature of Ms. R's presence in sessions. At times she would be overwhelmed by fatigue, whereas other times she would be engaging, funny, and analytical. She would often defend against undesirable thoughts or emotions by spending the session recounting the details of her day-to-day life in great detail. The disjunctions in self-states made it difficult at times to maintain continuity in the process, because Ms. R did not remember what happened from session to session.

A Kernbergian formulation (Kernberg 1967) of this patient was theoretically informative in describing some of her dynamics (defensive splitting had been one prominent theme in the treatment). However, the technical implications of this particular approach, with its direct confrontation of aggression in the transference early in the treatment (Kernberg 1987) would have endangered the sometimes fragile working alliance being forged. In fact, a few times when transference interpretations were attempted in the first phase of treatment, Ms. R became confused and distressed, quickly changing the subject away from a discussion of her relationship with the therapist, talking about

ending treatment, or becoming very sleepy and shut down for several sessions. On one occasion early on when an attempt was made by the therapist to address something in their relationship, Ms. R became very angry and said, "Why is any of this about here? These are my problems and I don't see what any of this has to do with you!" Clearly, in the beginning phase of treatment with some patients, one needs a different way of entering the patient's psychic world (Ellman 1998). On the other hand, Ms. R was responsive to gentle interpretations of her defenses, such as the therapist pointing out to her that her self-harm behaviors were a way of "being mean" to herself instead of channeling anger toward those who had upset her.

Thus, for most of the first 3–4 years of this treatment, the primary tasks were to develop a working alliance and establish a "holding environment" (Winnicott 1965) within which Ms. R could begin to feel safe to explore her history, her feelings, and her own mind. This approach paid off, because it eventually became possible to uncover, in ways that were meaningful and transformative to Ms. R, some of the split-off rage and despair underlying the identity instability and distorted cognitive functioning. Deeper experience and exploration of these feelings paved the way for further integration and less disjunctive experiences in her life and from session to session, and working with the transference increasingly became both possible and very productive. Ms. W has not been depressed for years and no longer meets any borderline criteria.

Cognitive-Behavioral Therapies

In recent years, work has been done to apply to personality disorders cognitive and cognitive-behavioral treatments that have typically been used to treat Axis I symptoms. However, Tyrer and Davidson (2000) observed that the approaches generally taken in these therapies for Axis I "mental state disorders" cannot be simply transferred to treating personality disorders without certain adjustments. Most cognitive and cognitive-behavioral therapies are based prominently on a therapist–patient collaboration that is assumed to be present from very early in the treatment. Such a collaboration, which revolves around the patient undertaking specific activities and assignments, depends on the establishment of a solid working alliance; however, it is sometimes very difficult to engage certain personality disorder patients in the therapeutic tasks. To facilitate this alliance when working with personality disorder patients—in addition to requiring lengthier periods to complete these treatments—work needs to directly address patient–therapist collaboration with clearly set boundaries and to focus on the therapeutic relationship itself when appropriate (Tyrer and Davidson 2000).

For example, in using the initial sessions of dialectical behavior therapy (DBT) (see Chapter 12, "Dialectical Behavior Therapy") to begin establishing a working relationship, Marsha Linehan (1993) observed: "These sessions offer an opportunity for both patient and therapist to explore problems that may arise in establishing and maintaining a therapeutic alliance" (p. 446). Even though DBT is a manualized treatment with clearly elaborated therapeutic tasks, it is quickly evident, particularly in working with patients with borderline personality disorder, that a great deal of flexibility must be maintained within this paradigm to achieve an alliance. More specifically, there may be frequent occurrences of therapy-interfering behaviors ranging from ambivalence causing missed sessions to multiple suicide attempts that prevent the treatment from progressing as the method outlines.

Case Example

Ms. S, a young woman with dependent personality disorder, was referred for behavioral treatment of a phobia of all forms of transportation (her other issues were already being addressed in an ongoing psychotherapy). The therapist spent several sessions with Ms. S outlining the exposure techniques recommended for treating her phobia, but she was resistant to beginning any of the activities described. At the same time, while trying to pursue a classically behavioral approach, the therapist realized that it was very important for Ms. S to spend some of the time talking about her life and the impact the phobia symptoms had for her. This approach helped Ms. S to feel a connection to the therapist. The therapist made this relationship-building aspect explicit with Ms. S by agreeing to take a part of each session to talk about her situation, but the therapist also made it clear that it was necessary to reserve enough time for the exposure activities. This approach fostered an alliance sufficiently to begin the behavioral tasks. By being flexible, while setting clear tasks and boundaries, the therapist was able to engage Ms. S in the treatment, and she began taking short rides with the therapist on the bus, eventually overcoming these fears completely.

Psychopharmacology Sessions

One large-scale depression study (Krupnick et al. 1996) comparing several different psychotherapies with medication and placebo showed that the quality of the alliance was significantly related to outcome for all of the study groups. This finding demonstrates the importance of considering the alliance not only in psychotherapies but in medication sessions as well. Gutheil (1982) suggested that there is a particular aspect of the therapeutic alliance—what he calls the *pharmaco-therapeutic alliance*—that is relevant to the prescription of medications. In this formulation of the alliance, it is recommended that the physician adopt the stance of *participant prescribing*—that is, rather than adopting an authoritarian role, the clinician should make every effort to involve the patient as a collaborator who engages actively in goal-setting and observing and evaluating the experience of using specific medications. Such collaboration, like other therapeutic processes, may be affected by the patient's transference distortions of the clinician.

This latter notion can be more broadly applied in transtheoretical terms to personality disorders, where it is appropriate to consider how the patient's characteristic style may influence his or her attitudes and behaviors toward taking psychiatric medications. Some patients may become upset if medication is not prescribed, feeling slighted because they think their problems are not being taken seriously. Others with paranoid tendencies may think the physician is trying to put something over on them, or worse. Some patients who are prone to somaticizing, such as those with borderline or histrionic tendencies, might be hypersensitive to any possible side effects (real or imagined) and argue with the prescriber about his or her competence. The following is another example (Benjamin 1993) illustrating the importance of being mindful of how personality disorder patients might react around issues of medication:

> A patient [with avoidant personality disorder] overdosed one evening on the medicine her doctor had prescribed for her persistent depression. She liked and respected him a lot. She was discovered comatose by a neighbor who wondered why her cat would not stop meowing. The neighbor was the patient's only friend. It turned out that that morning her doctor had wondered aloud whether she had a personality disorder. The patient was deeply humiliated by that idea but secretly agreed with it. She felt extremely embarrassed and was convinced that her doctor now knew she was a completely foolish person.... Rather than endure the humiliation of facing him again, she decided to end it all. (p. 411)

Psychiatric Hospital Settings

Across the spectrum of personality disorders, psychiatric hospitalizations—both inpatient and day treatment programs—are most common for those with borderline personality disorder (Bender et al. 2001). The central consideration regarding the alliance in this treatment context is that there is always a team of individuals responsible for the patient. With patients with borderline issues, splitting tendencies frequently are quite pronounced. That is, as a way of trying to cope with inner turmoil, the patient's mental world is often organized in black/white, good/bad polarities, and through complicated (see explanation of projective identification in Chapter 10, "Psychoanalysis and Psychodynamic Psychotherapy") interaction patterns with various staff members, this internal world becomes replayed externally, dividing staff member against staff member.

Gabbard (1989) observed that this dynamic is often set up because the patient will present one self-representation to one or several team members and a very different representation to another. One of these staff factions may be viewed as the "good" one by the patient and the other as the "bad" one—although these designations can flip precipitously in the patient's mind—and this split becomes enacted among team members as they begin to work at cross-purposes. It can be seen rather readily that trying to develop a constructive alliance with such a patient can be extremely precarious, particularly given the ever-decreasing length of hospital stays under managed care. That means that communication and close collaboration among the members of the team are vital during every phase of the hospital treatment.

Matters are complicated further at times by the need to find a productive way for hospital staff to collaborate with clinicians providing ongoing outpatient psychotherapy and/or psychopharmacology treatments. Although the hospitalization may represent a significant rupture in the outpatient treatment alliance, this rupture does not necessarily indicate that the outpatient treatment was ineffective and must be terminated but that work will be needed to reestablish the continuity of the treatment relationship. However, it is not uncommon for the hospital staff, seeing the patient's current condition, to conclude that the outpatient clinicians were somehow not doing a competent job (this conclusion may, of course, be fueled by further splitting on the part of the patient). Moreover, at times it may be obvious that the outpatient treatment was inadequate or inappropriate. In any event, it becomes rather dicey for all parties concerned to sort out the proper role of hospital staff versus outpatient staff over the course of the inpatient or day treatment program.

Case Example

A young woman, Ms. T, with borderline personality disorder was admitted to a psychiatric inpatient unit after coming to the emergency department reporting acute suicidal ideation. This patient had been hospitalized several times previously, was in the mental health field, and "knew the ropes" quite well. She had been assigned a psychiatrist who was responsible for overall case management and a psychologist who was to provide short-term psychotherapy on the unit.

The initial psychotherapy session was extremely difficult, with Ms. T refusing to speak very much and regarding the therapist with rageful contempt. However, after several more encounters, there was some softening by Ms. T and she began to discuss the upsetting circumstances that led to her hospitalization. It appeared there might be the beginnings of a working alliance. Indeed, as she opened up more about her life, she reported feeling slightly more hopeful and less fragmented.

However, at the same time, she had created quite a bit of trouble with the rest of the staff by being very demanding and uncooperative and attempting to initiate discharge procedures even while refusing to deny that she would kill herself. Having reached a point of needing to take some action in the courts to keep Ms. T hospitalized, the psychiatrist hastily called a meeting including himself, the psychologist, and the patient. Having had no opportunity to confer with other team members on the matter, the psychiatrist proceeded to tell Ms. T that he was initiating legal proceedings to keep her in the hospital. Mindful of the splitting tendencies of such patients, the psychiatrist was careful to make it clear that he represented the viewpoint of the entire team, including the psychologist. However, he unwittingly created another split. Ms. T, feeling betrayed, stared hatefully at the psychologist, the fragile working alliance was shattered, and she subsequently refused to participate in psychotherapy or any other therapeutic activities for the rest of the hospitalization. It is possible this rupture could have been ameliorated had there been adequate consultation among treatment team members so that a less alienating approach could be formulated.

CONCLUSION

Establishing an alliance in any treatment paradigm requires a great deal of empathy and attunement to a patient's way of seeing the world. Attention to alliance building is even more important when working with patients with personality disorders, because these individuals often present with disturbed patterns of interpersonal relations. Research has shown not only the importance of building an alliance but also that this alliance is vital in the earliest phase of treatment. One cannot rigidly pursue the dictates of one's treatment paradigm without being prepared to make frequent adjustments to address the various ruptures that may occur. Gleaning clues from the patient's accounts of his or her relationships can serve to guide the clinician's general interpersonal stance. Furthermore, monitoring the therapeutic alliance in response to clinical interventions is a useful way to assess the effectiveness of one's approach and is informative in determining appropriate adjustments in the style and content of the therapist's interactions with the patient.

REFERENCES

Adler G: Transference, real relationship and alliance. Int J Psychoanal 61:547–558, 1980

Akhtar S: Broken Structures: Severe Personality Disorders and Their Treatment. Northvale, NJ, Jason Aronson, 1992

American Psychiatric Association: Diagnostic and Statistical Manual of Mental Disorders, 3rd Edition, Revised. Washington, DC, American Psychiatric Association, 1987

American Psychiatric Association: Diagnostic and Statistical Manual of Mental Disorders, 4th Edition. Washington, DC, American Psychiatric Association, 1994

American Psychiatric Association: Diagnostic and Statistical Manual of Mental Disorders, 4th Edition, Text Revision. Washington, DC, American Psychiatric Association, 2000

Bach S: The Language of Perversion and the Language of Love. Northvale, NJ, Jason Aronson, 1994

Bach S: On treating the difficult patient, in The Modern Freudians. Edited by Ellman CS, Grand S, Silvan M, et al. Northvale, NJ, Jason Aronson, 1998, pp 185–195

Barber JP, Morse JQ, Krakauer ID, et al: Change in obsessive-compulsive and avoidant personality disorders following time-limited supportive-expressive therapy. Psychotherapy 34:133–143, 1997

Bender DS, Dolan RT, Skodol AE, et al: Treatment utilization by patients with personality disorders. Am J Psychiatry 158:295–302, 2001

Bender DS, Farber BA, Sanislow CA, et al: Representations of therapists by patients with personality disorders. Am J Psychother 57:219–236, 2003

Benjamin LS: Interpersonal Diagnosis and Treatment of Personality Disorders. New York, Guilford, 1993

Bennett D, Parry G, Ryle A: Resolving threats to the therapeutic alliance in cognitive analytic therapy of borderline personality disorder: a task analysis. Psychol Psychother 79:395–418, 2006

Berliner B: The role of object relations in moral masochism. Psychoanal Q 27:38–56, 1947

Bond M, Banon E, Grenier M: Differential effects of interventions on the therapeutic alliance with patients with personality disorders. J Psychother Pract Res 7:301–318, 1998

Bordin ES: The generalizability of the psychoanalytic concept of the working alliance. Psychotherapy: Theory, Research and Practice 16:252–260, 1979

Diamond D, Stovall-McClough C, Clarkin JF, et al: Patient–therapist attachment in the treatment of borderline personality disorder. Bull Menninger Clin 67:227–259, 2003

Dickenson KA, Pincus AL: Interpersonal analysis of grandiose and vulnerable narcissism. J Personal Disord 17:188–207, 2003

Ellman SJ: Freud's Technique Papers: A Contemporary Perspective. Northvale, NJ, Jason Aronson, 1991

Ellman SJ: The unique contribution of the contemporary Freudian position, in The Modern Freudians. Edited by Ellman CS, Grand S, Silvan M, et al. Northvale, NJ, Jason Aronson, 1998, pp 237–268

Freud S: The dynamics of the transference (1912), in Collected Papers, Vol 2. Translated by Riviere J. London, Hogarth Press, 1946, pp 312–322

Gabbard GO: Splitting in hospital treatment. Am J Psychiatry 146:444–451, 1989

Gabbard GO: An overview of countertransference: theory and technique, in Countertransference Issues in Psychiatric Treatment. Edited by Gabbard GO (Review of Psychiatry Series, Vol 18; Oldham JM, Riba MB, series eds). Washington, DC, American Psychiatric Press, 1999, pp 1–25

Gabbard GO: Psychodynamic Psychiatry in Clinical Practice, 4th Edtion. Washington, DC, American Psychiatric Press, 2005

Gerstley L, McLellan AT, Alterman AI, et al: Ability to form an alliance with the therapist: a possible social marker of prognosis for patients with antisocial personality disorder. Am J Psychiatry 146:508–512, 1989

Gibbons MBC, Crits-Cristoph P, de la Cruz C, et al: Pretreatment expectations, interpersonal functioning, and symptoms in the prediction of the therapeutic alliance across supportive-expressive psychotherapy and cognitive therapy. Psychother Res 13:59–76, 2003

Gunderson JG: Psychodynamic psychotherapy for borderline personality disorder, in Psychotherapy for Personality Disorders. Edited by Gunderson JG, Gabbard GO (Review of Psychiatry Series, Vol 19; Oldham JM, Riba MB, series eds). Washington, DC, American Psychiatric Press, 2000, pp 33–64

Gunderson JG, Najavits LM, Leonhard C, et al: Ontogeny of the therapeutic alliance in borderline patients. Psychother Res 7:301–309, 1997

Gutheil TG: The psychology of psychopharmacology. Bull Menninger Clin 46:321–330, 1982

Gutheil TG, Havens LL: The therapeutic alliance: contemporary meanings and confusions. Int Rev Psychoanal 6:467–481, 1979

Hersoug AG, Monsen J, Havik OE, et al: Quality of working alliance in psychotherapy: diagnoses, relationship and intrapsychic variables as predictors. Psychother Psychosom 71:18–27, 2002

Hill CE, Thompson BJ, Cogar MC, et al: Beneath the surface of long-term therapy: therapist and client report of their own and each other's covert processes. J Couns Psychol 40:278–287, 1993

Horvath AO, Greenberg LS (eds): The Working Alliance: Theory, Research, and Practice. New York, Wiley, 1994

Horvath AO, Luborsky L: The role of therapeutic alliance in psychotherapy. J Consult Clin Psychol 61:561–573, 1993

Horvath AO, Symonds BD: Relation between working alliance and outcome in psychotherapy: a meta-analysis. J Couns Psychol 38:139–149, 1991

Horwitz L, Gabbard GO, Allen JG, et al: Borderline Personality Disorder: Tailoring the Psychotherapy to the Patient. Washington, DC, American Psychiatric Press, 1996

Kernberg OF: Borderline personality organization. J Am Psychoanal Assoc 15:641–685, 1967

Kernberg OF: Severe Personality Disorders: Psychotherapeutic Strategies. New Haven, CT, Yale University Press, 1984

Kernberg OF: An ego psychology–object relations theory approach to the transference. Psychoanal Q 56:197–221, 1987

Kohut H: The Restoration of the Self. New York, International Universities Press, 1977

Kohut H: How Does Analysis Cure? Chicago, IL, University of Chicago Press, 1984

Krupnick JL, Sotsky SM, Simmens S, et al: The role of the therapeutic alliance in psychotherapy and pharmacotherapy outcome: findings in the National Institute of Mental Health Treatment of Depression Collaborative Research Program. J Consult Clin Psychol 65:532–539, 1996

Linehan MM: Cognitive-Behavioral Treatment of Borderline Personality Disorder. New York, Guilford, 1993

Lingiardi V, Filippucci L, Baiocco R: Therapeutic alliance evaluation in personality disorders psychotherapy. Psychother Res 15:45–53, 2005

Masterson JF: The Search for the Real Self: Unmasking the Personality Disorders of Our Age. New York, Free Press, 1988

McGlashan TH, Grilo CM, Skodol AE, et al: The Collaborative Longitudinal Personality Disorders Study: baseline Axis I/II and II/II diagnostic co-occurrence. Acta Psychiatr Scand 102:256–264, 2000

Meissner WW: The Therapeutic Alliance. New Haven, CT, Yale University Press, 1996

Menaker E: Masochism: a defense reaction of the ego. Psychoanal Q 22:205–220, 1953

Orlinsky DA, Grawe K, Parks BK: Process and outcome in psychotherapy: noch einmal, in Handbook of Psychotherapy and Behavior Change, 4th Edition. Edited by Bergin AE, Garfield SL. New York, Wiley, 1994, pp 270–376

Piper WE, Azim HFA, Joyce AS, et al: Quality of object relations versus interpersonal functioning as predictors of therapeutic alliance and psychotherapy outcome. J Nerv Ment Dis 179:432–438, 1991

Safran JD, Muran JC: Negotiating the Therapeutic Alliance. New York, Guilford, 2000

Safran JD, Muran JC, Samstag LW, et al: Repairing alliance ruptures. Psychotherapy 38:406–412, 2001

Samstag LW, Batchelder S, Muran JC, et al: Predicting treatment failure from in-session interpersonal variables. J Psychother Pract Res 5:126–143, 1998

Shapiro D: Neurotic Styles. New York, Basic Books, 1965

Shea MT, Widiger TA, Klein MH: Comorbidity of personality disorders and depression: implications for treatment. J Consult Clin Psychol 60:857–868, 1992

Spinhoven P, Giesen-Bloo J, van Dyck R, et al: The therapeutic alliance in schema-focused therapy and transference-focused psychotherapy for borderline personality disorder. J Consult Clin Psychol 75:104–115, 2007

Stone MH: Abnormalities of Personality. New York, WW Norton, 1993

Strauss JL, Hayes AM, Johnson SL, et al: Early alliance, alliance ruptures, and symptom change in a nonrandomized trial of cognitive therapy for avoidant and obsessive-compulsive personality disorders. J Consult Clin Psychol 74:337–345, 2006

Tyrer P, Davidson K: Cognitive therapy for personality disorders, in Psychotherapy for Personality Disorders. Edited by Gunderson JG, Gabbard GO (Review of Psychiatry Series, Vol 19; Oldham JM, Riba MB, series eds). Washington, DC, American Psychiatric Press, 2000, pp 131–149

Waldinger RJ, Gunderson JG: Completed psychotherapies with borderline patients. Am J Psychother 38:190–202, 1984

Wallerstein RS: Forty-Two Lives in Treatment: A Study of Psychoanalysis and Psychotherapy. New York, Guilford, 1986

Wetzler S, Morey LC: Passive-aggressive personality disorder: the demise of a syndrome. Psychiatry 62:49–59, 1999

Winnicott DW: The Maturational Processes and the Facilitating Environment. London, Hogarth Press, 1965

16

Boundary Issues

Thomas G. Gutheil, M.D.

Experience teaches us that any discussion of boundary issues—boundary crossings and violations—must begin with certain caveats, best delivered in the form of axioms. First, only the professional member of the treatment dyad has a professional code to honor or violate; thus only the professional is responsible for setting and maintaining professional boundaries. Second, patients, having no professional code, may transgress or attempt to transgress professional boundaries; if they are competent adults, they are responsible or accountable for their *behavior*. However, the professional must hold the line. Third, to explore the dynamics of interaction between therapist and patient is neither to "blame the victim" (i.e., the patient) nor to exonerate the professional from responsibility for the boundaries.

Boundary issues in the treatment of psychiatric patients are universal, as are concerns about these issues. Therefore, to discuss boundary issues in relation to patients with personality disorders is not to imply that *all* or *only* personality-disordered patients experience or pose boundary problems. Instead, this chapter examines a subset of the wider universe of boundary-related potential problem areas.

According to my own evidence, the above caveats do not indicate obsessive caution. In 1989, I pointed out that patients with borderline personality disorder (BPD) presented particular challenges with regard to boundaries (Gutheil 1989). That article was based on my forensic caseload and thus drawn from empirical reality. As discussed therein, the topic of boundaries for patients with BPD is fraught with tension, confusion, and political incorrectness.

The profession as a whole has had its consciousness raised by the careful study of trauma victims, many of whom had become highly sensitive to boundary transgressions in their treaters; indeed, boundary issues within the nuclear families of these individuals may have constituted, or been a component of, the trauma. The frequent association of boundary problems as precursors to actual sexual misconduct also focused attention on the subject.

It is critically important to retain nonjudgmental clarity in the important area of boundary issues, because the consequences of confusion about this topic may be serious. This chapter aims to alleviate possible confusion. Before turning our attention to personality disorders and their implications for boundary theory, the basic elements are summarized.

BASIC ELEMENTS OF BOUNDARY THEORY

Just what is a boundary? A working definition might be that a *boundary* is the edge of appropriate, professional conduct. The definition is highly context dependent. The relevant contexts may be the treater's ideology, the stage of the therapy, the patient's condition or diagnosis, the geographical setting, or the cultural milieu, among others. Although attorneys, boards of licensure, and young clinicians may long for a checklist of approved and disapproved behaviors, the matter is not that simple. Context is a critical and determinative factor.

Besides complaint procedures and their aftermath, data about boundary issues come from consultations, supervision and training settings, the literature, professional meetings, informal remarks by colleagues, and formal studies. These data permit empirical examination of the varieties of boundary phenomena, the criteria for boundary assessment, and the clinical contexts in which problems arise. An extensive literature has grown up around this subject in recent decades, and the reader is directed to this literature for additional discussion beyond the narrower focus of this chapter (Celenza 2007; Epstein and Si-

mon 1990; Gabbard 1999; Gabbard and Lester 2002; Gutheil and Brodsky 2008; Gutheil and Gabbard 1993, 1998; Gutheil and Simon 2002; Ingram 1991; Langs 1976; Simon 1989, 1992; Smith 1977; Spruiell 1983; Stone 1976). In summary, boundary problems may emerge from role issues, time, place and space, money, gifts and services, clothing, language, and physical or sexual contact as elsewhere addressed (Gutheil and Gabbard 1993).

BOUNDARY CROSSINGS AND BOUNDARY VIOLATIONS

In an earlier publication, Gabbard and I proposed a distinction that has proved important both in theory and in litigation related to boundaries: the difference between boundary crossings and boundary violations (Gutheil and Gabbard 1993).

Boundary crossings are defined as transient, nonexploitative deviations from classical therapeutic or general clinical practice in which the treater steps out to a minor degree from strict verbal psychotherapy. These crossings do not hurt the therapy and may even promote or facilitate it. Examples might include offering a crying patient a tissue, helping a fallen patient up from the floor, helping an elderly patient on with a coat, giving a fragile patient a home telephone number for emergencies, giving a patient traveling on foot a lift in your car during a blizzard, writing cards to a patient during a long absence, visiting a patient at home based on his or her medical needs, answering selected personal questions, disclosing selected personal information, and so on. None of these actions is psychotherapy in its pure "talking" form; they constitute instead a mixture of manners, helpfulness, support, or social amity. No one could reasonably claim that these actions are exploitative of the patient or the patient's needs. Depending on the context, the appropriate response to such actions is for the therapist to explore their impact, maximize their therapeutic utility, and detect and neutralize any difficulties the patient may have as a result. Even the therapist's well-mannered gesture of putting out a hand for a handshake may be experienced as an attack or threat by a patient with a horrendous trauma history. An important point about boundary crossings is that when they occur, the therapist should review the matter with the patient on the next available occasion and fully document the rationale, the discussion with the patient, and the description of the patient's response.

Boundary violations, in contrast, constitute essentially harmful deviations from the normal parameters of treatment—deviations that *do* harm the patient, usually through some sort of exploitation that breaks the rule of "First, do no harm." Usually, the therapist's needs are gratified by taking advantage of the patient in some manner. The therapy is not advanced and may even be destroyed by such violations. Examples might include taking advantage of the patient financially, using the patient to gratify the therapist's narcissistic or dependency needs, using the patient for menial services (cleaning the office, getting lunch, running errands for the therapist), or engaging in sexual or sexualized relations or relationship with the patient. A useful test for distinguishing a boundary crossing from a violation is whether the event can be discussed in the therapy (Gutheil and Gabbard 1993). An even better test is whether the behavior in question can be discussed openly (hence, is admissible) with a colleague. Many violators have admitted that they did not seek consultations with a colleague because they knew the consultant would tell them to stop the behavior. In any case, the only proper response to boundary violations is not to do them in the first place.

As the next section illustrates, the difference between these two types of boundary issues is highly context dependent. However, forensic experience demonstrates that some agencies, such as the more punitive state boards of registration, tend to view all boundaries from a rigid "checklist" perspective that does violence to clinical flexibility and the essential relevance of context.

CONTEXT DEPENDENCE

In a conceptual vacuum, it may be impossible to distinguish clearly a boundary crossing from a boundary violation. A therapist who sends a dependent patient a reassuring postcard from his vacation is merely crossing the boundary; however, if the postcard is highly eroticized, contains inappropriate content, and is part of an extended sexual seduction, the same gesture carries entirely different weight.

Another element of context is the type and goal of the therapy. A favorite example is an analyst doing classical psychoanalysis, for whom no justification would exist for accompanying an adult patient into the bathroom; however, in the behaviorist treatment of paruresis (fear of urinating in public restrooms), the last step in a behavioral paradigm of treatment might well be the therapist accompanying the patient there. This example also implies that the context may be affected by issues such as informed consent to the type of therapy, the nature and content of the therapeutic contract, the patient's expectations, and so on.

POWER ASYMMETRY AND FIDUCIARY DUTY

The concepts of power asymmetry and fiduciary duty play an important theoretical role in analyzing boundary problems and are frequently used in discussing the consequences of boundary breaches. *Power asymmetry* refers to the unequal distribution of power between the two parties in the therapeutic dyad: the therapist has greater social and legal power than the patient. With this power comes the greater responsibility for directing and containing the therapeutic envelope. The occasional protest of "it's not my fault, the patient seduced me" carries little weight under this formulation.

A *fiduciary duty* is a duty based on trust and obligation. The doctor, as a fiduciary, owes a duty to the patient to place the latter's interests first; primarily, the doctor does what the patient needs, not what the doctor wants to do. Exploitative boundary violations are thus viewed as breaches of the doctor's fiduciary duty to the patient: the treater has placed his or her own gratification ahead of the patient's needs.

CONSEQUENCES OF BOUNDARY PROBLEMS

The consequences of boundary problems may be divided into those *intrinsic* to the therapy and those *extrinsic* to the therapy. As indicated earlier, a serious and exploitative boundary violation may doom the therapy and cause the patient accurately to feel betrayed and used. The clinical consequences of boundary violations, including sexual misconduct, may encompass the entire spectrum of emotional harms from mild and transient distress to suicide.

The extrinsic harms fall into three major categories: civil lawsuits (in some jurisdictions, criminal charges for overtly sexual activity); complaints to the board of registration, the licensing agency; and ethics complaints to the professional society (such as the district branch of the American Psychiatric Association), usually directed to the ethics committee of the relevant organization.

The above three types of complaints constitute the most common forms of negative consequence from boundary problems; alas for fairness, neither attorneys, boards, nor ethics committees may be sufficiently sophisticated to distinguish between boundary crossings and violations. Thus, any boundary issues should be clearly described in the records together with their rationales, readily discussed, and explored within the therapy itself. The major categories of extrinsic harms are discussed below.

Civil Litigation

A civil lawsuit for boundary problems is based on the concepts that the treater's devi-

ation(s) from the appropriate standard of care were occasioned by negligence and that the patient consequently sustained some form of damages (Gutheil and Appelbaum 2000; Gutheil and Brodsky 2008). This blunt legal analysis scants the commonly encountered clinical complexity of these claims. Although lawsuits for clinician sexual misconduct were a serious problem in past decades, observers have noted an increase in what might be termed "pure" boundary cases; that is, cases in which actual sexual intercourse has not occurred, but the patient is claiming harm from boundary violations short of that extreme.

Other factors may come into play in the litigation arena. The growing awareness of both boundary issues and their common precursor role in actual sexual misconduct has led some disgruntled patients to use a boundary claim as a means of taking revenge against a disliked clinician. A current joke holds that under the advent of managed care and the severe restrictions placed on length of treatment, no therapy will continue long enough for the patient to develop erotic transferences for the doctor.

On the one hand, a malpractice suit against the clinician will generally be defended and—in case of a loss—paid for by the malpractice insurer; on the other hand, many insurance policies contain exclusionary language that avoids coverage for the more sexualized forms of boundary violation.

Board of Registration/Licensure Complaint

A complaint to the board of registration challenges the physician's fitness to practice, as supposedly rendered questionable by the boundary problem in question. There are three serious problems with this form of complaint. First, boards in some areas are extremely punitive, seeking to meet quotas of de-licensed practitioners and ignoring both context and evidence. Second, unlike a malpractice case, a loss in these cases may cost the clinician his or her license and livelihood.

Finally, because a complaint to the board is not a malpractice issue, insurers often will not fund the defense, leaving the legal expenses to be met out-of-pocket by the doctor. One implication of this grim scenario is that board complaints should be taken very seriously and must include legal assistance, no matter how bizarre, overreactive, and trivial the complaint may seem.

Ethics Complaints

The field of ethics has produced a vast wealth of philosophical opinion and literature as to what does and does not constitute ethical conduct, but an ethics complaint to one's professional society has an extremely concrete denotation: it asserts that a specific section of the American Psychiatric Association Code of Ethics (American Psychiatric Association 2001b) has been violated by the boundary issue in question. What is ethical is what is in the "book." The outcome of a formal ethics complaint (informal complaints are not accepted) ranges from censure and warning (not reportable to the National Practitioner Data Bank) to suspension or expulsion from the professional society (both of which are reportable). Such reportage may plague every subsequent job application and usually also reaches the relevant board of registration.

SOME PERSONALITY TYPES ENCOUNTERED IN CLINICAL PRACTICE

We turn now to boundary issues that arise in relation to various personality disorders. As a reminder, the clinical correlation of boundary problems with patients with a personality disorder neither blames the victim nor exonerates the treater, nor does it remove from the latter the burdens of setting and maintaining boundaries. Indeed, it takes two to generate a true boundary problem. Thus, the following discussion addresses the interactions between patients with personality disorders and the clinicians attempting to treat them.

As might be inferred from the earlier discussion, no particular therapist, patient, or personality disorder should be considered immune from actual or potential boundary problems (Norris and Gutheil 2003). Indeed, both members of the dyad may present risk factors increasing the likelihood of boundary problems. Therapist issues may include life crises; transitions in a career; illness; loneliness and the impulse to confide in someone; idealization of a "special patient"; pride, shame, and envy; problems with limit setting; denial; and issues peculiar to being in a small-town environment wherein interaction with patients outside the office is unavoidable. Patient issues increasing vulnerability to boundary problems may include enmeshment with the therapist; retraumatization from earlier childhood abuse and felt helplessness from that earlier event; the repetition compulsion; shame and self-blame; feelings that the transference is "true love"; dependency; narcissism; and masochism (Norris and Gutheil 2003).

Empirically, the Cluster A group, marked by a tendency toward detachment, is less likely to be involved in a boundary issue than the other two clusters; however, individuals in the group with very poor social skills and poor perspective-taking of others may cross boundaries more out of social ineptness than other dynamics.

Histrionic and Dependent Personality Disorders

Consultative experience demonstrates that two symptoms manifested by patients with histrionic or dependent personality disorder—drama and neediness—tend to play roles in boundary excursions. A patient's intense need for contact, self-esteem, approval, or relief from anxiety or tension may pressure clinicians into hasty actions that cross boundaries.

A dependent patient who had been out drinking for an evening called her therapist in a panic and begged him to pick her up at the bar and drive her home. Feeling somewhat trapped and choiceless, the therapist did so. The situation, though presented by the patient as an emotional emergency, was clearly one merely of "urgency."

Although probably harmless, such an event may well be used by a board of registration as evidence of boundary problems in the treater. Appropriate responses may have included the therapist's calling a cab, recommending public transportation if available, or the therapist's calling the patient's family or friends.

Dramatic behavior may "trigger" a boundary problem because of the clinician's wish to "turn down the volume":

A patient with histrionic personality disorder, distraught after a session in which the therapist announced vacation plans, seated herself on the floor just outside the therapist's door and moaned loudly for a prolonged interval. The therapist, embarrassed by this scene taking place in full view of the clinic waiting room in front of other patients and staff, brought the patient back into the office and conducted an impulsive, prolonged session, intruding into other patients' appointments.

Patients are free to cross boundaries—but the limits must be set by the clinician. The patient in this vignette might have been told that the behavior was inappropriate and should be discussed at the next appointment. If the patient refused to leave, security might have been called and the matter explored at the next session.

Although supervisory data were lacking in this vignette, it appears likely that the dynamic operating therein was the therapist's countertransference-based inability to deal with his own sadistic feelings both about planning a vacation (and thus causing abandonment feelings in the patient) and about

being able to turn the patient away when the latter was behaving inappropriately. Conflicts about sadism are a common source of boundary difficulties, especially in younger therapists; the issue of countertransference is further addressed later in the chapter.

One of the earliest and most famous examples of histrionic (it would then have been called "hysterical") behavior was the hysterical pregnancy and pseudochildbirth of Anna O., who was in the throes of an erotic transference to Joseph Breuer, as described in the *Studies in Hysteria* (Breuer and Freud 1893–1895/1955). Although Breuer is not recorded as violating any boundaries, the point can be made that patient reactions in this disorder may operate independently of the clinician's actual behavior, a fact leading to confusion among decision-making bodies.

Antisocial Personality Disorder

Individuals with antisocial personality disorder may strain the boundary envelope with the intent of furthering manipulation of the therapist or, through the therapist, others in the environment. Examples might include getting the therapist to advocate for the patient at work, at school, and in other areas in which the therapist is induced to step out of the limits of the clinical role to abet the patient's purposes.

Another boundary issue seen with patients in this category is excessive familiarity and pseudocloseness designed to get the therapist to perform uncharacteristic actions that transgress boundaries:

Doctor (on first meeting): How do you do, I am Dr. Thomas Gutheil.
Patient (with warm handclasp): Very glad to meet you, Thomas.
Doctor (slightly nonplussed): Um, well, Thomas *is* my given name, but I go by "Doctor Gutheil."
Patient (affably): Whatever you say, Tommy.

As illustrated, the patient may shift on first acquaintance to a first-name or nickname basis to establish an artificial rapport designed to persuade the therapist to alter the rules of proper conduct. The therapist may feel silly or stuffy correcting this undue familiarity or even bringing it up at all, but the effort should probably be made in concert with attempts to explore the meaning of the behavior.

Some common goals of this tendency toward pseudocloseness are obtaining excusing or exculpatory letters sent to nonclinical recipients; obtaining prescriptions of inappropriate, or inappropriately large amounts of, controlled substances; and intervention in the patient's extratherapeutic reality ("I need you to meet with my parole officer to go easier on me; you know how ill I am").

From the patient's viewpoint, the boundaries, if even recognized, may be ignored in a goal-directed manner. From the clinician's viewpoint, the boundary transgressions may lead to trouble, especially if the patient's actions encompass illegal behavior (e.g., selling prescriptions) into which the doctor is drawn by association.

The following is an unfortunately common clinically observed constellation of boundary problems: a female psychotherapist is treating a male patient with antisocial personality disorder, but she misses the antisocial elements in the patient, seeing him as a needy infant who requires loving care to "get better." In the course of this rescue operation, boundary incursions occur and increase (Gabbard and Lester 2002).

Borderline Personality Disorder

As in the previous diagnostic category, patients with BPD may manifest conscious or unconscious manipulative tendencies for a number of reasons. Some scholars assert that these patients manipulate because their low self-esteem leaves them feeling unentitled to ask directly to have their needs met. It is a clinical truism that a sense of being unentitled may be masked by an overt attitude of entitlement; the patient operates from the position that he or she is special and deserving of extra attention. This demand for spe-

cialness can lead therapists to grant favors that transgress boundaries with these patients. (Because BPD empirically poses the greatest boundary difficulties, the reader may wish to review the axioms given at the outset of this chapter in order to maintain a properly nonjudgmental perspective.)

The surprising power of the manipulation to slip under the clinician's radar, as it were, is one of the more striking findings in the boundary realm. "I sensed that I was doing something that was outside my usual practice and, in fact, outside the pale," the therapist will lament to the consultant, "but somehow I just found myself making exceptions for this patient and doing it anyway."

In an earlier paper (Gutheil 1989), I described my experience with therapists seeking consultation who would begin their narratives with, "I don't ordinarily do this with my patients, but in *this* case I...[insert a broad spectrum of inappropriate behaviors here]." The patients' sense of entitlement and of being "special" may infect the therapist with the same view of their specialness, such that even inappropriate exceptions are made.

The patient's own boundary problems—both in the ego boundary sense (Gabbard and Lester 2002) and in the interpersonal space—may evoke comparable boundary blindness in the therapist:

> A therapist noted that a patient with very primitive BPD would sidle out of the office along the wall in a puzzling manner that seemed to convey a fearful state. On exploration the patient revealed that she was struggling with the fantasy that if she passed too close to the therapist she might accidentally fall forward and sink into the therapist's chest and be absorbed as though into quicksand. (D. Buie, personal communication, 1969)

We may be able to detect clinically the unconscious wishes for fusion hidden under this fear, but the point of the anecdote is that for some patients, the boundary even of the physical self may be extremely tenuous. Indeed, wishes for fusion in both patient and therapist may provide the stimulus to boundary transgressions.

The patient with BPD may manifest impulsivity that presses the therapist to act precipitously without forethought: "I need you to do this now, right now!" The patient may demand an immediate appointment, an immediate telephone contact, an immediate home visit, an immediate ride home, an extended session, a medication refill, or a fee adjustment. Note, of course, that any or all of these may be clinically indicated but may also constitute or lead to boundary problems.

> A patient with BPD in a subsequent psychotherapy commented out of the blue that she really felt her previous therapist should not have charged her a fee but should in fact have paid her, because her case was so interesting.

Research data indicate that patients with BPD often have a history of trauma; that is, they were at one time victims (Herman, cited in Gutheil and Gabbard 1993). Some of these patients adopt a posture of victimization (an element of entitlement distinguishable from narcissistic entitlement). This posture may mobilize rescue feelings, fantasies, or attempts in the therapist that lead the latter to "bend the rules" to achieve the rescue and thus transgress boundaries. Indeed, consultative experience leads to the conclusion that a number of cases of sexual misconduct spring from claimed attempts to rescue the patient, to prevent suicide, to elevate the patient's self-esteem, or to provide a "good" relationship to counter a string of bad ones that the patient has experienced.

"Borderline rage" is also a factor in leading to boundary problems, often through its power to intimidate:

> A 6-foot, 7-inch tall former college linebacker, now a therapist, was asked in consultation why he went along with a boundary violation that he knew was inappropriate but was demanded by the patient: why did he not simply refuse? Looking down from his height he stated, "I just didn't dare."

As noted elsewhere, borderline rage may leave therapists feeling pressured into inappropriate self-disclosure, conceding to inappropriate requests, and manifesting other signs of being "moved through fear" (Gutheil 1989, p. 598).

Disappointed in many past relationships, the patient with BPD may contrive to "test the therapist's care or devotion" in boundary-transgressing ways that often represent reenactments of earlier developmental stages. One source of this view is the patient's perception that therapy offers some form of promise, such as the inclusion in the therapist's idealized family (Gutheil 1989; Smith 1977). The patient may demand to sit on the therapist's lap or to be held or hugged, arguing that without this demonstration of caring, there can be no trust in the therapy. Herman (cited in Gutheil and Gabbard 1993) pointed out that because so many patients with BPD have histories of sexual abuse, they may have been conditioned to interact with significant others on whom they depend in eroticized or seductive ways.

Forensic experience reveals the sad truth of how often these primitive maneuvers actually succeed, to the detriment of the therapy and often to the censure of the therapist. As might well be expected, the wellspring of these deviations is commonly the countertransference in the dyad, our next topic.

COUNTERTRANSFERENCE ISSUES

The patient's need for help and the treater's membership in a helping profession ordinarily provide a salutary and symmetrical reciprocity, but it is not immune to distortion or miscarriage. The basic wish to help and heal, unfortunately, may inspire efforts that—no matter how well-intended—transgress professional boundaries in problematic ways. The patient's transferential neediness and dependency may evoke a countertransferential need in the therapist to rescue, save, or heal the patient at any cost. Wishes to save the patient from anxiety, depression, or suicide are common stimuli to boundary violations in the name of rescue.

An example of this problem is what I call the "brute force" attempt at cure. Frustrated by the difficulty of working with the patient and disappointed at the latter's lack of progress, the therapist sees the patient more and more often each week, for longer and longer session times; weekends, holidays, even vacations are no exception to this relentless crescendo. Therapists in this situation are being held hostage by the patient's insatiable need and are setting themselves the wholly unrealistic goal of meeting that need by "giving more."

Related to this, such patients' suicidal risk may lead the therapist to try desperate measures to prevent this outcome at all costs, including violating boundaries to achieve this rescue. Gabbard (2003) described this phenomenon in detail under the heading of the therapist's masochistic surrender, a dynamic issue closely linked to boundary problems.

This frustration may rise to the level of overt anger, in which the therapist acts out countertransference hostility by violating boundaries such as confidentiality. The therapist who angrily and inappropriately calls the patient's partner at home and rails at him or her to protest some action involving the patient has lost the compass that would keep one in bounds.

In a useful discussion Smith (1977) defined the "golden fantasy" entertained by some patients with BPD and others, the belief that all needs—relational, supportive, nurturing, dependent, and therapeutic—will be met by the treater. As the patient loses track of what constitutes the therapeutic aspect of the work, the therapist may begin to lose track of the actual parameters within which the treatment should take place.

The American Psychiatric Association (2001a) practice guideline stresses four basic points relating to patients with BPD and boundaries. First, monitor countertransference carefully; second, be alert to deviations from usual practice ("red flags"); third, always avoid boundary violations; and fourth, obtain consultation for "striking deviations from the usual manner of practice." These points are fully congruent with the material in this chapter.

In summary—because of borderline patients' own difficulties with boundaries, their capacity to evoke powerful countertransference reactions, and the particular elements of their interpersonal style—patients with BPD pose some of the most noteworthy examples of boundary problems and challenges to clinicians to maintain proper limits.

SOME CROSS-CULTURAL OBSERVATIONS

One might expect that boundary issues are a uniquely American problem, what with our litigious and entitled population and our active attention in the professional literature to boundary issues. However, a recent cross-cultural study (Commons et al. 2006) comparing boundary matters in the United States and Rio de Janeiro, Brazil, turned up some interesting findings.

The U.S. sample and the Brazilian sample agreed at the extremes—that is, in both countries overt sexual misconduct at one end of the spectrum was seen as proscribed, and trivial deviations at the other end were seen as harmless. In the middle ranges, however, divergence was revealed. For example, subjects in the U.S. sample believed hugging a patient was suspect and kissing was surely wrong, but it was fully acceptable to display licenses, certificates, and some honors on the walls of the office. The Brazilian cohort found kissing the cheek in greeting to be universally acceptable and an accepted manner of greeting patients, whereas display of certificates was considered a deviation.

It is likely that both cultural differences and personal data, such as trauma history, shape a patient's perception of boundary problems and the degree of their harmful effect, if any.

RISK MANAGEMENT PRINCIPLES AND RECOMMENDATIONS

Clearly, a rigid formalism and an icy demeanor are not the solution to boundary problems when dealing with patients with personality disorders; patients so treated will simply leave treatment. Rather, some basic guidelines may prove helpful to the clinician who desires to stay out of trouble while preserving the therapeutic effect of the work.

1. First, clinicians of any ideological stripe must obtain some basic understanding of the dynamic issues relating to transference and countertransference. Training programs that foolishly boast of having transcended "that Freudian stuff" do a serious disservice to their graduates. A patient with BPD in the idealizing phase of treatment may worship the therapist, but if the latter is untrained in the vagaries of transference, he or she is left to assume that his/her own natural gifts of person have evoked this reaction—a dangerous view, indeed.

2. Treaters of these patients must keep in mind the latter's capacity to distort or overreact. If you write to such a patient and sign the letter, "Love, Dr. Smith," you may intend agape (nonerotic love), but the patient may interpret eros and expect treatment consistent with that emotion. Even if the patient initially understands the meaning, the regulatory agencies may interpret that salutation as a sign that the clinician has lost objectivity and may assume that boundaries have been violated (note that this sequence of events is not speculative but empirical). Therapists should of course take responsibility for their actions, but these patients can evoke strong feelings of guilt that distort the clinician's perception of what happened and who is responsible.

   For example, in a board of registration complaint, the patient claimed to have been hurt by some action of the doctor. Instead of writing "I am sorry you feel hurt," the doctor wrote, "I am sorry I hurt you." This ill-chosen expression of inappropriate self-blame made it almost impossible to convince the board that the doctor had remained within proper boundaries.

   The learning point here: When in doubt, obtain forensic or legal consultation.

3. The therapist should develop a "red flag" warning response when finding him- or herself doing what "I do not usually do"—that is, making an exception to customary practice. The exception in question may be an act of laudatory creativity in treatment, but it may also be a boundary problem. Self-scrutiny and consultation may be most useful at such times.

4. Gutheil and Simon (1995) observed that the neutral space and time—when both parties rise from their chairs and move toward the door at the end of a session—represents an occasion when both parties may feel that the rules do not really apply anymore because the session is theoretically over. We recommended that therapists pay attention to their experiences and to the events and communications that occur during this "window"—because a tendency toward crossing or even violating boundaries may emerge in embryonic form during this period, allowing the therapist to open the subject for exploration in the following session and, one hopes, to deflate its problematic nature.

5. When in doubt, get consultation; doing so honors my favorite maxim: "Never worry alone." Although getting consultation before taking a step that might present boundary ambiguities is an excellent idea, the therapist should also begin presenting the case to a colleague or supervisor when boundary problems begin to appear on the horizon or when the transference becomes eroticized. Such

consultation will aid in keeping perspective and in ensuring that the standard of care is being met.

6. Any potential boundary excursion of uncertain meaning should be marked by three critical steps: professional behavior; discussion with the patient; and documentation. Under some circumstances, a tactful apology to the patient for misreading a situation may be in order. Failure to perform these steps casts the therapist in the light of one who wants to conceal wrongdoing.

   For example, driving home from a late last appointment, a therapist sees his patient slogging wearily homeward on foot through the 2-foot high drifts that a recent blizzard had deposited on the area. To prevent the patient from dying of exposure in the subfreezing weather, he offers her a ride home in his Jeep. In the car he continues to behave in a formal, professional manner, despite the odd circumstances. At the office the next day, he records a careful note outlining his reasoning and the risk-benefit analysis of the incident. At the patient's next appointment, he inquires how the patient felt about the incident, and its therapeutic significance is explored.

7. Finally, the majority of boundary difficulties may be averted by the following approach: "Explore before acting." Impulsive responses to patient demands are likely to go astray, and such responses may inappropriately model impulsivity.

REFERENCES

American Psychiatric Association: Practice Guideline for the Treatment of Patients with Borderline Personality Disorder. Washington, DC, American Psychiatric Association, 2001a

American Psychiatric Association: The Principles of Medical Ethics With Annotations Especially Applicable to Psychiatry, 2001 Edition. Washington, DC, American Psychiatric Association, 2001b

Breuer J, Freud S: Studies on hysteria (1893–1895), in Standard Edition of the Complete Psychological Works of Sigmund Freud, Vol 2. Translated and edited by Strachey J. London, Hogarth Press, 1955, pp 1–319

Celenza A: Sexual Boundary Violations: Therapeutic, Supervisory, and Academic Contexts. New York, Jason Aronson, 2007

Commons ML, Miller PM, Gutheil TG: Cross-cultural aspects of boundaries: Brazil and the United States. J Am Acad Psychiatry Law 33:33–42, 2006

Epstein RS, Simon RI: The exploitation index: an early warning indicator of boundary violations in psychotherapy. Bull Menninger Clin 54:450–465, 1990

Gabbard GO: Boundary violations, in Psychiatric Ethics, 3rd Edition. Edited by Bloch S, Chodoff P, Green SA. Oxford, England, Oxford University Press, 1999, pp 141–160

Gabbard GO: Miscarriages of psychoanalytic treatment with suicidal patients. Int J Psychoanal 84:249–261, 2003

Gabbard GO, Lester EP: Boundaries and Boundary Violations in Psychoanalysis, 2nd Edition. Washington, DC, American Psychiatric Publishing, 2002

Gutheil TG: Borderline personality disorder, boundary violations and patient-therapist sex: medicolegal pitfalls. Am J Psychiatry 146:597–602, 1989

Gutheil TG, Appelbaum PS: Clinical Handbook of Psychiatry and the Law, 3rd Edition. Baltimore, MD, Lippincott, Williams & Wilkins, 2000

Gutheil TG, Brodsky A: Preventing Boundary Violations in Clinical Practice. New York, Guilford, 2008

Gutheil TG, Gabbard GO: The concept of boundaries in clinical practice: theoretical and risk management dimensions. Am J Psychiatry 150:188–196, 1993

Gutheil, TG, Gabbard GO: Misuses and misunderstandings of boundary theory in clinical and regulatory settings. Am J Psychiatry 155:409–414, 1998

Gutheil TG, Simon RI: Between the chair and the door: boundary issues in the therapeutic "transition zone." Harv Rev Psychiatry 2:336–340, 1995

Gutheil TG, Simon RI: Non-sexual boundary crossings and boundary violations: the ethical dimension. Psychiatr Clin North Am 25:585–592, 2002

Ingram DH: Intimacy in the psychoanalytic relationship: a preliminary sketch. Am J Psychoanal 51:403–411, 1991

Langs R: The Bipersonal Field. New York, Jason Aronson, 1976

Norris DM, Gutheil TG, Strasburger LH: "This couldn't happen to me": boundary problems and sexual misconduct in the psychotherapeutic relationship. Psychiatr Serv 54:517–522, 2003

Simon RI: Sexual exploitation of patients: how it begins before it happens. Psychiatr Ann 19:104–122, 1989

Simon RI: Treatment boundary violations: clinical, legal and ethical considerations. J Am Acad Psychiatry Law 20:269–288, 1992

Smith S: The golden fantasy: a regressive reaction to separation anxiety. Int J Psychoanal 58:311–324, 1977

Spruiell V: The rules and frames of the psychoanalytic situation. Psychoanal Q 52:1–33, 1983

Stone MH: Boundary violations between therapist and patient. Psychiatr Ann 6:670–677, 1976

17

Collaborative Treatment

Abigail Schlesinger, M.D.
Kenneth R. Silk, M.D.

What Is Split or Collaborative Treatment?

Collaborative treatment can mean different things in different clinical practice settings. In this chapter, *collaborative treatment* refers to the treatment relationship that occurs when two (or more) treatment modalities are provided by more than one mental health or medical professional. This type of treatment arrangement has had many names, such as *split treatment, joint* (or *conjoint*) *treatment,* or in certain specific circumstances, *medication backup* (Riba and Balon 1999). We reserve use of the term *split treatment* to circumstances in which there is disagreement among or between the collaborators. Collaborative treatment can be contrasted with integrative treatment, in which one mental health care provider—most frequently a psychiatrist—performs all mental health modalities for a patient.

In the most common form of collaborative treatment, one clinician prescribes psychotropic medication (or somatic treatments) and another performs psychotherapy. In psychiatry, collaborative treatment often in-

volves a psychiatrist prescribing psychiatric medication and another clinician (e.g., psychiatrist, psychologist, social worker, therapist, case manager) performing the therapy. Increasingly, collaborative treatment has come to represent a situation in which a primary care physician (PCP) prescribes psychotropic medication while a nonpsychiatrist clinician conducts psychotherapy. In addition, treatment can be divided up in many ways among PCPs, psychoanalysts, specialty medical doctors, psychiatrists, specialty psychiatrists, therapists, clinical nurse therapists, visiting nurses, physician assistants, case managers, different people and disciplines on an inpatient unit or in a partial hospital program, and many others.

The term *collaborative* highlights the need for treating clinicians to communicate and work together, because there are many legal, ethical, and treatment issues and pitfalls that can arise when more than one provider is involved in a person's treatment. Patients with personality disorders, especially those with Cluster B traits, tend to "split" even without a "split" treatment relationship, and this propensity must be kept in mind when entering into a collaborative care model with another clinician for a patient with a personality disorder. *Splitting*, in its most formal psychoanalytic sense, is a defensive process wherein a patient appears to attribute good characteristics almost exclusively to one person (or one provider of treatment) while attributing the other treater with all bad or negative feelings. The patient appears to take the natural ambivalence one feels about almost all people and divide it into two packages—a positive package bestowed upon one person and a negative package bestowed upon another. Each package almost exclusively contains either good or bad attributes, rarely contaminated by the opposite attribute. Defensive splitting can be accompanied by *projective identification*, in which the patient projects different aspects of himself onto different treaters. The different treaters, in turn, unconsciously identify with those projected characteristics and may experience pressure to respond accordingly (Gabbard 1989; Gabbard and Wilkinson 1994; Ogden 1982).

Case Example

Ms. U, a young woman diagnosed with borderline personality disorder (BPD), was in psychotherapy with a psychologist and receiving medication from a psychiatrist. Ms. U had an extensive history of self-mutilating behavior. The psychologist was, even in his everyday interactions, quite restrained.

Ms. U was acutely aware of rejection, and she would call the psychiatrist to complain vociferously about her psychotherapist's lack of feeling or empathy. Every 6 or 9 months of this 5-year treatment, she would try to convince the psychiatrist, who she knew did psychodynamic psychotherapy, to take

over all of the treatment. The psychiatrist always sent Ms. U back to discuss these issues with her psychologist, even though the psychiatrist was aware that many of the accusations made about the therapist were, in some ways, not untrue.[1]

As the therapy progressed, Ms. U's self-destructive behavior diminished and then eventually ceased as her interpersonal relationships grew more stable. Longer periods elapsed between her complaints about her therapist, and eventually the complaints stopped. The treatment terminated successfully.

This chapter discusses collaborative treatment in general and then collaborative treatment of patients with personality disorders. Much of what is discussed applies to any collaborative treatment, regardless of the patient's diagnosis, but the issues of collaboration are heightened when the patient has a diagnosis of a personality disorder. Although the techniques, strategies, or issues presented are pertinent to many patients with personality disorders, they cannot be applied to all such patients because we often discuss treatments in which psychotherapy is conducted by one person and psychopharmacology is managed by another, and there are few data to support prescribing medications to patients with schizoid, antisocial, histrionic, narcissistic, and dependent personality disorders.

EVIDENCE FOR EFFECTIVENESS OF COLLABORATIVE CARE

Although collaborative treatment is increasingly common in mental health care, the ef-

---

[1] This situation may occur frequently in collaborative treatment. The patient presents an observation about the collaborating psychotherapist that may be an astute and accurate perception of the psychotherapist. Despite the face validity of the observation, the psychiatrist must refrain from agreeing or disagreeing with the patient. Each patient brings his or her unique history and transference into play when making such observations, and a comment at this point might undermine that particular transferential process occurring in the psychotherapy.

tectiveness of collaborative versus integrative treatment has not been well studied. There are no head-to-head efficacy studies comparing collaborative with integrative treatment, although there are studies that examine one treatment modality versus another modality versus both modalities together (Greenblatt et al. 1965; Klerman 1990).

Many patients with personality disorders have complex biological and psychosocial issues and do not respond as well to medications as would patients whose primary diagnosis is from Axis I (except perhaps those with schizotypal personality disorder [Duggan et al. 2008; Binks et al. 2006; Koenigsberg et al. 2003; Nose et al. 2006; Paris 2003; Soloff 1990, 1998]). Treatment modalities beyond psychopharmacological treatment are necessary, and often each modality is provided by a different mental health professional. Thus there are many clinical situations in which multimodal treatment implies and warrants collaboration between at least two mental health professionals.

Most current outcome studies in psychotherapy and psychopharmacology do not measure the effects of any treatment other than the one being studied. There are surprisingly few studies—and even fewer randomized controlled trials—comparing psychotherapy alone, medication alone, and psychotherapy and medicine in combination to determine the differential efficacy or effectiveness (Browne et al. 2002). Studies of cognitive-behavioral therapy and nefazodone for depression (Keller et al. 2000) and cognitive-behavioral therapy and tricyclic antidepressants for panic disorder (Barlow et al. 2000) have interesting findings about the course and continuation of response to specific interventions (Manber et al. 2003). De Jonghe et al. (2004) found equivalent results between groups of mild to moderately depressed patients treated with psychotherapy (short-term psychodynamic) or a combination of psychotherapy and psychopharmacology with antidepressants. Often patients with personality disorders are excluded from these studies, or personality disorders are not assessed. Thus, for patients with personality disorders, no clear conclusions can be made concerning the effectiveness of a medication versus psychotherapy; furthermore, no conclusions about effectiveness or efficacy can be made if these treatments are combined and performed by one provider versus being divided between two (or more) providers with one providing psychotherapy and the other prescribing medications. The exceptions are the study by Kool et al. (2003), which found that patients with personality pathology and depression responded best to a combined approach of both psychopharmacology and psychotherapy, although personality pathology of patients with Cluster C diagnoses responded better than that of patients with Cluster B diagnoses; the 12-week study by Soler et al. (2005) that found greater improvement in depression, anxiety, and impulsivity/aggression in patients assigned to dialectical behavior therapy plus olanzapine than in those assigned to dialectical behavior therapy alone; and the small study by Simpson et al. (2004) that randomly assigned patients to placebo or fluoxetine after completion of a course of dialectical behavior therapy and found that those assigned to placebo had more positive pre-/posttreatment differences than those assigned to fluoxetine.

IMPORTANCE OF COLLABORATIVE TREATMENT IN CURRENT PERSONALITY DISORDERS CARE

General Issues

A large proportion of antidepressants being prescribed in the United States is prescribed by PCPs (Lecrubier 2001). Serotonin reuptake inhibitors are less complicated to prescribe, with fewer general side effects and less lethality, than tricyclic antidepressants (Healy 1997). PCPs appear ready to provide the ongoing management of psychopharmacological medication in consultation with a psychiatrist. Although they do not always prescribe concurrent psychotherapy, a number of PCPs are collaborating with therapists of varying levels of training. An interesting triangular relationship can develop: a therapist, a PCP writing the prescriptions for psychotropic medication, and a psychiatrist for referral or collaboration. Smith (1989) wrote, "In contemporary treatment situations that include a patient, a therapist, a pharmacotherapist, and a pill, the transference issues can become more complex than the landing patterns of airplanes at an overcrowded airport" (p. 80). Add a managed care utilization reviewer to the picture, and things really get complicated.

Managed care companies often believe that patients with personality disorders use too much or at least more than their share of treatment. One of the challenges associated with providing collaborative care for these patients is convincing utilization reviewers that more than one modality of care is needed. To avoid divergent reports that negatively affect the reimbursed care for the patient, it is best to designate one member of the team to report the progress of treatment and the treatment plan to the reviewer. In general, this designated "reporter" should be the psychiatrist.

Increasing Prescription of Antidepressants

Despite the lack of hard evidence for the benefits of psychopharmacology in personality disorders, the practice of prescribing antidepressants for a wide array of symptom complexes suggestive of depression continues to increase (Healy 1997). Although depression is prevalent among patients with personality disorders (Skodol et al. 1999), quite often the nature of the depression, especially among patients with Cluster B disorders, is not the classic psychophysiological presentation frequently seen in a major depressive episode (Westen et al. 1992). There has been much debate about the type and nature of depression

in patients with personality disorders. The effectiveness of antidepressants in treating depression in such patients is moderate at best, even as their prescriptions are increasing (Duggan et al. 2008; Binks et al. 2006; Nose et al. 2006; Paris 2003). Many patients who may have been treated by psychotherapy alone in the past are now receiving psychopharmacological treatment as well. An emerging literature suggests that antidepressants can be helpful in the treatment of specific symptom complexes such as employing selective serotonin reuptake inhibitors or mood stabilizers for impulsivity, affect lability, and aggression in patients with BPD (Coccaro and Kavoussi 1997; Coccaro et al. 1989; Cowdry and Gardner 1988; Hollander et al. 2001, 2005; Loew et al. 2006; Markowitz 2001, 2004; Nickel et al. 2005; Rinne et al. 2002; Salzman et al. 1995; Sheard et al. 1976; Soloff 1998; Soloff et al. 1993; Tritt et al. 2005). The American Psychiatric Association practice guideline recommends treatment with selective serotonin reuptake inhibitors in a symptom-specific manner for patients with BPD; this recommendation is based on evidence from several double-blind, placebo-controlled studies; a number of open studies; and clinical experience in conjunction with a relatively benign side-effect profile and risk of overdose (American Psychiatric Association 2001). Also, some strong evidence suggests that neuroleptics and atypical antipsychotics can be effective for patients with schizotypal personality disorder and BPD (Bogenschutz and Nurnberg 2004; Goldberg et al. 1986; Koenigsberg et al. 2003; Markowitz 2001, 2004; Nickel et al. 2006; Schulz and Camlin 1999; Soloff et al. 1986b, 1993; Zanarini and Frankenburg 2001).

Patients with personality disorders present with a complex admixture of symptoms and problems, some of which appear to arise from psychosocial issues and interpersonal events, whereas others appear more related to expressions of underlying traits such as baseline anxiety, emotional lability, and impulsivity (Livesley 2000; Livesley et al. 1998; Putnam and Silk 2005). When treatment is divided among two providers, the psychotherapist may believe that all problems arise from psychosocial issues and subtly demean, undermine, or dismiss the psychopharmacological treatment. Conversely, the psychopharmacologist may think that difficulties are primarily due to "trait expression" and that once the right combination of medications is discovered, all symptoms will be alleviated.

STRENGTHS AND WEAKNESSES OF COLLABORATIVE TREATMENT

There are many positives to a collaborative treatment. Some of these positives have direct reference to patients with personality disorders.

1. Collaborative treatment can provide the patient with both a clinician to idealize and a clinician to denigrate within one treatment relationship. Although this situation might at first appear to be problematic, it can be useful if both providers confer with each other and work to have the patient develop a more balanced view of each of them. For example, both treaters may have an opportunity to model more appropriate coping mechanisms for the patient, or the idealized therapist might be able to work with the patient to modify or mollify the patient's denigration of the other treater and thus help keep the patient in treatment with the therapist being denigrated. The classic example is the patient with BPD, but patients with narcissistic personality disorder also contemptuously devalue and criticize treaters who do not treat them in the way in which they believe they are entitled. Feeling devalued can occur when faced with the moralistic, judgmental, and somewhat contemptuous attitude of the patient with obsessive-compulsive

personality disorder. In all these instances, the "good" therapist may be able to provide support to the criticized, or "bad," therapist. One way this support may occur is by the "good" therapist providing examples of other situations in which he or she had the misfortune of owning and bearing the "bad" therapist label and how difficult it was to bear at the time but how useful it was to the eventual outcome of the treatment. The "good" therapist may also try to minimize the negative countertransferential feelings the "bad" therapist is experiencing and may be able to ward off the "bad" therapist's wish to end treatment with the patient.

2. Collaborative treatment provides a basis for ongoing consultation between providers. It also provides the potential for multiple perspectives on complicated clinical and diagnostic situations. Such complex situations are not uncommon in patients with personality disorders, whose symptoms, behaviors, and interpersonal interactions can be so entwined that it is difficult to unravel the trait biological functioning from the interpersonally and experientially learned behaviors and maneuvers (Cloninger et al. 1993; Livesley et al. 1998).

3. When collaboration is with a PCP, the mental health professional can confer with someone who may have a longitudinal relationship with and understanding of the patient. The PCP often is viewed as fairly neutral by the patient and may be more impervious to the distortions of transference that appear frequently among patients with personality disorders. The PCP may be able to assist the patient in remaining medication compliant.

4. Patients with personality disorders can be very draining to treat. Patients with BPD can be demanding and threatening. Constant demands for attention from the patient with histrionic or narcissistic personality disorder can become exhausting. The

complaints of histrionic patients can be very difficult to listen to and to take seriously. Patients with dependent personality disorder can be draining and pulling, whereas the chronic anger and distrustfulness of patients with paranoid personality disorder can be quite difficult to tolerate. Therefore, a group of therapists and psychiatrists working as a team to provide overall patient management can support and confer with one another to reduce burnout.

Collaborative treatment can readily turn into a split treatment when the collaborators fail to collaborate. There can be many causes for this failure. Some patients with personality disorders have a tendency, as explained earlier, to split by attributing all good to one person and all bad to another. Although this splitting is most blatant among patients with BPD, it occurs in more subtle forms among patients with schizotypal, narcissistic, antisocial, and obsessive-compulsive personality disorders. Failure to collaborate in the treatment of these patients can lead to serious problems in the treatment. Table 17–1 presents specific issues that need to be considered in a collaborative treatment for each of the personality disorders.

Failure to collaborate or the end of collaboration can develop when the treaters identify with the projections of the patient. In this situation, each of the treaters begins to lose respect for the other treater as each begins to identify and psychologically own some of the negative projections of the patient (Gabbard 1989; Ogden 1982). Such events or situations are not uncommon on inpatient units where the split is often between the attending or resident psychiatrist and a member or members of the nursing staff, although they can occur between nurses as well (see Gabbard 1989; Gunderson 1984; Main 1957; Stanton and Schwartz 1954).

A ward staff member suddenly accuses another staff member of deliberately trying to jeopardize the treatment of a specific patient, while each staff member believes that she or he alone really knows best. The director of the ward, who has frequently encountered such sudden disagreements, decides to deal with these types of difficulties by bringing together the "warring parties" and wondering out loud with them why each has suddenly begun to despise his or her other colleague on the unit. The director emphasizes that prior to the disagreement, each person appeared to have great respect for and to enjoy working with the other person. The director moves to a discussion of the patient and tries to show the parties how each is really only seeing a part of the patient, upon which they have each constructed the idea that they alone know how best to treat the patient.

Collaboration in divided treatment is essential but does not always occur easily or frequently; a concerted effort must be made. Regularly scheduled phone calls or e-mail exchanges may be the best way to sustain the collaboration even when there is skepticism as to its value or a belief that another provider is causing difficulty.

COLLABORATIVE TREATMENT AND PERSONALITY DISORDERS

Treatment with psychopharmacology and psychotherapy is more common now in the treatment of all personality disorders than it has ever been. This probably is due to a number of factors:

1. Use of psychopharmacological agents among all psychiatric patients has increased, reflecting the general ascendancy of biological psychiatry (Siever and Davis 1991; Siever et al. 2002; Silk 1998; Skodol et al. 2002).

2. Since the early 1990s, there has been an expansion in specific types of psychotherapy for patients with personality disorders, such as dialectical behavior therapy (Linehan et al. 1993), transference-focused

psychotherapy (Clarkin et al. 1999; Kernberg et al. 2000), dynamic therapy (Bateman and Fonagy 1999, 2001), cognitive-behavioral therapy (Beck and Freeman 1990; Davidson et al. 2006), interpersonal reconstructive psychotherapy (Benjamin 2003), aand schema-focused cognitive-behavioral therapy (Young et al. 2003). None of these therapies opposes the concurrent use of psychopharmacological agents.

3. Psychopharmacological agents are in more common use in psychiatric treatment today, and the medications used are generally safer and have more tolerable side-effect profiles (Healy 2002). Safety is important among a group of patients, particularly patients with BPD, who have very high suicide rates (Paris 2002; Stone 1990).

4. Managed care companies play a significant role. They are reluctant to approve treatment sessions with seriously ill patients (including a significant number of patients with personality disorders) who are not receiving medication.

5. There is a growing appreciation of the role of biological and constitutional factors in the etiology of personality disorder symptoms. The nature-nurture dichotomy has been replaced by consideration of the subtle interplay of biological predisposition, resulting in traits that are expressed through behavior that is affected by experiential and environmental factors (both shared and nonshared) (Rutter 2002). Such a theory of interaction between biological predispositions and life experience supports a multimodal treatment approach (Paris 1994).

6. The comorbidity of both Axis I and Axis II disorders has received increased consideration. If one prefers to treat Axis II problems with psychotherapy, Axis I comorbidity still must be considered and treated, or it will likely worsen the clinical manifestation of the Axis II disorder (Yen at al. 2003; Zanarini et al. 1998). Axis I comorbid diagnoses may respond to pharmacological agents, and even in the absence of a clear Axis I comorbid diagnoses, the patient may have pharmacologically responsive symptom clusters that are reminiscent of Axis I and should be treated as such.

SITUATIONS OF COLLABORATIVE TREATMENT

Although *collaborative treatment* usually refers to the arrangement in which a nonmedical psychotherapist performs the psychotherapy and a psychiatrist or other medical doctor prescribes medication, variations on that arrangement still qualify as collaborative treatment. Some such variations occur regardless of the diagnosis, but others are more prone to occur in the treatment of patients with personality disorders.

Comorbid Substance Abuse Treatment

Collaboration should occur when the patient is in both substance abuse treatment and treatment with a psychiatrist for personality disorder issues. Continuous use of substances can exacerbate personality disorder psychopathology, and in these instances it is very important that the substance abuse counselor and/or psychotherapist and the treating psychiatrist immediately confer (Casillas and Clark 2002; de Groot et al. 2003). If an increase in or a resumption of substance use after a period of abstinence should occur, the counselor/psychotherapist needs to initiate contact with the psychiatrist. Sometimes a patient will feel embarrassed about resuming use of substances after a period of sobriety and may ask the counselor/psychotherapist not to inform the psychiatrist. Obviously this wish cannot be granted, because there would be 1) collusion between the counselor/psychotherapist and the patient to keep the psychiatrist in the

Table 17–1. Specific issues to address in collaborative treatment with specific personality disorders

Personality disorder	Classic features	Tips for providers of collaborative treatment
Paranoid	Distrust, suspiciousness	Be clear about frequency of contact among providers and be sure to inform patient whenever a contact between any of the providers has occurred. Regularly remind patient about sources of specific information and be sure that each treater knows whether the information he or she has about the patient comes from the patient or other sources (providers).
Schizoid	Detachment from emotional relationships	Work among providers to minimize redundancy of visits so that patient can come as infrequently as possible. Coordinate treatment visits so patient can visit all providers on the same day.
Schizotypal	Discomfort with close relationships, cognitive or perceptual distortions, eccentricities of behavior	Be prepared to contact other providers when increased distortions arise in sessions. Work together to minimize redundancy of visits (see schizoid above).
Antisocial	Disregard for rights of others	Convey clearly that all members of the treatment team will communicate regularly. Be prepared for misrepresentations of facts. Be prepared to verify information with providers. If different providers are getting very different facts from the patient, a designated provider needs to discuss the discrepancies with the patient.
Borderline	Instability in mood and interpersonal relationships, impulsivity	Provide support for the patient without becoming caught up in splitting among providers. Discuss strong countertransference feelings with other providers. Have a clear plan about roles and responses of all providers to emotional outbursts, threats, increased suicidality, other crises, and medication changes. Be careful that repeated crises or turmoil are not reinforced by increased attention from providers.
Histrionic	Excessive emotionality, attention seeking	Have a clear plan among providers as to how to handle emotional outbursts. Be prepared to contact other providers at periods of increasing physical symptoms and/or increasing attention-seeking behavior.

Table 17–1. Specific issues to address in collaborative treatment with specific personality disorders (continued)

Personality disorder	Classic features	Tips for providers of collaborative treatment
Narcissistic	Grandiosity, lack of empathy	Be prepared to contact other providers when overt or covert signs of increasing contempt toward one of the treaters occurs. Have a clear plan among providers regarding how to handle contemptuous behavior so that one of the providers addresses the issue even if the patient is expressing contempt toward only one of them.
Avoidant	Social inhibition, feelings of inadequacy, hypersensitivity to negative evaluation	Work among each other to encourage consistent treatment relationships and attitudes in all treatments involved in the collaboration. Be prepared to communicate with other providers whenever missed appointments with any provider occur. Coordinate treatment visits so patient can visit all providers on the same day.
Dependent	Submissive behavior, a need to be taken care of	Work with patient to minimize appointments and avoid overutilization of services. Work together to anticipate how to handle patient needs during vacations. Plan to ensure that increasing distress does not lead to increasing number of appointments.
Obsessive-compulsive	Preoccupation with order, cleanliness, control	Ensure that consistent recommendations are made by each provider. Be prepared to communicate with other providers when patient is having difficulty adhering to recommendations. Have a clear plan regarding how to confront a patient who constantly obsesses and complains about the lack of consistency or thoroughness of the treatment when the particular obsessing is a sign of disdain toward other people.

Note. In many personality disorders in which there is no clear indication or no data to support the use of medications, collaborative treatment might arise because there is psychopharmacological treatment of a comorbid Axis I disorder. This table provides tips with respect to how the patient's personality disorder might be dealt with in a collaborative treatment even if the medication is being administered for reasons other than the patient's personality disorder diagnosis.

dark and 2) a splitting between the counselor/psychotherapist and the psychiatrist.

Case Example

An engineer in his mid-50s, Mr. V was referred for substance abuse treatment after his second citation for driving while intoxicated. The substance abuse counselor referred Mr. V to a psychiatrist for treatment of narcissistic personality disorder. Whenever Mr. V increased his alcohol use, he would miss his appointments with the psychiatrist because he was embarrassed, although he *would* attend his substance abuse sessions. The psychiatrist called the substance abuse counselor whenever Mr. V missed an appointment, and the counselor always convinced Mr. V to return to and continue with the psychiatrist. The psychiatrist eventually concluded that Mr. V's shame about his substance abuse behavior related more to avoidance than narcissism in interpersonal functioning, and this information allowed the substance abuse counselor to modify his approach to Mr. V.

Somatic Complaints, the Primary Care Physician, and the Psychiatrist

Patients with personality disorders, particularly those with Cluster B and Cluster C personality disorders, have a tendency to be somatically preoccupied (Benjamin et al. 1989; Frankenburg and Zanarini 2006). Although the treating psychiatrist may suspect mere somatic preoccupation, one cannot make the mistake of not taking the complaint seriously. If complaints persist or if different somatic concerns frequently appear, it is important for the psychiatrist to share his concern with the physician working up the somatic issues. Together, the two physicians can decide how much physical exploration of somatic concerns should occur and coordinate a consistent therapeutic response to persisting somatic issues (Williams and Silk 1997).

SEVEN PRINCIPLES TO FOLLOW IN COLLABORATIVE TREATMENT

A number of principles can apply to any collaborative treatment, but they have special application in personality disorders. Adherence to these principles can lead to a smoother and more synergistic approach to collaborative treatment (Silk 1995).

Understanding and Clarifying the Relationship Between the Therapist and the Prescriber

The relationship between a psychotherapist and a pharmacotherapist, or "prescriber," has been described as the "pharmacotherapy-psychotherapy triangle" (Beitman et al. 1984). In managed care, psychiatrists may be expected to provide medical backup for therapists whose work they do not know, whose approach they may not agree with, or whom they do not respect (Goldberg et al. 1991). Conversely, the psychotherapist may have to deal with a psychiatrist whom he or she does not know or agree with. In the best of worlds, neither the psychiatrist nor the psychotherapist would feel obligated to collaborate with a treater whom he or she does not respect.

Patients with personality disorders are quite sensitive to disagreements among members of the treatment team (Main 1957; Stanton and Schwartz 1954). Without communication and knowledge about what other professionals involved in the case are doing, the patient can become caught in the middle of disagreement (Stanton and Schwartz 1954). Each treater should respect what the other is trying to accomplish. This respect for treatment modality should be separated from personal feelings (although it is always easier if there is mutual liking). Each provider should be free to conduct an open communication with the other so that treatment collaboration and coordination can occur (Koenigsberg 1993).

Ideally, the prescriber and the therapist will know each other or at least know something about each other's practice and practice reputation. The prescriber should have an appreciation for the basic psychological issues involved in treatment and a general understanding of how they may manifest in psychopharmacological treatment. The prescribing psychiatrist needs to be clear with the therapist as to his or her beliefs in the putative efficacy of psychotherapy in the personality disorder in general as well as for each patient specifically. Psychotherapy will not proceed constructively if the prescriber does not believe in the usefulness of psychotherapy, particularly with patients with personality disorders (especially those belonging to Cluster B). Maintenance of therapeutic boundaries between treaters is crucial in patients with personality disorders and must be clarified (Woodward et al. 1993). Some questions to ask are: Should between-session phone calls be permitted in the pharmacological treatment if they are not permitted or are frowned upon in the psychotherapy? In what quantities will pills be prescribed, and what course should the therapist take if there is a sudden increase in the suicidality of the patient? When the patient requests a change or an increase in dosage, will the prescriber contact the therapist beforehand to understand better what issues might be coming up in the psychotherapy? How frequently will discussions between the prescriber and the therapist take place? How will issues that belong primarily in the psychotherapy be dealt with if they are brought up in the psychopharmacological treatment? Will the psychopharmacologist notify the psychotherapist that he or she has directed some issue back to the psychotherapist?

The psychotherapist, in a similar manner, needs to have respect for the prescriber and for the intervention of psychopharmacology (Koenigsberg 1993). Although there is probably little need for nonmedical therapists to be experts in psychotropic drug usage, nonmedical psychotherapists should understand the general indications for pharmacotherapy and be aware of the specificity as well as the limitations of the psychopharmacological treatment. The therapist should have some rudimentary knowledge of both the expected therapeutic effects as well as the possible side effects of at least the broader classes of psychotropic medications. In the course of the psychotherapy, the therapist should be willing to discuss, albeit on a limited basis, the patient's experience (both positive and negative) of taking the medication. Additionally, the therapist needs to have some knowledge of medications so that he or she can have some appreciation of what might be subjective versus objective reactions of the patient to taking the medication.

As stated earlier, no psychotherapist or psychopharmacologist should feel obligated to work with a collaborative partner with whom they do not agree or respect. They each must respect the roles and competence of their co-treater. In this atmosphere of mutual respect, both the prescriber and the therapist need to appreciate the perceived efficacy as well as limitations of each of the interventions. Both need to be able to tolerate treatment situations where progress is often slow, punctuated by periods of improvement and regression, and where the long-range prognosis is often guarded but not necessarily negative. Appreciating each other's difficulties and those of the patient in the treatment may help each treater avoid blaming the other (or the patient) during difficult periods.

Appelbaum suggested that, to address both clarity of treatment and treatment expectations, as well as medicolegal issues, the therapist and prescriber draw up a formal contract that delineates their respective roles as well as the expected frequency and range of, or limitations on, their communication (Appelbaum 1991; Chiles et al. 1991). Such a contract works well when the two people share responsibility for a number of patients (Smith 1989). These ideas about contracts are merely suggestions and certainly may not be necessary or useful when the two collaborators work in the same clinic or the same health system.

Much of what we diagnose as personality disorder reflects a group of patients who have chronic maladaptive interpersonal functioning across a wide range of settings. Interpersonal dysfunction cannot and should not be ignored, dismissed, or denied, and whenever and wherever it occurs in the therapeutic endeavor, it should be discussed not only between the two therapists but among the treaters *and* the patient. Transference is not solely reserved for transference-oriented psychotherapy (Beck and Freeman 1990; Goldhamer 1984), and "pharmacotherapy is [also] an interpersonal transaction" (Beitman 1993, p. 538).

Understanding What the Medication Means to Both Therapist and Prescriber

Medications may play both a positive and a negative role in treatment. The therapist and the prescriber need to be attuned to what the initiation of medication means to each of them.

Although DSM-IV-TR (American Psychiatric Association 2000) lists 10 personality disorders, in clinical practice patients with personality disorders defy easy classification and do not always fit neatly into any of these DSM categories (Westen and Arkowitz-Westen 1998). In addition, no medications have yet been indicated for any specific personality disorder. Although there are algorithms with respect to the pharmacological treatment of personality disorders (particularly BPD [American Psychiatric Association 2001; Soloff 1998]), there are no clear-cut rules as to when or what medication should be used in any given Axis II diagnosis. In circumstances with prescriber self-doubt, ambivalence, and uncertainty about either the diagnosis or, more probably, the chosen pharmacological agent, a defensive and authoritarian posture might be assumed by the prescriber in an attempt to assure that the pharmacological decision was correct. The prescriber and/or the therapist may deny ambivalence about the medication, become intolerant of the patient's (or the other provider's) questions and concerns, and present the possible therapeutic effects of the medications in a more positive light than the evidence would imply. This idealization of the medication, similar to the patient's periodic idealization of the treatment, will usually be short-lived.

Pessimism about progress in the therapy was given as a reason to consider prescribing medications by 65% of the respondent psychotherapists in a study by Waldinger and Frank (1989). Given that some patients with personality disorders, particularly BPD, seem especially attuned to feelings, a treater's pessimism or frustration with the course of therapy may be inadvertently and unconsciously conveyed to the patient. Conversely, a referral to a psychopharmacologist could be viewed as an opportunity for consultation and second opinion (Chiles et al. 1991).

It is easy for treaters to develop anger and rage at patients with personality disorders, particularly with patients with substantial borderline, narcissistic, and paranoid personality disorder characteristics, when there is little apparent therapeutic progress (Gabbard and Wilkinson 1994). At these times, one treater may try to pull back from the treatment or, conversely, try to take over control of the entire treatment. The best way to handle these feelings is not to isolate oneself but to approach the other provider and be willing to share one's frustrations. More often than not, the first provider will discover that the other provider shares similar frustrations. This shared frustration not only will lead to less tension in each provider and in the therapy but also, at times, to a discussion and a review of the treatment.

When medication is being considered in a collaborative treatment, the following questions may be asked: Where is the impetus for the medication coming from? Does the therapist think the medication will affect or change the therapeutic relationship? In turn, the prescriber should be able to let the therapist know if he or she feels that the therapist's expectations for the medication are unrealistic and what might be a reasonable expected response.

Understanding What the Medication Means to the Patient

Beginning pharmacotherapy or changing medication may not always be seen as favorable by patients, and a negative reaction to the idea of medication needs to be anticipated. A propensity to put the most negative spin on interpersonal encounters or perceived intentions may cause patients with personality disorders to experience the introduction of medication as a failure of their role in treatment or as the psychotherapist giving up on them. Patients might also, albeit rarely, experience the introduction of medication as a hopeful sign, as an additional modality that might help speed the progress of the treatment (Gunderson 1984, 2001; Waldinger and Frank 1989). Whatever the patient's reaction, understanding what the medication means to the patient and how the patient understands the use of medication within the context of the therapy as well as in the context of his or her own life experience is crucial (Metzl and Riba 2003).

Understanding the patient's reaction to the introduction of medication can be important not only for the patient's cooperation and compliance but also for transferential issues. The patient may take medication in a spirit of collaboration with the therapist and the prescriber. The patient may disagree with the decision, but cooperate out of a strong need to please. A patient's reactions will depend on whether the therapist and prescriber are truly collaborating or at odds.

The introduction of medication into any therapy, even if by a conferring psychiatrist, has repercussions on the transference (Goldhamer 1984). If the idea of medication is in-

troduced early in the treatment process, the potential negative transferential reaction to the introduction of medications later may be minimized. It is important that the therapist and the prescriber be on the same page as to "how" medication will be chosen, introduced, continued, discontinued, and so on. Discussions at the beginning of treatment can model the ethos of an open forum for exchange of information about medications and other feelings.

Case Example

Mr. W, a 50-year-old man with histrionic personality disorder and panic disorder, was referred to an anxiety disorder clinic after several emergency department visits because of uncomfortable arousal symptoms precipitated by an antidepressant (Soloff et al. 1986a). He received cognitive-behavioral therapy and responded well, although he had trouble starting an antidepressant without having his panic symptoms increase. He did tolerate a low-dose benzodiazepine but was fearful of becoming "addicted" to the benzodiazepine and would intermittently reduce his dosage despite his therapist's attempts to discourage it. When Mr. W's insurance ran out, he stopped seeing his therapist because he was "doing so well," and he also stopped his medication. He began to have emotional outbursts and increased panic attacks and called the psychiatric emergency department inquiring about rehabilitation for drug abuse. Therapy was reinitiated after both the therapist and psychiatrist discussed Mr. W's concerns about medication and how these concerns were affecting his life. The providers developed clear plans as to whom Mr. W would call for "medication questions," whom for "exposure questions," and how they would respond to emotional upheavals.

Both therapist and prescriber should be aware that patients may use medications as transitional objects (particularly patients with borderline, histrionic, and perhaps severely dependent personality disorders

[Cardasis et al. 1997; Gunderson et al. 1985; Winnicott 1953]). In this context, the patient's attachment and/or resistance to changing or altering medications may seem out of proportion to the actual therapeutic benefit derived from the medication (Adelman 1985). It may also explain why the patient who has repeatedly complained about the medications is unwilling to change them even when there has been little clear evidence that the medications have been effective.

Understanding That the Medication Will Probably Have Limited Effectiveness

Therapists and prescribers need to appreciate the therapeutic benefits and limitations of medication. Therapists should inquire about their patient's medications at moments of calm, not during periods of crisis. Perhaps the most instructive and useful time for (ex)change is when things are actually going well and treatment does not seem bleak or hopeless.

The prescriber should describe what features of a specific medication may or may not be useful in this particular patient at this particular time. The prescriber should tell the therapist what unusual idiosyncratic reactions to the medication might occur (Gardner and Cowdry 1985; Soloff et al. 1986a), especially because these paradoxical reactions or tendencies toward dependency may not always be listed in the package insert or in the *Physician's Desk Reference*.

With effective collaboration, medication decisions will not be solely in the hands of the prescriber. A dialogue between therapist and prescriber should take place as to how each particular type or category of medication with the particular patient might work.

Case Example

Ms. X was referred by a psychiatrist from out of town for treatment of anxiety and depression. Ms. X had a long history of major depressive episodes. At the time of the evaluation, she was tak-

ing five medications: two mood stabilizers, a low-dose atypical antipsychotic, an antidepressant, and a benzodiazepine. She insisted that this combination was the correct regimen for her and that the new psychiatrist not tamper with her medications. She said it took many months and finally a referral to the most prominent psychopharmacologist in her region before the right combination was found. She also stated that she was going to remain in psychotherapy with her old therapist through weekly long-distance phone contacts.

The new psychiatrist, after seeing Ms. X five or six times, began to feel that Ms. X primarily had a narcissistic personality disorder and that her depressions were brought about by her extreme sensitivity to anything that could remotely represent a narcissistic injury. The psychiatrist called Ms. X's therapist, who acknowledged that although Ms. X did have some narcissistic issues, she really had experienced a number of major depressive episodes during their treatment together.

After a few months, Ms. X grew more depressed, but her depression was marked primarily by lethargy, absenteeism from work, and an inability to concentrate. She was, however, able to date and had no loss of libido or appetite. Instead of feelings of guilt or worthlessness, she had feelings of grandiosity and entitlement. Ms. X requested a psychostimulant to help with her concentration and lethargy. The psychiatrist balked and tried to address some of the ways in which he felt her depression was atypical. He pointed out that she seemed more invested in wanting the psychiatrist to figure out what pills would make her better rather than in exploring events in her life that might be leading to what she thought was depression. She stormed out of the office. Later that week, Ms. X called the psychiatrist to say that her therapist also believed that she could benefit from a psychostimulant, and she was going to find a psychiatrist who was an expert in depression and more up-to-date about treatment. Calls the psychiatrist made to Ms. X's long-distance therapist went unanswered.

Understanding How the Medication Fits Into the Overall Treatment and Treatment Plan for the Patient

If a psychotherapist considers using medications at some time during the course of treatment, it is hoped that he or she will have an ongoing arrangement with a prescriber or know ahead of time who the prescriber might be. It is never wise to begin searching for a prescriber during a time of pressing need for medications.

The goal of treatment for a patient with personality disorder cannot be cure. Deciding to use medications or changing medications should not imply that one is "going for the cure." The goal of treatment should be to try to improve the ways in which our patients cope, to help them develop increased awareness of their cognitive rigidity and distortions, to assist them in becoming somewhat less impulsive and less affectively labile, and to try to increase the distance between, while reducing the amplitude of, their interpersonal crises (Koenigsberg 1993). These goals are attributable to both the psychotherapy and psychopharmacology and need to be appreciated by both the therapist and the prescriber. A prescriber who conveys a powerful belief in finding the "right" medication will promote an unrealistic and difficult situation.

Any therapy for patients with character disorders must have realistic and limited goals set early in the therapy, lest any of the players begin to idealize another player or another modality. Such idealization can only lead to disappointment and the multiple repercussions that occur in the treatment as a result.

Understanding the Potential and Actual Lethality of the Medication

Many psychotropic medications can be lethal, particularly tricyclic antidepressants, lithium, and the mood stabilizers/anticonvulsants. The monoamine oxidase inhibitors and the benzodiazepines also have a significant morbidity and mortality associated with overdose, especially when combined with other agents. Suicide potential needs to be continually assessed, and when it increases, a plan should be enacted that takes into account when the therapist will contact the prescriber, whether the prescriber is going to limit the size of the prescription, which of the treating professionals might hold onto the medications if a decision is made to limit their administration, and so on. At a minimum, if the therapist believes there is an increase in suicide potential, then the prescriber should be notified. If the therapist is fearful that the patient may overdose, this issue should be discussed openly with the prescriber.

Patients with personality disorders, particularly BPD, are potentially volatile and can act out when they feel that relationships are threatened (Gunderson 1984). The therapist–patient relationship is one that, when complicated by transference, can increase the possibility of acting-out in ways that include suicidal and other self-destructive behaviors; the prescriber–patient relationship is another that also holds the potential for these types of dangers. Mutual respect and communication between the therapist and the prescriber are indispensable to ensuring that a crisis is defused.

Understanding That Interpersonal Crises and Affective Storms Cannot Be Relieved Simply Through Initiation or Modification of the Medication

Introducing medication into the treatment of a patient with personality disorder should not be a spur-of-the-moment decision. It should be done in a controlled manner with forethought and not in the midst of an interpersonal or transferential crisis. Our patients' lives and affects do not follow well-designed courses or even respond to well-designed plans. Even if careful plans are made, the interpersonal crises and affective storms that occur in treatment, combined with the interpersonal demandingness and/ or helplessness and passivity of the patient, put enormous pressure on the therapist to do something, to change something, to make the pain go away. There is a tendency to promise much more than can be accomplished, ultimately leading to idealization, disappointment, and subsequent devaluation. If there is a collaborative relationship, and it is very good and mutually supportive, then neither treater should deal with the patient's attacks and demands alone. Each can use the opportunity to think through and resolve the crisis.

In a crisis, all of the six points just described come into play. How well has there been open collaboration between the psychotherapist and the prescriber? How well do they work together, and can they trust each other and each other's judgment? How do they each, as well as the patient, understand the role of medication in the treatment and the medication's benefits and symbolic meaning? How well does each person understand the limits of the medication, and is one of the treaters overreacting, merely prescribing or wanting a prescription written for medication in order to feel that a crisis is being defused? What has been said about medications in the treatment in the past, and how and when have medications been used in the treatment? Have medications been employed successfully, and have they been used safely by the patient?

CONTRAINDICATIONS TO COLLABORATIVE TREATMENT

Before concluding, we need to make mention of situations in which collaborative treatment may be contraindicated. First, however, we must point out that when a patient needs both medication and psychotherapeutic treatment, it is very common that both treatments are provided by a single psychiatrist. We continue to urge treatment by one individual psychiatrist whenever possible if the psychiatrist feels capable of and competent in providing both the medication and the specific form of psychotherapy most useful to the patient.

There may be situations in which collaborative treatment is contraindicated. The first situation would be when the patient is extremely paranoid or psychotic. These types of patients may not agree to having people "talk about them" and thus would not sign a release of information for such exchanges to occur. Also, paranoid people often think that all or most other people are talking about them, and the therapist may not wish to reinforce this idea by means of an arrangement wherein people *are* talking about the patient.

There may also be instances in which patients have an admixture of serious medical and psychiatric problems. The medical problems may directly affect the patient's psychological problems and presentation as well as the patient's cognitive processes and ability to comprehend. A physician who understands the impact of medical conditions on psychological presentation and functioning and who can conduct the psychotherapy as well as manage the medications would be most helpful in these cases, especially if the medical condition or related psychological problems wax and wane. In this instance, drug–drug interactions may have a direct impact on psychological and medical well-being, and changes in medical condition may warrant repeated reevaluation of psychotropic drug regimens.

In other instances, practical reality issues may lead to treatment by a single provider rather than collaborative treatment. If a patient has a severe limit on the number of sessions of psychological or psychiatric treatment because of third-party payer restrictions, then the psychiatrist must consider how to use those sessions most efficiently and cost-effectively for the patient. In this instance, being able to manage medications and conduct psychotherapy in a single session may be important. A similar situation can occur when the patient has severely restricted financial resources or lives so far away that a trip to the psychotherapist and/or psychiatrist involves a significant expenditure of time or money. In this case, if both psychotherapy and psychopharmacology can be accomplished in a single trip or visit, then this approach should be seriously considered.

CONCLUSION

Collaborative treatment is increasing because of a number of factors, some economic, some because of advances in neuroscience and pharmacology, and some because of managed care and the way health care in the United States is delivered. The various combinations and permutations of collaborative treatment are growing beyond the standard combination of one person writing prescriptions for psychiatric medications while another person provides the psychotherapy. Psychiatrists, psychologists, PCPs, social workers, case managers, physician assistants, and visiting nurses are just some of the players involved in a collaborative treatment.

Advances in neuroscience and trends toward using psychotropic medications more regularly for patients with personality disorders have led to more such patients receiving collaborative treatment. Managed care puts pressure on psychiatrists to use medications for a "quicker" response, and patients, bolstered by direct-to-consumer advertising, assume a medication is available for every ailment. Given the co-occurrence of many Axis I disorders with personality disorders, it is not uncommon to find one provider managing medications while another directs or conducts psychodynamic, cognitive-behavioral, or interpersonal psychotherapy.

Patients with personality disorders have major difficulties in interpersonal relationships, and every visit with a psychopharmacologist or a psychotherapist is an interpersonal encounter. These interpersonal encounters must be managed carefully, and when there are two or more providers of treatment, the providers must communicate with each other on a regular basis. This communication is not only a hallmark of good psychiatric care but is also a method whereby two or more providers can coordinate their treatment approach and collaborate on decision making so that the experience can be a synergistic rather than a divisive one.

Collaborative treatment at its best occurs in an atmosphere of respect and results in open and free communication with fellow providers. An opportunity for collaborators to consult and learn from one another exists, and this collaboration has the potential to result in more comprehensive and thoughtful care for difficult-to-treat groups of patients.

REFERENCES

Adelman SA: Pills as transitional objects: a dynamic understanding of the use of medication in psychotherapy. Psychiatry 48:246–253, 1985

American Psychiatric Association: Diagnostic and Statistical Manual of Mental Disorders, 4th Edition, Text Revision. Washington, DC, American Psychiatric Association, 2000

American Psychiatric Association: Practice guideline for the treatment of patients with borderline personality disorder. Am J Psychiatry 158 (10 suppl):1–52, 2001

Appelbaum PS: General guidelines for psychiatrists who prescribe medications for patients treated by nonmedical psychotherapists. Hosp Community Psychiatry 42:281–282, 1991

Barlow DH, Gorman JM, Shear MK, et al: Cognitive behavioral therapy, imipramine, or their combination for panic disorder: a randomized controlled trial. JAMA 28:2529–2539, 2000

Bateman A, Fonagy P: Effectiveness of partial hospitalization in the treatment of borderline personality disorder: a randomized controlled trial. Am J Psychiatry 156:1563–1569, 1999

Bateman A, Fonagy P: Treatment of borderline personality disorder with psychoanalytically oriented partial hospitalization: an 18-month follow-up. Am J Psychiatry 158:36–42, 2001

Beck AT, Freeman A: Cognitive Therapy of Personality Disorders. New York, Guilford, 1990

Beitman BD: Pharmacotherapy and the stages of psychotherapeutic change, in American Psychiatric Press Review of Psychiatry, Vol 12. Edited by Oldham JM, Riba MB, Tasman A.

Washington, DC, American Psychiatric Press, 1993, pp 521–539

Beitman BD, Chiles J, Carlin A: The pharmacotherapy-psychotherapy triangle: psychiatrist, non-medical psychotherapist, and patient. J Clin Psychiatry 45:458–459, 1984

Benjamin J, Silk KR, Lohr NE, et al: The relationship between borderline personality disorder and anxiety disorders. Am J Orthopsychiatry 59:461–467, 1989

Benjamin LS: Interpersonal Reconstructive Therapy. New York, Guilford, 2003

Binks CA, Fenton M, McCarthy L, et al: Pharmacological interventions for people with borderline personality disorder. Cochrane Database of Systematic Reviews 2006, Issue 1. Art. No: CD005653. DOI: 10.1002/14651858.CD005653

Bogenschutz MP, Nurnberg GH: Olanzapine versus placebo in the treatment of borderline personality disorder. J Clin Psychiatry 65:104–109, 2004

Browne G, Steiner M, Roberts J, et al: Sertraline and/or interpersonal psychotherapy for patients with dysthymic disorder in primary care: 6-month comparison with longitudinal 2-year follow-up of effectiveness and costs. J Affect Disord 68:317–330, 2002

Cardasis W, Hochman JA, Silk KR: Transitional objects and borderline personality disorder. Am J Psychiatry 154: 250–255, 1997

Casillas A, Clark LA: Dependency, impulsivity, and self-harm: traits hypothesized to underlie the association between cluster B personality and substance use disorders. J Personal Disord 16:424–436, 2002

Chiles JA, Carlin AS, Benjamin GAH, et al: A physician, a nonmedical psychotherapist, and a patient: the pharmacotherapy-psychotherapy triangle, in Integrating Pharmacotherapy and Psychotherapy. Edited by Beitman BD, Klerman GL. Washington DC, American Psychiatric Press, 1991, pp 105–118

Clarkin JF, Yeomans FE, Kernberg OF: Psychotherapy for borderline personality. New York, Wiley, 1999

Cloninger CR, Svrakic DM, Przybeck TR: A psychobiological model of temperament and character. Arch Gen Psychiatry 50:975–990, 1993

Coccaro EF, Kavoussi RJ: Fluoxetine and impulsive aggressive behavior in personality-disordered subjects. Arch Gen Psychiatry 54:1081–1088, 1997

Coccaro EF, Siever LJ, Klar HM, et al: Serotonergic studies in patients with affective and personality disorders: correlates with suicidal and impulsive agressive behavior. Arch Gen Psychiatry 46:587–599, 1989

Cowdry RW, Gardner DL: Pharmacotherapy of borderline personality disorder: alprazolam, carbamazepine, trifluoperazine, and tranylcypromine. Arch Gen Psychiatry 45:111–119, 1988

Davidson K, Norrie J, Tyrer P, et al: The effectiveness of cognitive behavior therapy for borderline personality disorder: results from the borderline personality disorder study of cognitive therapy (BOSCOT) trial. J Personal Disord 20:450–465, 2006

de Groot MH, Franken IH, van der Meer CW, et al: Stability and change in dimensional ratings of personality disorders in drug abuse patients during treatment. J Subst Abuse Treat 24:115–120, 2003

de Jonghe F, Hendricksen M, van Aalst G, et al: Psychotherapy alone and combined with pharmacotherapy in the treatment of depression. Br J Psychiatry 185:37–45, 2004

Duggan C, Huband N, Smailagic N, et al: The use of pharmacological treatments for people with personality disorder: a systematic review of randomized controlled trials. Personalality and Mental Health 2:119–170, 2008

Frankenburg FR. Zanarini MC: Personality disorders and medical comorbidity. Curr Opin Psychiatry 19:428–431, 2006

Gabbard GO: Splitting in hospital treatment. Am J Psychiatry 146:444–451, 1989

Gabbard GO, Wilkinson SM: Management of Countertransference With Borderline Patients. Washington, DC, American Psychiatric Press, 1994

Gardner DL, Cowdry RW: Alprazolam induced dyscontrol in borderline personality disorder. Am J Psychiatry 142:98–100, 1985

Goldberg RS, Riba M, Tasman A: Psychiatrists' attitudes toward prescribing medication for patients treated by nonmedical psychotherapists. Hosp Community Psychiatry 42:276–280, 1991

Goldberg SC, Schulz SC, Schulz PM, et al: Borderline and schizotypal personality disorders treated with low-dose thiothixene vs. placebo. Arch Gen Psychiatry 43:680–686, 1986

Goldhamer PM: Psychotherapy and pharmacotherapy: the challenge of integration. Can J Psychiatry 38:173–177, 1984

Greenblatt M, Solomon MH, Evans A, et al (eds): Drug and Social Therapy in Chronic Schizophrenia. Springfield, IL, Charles C Thomas, 1965

Gunderson JG: Borderline Personality Disorder. Washington, DC, American Psychiatric Press, 1984

Gunderson JG: Borderline Personality Disorder: A Clinical Guide. Washington DC, American Psychiatric Press, 2001

Gunderson JG, Morris H, Zanarini MC: Transitional objects and borderline patients, in The Borderline: Current Empirical Research. Edited by McGlashan TH. Washington, DC, American Psychiatric Association, 1985, pp 43–60

Healy D: The Anti-Depressant Era. Cambridge, MA, Harvard University Press, 1997

Healy D: The Creation of Psychopharmacology. Cambridge, MA, Harvard University Press, 2002

Hollander E, Allen, A, Lopez, RP, et al: A preliminary double-blind, placebo-controlled trial of divalproex sodium in borderline personality disorder. J Clin Psychiatry 62:199–203, 2001

Hollander E, Swann AC, Coccaro EF, et al: Impact of trait impulsivity and state aggression on divalproex versus placebo response in borderline personality disorder. Am J Psychiatry 162:621–624, 2005

Keller MB, McCullough JP, Klein DN, et al: A comparison of nefazodone, the cognitive behavioral-analysis system of psychotherapy, and their combination for the treatment of chronic depression. N Engl J Med 342:1642–1670, 2000

Kernberg O, Koenigsberg H, Stone M, et al: Borderline Patients: Extending the Limits of Treatability. New York, Basic Books, 2000

Klerman GL: The psychiatric patient's right to effective treatment: implications of Osheroff vs. Chestnut Lodge. Am J Psychiatry 147:409–418, 1990

Koenigsberg HW: Combining psychotherapy and pharmacotherapy in the treatment of borderline patients, in American Psychiatric Press Review of Psychiatry, Vol 12. Edited by Oldham JM, Riba MB, Tasman A. Washington, DC, American Psychiatric Press, 1993, pp 541–563

Koenigsberg HW, Reynolds D, Goodman M, et al: Risperidone in the treatment of schizotypal personality disorder. J Clin Psychiatry 64:628–634, 2003

Kool S, Dekker J, Duijsens IJ, et al: Changes in personality pathology after pharmacotherapy and combined therapy for depressed patients. J Personal Disord 17:60–72, 2003

Lecrubier Y: Prescribing patterns for depression and anxiety worldwide. J Clin Psychiatry 62 (suppl 13):31–36, 2001

Linehan MM, Heard HL, Armstrong HE: Naturalistic follow-up of a behavioral treatment for chronically parasuicidal borderline patients. Arch Gen Psychiatry 50:971–974, 1993

Livesley WJ: A practical approach to the treatment of patients with borderline personality disorder. Psychiatr Clin North Am 23:211–232, 2000

Livesley WJ, Jang KL, Vernon PA: Phenotypic and genetic structure of traits delineating personality disorder. Arch Gen Psychiatry 55:941–948, 1998

Loew TH, Nickel MK, Muehlbacher M, et al: Topiramate treatment for women with borderline personality disorder: a double-blind, placebo-controlled study. J Clin Psychopharmacol 26:61–66, 2006

Main TF: The ailment. Br J Med Psychol 30:129–145, 1957

Manber R, Arnow B, Blasey C, et al: Patient's therapeutic skill acquisition and response to psychotherapy, alone or in combination with medication. Psychol Med 33:693–702, 2003

Markowitz P: Pharmacotherapy, in Handbook of Personality Disorders: Theory, Research and Treatment. Edited by Livesley WJ. New York, Guilford, 2001, pp 475–493

Markowitz PJ: Recent trends in the pharmacotherapy of personality disorders. J Personal Disord 18:90–101, 2004

Metzl JM, Riba M: Understanding the symbolic value of medications: a brief review. Prim Psychiatry 10:1–4, 2003

Nickel MK, Nickel C, Kaplan P, et al: Treatment of aggression with topiramate in male borderline patients: a double-blind, placebo-controlled study. Biol Psychiatry 57:495–499, 2005

Nickel MK, Muehlbacher M, Nickel C, et al: Aripiprazole in the treatment of patients with borderline personality disorder: a double-blind, placebo-controlled study. Am J Psychiatry 163:833–838, 2006

Nose M, Cipriani A, Biancosino B, et al: Efficacy of pharmacotherapy against core traits of borderline personality disorder: meta-analysis of randomized controlled trials. Int Clin Psychopharmacol 21:345–353, 2006

Ogden TH: Projective Identification and Psychotherapeutic Technique. New York, Jason Aronson, 1982

Paris J: Borderline Personality Disorder: A Multidimensional Approach. Washington, DC, American Psychiatric Press, 1994

Paris J: Chronic suicidality among patients with borderline personality disorder. Psychiatr Serv 53:738–742, 2002

Paris J: Personality Disorders Over Time: Precursors, Course, and Outcome. Washington, DC, American Psychiatric Publishing, 2003

Putnam KM, Silk KR: Emotion dysregulation and the development of borderline personality disorder. Dev Psychopathol 17:899–925, 2005

Riba M, Balon R (eds): Psychopharmacology and Psychotherapy: A Collaborative Approach. Washington, DC, American Psychiatric Press, 1999

Rinne T, van de Brink W, Wouters I, et al: SSRI treatment of borderline personality disorder: a randomized, placebo-controlled clinical trial for female patients with borderline personality disorder. Am J Psychiatry 159: 2048–2054, 2002

Rutter M: The interplay of nature, nurture, and developmental influences: the challenge ahead for mental health. Arch Gen Psychiatry 59:996–1000, 2002

Salzman C, Wolfson AN, Schatzberg A, et al: Effect of fluoxetine on anger in symptomatic volunteers with borderline personality disorder. J Clin Psychopharmacol 15:23–29, 1995

Schulz SC, Camlin KL: Treatment of borderline personality disorder: potential of the new antipsychotic medications. Journal of Practical Psychiatry and Behavioral Health 5:247–255, 1999

Sheard M, Marini J, Bridges C, et al: The effect of lithium on impulsive aggressive behavior in man. Am J Psychiatry 133:1409–1413, 1976

Siever LJ, Davis KL: A psychobiological perspective on the personality disorders. Am J Psychiatry 148:1647–1658, 1991

Siever LJ, Torgersen S, Gunderson JG, et al: The borderline diagnosis, III: identifying endophenotypes for genetic studies. Biol Psychiatry 51:964–968, 2002

Silk KR: Rational pharmacotherapy for patients with personality disorders, in Clinical Assessment and Management of Severe Personality Disorders. Edited by Links P. Washington, DC, American Psychiatric Press, 1995, pp 109–142

Silk KR (ed): Biology of Personality Disorders. Washington, DC, American Psychiatric Press, 1998

Simpson EB, Yen S, Costello E, et al: Combined dialectical behavior therapy and fluoxetine in the treatment of borderline personality disorder. J Clin Psychiatry 65:379–385, 2004

Skodol AE, Stout RL, McGlashan TH, et al: Co-occurrence of mood and personality disorders: a report from the Collaborative Longitudinal Personality Disorders Study (CLPS). Depress Anxiety 10:175–182, 1999

Skodol AE, Siever LJ, Livesley WJ, et al: The borderline diagnosis, II: biology, genetics, and clinical course. Biol Psychiatry 51:951–963, 2002

Smith JM: Some dimensions of transference in combined treatment, in The Psychotherapist's Guide to Pharmacotherapy. Edited by Ellison JM. Chicago, IL, Year Book Medical, 1989, pp 79–94

Soler J, Pascual JC, Campins J, et al: Double-blind, placebo-controlled study of dialectical behavior therapy plus olanzapine for borderline personality disorder. Am J Psychiatry 162:1221–1224, 2005

Soloff PH: What's new in personality disorders? An update on pharmacologic treatment. J Personal Disord 4:233–243, 1990

Soloff PH: Algorithms for pharmacological treatment of personality dimensions: symptom-specific treatments for cognitive-perceptual, affective, and impulsive-behavioral dysregulation. Bull Menninger Clin 62:195–214, 1998

Soloff PH, George A, Nathan RS, et al: Paradoxical effects of amitriptyline in borderline patients. Am J Psychiatry 143:1603–1605, 1986a

Soloff PH, George A, Nathan RS, et al: Progress in pharmacotherapy of borderline disorders: a double-blind study of amitriptyline, haloperidol, and placebo. Arch Gen Psychiatry 43:691–697, 1986b

Soloff PH, Cornelius J, George A, et al: Efficacy of phenelzine and haloperidol in borderline personality disorder. Arch Gen Psychiatry 50:377–385, 1993

Stanton AH, Schwartz MS: The Mental Hospital: A Study of Institutional Participation in Psychiatric Illness and Treatment. London, Tavistock, 1954

Stone MH: The Fate of Borderline Patients: Successful Outcome and Psychiatric Practice. New York, Guilford, 1990

Tritt K, Nickel C, Lahmann C, et al: Lamotrigine treatment of aggression in female borderline patients: a randomized, double-blind, placebo-controlled study. J Psychopharmacol 19:287–291, 2005

Waldinger RS, Frank AF: Clinicians' experiences in combining medication and psychotherapy in the treatment of borderline patients. Hosp Community Psychiatry 40:712–718, 1989

Westen D, Arkowitz-Westen L: Limitations of Axis II in diagnosing personality pathology in clinical practice. Am J Psychiatry 155:1767–1771, 1998

Westen D, Moses M, Silk KR, et al: Quality of depressive experience in borderline personality disorder and major depression: when depression is not just depression. J Personal Disord 6:382–393, 1992

Williams BC, Silk KR: "Difficult" patients, in Primary Care Psychiatry. Edited by Knesper DJ, Riba MB, Schwenk TL. Philadelphia, PA, WB Saunders, 1997, pp 61–75

Winnicott D: Transitional objects and transitional phenomena. Int J Psychoanal 34:89–97, 1953

Woodward B, Duckworth KS, Gutheil TG: The pharmacotherapist-psychotherapist collaboration, in American Psychiatric Press Review of Psychiatry, Vol 12. Edited by Oldham JM, Riba MB, Tasman A. Washington, DC, American Psychiatric Press, 1993, pp 631–649

Yen S, Shea MT, Pagano M, et al: Axis I and Axis II disorders as predictors of prospective suicide attempts: findings from the collaborative longitudinal personality disorders study. J Abnorm Psychol 112:375–381, 2003

Young JE, Klosko JS, Weishaar ME: Schema Therapy: A Practitioner's Guide. New York, Guilford, 2003

Zanarini MC, Frankenburg FR: Olanzapine treatment of female borderline personality disorder patients: a double-blind, placebo-controlled pilot study. J Clin Psychiatry 62:849–854, 2001

Zanarini MC, Frankenburg FR, Dubo ED, et al: Axis I comorbidity of borderline personality disorder. Am J Psychiatry 155:1733–1739, 1998

18

Assessing and Managing Suicide Risk

Paul S. Links, M.D., F.R.C.P.C.
Nathan Kolla, M.D.

Robins and colleagues in 1959 demonstrated the strong association between mental disorders and suicide, but the relationship between suicidal behavior and personality disorders (Axis II disorders) has only been systematically studied since the mid-1980s. The purpose of this chapter is threefold. First, the epidemiological evidence for the association between suicidal behavior and suicide in individuals diagnosed with personality disorders is reviewed. Second, we examine whether any potentially modifiable risk factors are associated with these diagnoses, based on existing empirical evidence. Last, clinical approaches to the assessment of the uncommunicative patient and patients with antisocial, borderline, and narcissistic personality disorders presenting at risk for suicide are discussed.

DEFINITION OF TERMS AND METHODOLOGY

For purposes of this review, *suicidal behavior* is defined through three components: suicide, suicide attempts, and self-injurious behaviors. The definitions of O'Carroll et al. (1996) have been adopted. They defined *suicide* as self-injurious behavior with a fatal outcome

This chapter is adapted with permission from Links PS, Gould G, Ratnayake R: "Assessing Suicidal Youth With Antisocial, Borderline, or Narcissistic Personality Disorder." *Canadian Journal of Psychiatry* 48:301–310, 2003.

for which there is evidence (either explicit or implicit) that the individual intended at some (nonzero) level to kill him- or herself. A *suicide attempt* is defined as self-injurious behavior with a nonfatal outcome for which there is evidence (either explicit or implicit) that the individual intended at some (nonzero) level to kill him- or herself. A definition of *self-injurious behavior* not intended to be fatal has also been utilized. Simeon and Favazza (2001) defined *self-injurious behavior* as all behaviors that involve deliberate infliction of direct physical harm to one's body with zero intent to die as a consequence of this behavior.

Our discussion of suicide risk focuses on the clinical entities known as personality disorders. Primarily, the diagnoses from DSM-III, DSM-III-R, DSM-IV, and DSM-IV-TR (American Psychiatric Association 1980, 1987, 1994, 2000) are discussed; however, we also include studies employing ICD-9 and ICD-10 diagnoses (World Health Organization 1977, 1992) for completeness. Personality or personality traits are often discussed from a dimensional approach. These dimensions have inherent advantages for measurement and statistical purposes, describing cases at categorical borders and connecting with the large body of normal personality research. A diagnostic or categorical approach has certain advantages for the practicing clinician, because a considerable body of research related to risk assessment exists based on psychiatric and personality disorder diagnoses. As discussed later, there is a lesser body of clinical research and little consensus related to personality dimensions and suicide risk assessment.

This review is based on the English-language literature from 1991 to 2003 using the search terms of all personality disorders and suicide and suicidal behavior. In particular, this chapter focuses on research that examined potential risk factors for these diagnoses compared with those for other psychiatric disorders. The final section of this chapter describes clinical approaches to patients at risk for suicidal behavior who are uncommu-

nicative and patients with antisocial, borderline, and/or narcissistic personality disorder. These observations are based on clinical experience and not on empirical evidence. The observations would not replace the need for doing a comprehensive suicide risk assessment based on formats such as those described by Jacobs et al. (1999), Rudd and Joiner (1998), and the American Psychiatric Association's (2003) practice guideline for assessing and treating patients with suicidal behavior. The difficult decisions that arise during a suicide risk assessment—such as whether the patient should be admitted to hospital, whether such admission should be involuntary, or whether the person's risk of suicide should be communicated to the family—are most soundly based on careful clinical assessment, because there is no measurement scale that can replace clinical expertise.

PERSONALITY, PERSONALITY DISORDERS, AND SUICIDE RISK ASSESSMENT

Goldsmith et al. (1990) articulated modern conceptualizations of the causal relationship between personality and/or personality disorder and suicidal behavior, but most importantly, they asked whether personality disorders directly predispose to suicidal behavior independent of other risk factors. Although the causal relationship between personality and/or personality disorders and suicidal behavior is likely complex, research since 1990 has suggested that certain personality features and/or disorders are related to suicidal behavior and are independent of other known risk factors.

Conner et al. (2001) thoroughly reviewed the empirical literature to determine whether psychological vulnerability was a risk factor for completed suicide. The authors argued that *personality traits* was too narrow a concept and that psychological vulnerabilities encompassed dysfunctional cognitions, behavior, and emotions. For example, hopelessness was examined as a form of psychological vulnerability, although it remains unclear whether hopelessness is best considered a personality trait, an affect, or a part of a psychiatric illness.

Reviewing databases from January 1966 to February 2000 and including only constructs found to be associated with suicide by at least two independent teams, Conner et al. (2001) identified five dimensions: impulsivity/aggression, depression, hopelessness, anxiety, and self-consciousness/social disengagement. The proportion of significant findings out of the studies testing the constructs did not differ significantly across the five dimensions: impulsivity/aggression (14/20, 70%); hopelessness (11/16, 69%); depression (13/22, 59%); anxiety (13/22, 59%); and self-consciousness/social disengagement (18/24, 75%). Given the breadth of concepts identified by their review, the authors concluded that "no single conceptual or empirically derived model of personality constructs" (p. 371) was sufficient to explain the relationship of psychological vulnerabilities to suicide. No such comprehensive review was found relating personality traits and suicide attempts.

Johnson et al. (1999) reviewed the empirical literature to determine the value of objective personality inventories for predicting assessment of "long-term" suicide risk. The authors searched PsychLit journal databases from January 1974 to March 1996 and restricted their inquiry to self-reported inventories and reports on entire measures rather than focusing on subscales. The measures reviewed included the California Personality Inventory; Edwards Personal Preference Schedule; Eysenck Personality Tests; Millon Clinical Multiaxial Inventory, versions I–III; Minnesota Multiphasic Personality Inventory (MMPI), versions 1 and 2; Myers-Briggs Type Indicator; 16 Personality Factors Test; Neuroticism, Extroversion, Openness Personality Inventory; and the Personality Diagnostic Questionnaire.

Based on the review, the MMPI was considered the most empirically investigated objective personality measure; however, the authors found no "support of the notion that any MMPI item(s), scale or configural profile consistently differentiates suicidal from nonsuicidal patients" (p. 178). Overall, Johnson et al. (1999) concluded there was little indication of the utility for any single inventory, scale, or item in the prediction of long-term suicide risk.

These two authoritative reviews expose the limits of our current understanding of the relationship between personality and suicide. However, research continues, and three personality characteristics are highlighted as uniquely related to suicidal behavior and as principal areas for further study. Impulsive aggressiveness has been shown to have a unique relationship to a history of suicidal behavior, and Mann et al. (1999) demonstrated that impulsive aggressiveness was more strongly associated with a history of suicide attempts than was the strength of psychiatric symptomatology. In addition, various biological research strategies have demonstrated that low serotonergic function was specifically related to impulsive aggressiveness, providing evidence for the biological bridge between suicide and personality traits (Mann et al. 1999).

At the other extreme, the individual who appears perfectionistic and vulnerable to narcissistic injury might be at risk for suicidal behavior. Hewitt et al. (1998) demonstrated that perfectionism was significantly related to suicide risk even after controlling for the level of hopelessness and depression. In particular, perceiving oneself as not meeting others' expectations was significantly related to increased suicide risk. Finally, emotional dysregulation, characterized as rapidly shifting mood states, has been theoretically and empirically linked to suicidal behavior. Linehan (1993) hypothesized that emotional dysregulation in conjunction with an invalidating environment explained the suicidal behavior characteristic of individuals with borderline personality disorder (BPD). Fawcett et al. (1990) found that *depressive turmoil*, defined as rapid shifts from one dysphoric state to another without persistence of one affect, was significantly predictive of suicide in their cohort of individuals with major affective disorders. Although emotional dysregulation should be a primary focus of research, the precise definition of this characteristic requires further refinement. Emotional dysregulation is often subsumed within the concept of neuroticism; however, we have suggested that emotional dysregulation or affective lability might encompass four elements: cyclicity, intensity, variability, or hyperreactivity of mood to external stimuli. Because suicidal behavior is undoubtedly multidetermined, complex modeling of various personality characteristics with other distal and proximal risk factors and utilizing multilevel analyses will be required to explain suicide or suicidal behavior as the outcome.

EPIDEMIOLOGICAL EVIDENCE

Most of the evidence points to the relationship between antisocial and borderline personality disorders and suicidal behavior. Therefore, we begin by reviewing the epidemiological evidence for each of the Cluster B personality disorders. The more limited literature related to Clusters A and C and suicidal behavior is reviewed according to the respective clusters rather than the individual personality disorders. To organize the literature, we discuss the rates of the various personality disorders in individuals who completed suicide or made suicide attempts. Then we present the rates of suicide and suicide attempts in samples of individuals with the various personality disorders.

Cluster B

Studies have been done of the rates of personality disorders in adolescents who died by suicide. Marttunen et al. (1991), from the Comprehensive Psychological Autopsy Study in Finland, estimated that 17% of adolescents ages 13–19 who died by suicide met criteria for conduct disorder or antisocial personality disorder (ASPD). When Marttunen et al. (1994) examined adolescents with nonfatal suicidal behavior, approximately 45% of males and one-third of females were characterized by antisocial behavior. In other research, suicidal behavior was found to be higher among adolescents with conduct disorders than in the comparison groups even after controlling for major depression (Brent et al. 1993b). Beautrais et al. (1996) studied individuals who had made medically serious suicide attempts and compared them with community comparison subjects. After controlling for the intercorrelations between mental disorders, these researchers found the risk of a serious suicide attempt was 3.7 times higher for individuals with ASPD than for those without. When they examined men under age 30, the risk of a serious suicide attempt was almost nine times more likely among individuals with ASPD than among those without the disorder; for women, the risk of a serious suicide attempt was 2.3 times higher.

A few studies have documented the lifetime risk of suicide in samples of individuals with ASPD. Maddocks (1970), in a 5-year follow-up of a small sample of 59 persons with the disorder, estimated a 5% lifetime risk of suicide. Laub and Vaillant (2000) examined causes of death of 1,000 delinquent and nondelinquent boys followed up from ages 14 to 65 years. Deaths due to violent causes (accident, suicide, or homicide) were significantly more common in delinquent compared with nondelinquent boys; however, equal proportions of both groups died by suicide.

Patients with BPD represent 9%–33% of all suicides (Kullgren et al. 1986; Runeson and Beskow 1991). Bongar et al. (1990) studied chronically suicidal patients with four or more visits in a year to a psychiatric emergency department, and most often these patients met criteria for BPD. These patients accounted for over 12% of all psychiatric emergency department visits during the year studied. Crumley (1979) showed a high incidence of BPD in adolescents and young adults age 15–24 years who engaged in suicidal behavior. Paris and Zweig-Frank (2001) indicated that this diagnosis significantly increases the risk of eventual suicide. Depending on the study, the lifetime risk of suicide among patients with BPD patients is between 3% and 10% (Paris and Zweig-Frank 2001). Those at highest risk appeared to be young, ranging from adolescence into the third decade (Berman 1985; Friedman and Corn 1987; Stone 1990), which likely reflects a decrease in severity of symptoms later in adulthood in the majority of patients (Crumley 1979; Stone 1990). The high rates of suicidal behavior in patients with BPD are reflected by, or some would say result from, the inclusion of recurrent suicidal behavior, gestures, threats, or self-mutilating behavior as a diagnostic criterion in DSM-IV-TR. A history of suicidal behavior is found in 55%–70% of individuals with a personality disorder (Casey 1989; Clarkin et al. 1984; Gomez et al. 1992) and in 60%–78% of individuals with BPD (Gunderson 1984; Kjellander et al. 1998).

Narcissistic personality disorder is an uncommon diagnosis in community samples compared with ASPD and BPD, and few data exist regarding the risk of suicide in individuals with this disorder. In samples of suicide victims studied with the psychological autopsy method, narcissistic personality is infrequently identified. However, Apter et al. (1993) studied 43 consecutive suicides by Israeli males ages 18–21 that occurred during their compulsory military service. Psychological autopsies were carried out using preinduction assessment information, service records, and extensive postmortem interviews. Based on this methodology, the most common Axis II personality disorders were schizoid personality in 16 of 43 (37.2%) and narcissistic personality in 10 of 43 (23.3%). Stone's (1990) extensive follow-up study of 550 patients admitted to the general clinical service of the New York State Psychiatric Institute provided some information on this outcome for individuals hospitalized with the diagnosis of narcissistic personality disorder. According to the 15-year follow-up, patients with the disorder or narcissistic traits were significantly more likely to have died by suicide compared with patients without the disorder or traits (14% versus 5%; $P<0.02$).

Few studies have reported on the risk of suicide or suicide attempts in individuals with histrionic personality disorder, and studies that do comment on the relationship between this diagnosis and suicidal behavior have rarely controlled for the presence of BPD. Although histrionic personality disorder has been diagnosed in 1%–17% of all adult suicide attempters being assessed at hospital emergency departments (Braun-Scharm 1996; Dirks 1998; Ferreira de Castro et al. 1998; Gupta and Trzepacz 1997; Markar et al. 1991; Soderberg 2001) as well as in 16% of individuals forming a sample of adolescent inpatient suicide attempters (Brent et al. 1993a), Ferreira de Castro et al. (1998) noted that histrionic personality disorder was the most common personality disorder diagnosis (22% of all subjects) in their sample, comprising individuals who engaged in self-injurious behavior but whose intention was not death. Other studies examining the connection between histrionic personality disorder and completed suicide include one by Harwood et al. (2001), who observed that 4% of their sample of individuals over age 60 years had the disorder. The prevalence of suicidal tendencies in a sample of patients diagnosed with hysterical personality disorder, the ICD-9 equivalent of histrionic personality disorder, has been found to be approximately 39% (Ahrens and Haug 1996).

Clusters A and C

Epidemiological evidence for the risk of suicide or suicide attempts among individuals with either Cluster A or Cluster C personality disorders is relatively scarce. Again, most studies do not control for the possibility of coexisting BPD mediating the observed suicidal behavior in the subjects examined. Depending on the study, the prevalence of Cluster A or C personality disorders in adults presenting to an emergency department following a suicide attempt or self-injury ranges from 3% to 5% for schizoid personality disorder (Braun-Scharm 1996; Dirks 1998; Ferreira de Castro et al. 1998), 9% for schizotypal personality disorder (Markar et al. 1991), 8%–10% for paranoid personality disorder (Persson et al. 1999; Soderberg 2001), 6%–20% for avoidant personality disorder (Persson et al. 1999; Soderberg 2001), 30% for anxious personality disorder (Dirks 1998), 1%–9% for dependent personality disorder (Braun-Scharm 1996; Dirks 1998; Gupta and Trzepacz 1997), 6% for obsessive-compulsive personality disorder (Soderberg 2001), and 13% for anankastic personality disorder (Dirks 1998). In their study of inpatient suicide attempters between ages of 13 and 19 years, Brent et al. (1993a) reported that 27% fulfilled criteria for any Cluster A personality disorder and 70% for any Cluster C personality disorder. However, only a diagnosis of BPD or any personality disorder was significant in this sample of adolescent suicide attempters when compared with a group of psychiatric nonsuicidal control subjects.

Similar to the studies just cited, Haw et al. (2001) reported on the prevalence of ICD-10 personality disorders among individuals admitted to a British hospital following an episode of deliberate self-harm and diagnosed on follow-up approximately 12–16 months later. These researchers found that 5% of their sample fulfilled criteria for schizoid personality disorder, 15% for paranoid personality disorder, 21% for anxious personality disorder, 13% for dependent personality disorder, and 20% for anankastic personality disorder.

Several studies have employed the psychological autopsy method of retrospectively diagnosing personality disorders in completed suicides. Among individuals older than 23 whose deaths received a verdict of suicide or unknown cause, Houston et al. (2001) reported that 4% of the victims had a primary paranoid personality disorder, 4% a primary anxious personality disorder, and 7% a primary anankastic personality disorder, whereas 4% had secondary paranoid,

anxious, and anankastic personality disorders. Analyzing data from the National Suicide Prevention Project in Finland, Isometsä et al. (1996) determined that 1% of their sample fulfilled criteria for paranoid personality disorder, 6% for avoidant personality disorder, 7% for dependent personality disorder, 3% for obsessive-compulsive personality disorder, and 18% for Cluster C personality disorders not otherwise specified. Harwood et al. (2001) examined individuals over the age of 60 whose deaths received a verdict of suicide and found that 4% of their sample had had anankastic personality disorder during their lifetimes. Finally, data from a psychological autopsy study comprising 163 subjects revealed that Cluster A and Cluster C personality disorders were associated with completed suicide (Schneider et al. 2006). Significantly higher frequencies of isolated Cluster C personality disorders were also observed among male but not female suicide victims.

Studies have also reported on rates of attempted and completed suicides among individuals diagnosed with personality disorders. Fenton et al. (1997) located patients from the Chestnut Lodge Follow-Up Study who were originally diagnosed with schizotypal personality disorder and found that 3% had committed suicide, 24% had attempted suicide, and 45% had expressed suicidal ideation at some point during the previous 19 years. Among patients admitted to the psychiatric department of a German hospital between 1981 and 1994 who were assigned a primary diagnosis of personality disorder upon admission, Ahrens and Haug (1996) found that 44% of individuals diagnosed with schizoid personality disorder displayed suicidal tendencies, as did 47% of the patients with paranoid personality disorder or anankastic personality disorder.

Summary

Modestin et al. (1997) noted that suicidal behavior in women is independently correlated with each of the three personality disorder clusters, whereas suicidal behavior in men only correlates with the clusters as a group. Thus, although evidence suggests that Cluster A and C personality disorders are associated with the risk of suicide or suicide attempts, the relationship between Cluster B personality disorders and suicidal behavior has been well documented and appears to be more robust.

RISK FACTORS FOR SUICIDE AND SUICIDAL BEHAVIOR

Many studies have identified factors at a population level that alone or in combination increase the risk of suicide. Although extrapolating these risk factors to an individual allows for categorization of risk, it does little to predict which individual will commit suicide and when. "The goal of a suicide assessment is not to predict suicide, but rather to place a person along a putative risk continuum, to appreciate the bases of suicidality, and to allow for a more informed intervention" (Jacobs et al. 1999; p. 4). Many risk factors are fixed (age, race, gender), providing little opportunity to intervene. However, several of the most significant risk factors are modifiable. Forster and Wu (2002) captured the concept eloquently in the following statement, "Suicide is almost always the catastrophic result of inadequately treated psychiatric illness" (p. 105). Forster and Wu suggested concentrating on modifiable risk factors. Therefore, the purpose of this review is to discuss risk factors that place patients with personality disorders at a higher risk relative to other individuals with like disorders or place them at higher risk relative to other times in the course of their illness. In addition, purportedly modifiable risk factors are discussed because they might present opportunities for interventions. By far, the majority of the studies have focused on subjects with BPD, with little or no research on patients with other personality disorders. This chapter reviews each of the major risk factors and discusses, in some detail, findings from

key studies—those employing carefully characterized comparison groups and controlling for potential confounding factors.

Comorbid Disorders

The presence of two or more psychiatric disorders appears to substantially increase the suicide attempt rate compared with the presence of a single disorder, and comorbidity is found to be higher in adolescents than in adults (Lewinsohn et al. 1995). Most of the research has been done with regard to BPD, and the following studies indicate that certain specific comorbidities may increase the risk for suicidal behavior in patients with BPD.

Major Depressive Episode

Several studies have documented that the existence of depression plus BPD may confer an increased risk for suicidal behavior. In adolescents, coexistence of disruptive behavior plus depression is felt to be a particularly "dangerous" combination (McCracken et al. 1993). The most careful study of this combination was completed by Soloff et al. (2000). They examined a well-characterized group of patients with BPD comorbid with major depressive episodes and compared them with subjects with BPD without a major depressive episode and with subjects with current major depressive episode only. The number of lifetime suicide attempts significantly differentiated the comorbid patients from the other two comparison groups, with a mean of 3.0 lifetime attempts among the comorbid group versus 1.9 lifetime attempts for subjects with pure BPD and 0.8 lifetime attempts for subjects with major depressive episodes only. Comorbid patients reported significantly higher levels of objective planning based on the most serious lifetime attempt than the other comparison groups. Using regression analysis, the researchers demonstrated that the number of lifetime attempts was predicted by BPD diagnosis and comorbidity, history of aggression, and the level of hopelessness. Overall, the patients with comorbidity demonstrated an increased risk for suicidal behavior, particularly with a higher number of lifetime attempts and evidence for more objective planning. The authors concluded that suicidal behavior in inpatients with BPD should not be considered "less serious" than the suicidal behavior of inpatients with a major depressive episode. In a five-year prospective follow-up study, Soloff and Fabio (2008) found that comorbid major depressive disorder increased the risk of suicide attempts in the first year of follow-up while poor social adjustment predicted increased risk across the whole follow-up period. There is also some evidence to suggest that major depressive disorder increases risk of suicidal behavior among individuals with pure Cluster C personality disorders (Dervic et al. 2007).

Substance Abuse Disorder

Comorbidity of substance abuse disorder with BPD has also been found to be related to increased suicidal behavior (Runeson and Beskow 1991; Soloff et al. 1994). Links et al. (1995) examined the prognostic significance of comorbid substance abuse in BPD patients. These patients were followed prospectively over a 7-year period. The researchers found that patients comorbid for substance abuse and BPD perceived themselves at significantly more risk for the likelihood of killing themselves than the comparison groups of BPD patients without comorbidity, patients with substance abuse without BPD, and patients with borderline traits only. The comorbid patients also demonstrated a more frequent pattern of self-mutilative behavior and reported a more frequent pattern of suicide threats and attempts than the noncomorbid patients. Yen et al. (2003) prospectively studied the diagnostic predictors of suicide attempts using the Collaborative Longitudinal Personality Disorders sample made up of four personality-disordered groups—schizotypal, borderline, avoidant, and obsessive-compulsive—and a group with major depressive disorder without personality disorder.

The baseline diagnosis of a drug use disorder and BPD was predictive of suicide attempts during the follow-up interval; however, alcohol use disorder did not significantly add to the model once the BPD diagnosis was entered. McGirr et al. (2007) demonstrated that individuals with BPD who died by suicide were significantly more likely to have had alcohol dependence and Cluster B comorbidity than living individuals with BPD. Evidence also indicates that comorbidity between substance abuse disorder and conduct disorder increases the risk for suicidal behavior in youth (Kelly et al. 2002; Marttunen et al. 1991).

Recent Life Events

Adverse life events may push high-risk patients into actual suicidal crises. Kelly et al. (2000) studied the impact of recent life events and the level of social adjustment in patients with major depression, patients with BPD, and patients comorbid for major depression and BPD. Kelly et al. (2000) found that the suicide attempters within this sample had experienced more adverse life events recently, particularly in the area of stressful events at home, either family or financially related. In addition, the total number of life events was related to increased risk of suicidal behavior. When the authors did a regression analysis to predict suicide attempter status, the diagnosis of BPD was predictive, as was the level of social adjustment in the family unit. However, once these variables were accounted for in the model, the level of recent life events was not predictive. Patients characterized by the presence of low social adjustment and the BPD diagnosis were found to be 16 times more likely to be classified as suicide attempters than the patients with major depressive episodes. Heikkinen et al. (1997) similarly reported that life events such as job problems, family discord, financial trouble, unemployment, and interpersonal loss were more common among suicide victims with personality disorders than among suicide victims without personality disorders. Interestingly, these researchers also concluded that interpersonal and job-related or financial problems most closely preceded suicide among individuals with personality disorders. On the other hand, rates of financial trouble and unemployment among individuals with Cluster C personality disorders were found to be no different from rates for suicide victims without a diagnosis of personality disorder. Runeson and Beskow (1991) also found the number of stressful life situations was related to death by suicide for adolescents with BPD versus others without BPD. These situations included such things as unstable employment, financial problems, lack of a permanent residence, and a sentence by a court of law.

Discharge from hospital should be considered a stressful event. Kullgren (1988) found that patients with BPD were at somewhat increased risk for suicide around the time of imminent discharge from hospital and that suicides of such patients occurred during the period of inpatient care and in the weeks following discharge. Kjelsberg et al. (1991) noted that patients with BPD who died by suicide during or following hospitalization were more frequently discharged after violating an in-hospital contract than were the surviving borderline patients.

History of Childhood Abuse

A history of childhood abuse needs to be mentioned because its association with suicidal behavior has been documented by several investigators (Dubo et al. 1997; Runeson and Beskow 1991; Stone 1990); however, it is debatable whether childhood abuse is a modifiable risk factor. Soloff et al. (2002) completed a key study examining the relationship between childhood abuse and suicidal behavior in a sample of patients with BPD. They found that suicidal behavior, in terms of the number of attempts, was predicted by a history of childhood sexual abuse, by the severity of BPD, and by the level of hopelessness. In fact, childhood sexual abuse continued to predict the number of attempts independently, even after entering a number of other selected risk factors into the analysis. The severity of childhood sexual abuse was associated with the severity of comorbid depression in these patients, the presence of antisocial traits, and a trend toward greater hopelessness. Childhood sexual abuse as a risk factor for suicidal behavior may be mediated by these factors. Soloff et al. (2002) indicated that patients with a history of childhood sexual abuse had a 10-fold greater risk of suicidal behavior versus those patients without such a history.

Case Example

Ms. Y, a 28-year-old single female, presented herself to the emergency department complaining that she felt terrible. "I am close to overdosing," she explained. For the last 2 days, she had medicated herself by binging on cocaine and alcohol. The patient was clear about her distress. Two days prior to presentation, her gynecologist had informed Ms. Y that she needed a hysterectomy and that the surgery could not be put off any longer. Although the precipitating events were plain, a more complete picture emerged after the patient was hospitalized. She and her colleagues at work reported a 2-month history of declining work performance, increasing depression with suicidal ideation, and heightened irritability. Ms. Y had not been under psychiatric care for several years; however, she had a history of three previous suicide attempts, very stormy relationships, impulsivity including periodic binging on alcohol and cocaine, and chronic feelings of dysphoria. Her previous therapist had given her a diagnosis of BPD. During her worst bout of depression, Ms. Y carefully planned her first suicide attempt. She acquired several months' worth of prescription tricyclic antidepressants and made arrangements to be unavailable to her family for the weekend. While taking a hot bath, she ingested all of the pills and waited for her outcome. Fortunately, her stomach was the first organ affected, and she became violently ill and unable to keep her death potion down.

This case demonstrates the association between major depression and BPD and how it can lead to heightened risk for suicide. The underlying depression could have been missed if the time had not been taken to elicit a careful history of the last few weeks and months leading to Ms. Y's presentation. Collateral sources of information were extremely beneficial in confirming the patient's deteriorating mood. One should always look for the effects on functioning that comorbid depression most often has on BPD patients. Although anger is part of the BPD diagnosis, for this woman anger was an indication of her comorbid depression.

In summary, patients with ASPD or BPD are likely to be at increased risk when they demonstrate the risk factors described. In particular, patients with these disorders are likely to be at increased risk when they demonstrate a confluence of risk factors. The presence of comorbidity, particularly when it is acutely evident, may lead high-risk patients into episodes of acute suicidal behavior. The accumulation of recent life events and/or the lack of intimate or family support also indicates times of high risk for these patients. If factors such as a history of childhood sexual abuse and the associated psychopathological deficits, the level of hopelessness, or a history of impulsivity are modifiable based on clinical interventions, then potentially these interventions could reduce the ongoing risk in these patients.

CLINICAL APPROACH TO THE UNCOMMUNICATIVE PATIENT AND PATIENTS WITH ANTISOCIAL, BORDERLINE, AND NARCISSISTIC PERSONALITY DISORDERS

Uncommunicative Patients

Uncommunicative patients are among the most difficult to assess for the risk of suicide. The presence or absence of suicidal ideation should be elicited if possible. However, the denial of suicidal ideation does not negate the risk of suicide. Duberstein and colleagues (Conner et al. 2001) found that individuals who committed suicide lacked an openness to experience, and the authors connected this personality feature to the interpersonal process of individuals who, when assessed, are less likely to feel and report feeling suicidal. Fawcett et al. (1990) found that suicidal ideation was not predictive of suicide in the short term, within 1 year of the assessment, but was related to suicide in the longer term. When questions related to suicidal ideation are denied or not responded to, the clinician must judge the level of risk based on the inference of all available risk and protective factors.

In assessing the uncommunicative patient, the clinician has to pay particular attention to the interview process. What is the patient communicating through his or her lack of verbal communication? For many uncommunicative patients, their failure to respond expresses the lack of personal safety they feel during the assessment encounter. Creating some sense of safety may facilitate more verbal communication. For suicidal men, in particular, the clinician must attend to the process of the assessment interview. Suicidal men may enter a clinical encounter with the expectation that no help is available. Therefore, from a single question or comment the patient may interpret the clinician as being uninterested or dismissive, and the patient will terminate his willingness to be frank and truthful. The clinician must carefully attend to such lapses in cooperation. Finally, the clinician should remember that uncooperativeness is a patient characteristic that is predictive of the need for hospitalization, and sometimes this is the necessary outcome for such patients.

Case Example

Mr. Z, an 18-year-old man called "the Street Kid" by the emergency staff, presented himself to hospital stating "I'm suicidal. I don't feel safe." After uttering those few words, the patient remained mute and huddled in the corner of the examination room. When I entered the room, the patient was sitting cross-legged on the stretcher with his jacket hood covering almost all of his face. In spite of the winter jacket, scars from previous self-attacks were apparent on his wrists, hands, and neck.

"I'm the doctor with the Crisis Team. They asked me to speak with you. You are feeling suicidal?" No response. No acknowledgment at all.

"Can you tell me your name and where you're living?" No response.

"Have you ever been to this hospital before?" No response. Several questions later, I stated the following:

"You're obviously not feeling safe and not safe enough to speak with someone that you have never met before. Is there something I could do to make you feel safer while you're here in the hospital?" He made no response, although he moved his hooded head up as if to catch a glance of my face.

"Is there someone I could talk with who knows about your problems and can help me understand why you've come to the hospital today?"

"Angela, at Streetview, knows why I'm here," the patient abruptly responded.

"Is Angela a counselor at Streetview?"

"Yea. She told me to get lost…so I came here."

"That sounds pretty hurtful. Can you tell me more about what happened?"

For Mr. Z, identifying his hurt feelings allowed the interview to progress. The patient gave permission for the psychiatrist to speak with his counselors and the staff at Streetview.

For the immediate management of individuals at risk for suicide, involvement of significant others including family members is crucial. The patient's primary care physician or family doctor should be another resource included in the aftercare plan. The family members or significant others need to understand the likelihood of future suicidal behavior to be able to monitor the risk effec-

tively. They need to be involved in encouraging the patient to attend follow-up appointments. Family members or significant others need to be educated to take action and remove the patient's access to means of suicide; for example, disposing of firearms or large quantities of pills. Evidence has established that simple educational interventions significantly increase the chances that families will remove access to means (Brent et al. 2000; Kruesi et al. 1999).

In most cases when the patient is deemed a risk to him- or herself and will not provide consent to speak to family or significant others, the psychiatrist is well advised to attenuate confidentiality to the extent needed to address the safety of the patient (see American Psychiatric Association 2003). In the case of Mr. Z, we were able to resolve some of the miscommunication between himself and "Angela," which helped lessen his risk of suicide. He became more cooperative and agreed to a referral to a safe house. The safe house was able to offer Mr. Z a nonmedical community crisis bed for a few days to help resolve the situation.

Patients With Antisocial Personality Disorder

Patients with ASPD or conduct disorder present a unique challenge to the clinician. When these patients present in crisis, the clinician is faced with the risk of assessing the potential for violence in addition to the risk of suicide or suicidal behavior. For example, Marttunen et al. (1994) reported that 10 of 23 patients with antisocial behavior had a history of violence against others. In fact, all of the patients that met criteria for conduct disorder or ASPD had had a history of violence. Clinicians need to carefully consider interventions, such as hospitalization, based on the potential risk to the patient versus the risk this individual might represent to other patients.

Besides the usual factors involved in a risk assessment, when the clinician is trying to balance the risks to the patient versus others, the psychopathy concept can be clinically of value. Cleckley's (1976) classic description of *psychopathic personality disorder* described that these patients had a "disinclination" toward suicide. Clinically, he observed that among ward patients, suicidal behavior was much rarer among psychopathic patients than other patients. Cleckley wrote "instead of a predilection for ending their own lives, psychopaths, on the contrary, show much more evidence of a specific and characteristic immunity for such an act" (p. 359).

Cleckley's clinical observation has had some support from empirical research. Hare (1991) developed the Psychopathy Checklist—Revised to capture the aspects of Cleckley's psychopathic concept. Research has shown that the concept is composed of two underlying dimensions. The first dimension, called Factor 1 or "emotional detachment," includes the affective component of psychopathy: the glibness, superficial charm, grandiose sense of self-worth, pathological lying, cunning and manipulativeness, lack of remorse or guilt, shallow affect, callousness, lack of empathy, and failure to accept responsibility. Factor 2 relates to antisocial behavior; in this factor, items such as a proneness to boredom, poor behavioral controls, early problematic behavior, lack of realistic long-term goals, impulsivity, irresponsibility, juvenile delinquency, and revocation of conditional release were found (Hare 1991). In a direct examination of the relationship between the factors of psychopathy, ASPD, and suicide risk, Verona et al. (2001) attempted to determine whether a suicidal history was differently related to Factors 1 and 2. The authors found that suicidal history was significantly related to Factor 2. However, Factor 1 was negatively related to a history of suicidal behavior, although this relationship was not statistically significant.

The mechanism by which Factor 1 might work to lessen the risk of suicide seems related to the emotional deficit found in some psychopaths. Physiological studies have demonstrated that psychopathic individuals have reduced startle response when processing adverse stimuli (Herpertz et al. 2001; Patrick 1994). This deficit may indicate a temperamental difficulty in their capacity to reflect negative affect or to experience depression or dysphoric states (Lovelace and Gannon 1999). Therefore, the psychopathic Factor 1 might assist the clinician deciding on the relative risk a patient presents for himself or herself versus others. It appears that patients demonstrating elements of the Factor 1 "emotional detachment" are more likely to be a risk to others than to themselves. In making particular decisions to admit such patients to an inpatient psychiatric environment, one must be careful to weigh the risks to vulnerable others versus the risk to the patient him- or herself.

Patients With Borderline Personality Disorder

The clinical assessment of the BPD patient in crisis is complicated. Often these patients have made multiple suicide attempts, and it is unclear whether a short-term admission will have any impact on the ongoing risk of suicidal behavior. These patients typically are at a chronically elevated risk of suicide much above that of the general population. This risk exists because of a history of multiple attempts; in addition, these patients' history of self-injurious behavior also increases the risk for suicide (Linehan 1993; Stanley et al. 2001). Stanley et al. (2001) found that patients with self-injurious behavior were at risk for suicide attempts because of their high level of depression, hopelessness, and impulsivity and also because they misperceive and underestimate the lethality of their suicidal behaviors. The patient's level of chronic risk can be estimated by taking a careful history of the previous suicidal behavior and focusing on the times when the patient may have demonstrated attempts with the greatest intent and medical lethal-ily. By documenting the patient's most serious suicide attempt, one can estimate the severity of the patient's ongoing chronic risk for suicide.

In patients with BPD, the acute-on-chronic level of risk (i.e., the acute risk that occurs over and above the ongoing chronic risk) is related to several factors. An acute-on-chronic risk will be present if the patient has comorbid major depression or if the patient is demonstrating high levels of hopelessness or depressive symptoms, as reviewed earlier. The study by Yen et al. (2003) supported the need to look for an acute-on-chronic change in status; the authors demonstrated that a worsening of depression or substance use occurred in the month preceding a suicide attempt relative to the general levels of change in all other months. In addition, patients with BPD are known to be at risk for suicide around times of hospitalization and discharge. The clinical scenario of a patient presenting in crisis shortly after discharge from an inpatient setting illustrates a time when the risk assessment must be very carefully completed to ensure that a proper disposition is made. This patient is potentially at an acute-on-chronic risk and the assessment cannot be truncated because of the recent discharge from hospital. Proximal substance abuse can increase the suicide risk in a patient with BPD. Of course, the existence of a diagnosis of substance abuse increases the chronic risk for suicidal behavior. The risk is acutely elevated in patients who have less immediate family support or who have lost or perceive the loss of an important relationship.

Gunderson (1984) made the distinction that the BPD patient who is attempting to manipulate the environment is at less risk than the BPD patient who presents in a highly regressed dissociative state. At these times, interventions frequently have to be put in place acutely to reduce the risk of suicide attempts or self-harm. Using the acute-on-chronic model can be very effective for communicating in the medical record the de-

cisions regarding interventions. For example, if a patient is felt to be at a chronic but not acute-on-chronic risk for suicide, one can document and communicate that a short-term hospital admission will have little or no impact on a chronic risk that has been present for months and years. However, an inpatient admission of a patient demonstrating an acute-on-chronic risk might well be indicated. In this circumstance, a short-term admission may allow the level of risk to return to chronic preadmission levels. Managing the chronic level of suicide risk in patients with BPD often involves strategic outpatient management such as dialectical behavior therapy, which has been shown to be effective in reducing suicidal behavior (Koerner and Linehan 2000; Linehan 1993).

Patients With Narcissistic Personality Disorder

Assessing patients with narcissistic personality disorder for suicidal risk presents a unique clinical challenge. Ronningstam and Maltsberger (1998) thought-provokingly described how narcissistic patients can be at risk for suicide at times when they are not depressed. Certainly, narcissistic patients will be at increased risk during episodes of comorbid depression (Perry 1990). However, these patients present a unique clinical challenge because they can become acutely suicidal outside of episodes of clinical depression. Suicide attempts in narcissistic patients can arise because of their very fragile self-esteem and in response to perceived narcissistic injury. Ronningstam and Maltsberger (1998) described that suicidal behavior can have several meanings in these patients, including an attempt to raise self-esteem through a sense of mastery; as a way to protect themselves against anticipated narcissistic threats—"death before dishonor"; as a revengeful act against a narcissistic trauma; the false belief of indestructibility; and the expression of a wish to destroy or attack an imperfect self. Narcissistic individuals, therefore, can demonstrate a "Richard Corey suicide"—that is, like the title character in the poem by Edwin Arlington Robinson, they are individuals who take their lives in spite of seeming to have every happiness and good fortune.

The clinician can take four steps to monitor the risk of suicide and suicidal behavior in patients with narcissistic personality disorder. First, the patient should be routinely monitored for evidence of coexisting major depression or for an acute episode of lowered self-esteem resulting from a felt narcissistic injury. Because suicide attempts in narcissistic individuals tend to arise abruptly, the risk can be lessened by preventing the patient from having access to a means of suicide. Therefore, attention should be paid to ensure the patient has no access to highly lethal means of suicide such as guns or large quantities of pills. The patient's family and other significant supports should be aware of the potential for an acute onset of suicidal feelings and the need to avoid access to lethal means. Finally, Kohut (1972) suggested that narcissistic patients may be at less risk of acting out suicidal behavior once they have established a stable transference within a therapeutic relationship and the therapist has established some empathic closeness to the patient's fragmented self. The creation of a stable therapeutic relationship seems to be an important factor that can lessen the risk of suicide in patients with narcissistic personality disorder and should be a consideration in their ongoing outpatient management.

Conclusion

The uncommunicative patient and patients with antisocial, borderline, and narcissistic personality disorder present unique challenges to clinicians. First, these diagnoses clearly identify individuals at increased risk for suicidal behavior and death by suicide. Second, the assessment of their risk of suicide is problematic. When patients deny or

refuse to respond to questions regarding suicidal ideation or intent, the assessment needs to be carefully based on the balance of other risk and protective factors. For the ASPD patient, the risk of violence has to be judged in addition to the risk of suicide or self-harm. For BPD patients, one has to differentiate an acute from chronic risk and determine interventions based on this approach. Finally, patients with narcissistic personality disorder can be at high risk of suicide outside of times of clinical depression. These episodes can seem to arise in an unpredictable fashion. This chapter provides some clinical approaches to the assessment of these patients. However, in the future we hope that empirical evidence will provide a more sound footing for assessing and managing suicide risk in patients with antisocial, borderline, narcissistic, and other personality disorders.

References

Ahrens B, Haug HJ: Suicidality in hospitalized patients with a primary diagnosis of personality disorder. Crisis 17:59–63, 1996

American Psychiatric Association: Diagnostic and Statistical Manual of Mental Disorders, 3rd Edition. Washington, DC, American Psychiatric Association, 1980

American Psychiatric Association: Diagnostic and Statistical Manual of Mental Disorders, 3rd Edition, Revised. Washington, DC, American Psychiatric Association, 1987

American Psychiatric Association: Diagnostic and Statistical Manual of Mental Disorders, 4th Edition. Washington, DC, American Psychiatric Association, 1994

American Psychiatric Association: Diagnostic and Statistical Manual of Mental Disorders, 4th Edition, Text Revision. Washington, DC, American Psychiatric Association, 2000

American Psychiatric Association: Practice Guideline for the Assessment and Treatment of Patients With Suicidal Behavior. Washington, DC, American Psychiatric Association, 2003

Apter A, Bleich A, King RA, et al: Death without warning? a clinical postmortem study of suicide in 43 Israeli adolescent males. Arch Gen Psychiatry 50:138–142, 1993

Beautrais AL, Joyce PR, Mulder RT, et al: Prevalence and comorbidity of mental disorders in persons making serious suicide attempts: a case-control study. Am J Psychiatry 153:1009–1014, 1996

Berman AL: The teenager at risk for suicide. Med Aspects Hum Sex 19:123–129, 1985

Bongar B, Peterson LG, Golann S, et al: Self-mutilation and the chronically "suicidal" emergency room patient. Ann Clin Psychiatry 2:217–222, 1990

Braun-Scharm H: Suicidality and personality disorders in adolescence. Crisis 17:64–68, 1996

Brent DA, Johnson B, Bartle S, et al: Personality disorder, tendency to impulsive violence and suicidal behavior in adolescents. J Am Acad Child Adolesc Psychiatry 32: 69–75, 1993a

Brent DA, Perper JA, Moritz G, et al: Psychiatric risk factors for adolescent suicide: a case-control study. J Am Acad Child Adolesc Psychiatry 32:521–529, 1993b

Brent DA, Baugher M, Birmaher B, et al: Compliance with recommendations to remove firearms in families participating in a clinical trial for adolescent depression. J Am Acad Child Adolesc Psychiatry 39:1220–1226, 2000

Casey PR: Personality disorder and suicide intent. Acta Psychiatr Scand 79:290–295, 1989

Clarkin JF, Friedman RC, Hurt SW, et al: Affective and character pathology of suicidal adolescent and young adult inpatients. J Clin Psychiatry 45:19–22, 1984

Cleckley H: The Mask of Sanity. St. Louis, MO, Mosby, 1976

Conner KR, Duberstein PR, Conwell Y, et al: Psychological vulnerability to completed suicide: a review of empirical studies. Suicide Life Threat Behav 31:367–385, 2001

Crumley FE: Adolescent suicide attempts. JAMA 241:2404–2407, 1979

Dervic K, Grunebaum MF, Burke AK, et al: Cluster B personality disorders in major depressive episodes: the relationship between hostility and suicidality. Arch Suicide Res 11:83–90, 2007

Dirks BL: Repetition of parasuicide: ICD-10 personality disorders and adversity. Acta Psychiatr Scand 98:208–213, 1998

Dubo ED, Zanarini MC, Lewis RE, et al: Childhood antecedents of self-destructiveness in borderline personality disorder. Can J Psychiatry 42:63–69, 1997

Fawcett J, Scheftner WA, Fogg L, et al: Time-related predictors of suicide in major affective disorder. Am J Psychiatry 148:1189–1194, 1990

Fenton WS, McGlashan TH, Victor BJ, et al: Symptoms, subtype, and suicidality in patients with schizophrenia spectrum disorders. Am J Psychiatry 154:199–204, 1997

Ferreira de Castro E, Cunha MA, Pimenta F, et al: Parasuicide and mental disorders. Acta Psychiatr Scand 97:25–31, 1998

Forster PL, Wu LH: Assessment and treatment of suicidal patients in an emergency setting, in Emergency Psychiatry (Review of Psychiatry Series, Vol 21; Oldham JM, Riba MB, series eds). Edited by Allen MH. Washington, DC, American Psychiatric Publishing, 2002, pp 75–113

Friedman RC, Corn R: Suicide and the borderline depressed adolescent and young adult. J Am Acad Psychoanal 15:429–448, 1987

Goldsmith SJ, Fyer M, Frances A: Personality and suicide, in Suicide Over the Life Cycle: Risk Factors, Assessment, and Treatment of Suicidal Patients. Edited by Blumenthal SJ, Kupfer DJ. Washington, DC, American Psychiatric Press, 1990, pp 155–176

Gomez A, Lolas F, Martin M, et al: The influence of personality on suicidal behavior. Actas Luso Esp Neurol Psiquiatr Cienc Afines 20:250–256, 1992

Gunderson JG: Borderline Personality Disorder. Washington, DC, American Psychiatric Press, 1984

Gupta B, Trzepacz PT: Serious overdosers admitted to a general hospital: comparison with nonoverdose self-injuries and medically ill patients with suicidal ideation. Gen Hosp Psychiatry 19:209–215, 1997

Hare RD: The Hare Psychopathy Checklist—Revised. Toronto, ON, Canada, Multi-Health Systems, 1991

Harwood D, Hawton K, Hope T, et al: Psychiatric disorder and personality factors associated with suicide in older people: a descriptive and case-control study. Int J Geriatr Psychiatry 16:155–165, 2001

Haw C, Hawton K, Houston K, et al: Psychiatric and personality disorders in deliberate self-harm patients. Br J Psychiatry 178:48–54, 2001

Heikkinen ME, Henriksson MM, Isometsa ET, et al: Recent life events and suicide in personality disorders. J Nerv Ment Dis 185:373–381, 1997

Herpertz SC, Werth U, Lukas G, et al: Emotion in criminal offenders with psychopathy and borderline personality disorder. Arch Gen Psychiatry 58:737–745, 2001

Hewitt PL, Norton GR, Flett GL, et al: Dimensions of perfectionism, hopelessness, and attempted suicide in a sample of alcoholics. Suicide Life Threat Behav 28:395–406, 1998

Houston K, Hawton K, Shepperd R: Suicide in young people aged 15–24: a psychological autopsy study. J Affect Disord 63:159–170, 2001

Isometsä ET, Henriksson MM, Heikkinen ME, et al: Suicide among subjects with personality disorders. Am J Psychiatry 153:667–673, 1996

Jacobs DG, Brewer M, Klein-Benheim M: Suicide assessment: an overview and recommended protocol, in The Harvard Medical School Guide to Suicide Assessment and Intervention. Edited by Jacobs DG. San Francisco, CA, Jossey-Bass, 1999, pp 3–39

Johnson WB, Lall R, Bongar B, et al: The role of objective personality inventories in suicide risk assessment: an evaluation and proposal. Suicide Life Threat Behav 29:165–185, 1999

Kelly TM, Soloff PH, Lynch KG, et al: Recent life events, social adjustment, and suicide attempts in patients with major depression and borderline personality disorder. J Personal Disord 14:316–326, 2000

Kelly TM, Cornelius JR, Lynch KG: Psychiatric and substance use disorders as risk factors for attempted suicide among adolescents: a case control study. Suicide Life Threat Behav 32:301–312, 2002

Kjellander C, Bongar B, King A: Suicidality in borderline personality disorder. Crisis 19:125–135, 1998

Kjelsberg E, Eikeseth PH, Dahl AA: Suicide in borderline patients: predictive factors. Acta Psychiatr Scand 84:283–287, 1991

Koerner K, Linehan MM: Research on dialectical behavior therapy for patients with borderline personality disorder. Psychiatr Clin North Am 23:151–167, 2000

Kohut H: Thoughts on narcissism and narcissistic rage. Psychoanal Study Child 27:360–400, 1972

Kruesi MJP, Grossman J, Pennington JM, et al: Suicide and violence prevention: parent education in the emergency department. J Am Acad Child Adolesc Psychiatry 38: 250–255, 1999

Kullgren G: Factors associated with completed suicide in borderline personality disorder. J Nerv Ment Dis 176:40–44, 1988

Kullgren G, Renberg E, Jacobsson L: An empirical study of borderline personality disorder and psychiatric suicides. J Nerv Ment Dis 174:328–331, 1986

Laub JH, Vaillant GE: Delinquency and mortality: a 50-year follow-up study of 1,000 delinquent and nondelinquent boys. Am J Psychiatry 157:96–102, 2000

Lewinsohn PM, Rohde P, Seeley JR: Adolescent psychopathology, III: the clinical consequences of comorbidity. J Am Acad Child Adolesc Psychiatry 34:510–519, 1995

Linehan MM: Cognitive-Behavioral Treatment of Borderline Personality Disorder. New York, Guilford, 1993

Links PS, Heslegrave RJ, Mitton JE, et al: Borderline personality disorder and substance abuse: consequences of comorbidity. Can J Psychiatry 40:9–14, 1995

Lovelace L, Gannon L: Psychopathy and depression: mutually exclusive constructs? J Behav Ther Exp Psychiatry 30:169–176, 1999

Maddocks PD: A five year follow-up of untreated psychopaths. Br J Psychiatry 116:511–515, 1970

Mann JJ, Waternaux C, Haas G, et al: Toward a clinical model of suicidal behavior in psychiatric patients. Am J Psychiatry 156:181–189, 1999

Markar HR, Williams JM, Wells J, et al: Occurrence of schizotypal and borderline symptoms in parasuicide patients: comparison between subjective and objective indices. Psychol Med 21:385–392, 1991

Marttunen MJ, Aro HM, Henriksson MM, et al: Mental disorders in adolescent suicides: DSM-III-R axes I and II diagnoses in suicides among 13- to 19-year-olds in Finland. Arch Gen Psychiatry 48:834–839, 1991

Marttunen MJ, Aro HM, Henriksson MM, et al: Antisocial behaviour in adolescent suicide. Acta Psychiatr Scand 89:167–173, 1994

McCracken JT, Cantwell DP, Hanna GL: Conduct disorder and depression, in Monographs in Clinical Pediatrics, Vol 6: Depression in Children and Adolescents. Edited by Koplewicz HS, Klass E. New York, Harwood Academic, 1993, pp 121–132

McGirr A, Paris J, Lesage A, et al: Risk factors for suicide completion in borderline personality disorder: a case-control study of cluster B comorbidity and impulsive aggression. J Clin Psychiatry 68:721–729, 2007

Modestin J, Oberson B, Erni T: Possible correlates of DSM-III-R personality disorders. Acta Psychiatr Scand 96:424–430, 1997

O'Carroll PW, Berman AL, Maris RW, et al: Beyond the Tower of Babel: a nomenclature for suicidology. Suicide Life Threat Behav 26:237–252, 1996

Paris J, Zweig-Frank H: A 27-year follow-up of patients with borderline personality disorder. Compr Psychiatry 42:482–487, 2001

Patrick CJ: Emotion and psychopathy: startling new insights. Psychophysiology 31:319–330, 1994

Perry CJ: Personality disorders, suicide and self-destructive behavior, in Suicide: Understanding and Responding. Edited by Jacobs D, Brown H. Madison, CT, International Universities Press, 1990, pp 157–169

Persson ML, Runeson BS, Wasserman D: Diagnoses, psychosocial stressors and adaptive functioning in attempted suicide. Ann Clin Psychiatry 11:119–128, 1999

Robins E, Murphy GE, Wilkinson RH, et al: Some clinical considerations in the prevention of suicide based on a study of 134 successful suicides. Am J Public Health 49:888–899, 1959

Ronningstam EF, Maltsberger JT: Pathological narcissism and sudden suicide-related collapse. Suicide Life Threat Behav 28:261–271, 1998

Rudd MD, Joiner T: The assessment, management, and treatment of suicidality: toward clinically informed and balanced standards of care. Clin Psychol Sci Pract 5:135–150, 1998

Runeson B, Beskow J: Borderline personality disorder in young Swedish suicides. J Nerv Ment Dis 179:153–156, 1991

Schneider B, Wetterling T, Sargk D, et al: Axis I disorders and personality disorders as risk factors for suicide. Eur Arch Psychiatry Clin Neurosci 256:17–27, 2006

Simeon D, Favazza AR: Self-injurious behaviors: phenomenology and assessment, in Self-Injurious Behaviors: Assessment and Treatment. Edited by Simeon D, Hollander E. Washington, DC, American Psychiatric Publishing, 2001, pp 1–28

Soderberg S: Personality disorders in parasuicide. Nord J Psychiatry 55:163–167, 2001

Soloff PH, Fabio A: Prospective predictors of suicide attempts in borderline personality disorder at one, two and two-to-five year follow-up. J Personal Disord 22:123–134, 2008

Soloff PH, Lis JA, Kelly T, et al: Risk factors for suicidal behavior in borderline personality disorder. Am J Psychiatry 151:1316–1323, 1994

Soloff PH, Lynch KG, Kelly TM, et al: Characteristics of suicide attempts of patients with major depressive episode and borderline personality disorder: a comparative study. Am J Psychiatry 157:601–608, 2000

Soloff PH, Lynch KG, Kelly TM: Childhood abuse as a risk factor for suicidal behavior in borderline personality disorder. J Personal Disord 16:201–214, 2002

Stanley B, Gameroff MJ, Michalsen V, et al: Are suicide attempters who self-mutilate a unique population? Am J Psychiatry 158:427–432, 2001

Stone MH: The Fate of Borderline Patients. New York, Guilford, 1990

Verona E, Patrick CJ, Joiner TE: Psychopathy, antisocial personality and suicide risk. J Abnorm Psychol 110:462–470, 2001

World Health Organization: International Classification of Diseases, 9th Revision. Geneva, World Health Organization, 1977

World Health Organization: International Statistical Classification of Diseases and Related Health Problems, 10th Revision. Geneva, World Health Organization, 1992

Yen S, Shea TM, Pagano M, et al: Axis I and Axis II disorders as predictors of prospective suicide attempts: findings from the Collaborative Longitudinal Personality Disorders Study. J Abnorm Psychol 112:375–381, 2003

19

Substance Abuse

Roel Verheul, Ph.D.
Louisa M.C. van den Bosch, Ph.D.
Samuel A. Ball, Ph.D.

Since the introduction of DSM-III in 1980, there has been a growing interest in the study of personality disorder comorbidity among patients with substance use disorders (American Psychiatric Association 1980). The driving force behind this interest has been and still is the difficult clinical management of these dual-diagnosis patients as well as their high comorbidity. Although the evaluation of co-occurring personality disorders has been the subject of countless studies by addiction researchers, very little attention is paid by personality disorder researchers to the co-occurrence of substance abuse. This state of affairs is difficult to understand when one considers that substance abuse and personality disorders are far and away the most common form of dual diagnosis. In most personality disorder books, the topic of sub-stance abuse is rarely given any coverage. Several reasons might account for this. First, the field of personality disorder research started relatively recently in the 1980s, whereas the field of addiction has long recognized the interconnection with personality dysfunction—if for no other reason than because the first two editions of DSM embedded alcohol and drug addiction under sociopathy. Second, institutes and therapists specializing in the treatment of personality disorder, particularly out of a psychodynamic tradition, traditionally excluded patients with comorbid substance abuse from programs because they were considered to have little potential for change, could not be analyzed, and were at high risk for dropout. Finally, funding possibilities for personality disorder research has been limited, at least when compared with funding for research on Axis I. Thus, the major part of personality disorder studies has actually been conducted in samples of patients referred for treatment of Axis I disorders such as substance abuse.

An inevitable consequence of this situation is that this chapter is mostly based on studies focusing on the occurrence and implications of personality disorder in patients with substance use disorder. In addition, evidence from the literature on (normal) personality traits will be "borrowed" whenever informative. The primary focus in this chapter is on causal pathways and treatment issues, supplemented by some attention to epidemiology and diagnostic issues.

EPIDEMIOLOGY

Substance abuse is highly prevalent among individuals with personality disorders. For example, in a nonpatient sample, the lifetime prevalence of alcohol use disorders was found to range from 43% to 77% among patients with various personality disorders (Zimmerman and Coryell 1989). In a sample of more than 500 patients, Zanarini et al. (1998) reported substance use disorder to be prevalent in 64% of patients with borderline personality disorder (BPD) and in 54% of patients with other personality disorders.

A much larger number of studies has investigated prevalence of personality disorders among patients with substance use disorder. Verheul et al. (1995, 1998a) have provided the most comprehensive overview to date. The best estimate of personality disorder prevalence ranged from 44% among alcoholic patients to 79% among opiate abusers. The two most prevalent personality disorders among patients with substance use disorder are antisocial personality disorder (ASPD) and BPD, with reported best estimates of 22% for ASPD and 18% for BPD. Other personality disorders are usually prevalent among patients with substance use disorder in the range of 1%–10%. Thus high joint comorbidity is evident for ASPD and BPD and perhaps paranoid and avoidant personality disorders.

Reported prevalence rates of personality disorders in nonpatient samples of individuals with substance use disorder are at least three times higher than in normal individuals (i.e., those without mental disorders including substance use disorder) (Verheul et al. 1998a). The interpretation of these comorbidity figures is hampered because little knowledge is available about the extent to which a high personality disorder prevalence among individuals with substance use disorder is attributable to conceptually overlapping diagnostic criteria and measurement issues such as trait-state artifacts. Clearly overlapping criteria seem to be restricted to only a few of the criteria for ASPD and BPD. The possibility of trait-state artifacts in patients with substance use disorder is discussed later.

ASSESSMENT AND DIAGNOSIS

Semistructured interviews and self-report questionnaires for the assessment of DSM-IV (American Psychiatric Association 1994) personality disorders provide diagnoses with reliability that is comparable with diagnoses of Axis I disorders obtained using standardized procedures (Ball et al. 2001). There is some consensus that self-reports overdiagnose personality disorders. This tendency might be especially relevant in patients with substance use disorder, because these instruments do not ask respondents to differentiate personality traits from the effects of substance abuse or other prolonged changes in mental status. Thus, diagnostic interviews may have greater specificity because questions and answers can be clarified to tease out whether a symptom is chronic and pervasive, more situation-specific, or related to substance abuse. Further clinical inquiry can also determine whether other behavioral examples of the trait exist that are not specifically related to substance abuse. An Interview also provides important behavioral observations of the patient's interpersonal style that may inform clinical judgment (Zimmerman 1994). Some studies have shown promising findings in favor of the validity of personality disorder diagnoses in substance abusers obtained using a semi-structured interview schedule. First, Skodol et al. (1999) reported similar prevalence rates of personality disorders among patients with a current substance use disorder and patients with a lifetime substance use disorder. Second, in a sample of 273 patients with substance use disorder, remission of the disorder was not significantly associated with remission of personality pathology, suggesting that the two conditions follow an independent course (Verheul et al. 2000).

Part of the reliability and validity issue for personality disorder diagnosis in patients with substance use disorder centers on whether to include or exclude personality disorder symptoms that seem to be substance related (i.e., behaviors directly related to intoxication and/or withdrawal or other behaviors required to maintain an addiction). The magnitude of the effect of exclusion on the prevalence estimate seems partly attributable to the strategy used for exclusion. Measures with more stringent criteria exclude any symptom that has ever been linked to substance abuse and yield significantly reduced rates. Measures that exclude symptoms only if they were completely absent before substance abuse or during periods of extended abstinence show minimal effects on rates. It is important to realize that the more stringent strategy will probably exclude all secondary personality pathology and may even exclude primary personality pathology. The less stringent strategy is meant to exclude behaviors and/or symptoms that do not persist beyond periods of abuse and do not qualify for a personality disorder diagnosis. Consequently, the less stringent approach will probably not exclude primary personality pathology and will have only a limited impact on the diagnosis of secondary personality disorder.

Intuitively, one might suggest that excluding substance-related symptoms (at least following the less stringent strategy) would result in more valid diagnoses. Diagnosing personality disorders independent of substance use disorder is consistent with guidelines suggested by DSM-IV-TR (American Psychiatric Association 2000). However, the task of differentiating substance-related symptoms from personality traits is not easy for patients or clinical interviewers and thus may not be reliable. This task becomes almost impossible when the patient's entire adolescent and adult life is characterized by chronic abuse of substances. Furthermore, although most patients with substance use disorder can distinguish behaviors that are only related to substance intoxication or withdrawal, they have greater difficulty making the same distinction for other activities, such as lying or breaking the law, that may be related to obtaining substances. Such a distinction requires a high level of introspection and cognitive competence in making the judgment necessary to differentiate a trait from a situation or state. It also requires an empathic awareness of the impact of one's behavior on self and others and a willingness to accept responsibility for one's actions (Zimmerman 1994).

Patients with substance use disorder may be particularly impaired in the skills necessary to make these distinctions. Consistent with this view, Rounsaville et al. (1998) found that excluding substance-related symptoms reduced the reliability of ASPD diagnoses (but not of BPD diagnoses). Furthermore, they found that patients with independent diagnoses had a rather similar clinical profile compared with patients with substance-related diagnoses, thereby questioning the feasibility and clinical utility of exclusion. If one chooses to exclude substance-related symptoms from the measurement of any personality disorder, several considerations are in order:

- It is probably more reliable to determine whether a symptom should be eliminated as substance related on an item-by-item basis and not wait until the end of the interview or until all items relating to a specific disorder are administered.
- Criteria in which substance dependence is an inherent part should be scored as due to substance abuse unless non-substance-related behavioral indicators of the trait (e.g., impulsivity, unlawful behaviors) are also present.
- The interviewer should periodically remind patients that questions refer to the way the patients usually are—that is, when they are not symptomatic with either substance abuse or another Axis I disorder.

CAUSAL PATHWAYS

High (joint) comorbidity that cannot be explained by conceptual or measurement artifacts strongly suggests that the co-occurrence of substance use disorder and personality disorders is not due solely to random or coincidental factors. It seems reasonable to explore the assertion that substance use and personality disorders are in some way causally linked. Evidence for causal relationships between substance use and personality disorders can be derived from long-term longitudinal studies, epidemiological findings, genetic epidemiology, and retrospective studies that account for the order of onset of each disorder. Three superordinate meta-models of comorbidity can be distinguished: the primary substance use disorder model, the primary personality disorder model, and the common factor model.

Primary Substance Use Disorder Model

The primary substance use disorder model postulates that substance abuse contributes to the development of personality pathology. This pathway has received relatively little empirical attention. Bernstein and Handelsman (1995) tentatively proposed three mechanisms: 1) substance abuse often occurs within the context of a deviant peer group, and antisocial behaviors might be shaped and reinforced by social group norms (social learning hypothesis); 2) some Cluster A traits (e.g., suspiciousness, eccentric behaviors, ideas of reference, magical thinking), Cluster B traits (e.g., exploitativeness, egocentrism, manipulativeness), and Cluster C traits (e.g., passivity, social avoidance) may be shaped and maintained by the reinforcing and conditioning properties of psychoactive substances (behavioristic learning hypothesis); and 3) chronic substance abuse or withdrawal may alter personality through neuroadaptive changes or a direct effect on brain chemistry (neuropharmacological hypothesis).

As Bernstein and Handelsman (1995) pointed out, it is unclear to what extent these effects can "overwrite" or interact with pre-existing personality patterns to form new personality configurations. Considering the primary substance use disorder model, it is important to distinguish new enduring personality patterns from temporary behavior patterns that disappear with reductions of substance use. The latter should not be taken into account for a diagnosis of personality disorder. According to DSM-IV-TR, it is only when the consequences of substance abuse persist beyond the period of alcohol and/or drug consumption that these features constitute personality pathology. To the best of our knowledge, there are currently no studies yielding substantive evidence in favor of the primary substance use disorder model; on the contrary, some indirect evidence refutes the model. For example, personality disorder diagnoses in adults with alcoholism have been found to be associated with maladjustment in childhood, even after partialling out the current and cumulative effects of substance use (Bernstein et al. 1998; Morgenstern et al. 1997).

In summary, there is currently no direct evidence supporting the primary substance use disorder model, and there is some indirect evidence against the model. However, it would be premature to fully preclude the possibility that some symptoms in some individual patients with substance use disorder are shaped and maintained by the reinforcing and conditioning properties of psychoactive substances.

Primary Personality Disorder Model

The primary personality disorder model describes comorbid relationships in which (pathological) personality traits contribute to the development of substance use disorder. Since the 1990s, many studies have yielded empirical support for this model. It has been proposed that the available evidence suggests at least two or three different developmental pathways from personality to addiction (Finn et al. 2000; Verheul and van den Brink 2000). These pathways have been defined as the behavioral disinhibition pathway, the stress reduction pathway, and the reward sensitivity pathway.

Behavioral Disinhibition Pathway

The behavioral disinhibition pathway to substance abuse predicts that individuals scoring high on traits such as antisociality and impulsivity and low on constraint or conscientiousness have lower thresholds for deviant behaviors such as alcohol and drug abuse. This pathway might account for the association of ASPD and, to some extent, BPD with substance abuse. Of the three proposed pathways, this one is the best documented. First, high relative comorbidity is observed between substance use disorder and Axis I and Axis II disorders from the impulse control spectrum. For example, in a large sample recruited from the general population, individuals with substance use disorder were 17.2 times more likely to have ASPD than those without (Zimmerman and Coryell 1989). Second, several longitudinal studies have shown

that teachers' ratings of low constraint, low harm avoidance, lack of social conformity, unconventionality, antisociality, and aggression in children, particularly boys, predicted alcohol and drug abuse in adolescence and young adulthood (Caspi et al. 1997; Cloninger et al. 1988; Krueger et al. 1996; Masse and Tremblay 1997). The same pattern was observed in university students (Sher et al. 2000). More direct evidence can be derived from a study by Cohen et al. (2007), which found that personality disorders, especially those from Cluster B, were diagnosed on average for patients age 13 years to be highly predictive of diagnoses and symptoms of substance use disorders and their effects were independent of correlated family risks, participant sex, and other Axis I disorders. Third, Bahlman et al. (2002) found that the onset of ASPD characteristics preceded that of alcohol dependence by approximately 4 years. The relationship between behavioral disinhibition and early-onset addictive behaviors is probably mediated through deficient socialization, school failure, and affiliation with deviant peers (Sher and Trull 1994; Tarter and Vanyukov 1994; Wills et al. 1998). The behavioral disinhibition pathway is associated with an early onset of drinking, a more rapid development of alcohol dependence once drinking begins, and more severe symptoms than nonantisocial subjects (Verheul et al. 1998a).

Stress Reduction Pathway

The stress reduction pathway to substance abuse predicts that individuals scoring high on traits such as stress reactivity, anxiety sensitivity, and neuroticism are vulnerable to stressful life events. This pathway might account for the comorbidity of borderline, avoidant, dependent, and schizotypal personality disorders. These individuals typically respond to stress with anxiety and mood instability, which in turn can become a motive for substance use as self-medication. Longitudinal studies have shown that teachers' ratings of negative emotionality, stress reactivity, and low harm avoidance in children predicted substance abuse in adolescence and young adulthood (Caspi et al. 1997; Cloninger et al. 1988; Wills et al. 1998). Furthermore, Conrod et al. (1998) showed that coping motives for drinking as well as the fear-dampening properties of alcohol were far more pronounced among men scoring high on anxiety sensitivity than among their low-scoring counterparts. The self-medication pathway, which has most frequently been investigated for alcoholism, typically accounts for late-onset alcohol use disorders and is more prevalent among women than among men.

Reward Sensitivity Pathway

The reward sensitivity pathway predicts that individuals scoring high on traits such as novelty seeking, reward seeking, extraversion, and gregariousness will be motivated to substance use for its positive reinforcing properties. This pathway might account for the comorbidity of antisocial, histrionic, and narcissistic personality disorder. Consistent with this hypothesis, some longitudinal studies (Cloninger et al. 1988; Masse and Tremblay 1997; Wills et al. 1998) have shown that novelty seeking as a temperamental trait in childhood predicts later substance use problems. Furthermore, some evidence suggests that students' scores of extraversion, at least among those without a family history of alcoholism, predict alcohol dependence at age 30 years (Schuckit et al. 1994). As observed in animal studies, hyperresponsiveness to the positive reinforcing or rewarding effects of substances is partly accounted for by the sensitization processes initiated by the repetitive use of the substances themselves (Robinson and Berridge 1993) and to that extent is not precipitated by premorbid personality factors. However, this hyperresponsiveness or hypersensitivity might develop most strongly among individuals characterized by a more general sensitivity to positive reinforcements (Zuckerman 1999). Conrod et al. (1998) demonstrated that men with multigenerational

family histories of alcoholism demonstrated elevated resting heart rates (index of psychostimulation) in response to alcohol intake, suggesting that this pathway partly mediates the role of genetic vulnerability in the etiology of alcoholism.

Common Factor Model

The common factor model assumes that both personality pathology and substance abuse are linked to an independent third factor that contributes to the development of both disorders. This model is more likely for personality disorders that show relatively high joint comorbidity, such as ASPD and BPD. This hypothesis is consistent with a psychobiological perspective on personality disorders suggesting that BPD and ASPD are phenomenologically, genetically, and/or biologically related to Axis I impulse disorders such as substance abuse (Siever and Davis 1991; Zanarini 1993).

Family, twin, and adoption studies are generally considered most appropriate to evaluate whether a common risk factor is transmitted genetically or otherwise. Evidence from several adoption studies suggests that alcoholism and ASPD are genetically separate disorders (Cadoret et al. 1985). Furthermore, Loranger and Tulis (1985) reported that family members of patients with BPD were at greater risk for alcoholism than those of schizophrenic or bipolar-affective patients, but when patients were further subdivided based on their own level of alcohol consumption, family risk differences for alcoholism almost disappeared. A study by Fu et al. (2002) reported that the shared genetic risk between major depression and alcohol and marijuana dependence was largely explained by genetic effects on ASPD, which in turn was associated with increased risk of each of the other disorders. These data presented no evidence for cross-transmission of pure forms and no support for the shared-etiology model. However, the available studies do not preclude the possibility of common factors that, for example, are less specific to ASPD. For example,

Slutske et al. (2002) reported that genetic influences contributing to variation in behavioral undercontrol accounted for about 40% of the genetic variation in alcohol dependence and conduct disorder risk and about 90% of the common genetic risk for alcohol dependence and conduct disorder. This and other studies (e.g., Krueger et al. 2002) suggest that genetic factors contributing to variation in dimensions of personality, particularly behavioral undercontrol or impulsivity, account for a substantial proportion of the genetic diathesis for alcohol dependence and most of the common genetic diathesis for alcohol dependence and conduct disorder among men and women.

Another approach in the search for common factors has relied on high-risk strategies, with the aim of identifying markers of biological vulnerability for both conditions. Justus et al. (2001) found that a reduced amplitude of the P300 component of the scalp-recorded event-related brain potential in men is strongly associated with a general tendency toward antisocial, defiant, and impulsive traits, which in turn increase the risk for alcohol abuse. Furthermore, some reviewers (Bernstein and Handelsman 1995; Siever and Davis 1991) have concluded that abnormalities in serotonergic function may form a biological substrate underlying both substance abuse and impulsive/aggressive behavior.

Comment

It is important to note that the different meta-models are not necessarily mutually exclusive. In any individual case, more than one model may have explanatory value. Furthermore, it is possible that one model best describes the initiation of a comorbid disorder, whereas another describes long-term maintenance of the same comorbid association. For example, a borderline patient may use stimulants to reduce feelings of boredom and use alcohol to regulate affective instability. After a while, the patient becomes addicted to both substances, which in turn aggravates the impulsivity and sets the con-

ditions for aggressive suicide attempts. Simultaneously, the patient may get entangled with a deviant peer group, leading to both increased antisocial behavior and additional substance abuse.

TREATMENT OUTCOME

Outcomes of Treatments Focusing on Substance Abuse

Personality pathology has been found to be significantly related to poor treatment response and outcome in patients with affective and anxiety disorders (Reich and Vasile 1993). In the early 1990s it was generally believed that the same applied to patients with substance abuse. However, the available studies at the time had many methodological and interpretative problems, making it difficult to draw conclusions. Consequently, it was often unclear whether the reported effects on outcome were attributable to a poor treatment response of comorbid patients or to differences in pretreatment characteristics. Several studies published later on showed convincingly that personality pathology is associated with pre- and posttreatment problem severity but is not a robust predictor of the amount of improvement (e.g., Cacciola et al. 1995, 1996; Verheul et al. 1999). Furthermore, some studies showed that Axis II comorbidity is not associated with premature drop-out or a shorter time-in-program (Kokkevi et al. 1998; Marlowe et al. 1997; Verheul et al. 1998b), nor with less motivation to change (Verheul et al. 1998b) or outcomes in pharmacotherapy (Ralevski et al. 2007). In the late 1990s, some authors concluded that the available studies did not allow any firm conclusions about the prognosis of patients with both substance use disorder and personality disorders. This conclusion from empirical studies was in sharp contrast to clinical experiences and knowledge.

A number of other studies have yielded results that provide somewhat more clarity. For example, two studies showed that personality disorders predict a shorter time to relapse after discharge (Thomas et al. 1999), even when controlling for the baseline severity of alcohol problems (Verheul et al. 1998b). Thus it seems that "an equal amount of improvement" does not resemble a similar risk of relapse. A possible explanation for this apparent discrepancy is that patients without personality pathology improve to a level of problem severity that no longer leaves them at risk for relapse, whereas patients with personality pathology are at risk for relapse despite their improvement. Other studies focused on "normal" personality traits and reported that low persistence (Cannon et al. 1997; Janowsky et al. 1999; Sellman et al. 1997) and high novelty seeking (Meszaros et al. 1999) are strong predictors of time to relapse. Finally, it was found that high neuroticism and low conscientiousness predicted the time to relapse after discharge and that the combination of these two features was associated with the highest odds of relapse (Fischer et al. 1998).

Early studies typically examined the impact of personality pathology separately from other patient characteristics, although this approach might have failed to identify possible interactions with other important characteristics. For example, one study examined motivation for change and time in program as potential moderators and mediators of the relationship between personality disorders and relapse (Verheul et al. 1998b). It appeared that although motivation for change was unrelated to personality pathology, it moderated the relationship between personality disorders and relapse so that personality pathology was a strong predictor of relapse among less motivated individuals but not among their more motivated counterparts. In addition, two studies suggest that personality pathology interferes with the patient–therapist working alliance, thereby resulting in poorer outcomes or a higher risk for relapse (Gerstley et al. 1989; Verheul et al. 1998b). Finally, Pettinati et al. (1999) found that the combination of Axis I

and Axis II psychopathology was the best predictor of a return to substance use at 1 year posttreatment compared with those factors alone.

An alternative explanation of the available data that seems to refute common clinical knowledge with respect to the prognosis of ASPD is that the disorder's criteria set identifies a heterogeneous group of patients that includes both individuals with only antisocial behaviors and individuals with both antisocial and psychopathic personality traits, such as shallow affect, grandiosity, and lack of empathy and remorse. The latter group might be particularly at risk of poor treatment response and outcome. Consistent with this view, Woody et al. (1985) have shown that opiate addicts with ASPD and a lifetime diagnosis of major depression were able to benefit about as much from individual psychotherapy as patients without ASPD. This finding is in comparison with "pure" ASPD subjects, who experienced very little benefit from psychotherapy. Another interesting study found that antisocial patients who were able to form a working alliance with their therapists had better treatment response and outcome at follow-up than did antisocial patients who lacked this ability (Gerstley et al. 1989).

Outcomes of Treatments Focusing on Personality Disorder

Little is known about the impact of substance abuse on outcome for patients in treatment for personality problems; as noted earlier, this neglect in literature might be accounted for by the exclusion of dual-diagnosis patients from the treatment system. A similar phenomenon can also be observed in research. For example, patients with substance use disorder are often excluded from studies examining the efficacy of treatments designed to target borderline symptoms. The exclusion from research is often justified as a strategy to preserve the homogeneity in cohorts. This differential approach illustrates the limitations specific to a mental health system and a research policy oriented toward the treatment of single rather than multiple disorders (Ridgely et al. 1990).

To the best of our knowledge, only one study has investigated the impact of substance abuse on the outcome of a treatment focusing on personality disorders. In their randomized trial of dialectical behavior therapy (DBT) among Dutch women with BPD, Verheul et al. (2003) found no differences in effectiveness for patients with versus those without substance use problems. This finding is in obvious contrast with the tradition described earlier. Furthermore, studies of the efficacy of mentalization-based treatment (MBT) for severe BPD have typically included a large number of comorbid substance use disorders and have shown extremely favorable outcomes (Bateman and Fonagy 2001), including in the long run (Bateman and Fonagy 2008). MBT seems to be among the few promising programs for the treatment of comorbidity between severe BPD and substance use disorder.

Outcomes of Dual-Focus Treatments

Two psychotherapies developed for the treatment of personality disorders—schema-focused therapy and DBT—have been modified to meet the specific needs of dual-diagnosis patients.

Dual-Focus Schema Therapy

The only documented integrated dual-focus treatment for the broad range of personality disorders is dual-focus schema therapy (DFST), developed by Ball and Young (Ball 1998; Ball and Young 2000). DFST is a 24-week, manual-guided individual therapy including both symptom-focused relapse prevention and coping skills techniques and schema-focused techniques for maladaptive schemas and coping styles. Some preliminary empirical support can be derived from a randomized pilot study among 30 metha-

done maintenance patients comparing DFST with 12-step facilitation therapy (Ball 2007). Patients met criteria for an average of 3.3 personality disorders, with ASPD present in over 70% and BPD and avoidant personality disorder present in over 50% of the cases. Patients assigned to DFST reduced substance use frequency more rapidly over the 24-week treatment than did patients assigned to 12-step facilitation therapy. Further inspection of the data suggested that a difference began to emerge at month 3, which corresponds to a point in the manual at which the treatment shifts from an assessment and education focus to an active change focus. Furthermore, DFST patients reported an increase from a good early therapeutic alliance to a very strong alliance over the subsequent months of treatment, whereas the 12-step facilitation patients demonstrated no such increase. Consistent with this finding, DFST therapists reported feeling as though they had a stronger working alliance with patients than did 12-step facilitation therapists.

In a second randomized clinical trial, Ball et al. (2005) evaluated the treatment retention and utilization of 52 individuals with personality disorders who abused substances receiving services within a drop-in center for the homeless. Participants were randomly assigned either to receive DFST or a standard drug counseling group sessions for 24 weeks, both delivered on-site as enhancements to case management services. Results indicated superior utilization of DFST over drug counseling for participants overall. However, further analyses of separate Cluster A, Cluster B, and Cluster C symptoms scores favored drug counseling over DFST for therapy utilization by more severe Cluster A and C clients. Thus, the two published randomized trials of DFST suggest this is a promising approach, but one that needs further research with larger samples to determine what types of patients with personality disorder do well with this integrative model and what types do well (or better) with a single-focus addiction treatment.

Case Example

Mr. AA was a 36-year-old divorced male whose primary personality disorder diagnosis was obsessive-compulsive personality disorder. In addition to symptoms of depression, obsessive thoughts, compulsive behavior, and paranoid ideation, he had interpersonal problems related to being both exploitable and domineering as well as vindictive. He began using substances at the age of 14, had several prior substance abuse treatments, and had been on methadone for 1 year before starting individual therapy. His heroin dependence was in remission (on agonist medication), and his primary drug abuse problem was cocaine, with more sporadic use of a high-potency solvent to which his part-time job gave him ready accessibility. Mr. AA also met criteria for ASPD. This diagnosis does not frequently co-occur with obsessive-compulsive personality disorder; however, it was difficult to determine whether the ASPD diagnosis was independent of substance abuse given the very early age at onset and persistent use of multiple substances during adolescence and adulthood. In addition, Mr. AA met diagnostic criteria for depressive personality disorder, a category mentioned in the appendix of DSM-IV as needing further study.

Mr. AA was treated for 6 months as part of a research protocol evaluating DFST. His core early maladaptive schema was unrelenting standards/hypercriticalness (i.e., perfectionism, rigid rules, and preoccupation with time and efficiency), which appeared to originate from the seemingly contradictory combination of parental perfectionism (with physical or emotional abuse for Mr. AA's "failures" as child) and defeat secondary to both parents being torture survivors who escaped to the United States from another country. Mr. AA put a great deal of pressure on himself, and any minor deviation in his striving for perfection triggered a massive substance relapse, irresponsible giving up, and antisocial acting-out. He engaged in a number of maladaptive

coping behaviors that perpetuated this schema, including expecting too much of himself and others and being a perfectionistic workaholic. At other times, he sought relief from the pressures of these standards and would avoid occupational or social commitments, develop somatic symptoms, procrastinate, or give up on himself and use drugs when he could not get things to be perfect. These avoidance strategies actually reinforced his high standards even more because he would subsequently have to redouble his efforts to get desired outcomes.

Mr. AA began therapy in a loud, challenging manner, wanting to know for sure that therapy was going to help him and that he was going to get as much out of it as we got out of him as a research participant. Because he continued to abuse cocaine and inhalants for the first 3 months, therapy necessarily remained more relapse-prevention focused while he struggled to grasp cognitively any of the schema-focused psychoeducational material. By month 4, he had achieved complete abstinence from solvents and was using cocaine much less frequently. This had a significant positive effect on his personality (more agreeable and sociable, less depressed and agitated); however, his unrelenting standards/hypercriticalness schema was expressed even more strongly. Cognitively oriented interventions included cost-benefit analyses of his unrelenting standards and reducing the perceived risks of imperfection in his relationships. A core cognitive distortion targeted for dispute was "When I don't accomplish or get what I want, I should get enraged, give up, use drugs, and be dejected." Experiential techniques involved imagery dialogues with his parents about how they always made mistakes seem like catastrophes. Behavioral techniques included learning to accept "good enough" work from himself and others, accepting directions from people he did not respect, and redeveloping old leisure interests. Therapeutic relationship interventions included the therapist modeling acceptance of his own mistakes, processing homework noncompliance due to self-imposed rigid standards, and confronting his dichotomous views of the therapist. Much of the work in Mr. AA's outside relationships and in therapy involved helping him change his dichotomous view of other people as well as his own recovery (i.e., all good/sober vs. all bad/relapsed). Despite a rather turbulent course of treatment, Mr. AA appeared genuinely interested in improving himself and made some significant changes. In addition to his reduced substance abuse, he also experienced significant reductions in psychiatric symptoms and negative affect.

Dialectical Behavior Therapy

The second dual-focus treatment involves a modified version of DBT known as DBT-S. This program includes all of the components of standard DBT (i.e., weekly individual cognitive-behavioral psychotherapy sessions with the primary therapist, weekly skills training groups lasting 2–2.5 hours per session, weekly supervision and consultation meetings for the therapists, and phone consultation) plus application of dialectics to abstinence issues, application of a specific pharmacotherapy module, a treatment target hierarchy relevant to substance abuse, new strategies to keep difficult-to-engage and easily lost patients, the addition of six new and modified skills, an individual skills consultation mode, and increased emphasis on using natural and arbitrary reinforcers for maintenance of abstinence. There is some evidence from a randomized controlled trial that DBT-S is effective in reducing substance abuse in BPD patients with substance use disorder: Linehan et al. (1999) found that DBT-S yielded greater reductions in substance-related outcomes and psychiatric functioning (although not parasuicidality) when compared with referral for psychotherapy in the community for which poor retention and utilization provided potent explanations for differences in outcomes. Linehan et al. (2002) found few differences

between DBT-S and a comprehensive validation therapy incorporating 12-step facilitation in that both effectively promoted retention and reduced opiate use and psychopathology relative to standard L-α-acetyl-methadone treatment (although the lower follow-up in DBT-S complicated the findings). Likewise, van den Bosch et al. (2002) found that DBT was no more effective for reducing parasuicide or improving retention than an addiction-focused comparison intervention. The efficacy of DBT has been clearly established in a subgroup of patients with BPD and not with the wide range of personality disorders found in individuals who abuse substances, especially ASPD which has been described as a possible contraindication for DBT (Linehan and Korslund 2006).

Case Example

Ms. BB was a 27-year-old patient with BPD. Her first suicide attempt was at the age of 12; alcohol abuse began at 16, followed by cocaine and heroin. Her first admission into a psychiatric hospital was at age 12, and she had had a criminal record since age 16. In addition to interpersonal problems, anger outbursts, parasuicidal behaviors, and aggressive impulsiveness, she abused heroin, cocaine, cannabis, and alcohol. Previously, she had been in psychiatric and addiction treatments on both an outpatient and an inpatient basis. Among her typical therapy-interfering behaviors was attempting to invite the therapist into a very special and sometimes intimate relationship. She usually dropped out each time she failed to seduce a therapist. At the time of admission to the DBT program, she was in an addiction-oriented day hospital program.

Soon after the start of therapy, a basic behavior pattern became clear: after work on Friday evening, she would start to feel lonely. The thought "I need to comfort myself" would pop up. She would close the curtains, drink a glass of wine, and smoke cannabis while listening to "good old days" music.

Around 10 P.M. she would become restless, followed by feeling angry because she also deserved "some company." Then she would dress up in sexy clothes and go out for a drink. In the pub, she would often meet familiar drug dealers. After having had a few drinks together, the drug dealers would offer her cocaine. Because she could not afford to buy it, she would agree to have sex with them. Feelings of guilt would lead to more substance abuse, and finally she would lose contact with reality. The next morning, she would awake next to a stranger and would become self-destructive.

The behavior pattern described was targeted for treatment. Because of its threshold-lowering capacities for impulsive and self-destructive behavior, the alcohol abuse was given high priority early in treatment. Telephone consultation was of utmost importance in this stage. After 3 months, Ms. BB succeeded for the first time in not acting on the impulse to go to the bars late at night. Her contact with her father, mother, and sisters was restored. Because communication improved, reinforcement contingencies were changed. She resumed contact with a network of old friends who were not involved in drug abuse, and she accepted a new, more challenging job.

The cannabis use appeared to be the most change-resistant behavior. Reminding her of her own commitment (no hard or soft drugs), the therapist insisted that she practice her mindfulness skills every time she was tempted to use again. After 8 months she was clean and was able to "surf the craving." Then, finally, her attachment problems were targeted in treatment. Efforts to become more intimate with the therapist failed, as well as all efforts to make the therapist reject her (e.g., stalking by telephone, anger outbursts). The therapist was able to validate her behavior as fear of abandonment, and she finally recognized that she was more afraid of saying goodbye than of being rejected. After 54 sessions she left the program and the therapist by mutual agreement; she left a bouquet of flowers, combined with the words "this relationship is the most horrible thing that has ever happened to me in my life. Thanks so much."

Comment on Treatment Outcome

In summary, we have seen that 1) personality pathology has a strong impact on the course of addictive problems after discharge from addiction treatment, 2) individuals with substance use disorder are usually—without a proper theoretical or empirical basis—excluded from personality disorder treatments, and 3) some preliminary data are supportive of treatments with a dual focus. Together, these data provide strong support for the current movement toward treatment approaches that pay simultaneous attention to both addictive and personality problems, such as DFST and DBT-S. However, we need more empirical evidence that these treatments really have improved effectiveness over existing approaches. Attention to the feasibility of these treatments is also required. As currently developed, DFST and DBT-S require additional or separate clinical training beyond the standard programs from which they are derived. The focus on one target behavior seems to be a common characteristic of the different DBT programs. The question is to what extent this approach is useful for common clinical practice, which includes patients who have multiple symptoms. It would therefore be worthwhile to examine the possibility of integrated, multi-targeted treatment programs, rather than separate symptom-specific programs. This might imply that therapists are trained to address a range of symptomatic manifestations of personality pathology in the impulse control spectrum, including suicidal and self-damaging behavior, binge eating, and substance abuse.

TREATMENT GUIDELINES

In general, clinical guidelines for the treatment of personality disorders recommend psychotherapy whenever possible, complemented by symptom-targeted pharmacotherapy whenever necessary or useful. We see no reason to substantially deviate from this recommendation in dual-diagnosis patients, although effective treatment of these patients often requires modifications to traditional programs and methods. In the remainder of this chapter, some clinical recommendations for psychotherapy and pharmacotherapy, respectively, are formulated.

Psychotherapy

Dual Focus

Dual focus does not necessarily mean that attention to both foci should always take place simultaneously but rather that the program should consist of an integrated package of these elements. During the earlier sessions, it is often best to place the greatest emphasis on the establishment and maintenance of abstinence but with a secondary focus on identification of and psychoeducation about maladaptive personality traits. During later sessions, a greater emphasis can be placed on confronting and changing maladaptive traits, cognitive-affective processes, or interpersonal relationships.

Clinical Setting

Psychotherapy with patients with both substance use disorder and personality disorder probably should not be provided as a stand-alone treatment. Psychotherapy is likely to have greater success if it is provided in the context of a relatively long-term treatment program that provides sufficient structure and safety (e.g., day hospital, residential treatment, or methadone maintenance program).

Duration and Treatment Goals

The treatment of individuals with personality disorders can be a long-term process. The added problems of limited treatment reten-tion and compliance associated with substance abuse raise questions of what the appropriate treatment goals are for this group. In most cases, the goal will not be to accomplish deep and permanent change in personality structure within a relatively short term. If facilities or resources are limited, a more practical aim may be to improve substance abuse treatment outcome by teaching patients how to cope with or modulate maladaptive personality processes.

Required Therapist Training

Patients with substance use disorder and severe personality disorders are commonly seen in treatment programs and consume a disproportionate amount of staff time. They tend to be admitted into treatment repeatedly and exhaust the resources of one counselor after another. Therapists treating these dual-disorder patients probably should be professional or highly skilled therapists with extensive education and training in psychotherapy, psychopathology, personality disorders, and addiction. Drug counselors with limited training and supervision may not be as effective treating the complex psychopathology of these patients, although this has not been studied to date. Given the challenges of treating this population, all therapists should have some forum for supervision.

Essential Ingredients

Effective treatment of patients with both substance use disorder and personality disorders requires special and professional attention from the very beginning. Particular emphasis on motivational interviewing (Martino et al. 2002) during the admission phase and throughout the entire treatment process may be necessary with these dual-diagnosis patients. In addition to the regular program modules, intensive individual counseling is recommended to establish a working alliance and to prevent these patients from leaving treatment early. Direct therapeutic attention to maladaptive personality traits may increase cognitive and coping skills, which in turn may improve symptomatology and reduce the risk for relapse. Finally, participation in an appropriate aftercare program is highly recommended.

Pharmacotherapy

Pharmacotherapy may have an important role in the treatment of dual-diagnosis patients. Medications may ameliorate some personality disorder symptoms while simultaneously improving the outcome of substance use disorder. It should be noted, however, that the co-occurrence of these disorders is also associated with high rates of noncompliance and an increased risk of lethal overdose as well as the potential for dependence on the medication. The pharmacotherapy of personality disorders is discussed in detail in Chapter 14 of this volume, "Somatic Treatments."

Neuroleptics

Low doses of neuroleptics have been reported to be associated with a range of beneficial effects in patients with borderline, schizotypal, or paranoid personality disorders (Rocca et al. 2002; Soloff 1998) as well as with a decrease in craving in cocaine abusers (Gawin et al. 1989). However, recent studies do not support the anticraving or abstinence-promoting effect of neuroleptics (e.g., Dackis and O'Brien 2002).

Selective Serotonin Reuptake Inhibitors

Selective serotonin reuptake inhibitors have been shown to reduce aggression/impulsivity in patients with BPD and ASPD (Coccaro and Kavoussi 1997; Soloff 1998) and may have some positive effect on substance abuse in alcohol- and cocaine-dependent patients (Cornelius et al. 1997). However, a more recent study showed that fluvoxamine, as compared with placebo, produced a robust and long-lasting reduction in rapid mood shifts

in female borderline patients but had no effect on impulsivity or aggression (Rinne et al. 2002).

Mood Stabilizers

Lithium and other mood stabilizers (e.g., carbamazepine, divalproex sodium) have been reported to reduce aggressive and violent behaviors in prison inmates with ASPD and to decrease "within-day mood fluctuations" in BPD patients (Cowdry and Gardner 1988; Stein 1992). Early anecdotal reports and a small double-blind, placebo-controlled study also suggested that lithium may be efficacious in the treatment of alcohol dependence. However, a large Veterans Administration study showed no benefits of lithium over placebo for alcohol-dependent patients with or without depressive symptoms (Dorus et al. 1989). Similar negative findings are now available for the treatment of cocaine dependence with mood stabilizers (Silva de Lima et al. 2002).

Benzodiazepines

Benzodiazepines are generally contraindicated for this group because of the risk of addiction and of paradoxical reactions involving behavioral disinhibition (Cowdry and Gardner 1988).

Buspirone

The partial serotonin agonist buspirone seems to combine a lack of abuse potential with a positive effect on social phobia and avoidant personality disorder (Zwier and Rao 1994) and a delay in the return to heavy alcohol consumption in anxious alcohol-dependent patients (Kranzler et al. 1994).

Stimulants

Various stimulants, including methylphenidate, pemoline, dexamphetamine, and levodopa, have been reported to reduce impulsivity in BPD and ASPD patients with a history of attention-deficit/hyperactivity disorder. It has been claimed that childhood hyperactivity and a history of drug abuse are predictors of a favorable response to both psychostimulants and monoamine oxidase inhibitors among patients with personality disorders (Stein 1992). However, stimulants are known for their addictive and abuse potential, and restraint should be used in prescribing these drugs.

Naltrexone

It has been reported that the opioid antagonist naltrexone is effective in the treatment of alcohol and opiate dependence as well as in the prevention of self-mutilation in a BPD patient (Griengl et al. 2001; Soloff 1993).

CONCLUSION

Substance abuse is highly prevalent among patients with personality disorder, irrespective of type, with prevalences of 50% and beyond. Among patients with substance use disorder, ASPD and BPD are the predominant Axis II diagnoses, with prevalences of approximately 20%. Thus, high joint comorbidity is evident for ASPD/BPD and substance use disorder.

Personality disorders can be reliably and validly measured in patients with substance use disorder, but assessment and diagnosis require careful attention to disentangling substance-related and independent personality pathology.

With respect to causal pathways, the primary personality disorder model and common factor model have received the strongest empirical support. These models describe comorbid relationships in which personality traits contribute to the development of substance use disorder and in which both conditions are linked to an independent factor, respectively. Within the primary personality disorder model, the evidence supports multiple pathways from personality to

substance use disorder—that is, the behavioral disinhibition, stress reduction, and reward sensitivity pathways. With respect to the common factor model, evidence suggests that genetic factors contributing to variation in personality dimensions, particularly behavioral undercontrol, might account for a substantial proportion of the comorbidity of ASPD and substance use disorder.

Contrary to expectations, evidence has convincingly shown that comorbid patients usually benefit from addiction treatments. However, they often only improve to a level of problem severity that leaves them at considerable risk for relapse. In addition, the maladaptive personality traits remain untreated and also contribute to higher odds of relapse. Also contrary to expectations, some evidence suggests that comorbid patients benefit from treatments focusing on the personality disorder as much as do those without substance use disorder. Yet the current clinical consensus is that, if possible, so-called dual-focus treatments consisting of an integrated package of elements targeting both the substance use disorder and the maladaptive traits are preferable over strategies with a single focus. Some preliminary data are supportive of dual-focus treatments.

Clinical guidelines for the treatment of personality disorder recommend psychotherapy whenever possible, complemented by symptom-targeted pharmacotherapy whenever necessary or useful. We see no reason to substantially deviate from this recommendation in dual-diagnosis patients, although effective treatment of these patients often requires modifications to traditional programs and methods.

REFERENCES

American Psychiatric Association: Diagnostic and Statistical Manual of Mental Disorders, 3rd Edition. Washington, DC, American Psychiatric Association, 1980

American Psychiatric Association: Diagnostic and Statistical Manual of Mental Disorders, 4th

Edition. Washington, DC, American Psychiatric Association, 1994

American Psychiatric Association: Diagnostic and Statistical Manual of Mental Disorders, 4th Edition, Text Revision. Washington, DC, American Psychiatric Association, 2000

Bahlman M, Preuss UW, Soyka M: Chronological relationship between antisocial personality disorder and alcohol dependence. Eur Addict Res 8:195–200, 2002

Ball SA: Manualized treatment for substance abusers with personality disorders: dual focus schema therapy. Addict Behav 23:883–891, 1998

Ball SA: Comparing individual therapies for personality disordered opioid dependent patients. J Personal Disord 21:305–321, 2007

Ball SA, Young JE: Dual focus schema therapy for personality disorders and substance dependence: case study results. Cogn Behav Pract 7:270–281, 2000

Ball SA, Rounsaville BJ, Tennen H, et al: Reliability of personality disorder symptoms and personality traits in substance-dependent inpatients. J Abnorm Psychol 110:341–352, 2001

Ball SA, Cobb-Richardson P, Connolly AJ, et al: Substance abuse and personality disorders in homeless drop-in center clients: Symptom severity and psychotherapy retention in a randomized clinical trial. Compr Psychiatry 46:371–379, 2005

Bateman A, Fonagy P: Treatment of borderline personality disorder with psychoanalytically oriented partial hospitalization: an 18-month follow-up. Am J Psychiatry 158:36–42, 2001

Bateman A, Fonagy P: Eight-year follow-up of patients treated for borderline personality disorder: mentalization-based treatment versus treatment as usual. Am J Psychiatry 165:556–559, 2008

Bernstein DP, Handelsman L: The neurobiology of substance abuse and personality disorders, in Neuropsychiatry of Personality Disorders. Edited by Ratey J. Cambridge, England, Blackwell Science, 1995

Bernstein DP, Stein JA, Handelsman L: Predicting personality pathology among adult patients with substance use disorders: effects of childhood maltreatment. Addict Behav 23:855–868, 1998

Cacciola JS, Alterman AI, Rutherford MJ, et al: Treatment response of antisocial substance abusers. J Nerv Ment Dis 183:166–171, 1995

Cacciola JS, Alterman AI, Rutherford MJ, et al: Personality disorders and treatment outcome in methadone maintenance patients. J Nerv Ment Dis 184:234–239, 1996

Cadoret RJ, O'Gorman TW, Troughton E, et al: Alcoholism and antisocial personality: interrelationships, genetic and environmental factors. Arch Gen Psychiatry 42: 161–167, 1985

Cannon DS, Keefe CK, Clark LA: Persistence predicts latency to relapse following inpatient treatment for alcohol dependence. Addict Behav 22:535–543, 1997

Caspi A, Begg D, Dickson N, et al: Personality differences predict health-risk behaviors in young adulthood: evidence from a longitudinal study. J Pers Soc Psychol 73:1052–1063, 1997

Cloninger CR, Sigvardsson S, Bohman M: Childhood personality predicts alcohol abuse in young adults. Alcohol Clin Exp Res 12:494–505, 1988

Coccaro EF, Kavoussi RJ : Fluoxetine and impulsive aggressive behavior in personality-disordered subjects. Arch Gen Psychiatry 54:1081–1088, 1997

Cohen P, Chen H, Crawford TN, et al: Personality disorders in early adolescence and the development of later substance use disorders in the general population. Drug Alcohol Depend 88 (Suppl 1):S71–S84, 2007

Conrod PJ, Pihl RO, Vassileva J: Differential sensitivity to alcohol reinforcement in groups of men at risk for distinct alcoholism subtypes. Alcohol Clin Exp Res 22:585–597, 1998

Cornelius JR, Salloum IM, Ehler JG, et al: Fluoxetine in depressed alcoholics: a double-blind, placebo-controlled trial. Arch Gen Psychiatry 54:691–694, 1997

Cowdry RW, Gardner DL: Pharmacotherapy of borderline personality disorder: alprazolam, carbamazepine, trifluoperazine and tranylcypromine. Arch Gen Psychiatry 45:111–119, 1988

Dackis CA, O'Brien CP: Cocaine dependence: the challenge for pharmacotherapy. Curr Opin Psychiatry 15:261–267, 2002

Dorus W, Ostrow D, Anton R, et al: Lithium treatment of depressed and non-depressed alcoholics. JAMA 262:1646–1652, 1989

Finn PR, Sharkansky EJ, Brandt KM, et al: The effects of familial risk, personality, and expectancies on alcohol use and abuse. J Abnorm Psychol 109:122–133, 2000

Fischer LA, Elias JW, Ritz K: Predicting relapse to substance abuse as a function of personality dimensions. Alcohol Clin Exp Res 22:1041–1047, 1998

Fu Q, Heath AC, Bucholz KK, et al: Shared genetic risk of major depression, alcohol dependence, and marijuana dependence: contribution of antisocial personality disorder in men. Arch Gen Psychiatry 59:1125–1132, 2002

Gawin FH, Allen D, Humblestone B: Outpatient treatment of crack cocaine smoking with flupenthixol decanoate: a preliminary report. Arch Gen Psychiatry 46:322–325, 1989

Gerstley L, McLellan AT, Alterman AI, et al: Ability to form an alliance with the therapist: a possible marker of prognosis for patients with antisocial personality disorder. Am J Psychiatry 146:508–512, 1989

Griengl H, Sendera A, Dantendorfer K: Naltrexone as a treatment of self-injurious behavior: a case report. Acta Psychiatr Scand 103:234–236, 2001

Janowsky DS, Boone A, Morter S, et al: Personality and alcohol/substance-use disorder patient relapse and attendance at self-help group meetings. Alcohol Alcohol 34:359–369, 1999

Justus AN, Finn PR, Steinmetz JE: P300, disinhibited personality, and early-onset alcohol problems. Clin Exp Res 25:1457–1466, 2001

Kokkevi A, Stefanis N, Anastasopoulou E, et al: Personality disorders in drug abusers: prevalence and their association with Axis I disorders as predictors of treatment retention. Addict Behav 23:841–853, 1998

Kranzler HR, Burleson JA, Del Boca FK, et al: Buspirone treatment of anxious alcoholics: a placebo-controlled trial. Arch Gen Psychiatry 51:720–731, 1994

Krueger RF, Caspi A, Moffit TE, et al: Personality traits are differentially linked to mental disorders: a multitrait-multidiagnosis study of an adolescent birth cohort. J Abnorm Psychol 105:299–312, 1996

Krueger RF, Hicks BM, Patrick CJ, et al: Etiologic connections among substance dependence, antisocial behavior, and personality: modeling the externalizing spectrum. J Abnorm Psychol 111:411–424, 2002

Linehan MM, Korslund KE: Dialectical Behavior Therapy: From Soup to Nuts. Workshop presentation at the annual meeting of the Association for Behavioral and Cognitive Therapies, Chicago, IL, November 15–16, 2006

Linehan MM, Schmidt H, Dimeff LA, et al: Dialectical behaviour therapy for patients with borderline personality disorder and drug-dependence. Am J Addict 8:279–292, 1999

Linehan MM, Dimeff LA, Reynolds SK, et al: Dialectical behavior therapy versus comprehensive validation therapy plus 12-step for the treatment of opioid dependent women meeting criteria for borderline personality disorder. Drug Alcohol Drug Depend 67:13–26, 2002

Loranger AW, Tulis EH: Family history of alcoholism in borderline personality disorder. Arch Gen Psychiatry 42: 153–157, 1985

Marlowe DB, Kirby KC, Festinger DS, et al: Impact of comorbid personality disorders and personality disorder symptoms on outcomes of behavioral treatment for cocaine dependence. J Nerv Ment Dis 185:483–490, 1997

Martino S, Carroll K, Kostas D, et al: Dual Diagnosis Motivational Interviewing: a modification of Motivational Interviewing for substance-abusing patients with psychotic disorders. J Subst Abuse Treat 23:297–308, 2002

Masse LC, Tremblay RE: Behavior of boys in kindergarten and the onset of substance use during adolescence. Arch Gen Psychiatry 54:62–68, 1997

Meszaros K, Lenzinger E, Hornik K, et al: The Tridimensional Personality Questionnaire as a predictor of relapse in detoxified alcohol dependents. Alcohol Clin Exp Res 23:483–486, 1999

Morgenstern J, Langenbucher J, Labouvie E, et al: The comorbidity of alcoholism and personality disorders in a clinical population: prevalence rates and relation to alcohol typology variables. J Abnorm Psychol 106:74–84, 1997

Pettinati HM, Pierce JD, Belden PP, et al: The relationship of Axis II personality disorders to other known predictors of addiction treatment outcome. Am J Addict 8:136–147, 1999

Ralevski E, Ball S, Nich C, et al: The impact of personality disorders on alcohol-use outcomes in a pharmacotherapy trial for alcohol dependence and comorbid Axis I disorders. Am J Addict 16:443–449, 2007

Reich JH, Vasile RG: Effect of personality disorders on the treatment outcome of Axis I conditions: an update. J Nerv Ment Dis 181:475–484, 1993

Ridgely MS, Goldman HH, Willenbring M: Barriers to the care of persons with dual diagnoses: organizational and financing issues. Schizophr Bull 16:123–132, 1990

Rinne T, van den Brink W, Wouters L, et al: SSRI treatment of borderline personality disorder: a randomized, placebo-controlled clinical trial for female patients with borderline personality disorder. Am J Psychiatry 159:2048–2054, 2002

Robinson TE, Berridge KC: The neural basis of craving: an incentive-sensitization theory of addiction. Brain Res Rev 18:247–291, 1993

Rocca P, Marchiaro L, Cocuzza E, et al: Treatment of borderline personality disorder with risperidone. J Clin Psychiatry 63:241–244, 2002

Rounsaville BJ, Kranzler HR, Ball S, et al: Personality disorders in substance abusers: relation to substance use. J Nerv Ment Dis 186:87–95, 1998

Schuckit MA, Klein J, Twitchell G, et al: Personality test scores as predictors of alcoholism almost a decade later. Am J Psychiatry 151:1038–1043, 1994

Sellman JD, Muldert RT, Sullivan PF, et al: Low persistence predicts relapse in alcohol dependence following treatment. J Stud Alcohol 58:257–263, 1997

Sher KJ, Trull TJ: Personality and disinhibitory psychopathology: alcoholism and antisocial personality disorder. J Abnorm Psychol 103:92–102, 1994

Sher KJ, Bartholow BD, Wood MD: Personality and substance use disorders: a prospective study. J Consult Clin Psychol 68:818–829, 2000

Siever LJ, Davis KL: A psychological perspective on the personality disorders. Am J Psychiatry 148:1647–1658, 1991

Silva de Lima M, Garcia de Oliveira Soares B, Alves Pereira Reisser A, et al: Pharmacological treatment of cocaine dependence: a systematic review. Addiction 97:931–949, 2002

Skodol AE, Oldham JM, Gallaher PE: Axis II comorbidity of substance use disorders among patients referred for treatment of personality disorders. Am J Psychiatry 156:733–738, 1999

Slutske WS, Heath AC, Madden PA, et al: Personality and the genetic risk for alcohol dependence. J Abnorm Psychol 111:124–133, 2002

Soloff PH: Pharmacological therapies in borderline personality disorder, in Borderline Personality Disorder: Etiology and Treatment. Edited by Paris J. Washington, DC, American Psychiatric Press, 1993, pp 319–348

Soloff PH: Algorithms for pharmacological treatment of personality dimensions: symptom-specific treatments for cognitive-perceptual, affective, and impulsive-behavioral dysregulation. Bull Menninger Clin 62:195–214, 1998

Stein G: Drug treatment of the personality disorders. Br J Psychiatry 161:167–184, 1992

Tarter RE, Vanyukov M: Alcoholism: a developmental disorder. J Consult Clin Psychol 62:1096–1107, 1994

Thomas VH, Melchert TP, Banken JA: Substance dependence and personality disorders: comorbidity and treatment outcome in an inpatient treatment population. J Stud Alcohol 60:271–277, 1999

van den Bosch LMC, Verheul R, Schippers GM, et al: Dialectical behavior therapy of borderline patients with and without substance use problems: implementation and long-term effects. Addict Behav 27:911–923 2002

Verheul R, van den Brink W: The role of personality pathology in the etiology and treatment of substance use disorders. Curr Opin Psychiatry 13:163–169, 2000

Verheul R, van den Brink W, Hartgers C: Prevalence of personality disorders among alcoholics and drug addicts: an overview. Eur Addict Res 1:166–177, 1995

Verheul R, Ball SA, van den Brink W: Substance abuse and personality disorders, in Dual Diagnosis and Treatment: Substance Abuse and Comorbid Medical and Psychiatric Disorders. Edited by Kranzler HR, Rounsaville BJ. New York, Marcel Dekker, 1998a, pp 317–363

Verheul R, van den Brink W, Hartgers C: Personality disorders predict relapse in alcoholic patients. Addict Behav 23:869–882, 1998b

Verheul R, van den Brink W, Koeter MWJ, et al: Antisocial alcoholics show as much improvement at 14-month follow-up as non-antisocial alcoholics. Am J Addict 8:24–33, 1999

Verheul R, Kranzler HR, Poling J, et al: Axis I and Axis II disorders in substance abusers: fact or artifact? J Stud Alcohol 61:101–110, 2000

Verheul R, van den Bosch LMC, Koeter MWJ, et al: Efficacy of dialectical behavior therapy: a Dutch randomized controlled trial. Br J Psychiatry 182:135–140, 2003

Wills TA, Windle M, Cleary SD: Temperament and novelty seeking in adolescent substance use: convergence of dimensions of temperament with constructs from Cloninger's theory. J Pers Soc Psychol 74:387–406, 1998

Woody ME, McLellan T, Luborsky L, et al: Sociopathy and psychotherapy outcome. Arch Gen Psychiatry 42:1081–1086, 1985

Zanarini MC: Borderline personality disorder as an impulse spectrum disorder, in Borderline Personality Disorder: Etiology and Treatment. Edited by Paris J. Washington, DC, American Psychiatric Press, 1993, pp 67–86

Zanarini MC, Frankenburg FR, Dubo ED, et al: Axis I comorbidity of borderline personality disorder. Am J Psychiatry 155:1733–1739, 1998

Zimmerman M: Diagnosing personality disorders: a review of issues and research methods. Arch Gen Psychiatry 51:225–245, 1994

Zimmerman M, Coryell WH: DSM-III personality disorder diagnoses in a nonpatient sample: demographic correlates and comorbidity. Arch Gen Psychiatry 46:682–689, 1989

Zuckerman M: Vulnerability to psychopathology: a biosocial model. Washington, DC, American Psychological Association, 1999, pp 255–317

Zwier KJ, Rao U: Buspirone use in an adolescent with social phobia and mixed personality disorder (cluster A type). J Am Acad Child Adolesc Psychiatry 33:1007–1011, 1994

Part V

New Developments and Future Directions

20

Future Directions

Toward DSM-V

Andrew E. Skodol, M.D.
Donna S. Bender, Ph.D.
John M. Oldham, M.D., M.S.

Preparations for DSM-V began in 1999, when a DSM-V Research Planning Conference was held. As a result of that conference, 12 DSM-V Research Planning Work Groups were constituted, most of which met and produced "white papers" on the research needed to inform the revision process. In 2002, *A Research Agenda for DSM-V* was published (Kupfer et al. 2002), which contained the first series of these papers. In that book, the authors argued that the categorical approach to the diagnosis of mental disorders in general, and of personality disorders specifically, needed reexamination. No laboratory marker had been found to be specific for any DSM-defined Axis I or Axis II syndrome. Epidemiological and clinical studies showed high rates of comorbidity within and across axes, as well as short-term diagnostic instability. A lack of treatment specificity for individual disorders has been found to be the rule rather than the exception. Thus, the question of whether mental disorders, including personality disorders, should be represented by sets of dimensions of psychopathology and other features,

Sections of this chapter have been modified with permission from Oldham JM, Skodol AE: "Charting the Future of Axis II." *Journal of Personality Disorders* 14:17–29 2000.

rather than by multiple categories, was identified as one of seven basic nomenclature issues needing clarification for DSM-V.

In *A Research Agenda for DSM-V*, Rounsaville et al. (2002) elaborated: "There is a clear need for dimensional models to be developed and their utility compared with that of existing typologies in one or more limited fields, such as personality. If a dimensional system performs well and is acceptable to clinicians, it might be appropriate to explore dimensional approaches in other domains (e.g., psychotic or mood disorders)" (p. 13). Thus, personality disorders became a "test case" for the return to a dimensional approach to the diagnosis of mental disorders in DSM-V.

A DSM-V Research Planning Conference was held in 2004 on "Dimensional Models of Personality Disorder: Etiology, Pathology, Phenomenology, and Treatment." Two special issues of the *Journal of Personality Disorders* were published in 2005, containing the review papers prepared for this conference. Topics reviewed included alternative dimensional models of personality disorders, behavioral and molecular genetic contributions to a dimensional classification, neurobiological dimensional models of personality, developmental perspectives and childhood antecedents, cultural perspectives, the continuity of Axes I and II, coverage and cutoffs for dimensional models, clinical utility, and the problem of severity in personality disorder classification (Widiger and Simonsen 2005b, 2005c). These issues guided early deliberations of the DSM-V Personality and Personality Disorders Work Group.

PERSONALITY AND PERSONALITY DISORDERS WORK GROUP

In 2007, the Work Group was appointed to officially consider the future of personality and personality disorder assessment and classification for DSM-V. The Chair of the Work Group and first author of this chapter, Andrew E. Skodol, M.D., appointed 10 addi-

tional members in consultation with the DSM-V Task Force leadership. Individuals were chosen to represent the disciplines of both psychology and psychiatry, to have diverse theoretical perspectives, and to have specific research and clinical expertise. The Work Group members and their primary academic affiliations are listed in Table 20–1.

The initial task of the Work Group was to consider key questions to be addressed in order to inform potential revisions in DSM-V. Some of these questions are specific to the Personality and Personality Disorders Work Group itself, such as what is the core definition of a personality disorder that distinguishes it from other types of psychopathology? Is personality psychopathology better represented by diagnostic categories or by extremes on dimensions of general personality functioning? If dimensions are better, which dimensional system is preferable and why? Is there a value in retaining a separate Axis II for the assessment of personality disorders and traits? Other questions were addressed to the other DSM-V Work Groups. For example, can fundamental temperaments or personality traits be the basis for reorganizing disorders in DSM-V in a more clinically or empirically meaningful way? What is the clinical importance (e.g., risk or prognostic factor) of assessing personality or personality disorders in other diagnostic domains, such as mood, anxiety, substance use, or eating disorders? Of the Task Force, we asked what the criteria for making changes in DSM-V should be and under what circumstances would field trials of proposed revisions be indicated?

These questions then served as the focus for the formation of four working subgroups led by different Work Group members: 1) the core definition of personality disorder and evidence of its significance as a mental disorder that might justify inclusion of personality disorders on the same "axis" as other mental disorders (Donna S. Bender, Ph.D.); 2) the relative validity and clinical usefulness of alternative models of personality psychopathol-

Table 20–1. Personality and Personality Disorders Work Group membership

Renato A. Alarcon, M.D., M.P.H.	Mayo Clinic College of Medicine
Carl C. Bell, M.D.	University of Illinois at Chicago
Donna S. Bender, Ph.D.	University of Arizona College of Medicine
Lee Anna Clark, Ph.D.	University of Iowa
Robert Krueger, Ph.D.	Washington University St. Louis
W. John Livesley, M.D., Ph.D.	University of British Columbia
Leslie C. Morey, Ph.D.	Texas A&M University
John M. Oldham, M.D.	Baylor University College of Medicine
Larry J. Siever, M.D.	Mt. Sinai School of Medicine
Andrew E. Skodol, M.D. (Chair)	University of Arizona College of Medicine
Roel Verheul, Ph.D.	Viersprong Institute (The Netherlands)

ogy (Robert Krueger, Ph.D.); 3) personality as an organizing principle for the classification of psychopathology, integration of personality disorders and Axis I disorders, temperament and personality development over the life span, and personality as a risk or protective factor (Lee Anna Clark, Ph.D.); and 4) the validity of existing personality disorder categories (Larry J. Siever, M.D.).

A New Model of Personality Disorders

Recent longitudinal research in patient (Skodol et al. 2005a; Zanarini et al. 2005), nonpatient (Lenzenweger 2006), and general population samples (Cohen et al. 2005) indicates that personality disorders show consistency as syndromes over time but show rates of improvement that are inconsistent with their DSM-IV definitions (American Psychiatric Association 1994). Functional impairment in personality disorders is more stable than personality psychopathology itself (Skodol et al. 2005c). Some personality disorder criteria are more stable than others (McGlashan et al. 2005) and, in fact, personality traits are more stable than personality disorders, pre-

dict stability and change in personality disorders, and are associated with outcomes over time. Personality disorders, therefore, may be best conceptualized as hybrids of more stable personality traits and less stable symptomatic behaviors.

The implications of hybrid models are several. First, defining the core features of personality disorders, as distinct from personality traits or styles, is a high priority. One potential hybrid model would have a generic personality disorder diagnosis on Axis I with the types represented by dimensional trait structures or prototypes on Axis II. Other types of psychopathology, such as depression, anxiety, substance abuse, or suicidality that might become manifest secondary to stress or other life circumstances, would be noted separately. Functional impairment could continue to be rated on a separate axis, if a multiaxial system persisted in DSM-V, or by independent notations similar to those for psychopathology (see later section in this chapter, "Tripartite Model of Mental Disorder").

One initial attempt at redefining the core features of personality disorder was made by Krueger et al. (2007). According to this conceptualization, personality disorder is characterized by a persistent inability to accomplish one or more of the basic tasks of adult life: 1) the establishment of coherent and adaptive working models of self and others (e.g., is capable of formulating a clear and consistent sense of his or her goal in life and perceives other people as coherent entities); 2) establishment of intimate relationships and activities (e.g., is able to form long-term relationships that involve mutual emotional support); and 3) establishment of occupational relationships and activities (e.g., is able to maintain employment that provides a stable, independent source of income). This concept has been elaborated by Livesley and Jang (2005) in their proposed revised diagnostic criteria for personality disorder. According to these criteria, personality disorder is present when a person exhibits a persistent failure to develop adaptive solutions to life tasks as a result of impaired functioning in self and interpersonal domains, as a result of 1) a poorly differentiated self-structure (e.g., an impoverished self-concept manifested by difficulty in identifying or describing self attributes, or a confused self-concept manifested by poorly delineated interpersonal boundaries); 2) a poorly integrated self-structure (e.g., the lack of a sense of personal unity and continuity leading to the experience of being fragmented or experiences of marked different self-states and feeling like a different person on different occasions); 3) low self-directedness (e.g., difficulty with setting and attaining rewarding personal goals, or a lack of direction, meaning, and purpose to life); or 4) chronic interpersonal dysfunction (e.g., impaired capacity for close, intimate, attachment relationships, or impaired societal functioning due to the failure to develop the capacity for prosocial behavior). It is anticipated that a generic, unitary personality disorder diagnosis could be listed at the same level as other mental disorders in DSM-V and be diagnosed either alone or in combination with other psychopathology.

Borderline personality disorder is a classic example of a disturbance of self–other representations (Bender and Skodol 2007).

Borderline psychopathology emanates from impairment in the ability to maintain and use benign and integrated internal images of self and others, which leads to associated unstable interpersonal relationships, affective instability, and impulsivity. The centrality of self–other representational disturbance to borderline personality disorder is recognized across a wide theoretical spectrum spanning psychodynamic, interpersonal, cognitive-behavioral, and trait models.

An example of a trait-based description of borderline personality disorder features was also proposed by Krueger et al. (2007). Based on the traits derived by Livesley at al. (1998) from twin studies using the Dimensional Assessment of Personality Pathology (DAPP), the prototypical descriptive features of borderline personality disorder are the following: anxiousness, emotional reactivity, emotional intensity, attachment need, cognitive dysregulation, impulsivity, insecure attachment, pessimistic anhedonia, self-harming acts, and self-harming ideas. In order to meet the criteria for borderline personality disorder according to this type of hybrid model, a patient would need to meet the generic criteria for a personality disorder and to have extreme levels on a number of prototypical traits. The minimum number of extreme traits would need to be determined empirically. *Extreme* might be defined on a dimensional scale for traits characteristic of the patient ranging from highly characteristic (needed) to highly uncharacteristic.

Other trait-based models of personality (e.g., the five-factor model [FFM] or a three-factor model) with empirical support and clinical utility might substitute for the DAPP model in describing personality. Ratings of descriptive prototypes of personality styles and disorders are alternatives to trait-based descriptions (Westen et al. 2006a). Prototypes have been found to be user friendly and to receive high approval ratings from clinicians (Spitzer et al 2008)

Combining a categorical with a dimensional approach, the *Psychodynamic Diagnos-*

tic Manual (PDM; Psychodynamic Diagnostic Manual Task Force 2006) offers a method for personality assessment that addresses the importance of both identifying personality disorder types and designating the level of severity of personality impairment. The PDM Personality Axis (P-Axis) allows clinicians to characterize a patient by choosing from among 14 personality types, some which include subtypes. In addition, severity is addressed dimensionally by indicating where a patient falls on a spectrum ranging from healthy personality to neurotic level to borderline level. The PDM Mental Functioning Axis (M-Axis) includes nine dimensions used to rate a patient's level of functioning for specific psychological capacities such as defensive patterns, affective experience, and psychological mindedness.

Categorical Versus Dimensional Models: Advantages and Disadvantages

Considerable research has shown excessive co-occurrence among personality disorders diagnosed using the categorical system of DSM (Oldham et al. 1992; Zimmerman et al. 2005). In fact, most patients diagnosed with personality disorders meet criteria for more than one. In addition, use of the polythetic criteria of DSM, in which a minimum number (e.g., five) from a list of criteria (e.g., nine) are required, but no single one is necessary, results in extreme heterogeneity among patients receiving the same diagnosis. For example, there are 256 possible ways to meet criteria for borderline personality disorder in DSM-IV-TR (American Psychiatric Association 2000; Johansen et al. 2004). Furthermore, all of the personality disorder categories have arbitrary diagnostic thresholds (i.e., the number of criteria necessary for a diagnosis). There are no empirical rationales for setting the boundaries between pathological and "normal" personality functioning. Finally,

despite having criteria for 10 different personality disorder types, the DSM system still may not cover the domain of personality psychopathology adequately. This has been suggested by the observation that the most frequently used personality disorder diagnosis is personality disorder not otherwise specified (PDNOS) (Verheul and Widiger 2004), a residual category for evaluations indicating that a patient is considered to have a personality disorder but does not meet full criteria for any one of the DSM-IV-TR types, or is judged to have a personality disorder not included in the classification (e.g., depressive, passive-aggressive, or self-defeating personality disorders).

Dimensional models of personality psychopathology make the co-occurrence of so-called personality disorders and their heterogeneity more rational, because they include multiple dimensions that are continua on all of which people can vary. The configurations of dimensional ratings describe each person's profile of personality functioning, so many different multidimensional configurations are possible. Trait dimensional models were developed to describe the full range of personality functioning, so it should be possible to describe anyone.

Dimensional models, however, are unfamiliar to clinicians trained in the medical model of diagnosis, in which a single diagnostic concept is used to communicate a large amount of important clinical information about a patient's problems, the treatment needed, and the likely prognosis. Dimensional models are also more difficult to use; up to 30 dimensions (see the next section, "Alternative Proposals for a Dimensional Model of Personality Disorders") may be necessary to fully describe a person's personality. Finally, there is little empirical information on the treatment or other clinical implications of dimensional scale elevations and, in particular, where to set cut-points on dimensional scales to maximize their clinical utility. Thus, the advantages of both categorical and dimensional approaches are reciprocals of the other model's disadvantages. Proponents of dimensional models point out how extremes of some clinical phenomena in medicine that have continuous distributions, such as blood pressure, lead to meaningful categorical diagnoses (i.e., hypertension), once cut-points with significance for morbidity and a need for treatment are established. And, as an example from the realm of psychiatry, meaningful cut-points based on progressive degrees of functional impairment have been established for extreme (low) values of intelligence.

ALTERNATIVE PROPOSALS FOR A DIMENSIONAL MODEL OF PERSONALITY DISORDERS

Widiger and Simonsen (2005a) reviewed 18 alternative proposals for dimensional models of personality disorders. The proposals included 1) dimensional representations of existing personality disorder constructs; 2) dimensional reorganizations of diagnostic criteria; 3) integration of Axes II and I via common psychopathological spectra; and 4) integration of Axis II with dimensional models of general personality structure.

An example of dimensional representations of existing constructs was proposed by Oldham and Skodol (2000). This proposal converted each DSM-IV personality disorder into a six-point scale ranging from absent traits to prototypical disorder. Significant personality traits and subthreshold disorders could be noted, in addition to full diagnoses. This schema has been shown to be significantly associated with functional impairment of patients with personality disorders when seeking treatment, outperforming DSM categories and other dimensional systems based on diagnostic criteria or on general personality traits (Skodol et al. 2005a). Another example of this type of "person-centered" dimensional system is the prototype matching approach described by Shedler and Westen (Shedler and Westen 2004; Westen et al. 2006b). In this system, a patient is compared to a description of a prototypical patient with each disorder and the "match" is rated on a 5-point scale from "very good match" to "little or no match."

An example of a dimensional system in which criteria for personality disorders are arranged by trait dimensions instead of by categories is the assessment model of the Schedule for Nonadaptive and Adaptive Personality (SNAP) (Clark 1993). This model has three higher-order factors similar to Tellegen and Waller's (1987) model: negative temperament (or affectivity), positive temperament (or affectivity), and disinhibition (or constraint) (A. Tellegen, N.G. Waller: "Exploring Personality Through Test Construction: Development of the Multidimensional Personality Questionnaire," Minneapolis, MN, unpublished manuscript, 1987). In addition, there are 12 lower-order trait scales that measure traits such as dependency, aggression, and impulsivity. Another example of this approach is Livesley's DAPP (Livesley and Jackson 2000), with broad domains of emotional dysregulation, dissocial behavior, inhibition, and compulsivity, as well as 28 lower-order, primary traits.

Models designed to integrate Axis II and Axis I disorders based on shared spectra of psychopathology have been developed; Siever and Davis's (1991) model, for example, hypothesizes fundamental dimensions of cognitive/perceptual disturbance, affective instability, impulsivity, and anxiety that link related disorders across the DSM axes. Thus, schizophrenia and related psychotic disorders and schizotypal personality disorder (STPD) are on a spectrum of cognitive/perceptual disturbance, sharing some fundamental genetic and neurobiological processes, but also having differences that account for flagrant psychotic episodes in schizophrenic disorders and only psychotic-like symptoms in STPD (Siever and Davis 2004). Another integrative model has been proposed that hypothesizes only two fundamental dimensions: internalization and externalization (Krueger 2005; Krueger et al. 2001). Internalizing disorders include mood and anxiety disorders on Axis I and avoidant and dependent personality disorders on Axis II. Externalizing disorders include substance use disorders, for example, on Axis I and antisocial personality disorder (ASPD) on Axis II. Differences between Axis I and II disorders are a function of the extensiveness of the psychopathology, with personality disorders being more extensive and Axis I disorders more circumscribed.

Finally, the fourth group of alternatives hypothesizes that personality disorders are on a continuum of general personality functioning—extremes of normal personality traits. Three- and five-factor models have a long history. Three-factor models (Eysenck 1987; A. Tellegen, N.G. Waller: "Exploring Personality Through Test Construction: Development of the Multidimensional Personality Questionnaire," Minneapolis, MN, unpublished manuscript, 1987) usually include neuroticism, extroversion, and psychoticism (or disinhibition vs. constraint) as higher-order factors, and the FFM includes neuroticism, extroversion, agreeableness, openness, and conscientiousness (Costa and McCrae 1992). Each of the FFM factors is composed of six trait dimensions or "facets." Another model is the Temperament and Character Model (Cloninger 2000); this model consists of four dimensions of temperament (novelty seeking, harm avoidance, reward dependence, and persistence), originally hypothesized as genetic, and three dimensions of character (self-directedness, cooperation, and self-transcendence) that were believed to result from the environment, learning, or life experience.

Theoretical and empirical work has been done to describe personality disorders in terms of dimensional models (Trull 2005). For example, according to the FFM, personality disorders, in general, would be characterized by high neuroticism. A specific personality disorder, such as borderline personality dis-

order, would also be characterized by low agreeableness and low cooperativeness. According to the Temperament and Character Model, personality disorders would be characterized by low self-directedness and low cooperativeness. Personality disorders in Cluster B would also show high novelty seeking; those in Cluster C, high harm avoidance; and those in Cluster A, low reward dependence. Some research has suggested that it is easier to distinguish personality disorders from normality using these models than to distinguish specific personality disorders from each other (Morey et al. 2002).

With so many models from which to choose, attempts have been made to synthesize them into an overarching dimensional model. One such synthesis proposed that the alternative models could be integrated over four levels of specificity (Widiger and Simonsen 2005a). In this scheme, at the highest level, personality psychopathology is divided by the dimensions of internalization and externalization. Below these are three to five broad domains of personality functioning: extroversion versus introversion, antagonism versus compliance, impulsivity versus constraint, emotional dysregulation versus emotional stability, and unconventionality versus closed to experience. Below these are a number (25–30) of lower-order traits, each with behaviorally specific diagnostic criteria.

Despite this integration, questions remain. What is the evidence that personality psychopathology is best represented by categorical entities or by dimensions (Widiger and Samuel 2005)? If by dimensions, should these be abnormal constructs or are extremes of normal variation sufficient? Should personality psychopathology be described by the few (three to five) higher-order broad factors, or does the specificity of lower-order, more narrowly defined traits add to clinical utility? Finally, should personality psychopathology be conceptualized as static phenotypes or as dynamic processes?

COMPARISONS OF ALTERNATIVE MODELS

It remains to be seen how alternative models of personality psychopathology compare on important aspects of clinical utility to personality disorders and their dimensional representations. Testing the association of alternative models to a variety of antecedent (e.g., abuse, positive child experiences), concurrent (e.g., functioning, treatment utilization), and predictive (e.g., future functioning, course of Axis I disorders) validators has been the subject of ongoing studies in the Collaborative Longitudinal Personality Disorders Study (CLPS) (Skodol et al. 2005a).

In an initial study, Skodol et al. (2005b) compared DSM-IV personality disorder categories, dimensional representations (six-point continuous scales based on number of criteria met) of personality disorders, the FFM, and a three-factor model (positive affectivity, negative affectivity, disinhibition) derived from the SNAP on their associations to both interviewer-rated and self-reported domains of functional impairment. The DSM-IV dimensional representations had the strongest associations to employment, social, leisure, and global functioning.

A more elaborate study was undertaken by Morey et al. (2007). In this study, multiple antecedent, concurrent, and predictive markers of construct validity were examined for three major models of personality disorder: the FFM (five factors and 30 facets), the 15-trait SNAP model, and the DSM-IV personality disorders (both as categories and as criteria counts). Antecedent validity markers included various types of childhood abuse and neglect, positive childhood experiences reflecting resiliency, past history of medication use, and past history of psychiatric hospitalization. Concurrent markers included psychosocial functioning in multiple domains, co-occurring Axis I disorders, and current medications. Functioning, Axis I disorders, suicide attempts, hospitalizations,

and medication use over 2 years and 4 years of follow-up were the predicted outcome variables. All models showed substantial validity across marker variables over time. Dimensional models, especially the dimensionalized DSM personality disorders and the SNAP model, consistently outperformed DSM personality disorder categories and the FFM in predicting external validators. The SNAP model, which incorporates both normal and abnormal personality dimensions, seemed best, because it not only captured variables of clinical significance at baseline when most subjects were seeking treatment but also maintained its predictive power over time better than the DSM dimensions. The data demonstrated the importance of both stable trait and dynamic psychopathological influences in predicting external criteria over time.

TRIPARTITE MODEL OF MENTAL DISORDERS

Integrating work on the core features of personality disorder and on organizing psychopathology according to personality dimensions, Donna Bender, Ph.D. (2008, personal communication), proposed for the Work Group a "tripartite model of mental disorders," based on a model of patient assessment commonly used in clinical practice (Skodol and Bender 2008; Westen et al. 2006a) (Figure 20–1). The tripartite model consists of three fundamental assessment domains: functioning, personality, and psychopathology. Within the functional domain, strengths and challenges are assessed on cognitive, self, emotional, behavioral, physical, interpersonal, occupational, and recreational dimensions. These adaptive capacities encompass processes by which humans know about themselves and the world around them; how they think, learn, reason, and express themselves; how they feel and express these feelings; how they perceive their bodies, experience their sensations, and

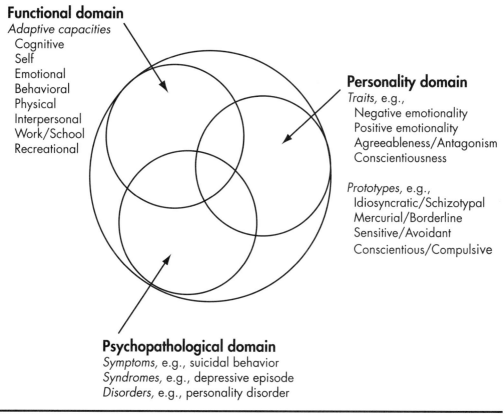

Functional domain
Adaptive capacities
  Cognitive
  Self
  Emotional
  Behavioral
  Physical
  Interpersonal
  Work/School
  Recreational

Personality domain
Traits, e.g.,
  Negative emotionality
  Positive emotionality
  Agreeableness/Antagonism
  Conscientiousness

Prototypes, e.g.,
  Idiosyncratic/Schizotypal
  Mercurial/Borderline
  Sensitive/Avoidant
  Conscientious/Compulsive

Psychopathological domain
Symptoms, e.g., suicidal behavior
Syndromes, e.g., depressive episode
Disorders, e.g., personality disorder

Figure 20–1.   Tripartite model of mental disorder.

perform essential functions; and how they act and react to both internal and external stimuli. Functioning constructs span adaptive to maladaptive functioning, integrating the assessment of dysfunctions with the assessment of functional strengths associated with mental health and the resilient personality (Vaillant 2003).

In support of a tripartite model, Westen and Arkowitz-Westen (1998) argued in favor of a "functional assessment of personality," resembling a case-formulation approach. They argued that instead of asking diagnostic questions such as "Does the patient cross the threshold for a personality disorder?" or "How low is the patient on the trait of agreeableness?" a functional assessment would ask, "Under what circumstances are which dysfunctional cognitive, affective, motivational, and behavioral patterns likely to oc-

cur?" Approaches such as these are appealing because they represent a return to the time-honored tradition of careful clinical assessment and formulation.

Once a functional assessment according to the tripartite model has been made, dysfunctions can be traced to personality problems, to psychopathology, or to both. The assessment of the personality domain may include personality traits, prototypes, or styles. Dimensional traits may range from normal to abnormal, and normal personality types that correspond to extreme forms (i.e., the DSM disorders) may be included (Oldham and Morris 1995). So, for example, an idiosyncratic type would be a normal variant of STPD, mercurial would correspond to borderline, sensitive to avoidant, and conscientious to compulsive. Of course, normal personality types would need to have dem-

Table 20–2.   Examples of associations of functional domains and psychopathology

Cognitive	Emotional
Psychotic spectrum	Affective disorders
Mental retardation	Anxiety disorders
Delirium	Behavioral
Dementia	Substance abuse
Self	Suicide/self-harm
Dissociative spectrum	Impulse control spectrum
Eating disorders	Physical
Personality disorders	Somatic concern disorders
Interpersonal	Sexual dysfunction
Pervasive developmental disorders	Sleep disorders
Personality disorders	

onstrated clinical utility. An empirically based set of prototypes, as described by Westen and Shedler (1999a, 1999b), could be adopted. These prototypes are derived from clinical constructs closely related to DSM-IV, based on clinician consensus.

Finally, the psychopathology domain would require assessment of any relevant symptoms, syndromes, or disorders. Thus, suicidality, major depressive episode, or personality disorder could be diagnosed in this domain. It is expected that the impairments in the specific adaptive capacities in the functional domain would map onto specific symptom disorders (see Table 20–2). For example, impairments in cognitive functioning would suggest mental retardation, delirium, dementia, or psychotic disorders. Impairment in emotional functions would suggest mood or anxiety disorders. Although most mental disorders have impairments in multiple domains, identification of the primary (and secondary) impairments is usually very helpful in the process of differential diagnosis.

Thus the tripartite model of mental disorders 1) provides a clinically useful assessment, grounded in the mental status examination; 2) eliminates the need for a multiaxial system of assessment; 3) provides a template for dimensional ratings of functioning, personality, and psychopathology for all patients; and 4) is consistent with empirical data on the classification of mental disorders according to developmental, latent trait, or spectrum criteria. It promotes a "whole person" approach to assessment that the five-axis DSM system often failed to do.

FUTURE DIRECTIONS

The implications of this growing body of evidence are several. In the future, personality disorders may need to be redefined in terms of their trait, symptom, and functional components. The course of personality disorders may need to be reconceptualized as waxing and waning, depending on life circumstances. Since personality disorders can improve, it may be possible to convey a more optimistic prognosis to patients and their families. Finally, it will be important to focus treatments on attaining adequate psychosocial functioning, in addition to symptom relief.

The simplest change in approach to Axis II in the future that would likely increase validity would be to rate (revised) personality disorder categories as dimensions, as proposed by Oldham and Skodol (2000) and others. Another possibility would be to move personality disorders as a class of disorders to Axis I, but to supplement their categorical diagnosis by rating personality traits on Axis II (Widiger et al. 2002). More dramatic revisions that include the reorganization of both Axis I and Axis II disorders according to temperamental dimensions (Clark 2005; Krueger 2005) and/or developmental stages (Kupfer 2005) are also possible. Any decisions to revise Axis II should be considered carefully, backed by empirical data, and tested for clinical utility (First 2005).

REFERENCES

American Psychiatric Association: Diagnostic and Statistical Manual of Mental Disorders, 4th Edition. Washington, DC, American Psychiatric Association, 1994

American Psychiatric Association: Diagnostic and Statistical Manual of Mental Disorders, 4th Edition, Text Revision. Washington, DC, American Psychiatric Association, 2000

Bender DS, Skodol AE: Borderline personality as a self-other representational disturbance. J Personal Disord 21:500–517, 2007

Clark LA: Schedule for Nonadaptive and Adaptive Personality (SNAP). Minneapolis, MN, University of Minnesota Press, 1993

Clark LA: Temperament as a unifying basis for personality and psychopathology. J Abnorm Psychol 114:505–521, 2005

Cloninger CR: A practical way to diagnose personality disorders: a proposal. J Personal Disord 14:99–108, 2000

Cohen P, Crawford TN, Johnson JG, et al: The Children in the Community study of developmental course of personality disorder. J Personal Disord 19:466–486, 2005

Costa PT, McCrae RR: Revised NEO Personality Inventory (NEO-PI-R) and NEO Five-Factor Inventory (NEO-FFI) Professional Manual. Odessa, FL, Psychological Assessment Resources, 1992

Eysenck HJ: The definition of personality disorders and the criteria appropriate for their description. J Personal Disord 1:211–219, 1987

First MB: Clinical utility: a prerequisite for the adoption of a dimensional approach in DSM. J Abnorm Psychol. 114:560–564, 2005

Johansen M, Karterud S, Pedersen G, et al: An investigation of the prototype validity of the borderline DSM-IV construct. Acta Psychiatrica Scand109:289–298, 2004

Krueger RF: Continuity of axes I and II: toward a unified model of personality, personality disorders, and clinical disorders. J Personal Disord 19:233–261, 2005

Krueger RF, McGue M, Iocono WG: The higher-order structure of common DSM mental disorders: internalization, externalization, and their connections to personality. Pers Individ Dif 30:1245–1259, 2001

Krueger RF, Skodol AE, Livesley WJ, et al: Synthesizing dimensional and categorical approaches to personality disorders: refining the research agenda for DSM-V Axis II. Int J Methods Psychiatr Res 16(S1):S65–S73, 2007

Kupfer DJ: Dimensional models for research and diagnosis: a current dilemma. J Abnorm Psychol. 114:557–559, 2005

Kupfer DJ, First MB, Regier DE, (eds): A Research Agenda for DSM-V. Washington, DC, American Psychiatric Association, 2002

Lenzenweger MF: The longitudinal study of personality disorders: history, design considerations, and initial findings. J Personal Disord 20:645–670, 2006

Livesley J, Jackson D: Dimensional Assessment of Personality Pathology. Port Huron, MI, Sigma Press, 2000

Livesley WJ, Jang KL: Differentiating normal, abnormal, and disordered personality. Eur J Pers 19:257–268, 2005

Livesley WJ, Jang KL, Vernon PA: Phenotypic and genetic structure of traits delineating personality disorder. Arch Gen Psychiatry 55:941–948, 1998

McGlashan TH, Grilo CM, Sanislow CA, et al: Two-year prevalence and stability of individual DSM-IV criteria for schizotypal, borderline, avoidant, and obsessive-compulsive personality disorders toward a hybrid model of Axis II disorders. Am J Psychiatry 162:883–889, 2005

Morey LC, Gunderson JG, Quigley BD, et al: The representation of borderline, avoidant, obsessive-compulsive, and schizotypal personality disorders by the five-factor model. J Personal Disord 16:215–234, 2002

Morey LC, Hopwood CJ, Gunderson JG, et al: Comparison of alternative models for personality disorders. Psychol Med 37:983–994, 2007

Oldham JM, Morris LB: The New Personality Self-Portrait. New York, Bantam, 1995

Oldham JM, Skodol AE: Charting the future of Axis II. J Personal Disord14:17–29, 2000

Oldham JM, Skodol AE, Kellman HD, et al: Diagnosis of DSM-III-R personality disorders by two structured interviews: patterns of comorbidity. Am J Psychiatry 149:213–220, 1992

Psychodynamic Diagnostic Manual (PDM) Task Force: Psychodynamic Diagnostic Manual. Silver Spring, MD, Alliance of Psychoanalytic Organizations, 2006

Rounsaville BJ, Alarcon RD, Andrews G, et al: Basic nomenclature issues for DSM-V, in A Research Agenda for DSM-V. Edited by Kupfer DJ, First MB, Regier DE. Washington, DC, American Psychiatric Association, 2002, pp 1–29

Shedler J, Westen D: Refining personality disorder diagnosis: integrating science and practice. Am J Psychiatry 161:1350–1365, 2004

Siever LJ, Davis KL: A psychobiological perspective on the personality disorders. Am J Psychiatry 148:1647–1658, 1991

Siever LJ, Davis KL: The pathophysiology of schizophrenia disorders: perspectives from the spectrum. Am J Psychiatry 161:398–413, 2004

Skodol AE, Bender DS: Psychopathology across the life span, in Psychiatry 3rd Edition. Edited by Tasman A, Kay J, Lieberman JA, et al. Chichester, England, John Wiley & Sons, 2008, pp 487–524

Skodol AE, Gunderson JG, Shea MT, et al: The Collaborative Longitudinal Personality Disorders Study (CLPS): overview and implications. J Personal Disord 19:487–504, 2005a

Skodol AE, Oldham JM, Bender DS, et al: Dimensional representations of DSM-IV personality disorders: relationships to functional impairment. Am J Psychiatry 162:1919–1925, 2005b

Skodol AE, Pagano ME, Bender DS, et al: Stability of functional impairment in patients with schizotypal, borderline, avoidant, or obsessive-compulsive personality disorder over two years. Psychol Med 35:443–451, 2005c

Spitzer RL, First MB, Schedler J, et al: Clinical utility of five dimensional systems for personality diagnosis: a "consumer preference" study. J Nerv Ment Dis 196:356–374, 2008

Trull TJ. Dimensional models of personality disorder: coverage and cutoffs. J Personal Disord 19:262–282, 2005

Vaillant GE: Mental health. Am J Psychiatry 160:1373–1384, 2003

Verheul R, Widiger TA: A meta-analysis of the prevalence and usage of personality disorder not otherwise specified (PDNOS). J Personal Disord 18:309–319, 2004

Westen D, Arkowitz-Westen, L: Limitations of Axis II in diagnosing personality pathology in clinical practice. Am J Psychiatry 155:1767–1771, 1998

Westen D, Shedler J: Revising and assessing Axis II, part I: developing a clinically and empirically valid assessment method. Am J Psychiatry 156:258–272, 1999a

Westen D, Shedler J: Revising and assessing Axis II, part II: toward an empirically based and clinically useful classification of personality disorders. Am J Psychiatry 156:273–285, 1999b

Westen D, Gabbard GO, Blagov P: Back to the future: personality structure as a context for psychopathology, in Personality and Psychopathology. Edited by Krueger RF, Tackett JL. New York, Guilford Press, 2006a, pp 335–384

Westen D, Shedler J, Bradley R: A prototype approach to personality disorder diagnosis. Am J Psychiatry 163:846–856, 2006b

Widiger TA, Samuel DB: Diagnostic categories or dimensions? A question for the Diagnostic and Statistical Manual of Mental Disorders– Fifth Edition. J Abnorm Psychol 114:494–504, 2005

Widiger TA, Simonsen E: Alternative dimensional models of personality disorder: finding a common ground. J Personal Disord 19:110–130, 2005a

Widiger TA, Simonsen E: Introduction to part two of the special section on the research agenda for the development of a dimensional classification of personality disorder. J Personal Disord 19:211, 2005b

Widiger TA, Simonsen E: Introduction to the special section: the American Psychiatric Association's research agenda for the DSM-V. J Personal Disord 19:103–109, 2005c

Widiger TA, Costa PT, McCrae RR: A proposal for Axis II: diagnosing personality disorders using the five-factor model, in Personality Disorders and the Five-Factor Model of Personality, 2nd edition. Edited by Costa PT, Widiger TA. Washington, DC, American Psychological Association, 2002, pp 431–456

Zanarini MC, Frankenburg FR, Hennen J, et al: The McLean Study of Adult Development (MSAD): overview and implications of the first six years of prospective follow-up. J Personal Disord 19:505–523, 2005

Zimmerman M, Rothchild L, Chelminski I: The prevalence of DSM-IV personality disorders in psychiatric outpatients. Am J Psychiatry 162:1911–1918, 2005

Appendix

DSM-IV-TR Diagnostic Criteria for Personality Disorders

General diagnostic criteria for a personality disorder

A. An enduring pattern of inner experience and behavior that deviates markedly from the expectations of the individual's culture. This pattern is manifested in two (or more) of the following areas:

(1) cognition (i.e., ways of perceiving and interpreting self, other people, and events)

(2) affectivity (i.e., the range, intensity, lability, and appropriateness of emotional response)

(3) interpersonal functioning

(4) impulse control

B. The enduring pattern is inflexible and pervasive across a broad range of personal and social situations.

C. The enduring pattern leads to clinically significant distress or impairment in social, occupational, or other important areas of functioning.

D. The pattern is stable and of long duration, and its onset can be traced back at least to adolescence or early adulthood.

E. The enduring pattern is not better accounted for as a manifestation or consequence of another mental disorder.

F. The enduring pattern is not due to the direct physiological effects of a substance (e.g., a drug of abuse, a medication) or a general medical condition (e.g., head trauma).

Personality disorder not otherwise specified

This category is for disorders of personality functioning (refer to the general diagnostic criteria for a personality disorder) that do not meet criteria for any specific personality disorder. An example is the presence of features of more than one specific personality disorder that do not meet the full criteria for any one personality disorder ("mixed personality"), but that together cause clinically significant distress or impairment in one or more important areas of functioning (e.g., social or occupational). This category can also be used when the clinician judges that a specific personality disorder that is not included in the classification is appropriate. Examples include depressive personality disorder and passive-aggressive personality disorder.

CLUSTER A

Diagnostic criteria for paranoid personality disorder

A. A pervasive distrust and suspiciousness of others such that their motives are interpreted as malevolent, beginning by early adulthood and present in a variety of contexts, as indicated by four (or more) of the following:

   (1) suspects, without sufficient basis, that others are exploiting, harming, or deceiving him or her

   (2) is preoccupied with unjustified doubts about the loyalty or trustworthiness of friends or associates

   (3) is reluctant to confide in others because of unwarranted fear that the information will be used maliciously against him or her

   (4) reads hidden demeaning or threatening meanings into benign remarks or events

   (5) persistently bears grudges, i.e., is unforgiving of insults, injuries, or slights

   (6) perceives attacks on his or her character or reputation that are not apparent to others and is quick to react angrily or to counterattack

   (7) has recurrent suspicions, without justification, regarding fidelity of spouse or sexual partner

B. Does not occur exclusively during the course of schizophrenia, a mood disorder with psychotic features, or another psychotic disorder and is not due to the direct physiological effects of a general medical condition.

Diagnostic criteria for schizoid personality disorder

A. A pervasive pattern of detachment from social relationships and a restricted range of expression of emotions in interpersonal settings, beginning by early adulthood and present in a variety of contexts, as indicated by four (or more) of the following:

   (1) neither desires nor enjoys close relationships, including being part of a family

   (2) almost always chooses solitary activities

   (3) has little, if any, interest in having sexual experiences with another person

   (4) takes pleasure in few, if any, activities

   (5) lacks close friends or confidants other than first-degree relatives

   (6) appears indifferent to the praise or criticism of others

   (7) shows emotional coldness, detachment, or flattened affectivity

B. Does not occur exclusively during the course of schizophrenia, a mood disorder with psychotic features, another psychotic disorder, or a pervasive developmental disorder and is not due to the direct physiological effects of a general medical condition.

CLUSTER A *(CONTINUED)*

Diagnostic criteria for schizotypal personality disorder

A. A pervasive pattern of social and interpersonal deficits marked by acute discomfort with, and reduced capacity for, close relationships as well as by cognitive or perceptual distortions and eccentricities of behavior, beginning by early adulthood and present in a variety of contexts, as indicated by five (or more) of the following:

   (1) ideas of reference (excluding delusions of reference)

   (2) odd beliefs or magical thinking that influences behavior and is inconsistent with subcultural norms (e.g., superstitiousness, belief in clairvoyance, telepathy, or "sixth sense"; in children and adolescents, bizarre fantasies or preoccupations)

   (3) unusual perceptual experiences, including bodily illusions

   (4) odd thinking and speech (e.g., vague, circumstantial, metaphorical, overelaborate, or stereotyped)

   (5) suspiciousness or paranoid ideation

   (6) inappropriate or constricted affect

   (7) behavior or appearance that is odd, eccentric, or peculiar

   (8) lack of close friends or confidants other than first-degree relatives

   (9) excessive social anxiety that does not diminish with familiarity and tends to be associated with paranoid fears rather than negative judgments about self

B. Does not occur exclusively during the course of schizophrenia, a mood disorder with psychotic features, another psychotic disorder, or a pervasive developmental disorder.

Cluster B

Diagnostic criteria for antisocial personality disorder

A. There is a pervasive pattern of disregard for and violation of the rights of others occurring since age 15 years, as indicated by three (or more) of the following:

(1) failure to conform to social norms with respect to lawful behaviors as indicated by repeatedly performing acts that are grounds for arrest

(2) deceitfulness, as indicated by repeated lying, use of aliases, or conning others for personal profit or pleasure

(3) impulsivity or failure to plan ahead

(4) irritability and aggressiveness, as indicated by repeated physical fights or assaults

(5) reckless disregard for safety of self or others

(6) consistent irresponsibility, as indicated by repeated failure to sustain consistent work behavior or honor financial obligations

(7) lack of remorse, as indicated by being indifferent to or rationalizing having hurt, mistreated, or stolen from another

B. The individual is at least age 18 years.

C. There is evidence of conduct disorder with onset before age 15 years.

D. The occurrence of antisocial behavior is not exclusively during the course of schizophrenia or a manic episode.

CLUSTER B *(CONTINUED)*

Diagnostic criteria for borderline personality disorder

A pervasive pattern of instability of interpersonal relationships, self-image, and affects, and marked impulsivity beginning by early adulthood and present in a variety of contexts, as indicated by five (or more) of the following:

(1) frantic efforts to avoid real or imagined abandonment
Note: Do not include suicidal or self-mutilating behavior covered in Criterion 5.

(2) a pattern of unstable and intense interpersonal relationships characterized by alternating between extremes of idealization and devaluation

(3) identity disturbance: markedly and persistently unstable self-image or sense of self

(4) impulsivity in at least two areas that are potentially self-damaging (e.g., spending, sex, substance abuse, reckless driving, binge eating)   **Note:** Do not include suicidal or self-mutilating behavior covered in Criterion 5.

(5) recurrent suicidal behavior, gestures, or threats, or self-mutilating behavior

(6) affective instability due to a marked reactivity of mood (e.g., intense episodic dysphoria, irritability, or anxiety usually lasting a few hours and only rarely more than a few days)

(7) chronic feelings of emptiness

(8) inappropriate, intense anger or difficulty controlling anger (e.g., frequent displays of temper, constant anger, recurrent physical fights)

(9) transient, stress-related paranoid ideation or severe dissociative symptoms

Diagnostic criteria for histrionic personality disorder

A pervasive pattern of excessive emotionality and attention seeking, beginning by early adulthood and present in a variety of contexts, as indicated by five (or more) of the following:

(1) is uncomfortable in situations in which he or she is not the center of attention

(2) interaction with others is often characterized by inappropriate sexually seductive or provocative behavior

(3) displays rapidly shifting and shallow expression of emotions

(4) consistently uses physical appearance to draw attention to self

(5) has a style of speech that is excessively impressionistic and lacking in detail

(6) shows self-dramatization, theatricality, and exaggerated expression of emotion

(7) is suggestible, i.e., easily influenced by others or circumstances

(8) considers relationships to be more intimate than they actually are

CLUSTER B *(CONTINUED)*

Diagnostic criteria for narcissistic personality disorder

A pervasive pattern of grandiosity (in fantasy or behavior), need for admiration, and lack of empathy, beginning by early adulthood and present in a variety of contexts, as indicated by five (or more) of the following:

(1) has a grandiose sense of self-importance (e.g., exaggerates achievements and talents, expects to be recognized as superior without commensurate achievements)

(2) is preoccupied with fantasies of unlimited success, power, brilliance, beauty, or ideal love

(3) believes that he or she is "special" and unique and can only be understood by, or should associate with, other special or high-status people (or institutions)

(4) requires excessive admiration

(5) has a sense of entitlement, i.e., unreasonable expectations of especially favorable treatment or automatic compliance with his or her expectations

(6) is interpersonally exploitative, i.e., takes advantage of others to achieve his or her own ends

(7) lacks empathy: is unwilling to recognize or identify with the feelings and needs of others

(8) is often envious of others or believes that others are envious of him or her

(9) shows arrogant, haughty behaviors or attitudes

CLUSTER C

Diagnostic criteria for avoidant personality disorder

A pervasive pattern of social inhibition, feelings of inadequacy, and hypersensitivity to negative evaluation, beginning by early adulthood and present in a variety of contexts, as indicated by four (or more) of the following:

(1) avoids occupational activities that involve significant interpersonal contact, because of fears of criticism, disapproval, or rejection

(2) is unwilling to get involved with people unless certain of being liked

(3) shows restraint within intimate relationships because of the fear of being shamed or ridiculed

(4) is preoccupied with being criticized or rejected in social situations

(5) is inhibited in new interpersonal situations because of feelings of inadequacy

(6) views self as socially inept, personally unappealing, or inferior to others

(7) is unusually reluctant to take personal risks or to engage in any new activities because they may prove embarrassing

Diagnostic criteria for dependent personality disorder

A pervasive and excessive need to be taken care of that leads to submissive and clinging behavior and fears of separation, beginning by early adulthood and present in a variety of contexts, as indicated by five (or more) of the following:

(1) has difficulty making everyday decisions without an excessive amount of advice and reassurance from others

(2) needs others to assume responsibility for most major areas of his or her life

(3) has difficulty expressing disagreement with others because of fear of loss of support or approval
Note: Do not include realistic fears of retribution.

(4) has difficulty initiating projects or doing things on his or her own (because of a lack of self-confidence in judgment or abilities rather than a lack of motivation or energy)

(5) goes to excessive lengths to obtain nurturance and support from others, to the point of volunteering to do things that are unpleasant

(6) feels uncomfortable or helpless when alone because of exaggerated fears of being unable to care for himself or herself

(7) urgently seeks another relationship as a source of care and support when a close relationship ends

(8) is unrealistically preoccupied with fears of being left to take care of himself or herself

Cluster C *(CONTINUED)*

Diagnostic criteria for obsessive-compulsive personality disorder

A pervasive pattern of preoccupation with orderliness, perfectionism, and mental and interpersonal control, at the expense of flexibility, openness, and efficiency, beginning by early adulthood and present in a variety of contexts, as indicated by four (or more) of the following:

(1) is preoccupied with details, rules, lists, order, organization, or schedules to the extent that the major point of the activity is lost

(2) shows perfectionism that interferes with task completion (e.g., is unable to complete a project because his or her own overly strict standards are not met)

(3) is excessively devoted to work and productivity to the exclusion of leisure activities and friendships (not accounted for by obvious economic necessity)

(4) is overconscientious, scrupulous, and inflexible about matters of morality, ethics, or values (not accounted for by cultural or religious identification)

(5) is unable to discard worn-out or worthless objects even when they have no sentimental value

(6) is reluctant to delegate tasks or to work with others unless they submit to exactly his or her way of doing things

(7) adopts a miserly spending style toward both self and others; money is viewed as something to be hoarded for future catastrophes

(8) shows rigidity and stubbornness

Index

*Page numbers printed in **boldface** type refer to tables or figures.*